THE EDWIN SMITH PAPYRUS

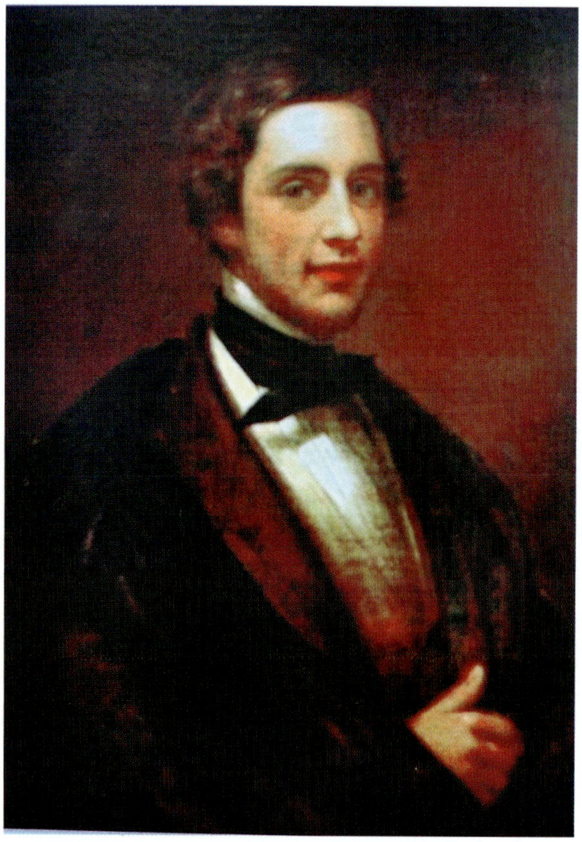

Edwin Smith. By Francesco Anelli, 1847.
With permission of the New York Historical Society.

THE EDWIN SMITH PAPYRUS

Updated Translation of the Trauma Treatise and Modern Medical Commentaries

Gonzalo M. Sanchez
and
Edmund S. Meltzer

LOCKWOOD PRESS
ATLANTA, GEORGIA

Published by
Lockwood Press
PO Box 133289
Atlanta, GA 30333
www.lockwoodpress.com

Printed in the United States of America

21 20 19 18 17 16 15 14 13 12 1 2 3 4 5

ISBN: 978-1-937040-01-7 (hardcover)

Library of Congress Control Number: 2012947516

This paper meets the requirements of ANSI/NISO Z39.48-1992 (Permanence of Paper).

Table of Contents

List of Illustrations

Visual Index

Figures

Foreword

Since the dawn of history, medical care has been a blend of magic and science. It is the curse of human nature that drives us to act according to our beliefs and disregard facts that fail to fit them. Much has been made of the role of magic in ancient Egyptian medicine, and its role was, indeed, very important. Were it not for the Edwin Smith papyrus, we might well believe that magic was the essence, if not the whole, of the ancient profession, and relied on exploiting the patient's belief in hope of generating a powerful placebo affect. That probably happened, but this amazing document shows that those physicians, called *swnw*, also practiced valid evidence-based medicine four millennia ago!

I look to a book's Foreword to tell me why I should read it. In this instance, it is widely recognized that James Henry Breasted produced a masterpiece in his translation of the Edwin Smith papyrus. But that was in 1930. The practice of medicine and our understanding of many conditions have taken massive leaps forward. Simultaneously, there has been steady progress by philologists in clarifying the ancient language. The production of the monumental *Grundriss der Medizin der alten Ägypter* (9 vols.; Hermann Grapow, Wolfart Westendorf, and Hildegard von Deines; Berlin: Akademie, 1954–1973) has provided an invaluable resource in subsequent studies.

We are fortunate to have the expertise of an outstanding neurosurgeon, Gonzalo Sanchez, combined with that of a dedicated and well-recognized scholar of the ancient text, Dr. Edmund Meltzer, to update our knowledge of this document. Their comprehensive new translation advances our understanding of ancient medical practice and further clarifies it as a thoroughly rational approach to assessing and managing the conditions presented.

The papyrus is primarily an ancient text book regarding trauma. In current parlance, most of these cases are neurosurgical problems, while the bulk of the remainder consists of orthopedic problems or simple trauma. The analysis of many of these complex skull injuries is relatively simple and straightforward for a skilled practicing neurosurgeon such as Gonzalo Sanchez. However, that analysis would require considerable research for me and my colleagues in other specialties, and be a truly imposing, nearly impossible challenge for those without medical training. Dr. Sanchez shows us the subtle distinctions between these injuries and how the ancient *swnw* similarly distinguished them to manage each in a rational manner. This could only have evolved from the *swnw* carefully and systematically observing a number of cases. No doubt trial and error informed them in their judgments of what to treat and how to treat it.

The cases that today would go to the hands of an orthopedic surgeon are more easily understood. The need to realign and stabilize broken bones to reduce pain and promote healing is obvious, as is the desirability of replacing dislocations. It is worthy of note that the *swnw* discerned important elements of these procedures that mirror those in use today. Furthermore, the limited pharmacopeia they utilized also reflects careful consideration of both benefit and avoidance of harm.

The inclusion of a Visual Index for the illustrations is a nice innovation. The illustrations are clear, well-labeled and to the point for each case. Figures also clarify some of the cases. This is especially important for the nonmedical reader.

As the text develops, a clear exposition of the thought processes leading to the identifications is clarified via voluminous footnotes. The footnotes also permit us to follow the authors' joint consideration of the work of other scholars in relation to their own and to present alternative interpretations. For the serious reader this is a refreshing approach lacking in many texts. As such, the work becomes accessible to the general public interested in all aspects of Egyptology rather than exiling it to the arena of arcane work for specialists.

The authors' collaboration has provided us important clarification of several terms that had been interpreted by Breasted in a manner that did not make good sense in the medical scenario. For example, in Case #6

Breasted interpreted the word *ryt* to mean "pus," but the new interpretation to mean "discharge" is more rational. Several other important words, such as *wbnw*, *mtw*, and *dgmy*, are now assessed in relation to their determinatives in the text to correlate with the different wounds, vessels/tendons, and particularly the subtle degrees of alteration of level of consciousness such as torpor, stupor, and coma.

In Case # 41 Breasted identified *bnf* as dung. If that were correct it would be the only instance in the text where a counterproductive and actually harmful medication was prescribed. The authors' new interpretation as "ox bile" brings the ancient pharmacopeia back to the realm of the rational as a strong case can be made for bile having therapeutic value.

Today we take scientific medicine for granted, but it took thousands of years before any significant advances were made from what the *swnw* practiced. We did not understand the human circulatory system any better than they did until the work of William Harvey in the seventeenth century. Yet the *swnw* did recognize a relationship between the heart and the pulse as seen in Case #1. They further recognized that the intact fused human skull of an adult prevents detection of the pulsation of the brain as can be found in the open fontanels of a baby or a disastrous injury exposing the brain as in Case #6.

The attention to detail of examination for each case permitted them to discern subtle differences to classify them. These distinctions then permitted them to make astute predictions for the outcome of each case. In fact it was not until well into the twentieth century that we have been able to improve on the treatments they recommended for the neurosurgical injuries cited and thus provide somewhat better prognoses.

We can only guess at the processes by which the ancient physicians reached their conclusions about the appropriate therapies for the forty-eight conditions discussed in this text. Some treatments, such as suturing a laceration, appear so obvious that anyone would accept them. Others, such as the skull injuries, would have required very careful observation to discern subtle differences. Perhaps most important is their avoidance of treatments that might aggravate the problem more than they would assist it. The latter are often found in magic-based therapies as in the Ebers Papyrus and others.

The medical profession did not understand the nature of the infection process until the mid-nineteenth century and even then could do nothing but provide little more than cleanliness and drainage until the dawn of the antibiotic era in the mid-twentieth century. Clearly the *swnw* knew as much and understood the need for cleanliness and the desirability to leave some wounds open or to provide a wick for drainage as in Cases #28 and #39. Furthermore, their limited pharmacopeia did serve to reduce risk or ameliorate infection. Even when the *swnw* following these instructions had little or nothing to offer, they still avoided doing harm. A nice example of this restraint is the demonstration of masterful non-intervention as seen in the patient with neurofibromatosis (Case #45).

The *swnw* who followed this text were often using what are best practices today. A good example is the reduction of a dislocated jaw. The concept is deceptively simple: just push the jaw down and back. But, the unaware therapist who puts his thumb on the back lower molars may be rewarded by a serious bite of the thumb as the jaw snaps shut in place! The directions for this case clearly indicate the operator must place his thumbs past the molars, thus avoiding this hazard.

The initial translation of this work by Henry Breasted from 1920–1930 was an enormous undertaking that transformed our thinking about the ancient practice of medicine. His work in converting the hieratic script to hieroglyphs and then laboriously translating the text is a monument to his scholarship and tenacity. In the intervening years great changes have occurred in the practice of medicine as well as in interpretation and understanding of the ancient Egyptian language.

Every subsequent consideration of this document has been based on Breasted's hieroglyphic translation. However, the authors of this new assessment have accepted the formidable challenge of returning to the original hieratic script. In the process they show us indications of subtle alterations in the scribe's work, suggesting fatigue, or the need for breaks to acquire a new pen, or haste, prompting the use of abbreviations or the introduction of an error that required subsequent revision. This new translation and commentary move our understanding forward to a significant degree.

Evidence-based medicine has become the mantra for medical care at the dawn of the twenty-first century. As the term implies, good medical care should be based on solid evidence. It is a sad fact that many of the practices of modern medicine are more hallowed by time and tradition than by factual data. For an example in my own specialty of gynecology, countless women suffered through uncomfortable Pap smear examinations because every text book stated that lubrication should not be used. When actually studied, it was found that the use of a lubricant had no adverse effect at all on the accuracy of the test. Following unverified advice has been part of medicine throughout history.

Were it not for the Edwin Smith papyrus, we would have a totally distorted view of ancient Egyptian medicine. We might consider them superstitious and naively incompetent, but the Edwin Smith papyrus shows us that the patients treated by the standards of this document received care that was as good or better than any place in the world prior to the last 150 years. The volume in hand enhances our appreciation of the sophistication of these ancient physicians in their evaluation and management of this remarkable variety of cases. We can be grateful that Edmund Meltzer and Gonzalo Sanchez were willing to tackle the extraordinary challenge of going back to the original hieratic text and doggedly following through to produce this splendid new addition to our corpus of texts on ancient Egyptian medicine.

W. Benson Harer, Jr., MD, FACOG

Acknowledgments

Dr. Edward Bleiberg, Curator of Egyptian, Classical and Ancient Middle Eastern Art, Brooklyn Museum, for facilitating the search for Edwin Smith's handwritten manuscript and giving us permission to publish it.

Ms. Kathy Zurek-Doule, Curatorial Assistant, ECAMEA, Brooklyn Museum, for sending us the Photostats and reversed images of the manuscript.

Ms. Sandy Wallace, Librarian, and Ms. Jessica Popkin, Graduate Intern, Brooklyn Museum, for searching and finding the Smith ms. in files which had belonged to the New York Historical Society.

Dr. Angela McDonald of Glasgow University, for generously discussing issues of hieratic and sending copies of several of her papers.

Dr. John Booss, Professor Emeritus of Neurology, Yale school of Medicine for his critical review of the manuscript and insightful observations.

Dr. James T. Goodrich, Professor of Clinical Neurological Surgery, Pediatrics, Plastic and Reconstructive Surgery at the Albert Einstein College of Medicine, for his enthusiastic support and constructive review of the manuscript.

Dr. Christian Tutundjian de Vartavan, Director of the Armenian Egyptology Centre, for generous correspondence about substances mentioned in the papyrus.

Mrs. Arlene Shaner, reference librarian of historical collections, The New York Academy of Medicine, for facilitating the use of the Edwin Smith Papyrus Recto photographic material.

The New York Historical Society for the use of Mr. Edwin Smith's portrait.

The Oriental Institute of the University of Chicago for the use of Prof. Breasted's photograph at his Haskell Hall office, with the Edwin Smith Surgical Papyrus plates, circa 1929.

The University of Michigan Museum of Art for the use of the painting "Medicine in Ancient Egypt" by Robert Thom, for the front cover.

The Royal Ontario Museum for their generosity in allowing us to use ancient Egyptian weapons photographs from their collection.

The Australian Centre for Egyptology, for permission to use extensive quotations from Dr. James E. Walker's *Studies in Ancient Egyptian Anatomical Terminology* (1996).

The Royal College of Surgeons, Edinburgh for the use of Sir Charles Bell's painting, "Tetanus following Gunshot Wounds."

The Army Medical Services Museum, Scotland, for their permission to use the painting, "Trooper 1st Royal Dragoons" by Sir Charles Bell.

Ms. Cinthya J. Coan, "Indexing by the Book," for her extremely efficient work in compiling the General and Medical Index.

Ian Stevens and Krista Zimmer of ISD for their encouragement and enthusiastic help and expertise in the distribution and marketing of the book.

And last but by no means least, Dr. Billie Jean Collins of Lockwood Press, for her confidence in us and in our project, her patience and expertise in working with an extremely complex manuscript and two demanding authors, and her indefatigable efforts in helping our work to become the book that she knew it could be.

We tender our most grateful thanks to all of the above colleagues and institutions. All opinions that we express in this work, and any remaining errors, are our own.

Note on Transliteration

The authors have adopted the following conventions for transliteration:

The single reedleaf is represented by *i*, the double reedleaf by *y*. The ending *y* is used on nisbe adjectives and the relative word *nty*.

The preposition "to, for," the genitival adjective in its simple form, and the negative arms as a particle are all transliterated *n*. Where written out, the feminine genitive word is transliterated *nt* and the masculine plural *nw*. It was decided that it would be too cumbersome to transliterate repeatedly *n(y)*, *n(y)t*, *n(y)w* for the inflected forms of the genitive word. As far as the negative arms are concerned, we decided that they should be rendered by a simple *n*, not *nj* or *ni*, especially in view of the use of the negative arms as a variant of the waterline *n* in hieratic of this period, including this document.

A dot is used to separate the formative (if any) and suffix-pronoun subject of a verbal complex (e.g., *sḏm.ḫr.f*) or mutatis mutandis the heavier endings of the Stative (*rḫ.kwi*, *ꜥnḫ.ti*), *sḏmty.fy* forms, etc. It is not used to separate feminine and plural endings (e.g., *ḏrt*, *ḏbꜥw*) or the initial augment or prefix added to a verbal stem (*išwy*, *sḫpr*).

A hyphen is used to separate elements of a compound word or name, for example, *ḥr-ib.f*, *mn-ḫpr-rꜥ*.

Angular brackets are used only to contain elements that are omitted in error by the scribe, not optional ones; thus *sḏm.<i>n.f*, *<m> bit*.

Curly brackets are used to contain elements that are added or included in error by the scribe, such as *gm.n.{n.}f*.

Square brackets are used only for restorations; e.g., *iwf* [*wꜣḏ*].

Parentheses are used sparingly to enclose optional elements that are not written in the Egyptian text. On the whole they have been avoided in the running transliteration, so as more closely to reflect the text, but used more freely in the notes.

Note on Column and Line Numbering

The present work employs the same numbering of the columns of the papyrus as Breasted and Allen. These scholars follow the same numbers as regards the Recto, but Breasted numbers the Verso consecutively with the Recto while Allen begins again with "Verso, Column 1" etc. We do not translate the Verso but in one regard we follow Breasted's practice more closely, as he used Roman numerals for the columns while Allen uses Arabic numerals. Breasted and Allen refer to the column that originally preceded what we now designate as Column I; this "lost column" (Breasted, *Edwin Smith*, 2:xi–xii) contained the title of the work and the very beginning of Case 1 (ibid.; cf. Allen *AM*, 70). Like Breasted, we use Arabic numerals for the lines.

When we received Smith's original handwritten manuscript, we found that he uses both Roman and Arabic numerals in the margin. His Roman numerals do not correspond to the columns but are his own numbering of the 48 cases and show how accurately he understood these subdivisions. His Arabic numerals are of the format "1.18" etc. It appears that the first number labels the column, and the number after the point designates the line. The lines are not numbered individually. Smith begins with "0.18" followed fairly closely by "1.1"; it is clear that "0" corresponds to the "lost column" mentioned above. There is, however, a discrepancy, because Smith concludes in his column "21" while there are twenty-two columns and Smith himself states that the Verso comprises five columns ("pages").

Abbreviations

Allen, *AM*	Allen, James P., *The Art of Medicine in Ancient Egypt*. New York: The Metropolitan Museum of Art; New Haven: Yale University Press, 2005
Allen, *ME*	Allen, James P., *Middle Egyptian: An Introduction to the Language and Culture of Hieroglyphs*. 2nd rev. edition. Cambridge: Cambridge University Press, 2010
Breasted, *Edwin Smith*	Breasted, James Henry, *The Edwin Smith Surgical Papyrus*. 2 vols. The University of Chicago. Oriental Institute Publications. Chicago: University of Chicago, 1930
Edel, *AG*	Edel, Elmar, *Altägyptische Grammatik*. 2 vols. Analecta Orientalia 34/39. Rome: Pontifico Istituto Biblico, 1955/1964
ESM	Edmund S. Meltzer
Faulkner, *CDME*	Faulkner, R. O., *A Concise Dictionary of Middle Egyptian*. Oxford: Griffith Institute Asmolean Museum, 1962. Repr. Frome and London: Butler & Tanner, 1996.
Gardiner, *EG*[3]	Gardiner, Alan H., *Egyptian Grammar*. 3rd ed. Oxford: Oxford University Press/ Griffith Institute, 1957
GEC	Lefebvre, Gustave, *Grammaire de l'égyptien classique*. 2nd ed. Le Caire: Institut français d'archéologie orientale, 1955
GMS	Gonzalo M. Sanchez
Grundriss	Grapow, Hermann, Wolfart Westendorf, and Hildegard von Deines, *Grundriss der Medizin der alten Ägypter*. 9 vols. Berlin: Akademie, 1954–1973
Grundriss 4/1	von Deines, Hildegard, Hermann Grapow, and Wolfhart Westendorf, *Übersetzung der medizinischen Texte*. Vol. 4/1 of *Grundriss der Medizin der alten Ägypter*. Berlin: Akademie, 1958
Grundriss 5	Grapow, Hermann, *Die Medizinischen Texte in hieroglyphischer Umschreibung Autographiert*. Vol. 5 of *Grundriss der Medizin der Alten Ägypter*. Berlin: Akademie, 1958
Grundriss 6	von Deines, Hildegard, and Hermann Grapow, *Wörterbuch der ägyptischen Drogennamen*. Berlin: Akademie, 1959
Grundriss 7	von Deines, Hildegard, and Wolfhart Westendorf, *Wörterbuch der Medizinischen Texte*. Vol. 7 of *Grundriss der Medizin der alten Ägypter*. 2 vols. Berlin: Akademie, 1961–62
Grundriss 8	Westendorf, Wolfhart, *Grammatik der medizinischen Texte*. Vol. 8 of *Grundriss der Medizin der alten Ägypter*. Berlin: Akademie, 1962
Hoch, *MEG*	Hoch, J. E., *Middle Egyptian Grammar*. SSEA Publications 15. Mississauga, Ontario: Benben, 1996
Urk.	Steindorff, Georg, ed., with Kurt Sethe and Heinrich Schäfer, *Urkunden des ägyptischen Altertums*. 8 vols. Leipzig: Hinrichs, 1904–
Wb.	Erman, Adolf, and Hermann Grapow, *Wörterbuch der ägyptischen Sprache*. 5 vols. Leipzig: Hinrichs, 1926–1931

General and Medical Introduction

Gonzalo M. Sanchez, M.D.

The Edwin Smith Papyrus is a didactic trauma treatise from ancient Egypt (ca. 1650–1550 BC) written in hieratic script, a cursive form of writing that developed alongside the hieroglyphic system. This rolled document was purchased in 1862 by Edwin Smith, an American who graduated from New York University and later became an antiquities dealer in Luxor. Knowledge of hieratic at this early time was scant. Smith was enthused with ancient Egypt, and he was dedicated to the study of ancient Egyptian scripts. Nine years prior to his acquisition of this medical text, which carries his name, Smith was recognized in a paper read before the Academy of Science of St Louis[1] where he was acknowledged as having devoted his leisure to Egyptian studies. When the French Egyptologist Théodule Devéria visited Smith in Luxor on March 19, 1862, he described him as "the hermit of Thebes ... devoting himself to the translation of a medical treatise written in beautiful hieratic."[2]

The papyrus was sold to Smith by a dealer named Mustapha Aga in three fragments (with the first column missing) between January 20th and March 17th, 1862. Smith recognized these fragments as belonging to a single scroll. Reconstituted as one, the papyrus measured 4.68 meters in length by 32.5 to 33 centimeters in width and consisted of recto and verso. The recto constitutes the trauma treatise, the subject of this work. There are seventeen columns of writing in 377 horizontal lines in the recto. The verso, not addressed in this work, has 92 lines and contains recipes and incantations akin to those found in other medical papyri, lacking the objectivity and rational approach to medical subjects and trauma found in the recto. In Breasted's opinion, the entire recto and the first three columns of the verso were written by the same individual. It will immediately be noted that in this edition we are including the 48 clinical cases, and not the mainly ritualistic and cosmetic material in the verso. This is not because we disparage such material as some other commentators do (including, alas, Edwin Smith himself), as our remarks in the Case 9 commentary should make clear. Our purpose in this work is to advance the understanding of the clinical/trauma section of the papyrus, and thus to arrive at a more definitive translation and explore what it reveals about the methodology of the Egyptian approach to trauma medicine. The verso material is similar in character to that seen in other Egyptian medical papyri and it is not the continuation of, nor is it related to, the trauma treatise in the recto of the Edwin Smith Papyrus. Although of scientific interest to the epidemiology of infectious disease, the verso does not require input from a medical specialist, nor does its renewed study provide the same degree of advancement in our understanding of ancient Egyptian medical methodology and knowledge, as does the study of the wounds section.

Edwin Smith referred to this papyrus as "my lesser Med. Pap." This papyrus was part of his private collection and not for sale. The larger medical papyrus, also in Smith's possession, was originally known as the Papyrus Smith and in 1872 was sold to Georg Ebers, who changed the papyrus's name and published it in 1873 as the "Ebers Papyrus." Meanwhile, Edwin Smith worked diligently in his papyrus's translation, taking the papyrus with him when he departed Luxor for Naples in 1876. After his death in 1906, his daughter donated the

1. F. G. Kilgour, "Locating Information in an Egyptian Text of the 17th Century B.C.," *Journal of the American Society for Information Sciences* 44 (1993): 292–97.

2. Théodule Devéria cited by ibid., 292.

papyrus to the New York Historical Society. It was later housed from 1938 to 1948 in the Brooklyn Museum. The New York Historical Society presented the papyrus to the New York Academy of Medicine in 1948, where it has resided to date, with the exception that the papyrus was publicly exhibited at the Metropolitan Museum of Art during "The Art of Medicine in Ancient Egypt" exhibit September 13, 2005, to January 15, 2006, under the expert direction of James P. Allen Ph.D., who also produced an updated translation for the Metropolitan Museum of Art published Catalogue.

Translation by James Henry Breasted

Professor James Henry Breasted, first chair in Egyptology and Oriental History in the United States, and founder of the Oriental Institute at the University of Chicago was requested in 1920 by the New York Historical Society to translate and publish the papyrus. After examining the document Breasted could not refuse. His preliminary report was published in the *New York Historical Society Quarterly Bulletin* Vol. 6(1) in April of 1922 and a more technical report was published as "The Edwin Smith Papyrus: Some Preliminary Observations," in *Recueil d'études égyptologiques dédiées à la mémoire de Jean-François Champollion* (Paris: Champion, 1922), 385–429.

The scroll contained a recto (front) forming approximately seven-eighths of the written papyrus and a verso (back). Although Breasted translated the entire document, he recognized the contents of the verso as being of great importance to Egyptology, medicine, and world history. The recto consisted of "incantations and recipes … a later addition, having no relation to the front."[3] Breasted's comprehensive work on this highly complex ancient medical document had no historical precedent and he admitted to possessing no competency in the medical field. Breasted then sought medical advice from his friend, Dr. Arno Luckhardt (American Physiologist, at the University of Chicago).[4]

Breasted identified the papyrus as a partial copy of a didactic medical text produced in the latter part of the seventeenth century BC, and determined that the complex structure and topographical organization address a series of trauma studies, "case types," organized anatomically from the head down and in order of increasing severity of injury. Breasted labeled the distinct segments he discerned within each case in the papyrus as: "Title," "Examination," "Diagnosis," and "Treatment." Recognizing that concepts and terminology appearing for the first time were explained at the end of that case, Breasted established these explanations as "glosses."[5] The terms, then, were used in later cases without further explanation. Text rubrics usually indicated the beginning of a new case (title), important elements of diagnosis and explanatory notes.

After ten years of meticulous work, Breasted's definitive work on the papyrus was published in two volumes by the University of Chicago Oriental Institute Publications as "The Edwin Smith Surgical Papyrus." With this work, Breasted gifted the world of medicine and history with the most outstanding medical document from antiquity.

Verdicts/Prognoses

Not unlike Greek and Roman medicine, the ancient Egyptian physician's diagnostic opinions were tied to treatment potential for each injury. Three verdicts are issued:

---

3. James Henry Breasted, *The Edwin Smith Surgical Papyrus* (2 vols; The University of Chicago. Oriental Institute Publications 3–4; Chicago: University of Chicago Press, 1930), 6.

4. Arno Benedict Luckhardt, 1885–1957. Online: http://www.the-aps.org/publications/tphys/legacy/1970/issue1/1.pdf.

5. Throughout the translation presented here, Breasted's "glosses" are described as "explanations."

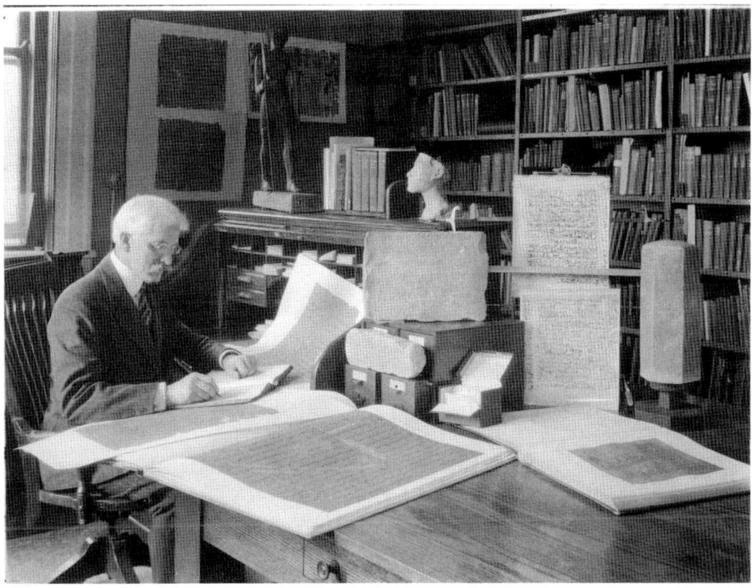

James Henry Breasted with plates of the Edwin Smith Papyrus in 1929 at his office, Haskell Hall, The Oriental Institute of the University of Chicago.

1. "a medical condition which I will handle/deal with"
2. "a medical condition I will fight with"
3. "a medical condition that cannot be handled/dealt with"

Verdict 1 is self-explanatory. Verdict 2 implies uncertainty about treatment results, but having "a fighting chance." Verdict 3 is exactly what it means, without implying that the patient will not be treated, but merely a declaration of their lack of expectation for successful treatment. Some cases were truly lethal, but some were not, the reality being that there was effective treatment that could be rendered as in a broken jaw, or fractured ribs. At first, these choices appear to be a sort of "triage." In reality the verdicts are expression of their realistic opinions and expectations of the patient's clinical course using the available treatments, with no equivalence in verdict 3 "a medical condition that cannot be handled/dealt with" to withholding, or delaying treatment. This is an important difference in our translation from Breasted's, who interpreted this verdict as: "An ailment not to be treated." The great majority of clinical situations in the Edwin Smith papyrus receiving verdict 3 were treated.

Our understanding today of basic sciences, medicine, surgery, and trauma is clearly much more complete. Four thousand years have passed since the Edwin Smith Papyrus was written, and, thus, the benefits of accumulated medical wisdom, antibiotics, anesthesia, surgery, and imaging studies. Yet, we face each trauma patient anew. In evaluation of these patients, we follow a clinical protocol, looking for those same important signs singled out by our predecessor, the Egyptian physician (*swnw*), so long ago. Medicine of ancient Egypt can pronounce as its most precious legacy the development and implementation of an elaborate clinical methodology to study each patient, the same methodology attributed by Plato to Hippocrates, but more than a thousand years after its actual origin with the Egyptian *swnw*.

This methodology established the grounds and facilitated progress in the rational knowledge of the human body, in health and in disease. Greek medicine was the direct beneficiary of the building blocks originated by the *swnw*, as we see here, which heralded the full future of medicine's development scientifically.

Of Special Interest to the Medical Field

The Edwin Smith Papyrus probably is a partial rendition of a comprehensive didactic medical treatise on trauma. No other copies have been found, nor have scholars determined its precise applications. The existence of established medicine and medical texts already in use by this time in ancient Egypt is recorded from the reign of Pharaoh Neferirkare, Fifth Dynasty (2450–2300 BC). The Vizier Ptahhotep suffered a stroke during an inspection of works with the King. The royal physicians were immediately summoned and the medical books were brought in and consulted. But unfortunately, there was nothing that could be done for the Vizier, and he died.

Of the forty-eight clinical cases in the Edwin Smith Papyrus, there are fourteen head injuries, seven cervical injuries, and one injury to the lower spine, all of which are of particular interest to the neurologist, neurosurgeon, and traumatologist. Injuries or lesions of the chest and arms constitute the rest of the treatise. Injuries are presented by the ancient Egyptian physician by key examination findings, given with sufficient clarity to allow us to form a medical opinion of the type of injury and of the patient's condition. The injuries described in this document for a specific anatomical area, are presented in order of increasing severity. Thus, it is possible to understand those factors that guided the Egyptian physician to reach a verdict (treatability assessment/prognosis) in cases that otherwise appear to be of similar gravity.

Breasted's original translation has been subject to various medically oriented interpretations, most notably by Courville in 1949,[6] Bardinet in 1995,[7] and Westendorf in 1966 and 1999.[8] In 2001, Brawanski first approached a full medical interpretation of the first eight cases of this document in modern terms.[9] Additionally, he has provided further valuable medical interpretation and commentaries of other selected cases. Further progress on philological and selective surgical issues has been made by many authors, most prominently by Grapow, von Deines, and Westendorf, the authors of the *Grundriss der Medizin der alten Ägypter*.[10] Other works have been presented by authors Walker,[11] Nunn,[12] Ghalioungui,[13] Chapman,[14] Majno,[15] Goodrich,[16] and, most recently, Allen's previously cited recent translation.[17] Despite point clarifications and better understanding of the Edwin Smith Papyrus, some passages still remained obscure. Some were considered to be scribal errors, and a few segments did not make clinical sense.

Brawanski called attention in 2001 to the fact that our modern clinical evaluation and treatment strategies in the management of head injury use comparable criteria to that existing at the time of the Edwin Smith

6. C. B. Courville, "Injuries to the Skull and Brain in Ancient Egypt," *Bulletin of the Los Angeles Neurological Society* 14/2 (1949): 53–82.

7. Thierry Bardinet, *Les papyrus médicaux de l'Égypte Pharaonique: traduction intégrale et commentaire* (Lyon: Fayard, 1995).

8. Wolfhart Westendorf, *Papyrus Edwin Smith: Ein medizinisches Lehrbuch aus dem alten Ägypten: Wund- und Unfallchirurgie, Zaubersprüche gegen Seuchen, verschiedene Rezepte*. Bern: Hans Huber,1966; Wolfhart Westendorf, *Handbuch der altägyptischen Medizin* (vol. 2; Leiden: Brill, 1999).

9. A. Brawanski, "Die Fälle 1–8 des Papyrus Edwin Smith," *Studien zur altägyptischen Kultur* 29 (2001): 7–39.

10. Hermann Grapow, Wolfart Westendorf, and Hildegard von Deines, *Grundriss der Medizin der alten Ägypter* (9 vols.; Berlin: Akademie, 1954–1973), esp. vols. 5 (Grapow, *Die medizinischen Texte in hieroglyphischer Umschreibung Autographiert*, 1958) and vol. 4 (von Deines, Grapow, and Westendorf, *Übertsetzung der medizinitschen Texte*, 1958).

11. James H. Walker, *Studies in Ancient Egyptian Anatomical Terminology* (The Australian Centre for Egyptology Studies 4; Warminster: Aris & Phillips, 1996),

12. John F. Nunn, *Ancient Egyptian Medicine* (Norman, OK: Oklahoma University Press, 1996).

13. Paul Ghalioungui, *Magic and Medical Science in Ancient Egypt* (Amsterdam: Israël, 1963).

14. P. H. Chapman, "Case Seven of the Smith Surgical Papyrus: The Meaning of *tp3w*," *Journal of the American Research Center in Egypt* 29 (1992): 35-42

15. Guido Majno, *The Healing Hand: Man and Wound in the Ancient World* (Cambridge, MA: Harvard University Press, 1975).

16. J. T. Goodrich, "History in Spine Surgery in the Ancient and Medieval Worlds," *Neurosurgical Focus* 16/1 (2004).

17. James P. Allen, *The Art of Medicine in Ancient Egypt* (New York: The Metropolitan Museum of Art; New Haven: Yale University Press, 2005).

Papyrus. The same observation struck me when I first became acquainted with this papyrus as a neurosurgical resident in Bellevue Hospital, New York City, in 1965. It was in that year that the book *Neurosurgical Classics* (ed. Robert H. Wilkins; New York: The Harvey Cushing Society, 1965) was published. Containing the neurosurgical classical works up to that time, *Neurosurgical Classics* began with an excerpt of James Henry Breasted's *The Edwin Smith Surgical Papyrus*. Reading on, I was astonished to realize that the ancient Egyptian physicians had faced thousands of years ago, challenges no different from ours, and, that their clinical approach to their injured patients was strangely familiar to me, because it followed the same rational clinical approach within their evaluation and treatment. At the Emergency Room, every head injury required us to follow a methodology and to have the clinical awareness to look for important examination findings, just as the Egyptian physician had practiced with his patients four thousand years before. This was the beginning of my life-long interest in the Edwin Smith Papyrus.

It was particularly through my study of Case #7 and the impasse I reached in understanding that case where the head injury is complicated by infection, that I fully understood the necessity of approaching the text as a physician, and that a succinct and thorough interpretation of the entire Edwin Smith Papyrus was awaiting realization. I initially sought the assistance of Ms. Alwyn L. Burridge, M.A. Egyptology, who also had a keen interest in this medical document, and who greatly contributed with her own interpretation of the hieratic text. Ms. Burridge has also collaborated with me in a medical-Egyptological publication on head injuries and with me and Dr. Joost van Middendrop in spinal trauma cases, both based on the Edwin Smith Papyrus.[18] The participation in the current work of Egyptologist and linguist Edmund S. Meltzer Ph.D. has produced the most updated and medically concordant translation of the original text. This work of Sanchez and Meltzer fulfills a need for both modern medical opinion and documentation with relevant medical scientific literature, as well as the exhaustive medically oriented philological analysis of the text.

In our methodology, we have given primacy to interpret the text in its medical context, restraining from speculation. However, given the wealth of data and the significance of this early medical document, we felt it to be critically important to say not more, but, to say no less than is written. Each case is interpreted on sound and reasonable clinical data. Where we digress from other authors' interpretations, it is merely on different clinical points of view, but always based on the textual evidence, the structure of the original document, or on comparable data from other medical papyri. To facilitate text analysis, the hieratic text belonging to each individual case has been isolated from surrounding material. Pertinent figures are included at the end of most cases, and, to fully display the quality of the clinical material contained in this papyrus and as a quick reference, a "Visual Index" section has been included at the back of the volume. Concise reference sections on Open and Closed Injuries (appendix 1), Neurological Symptoms and Signs (appendix 2), a compilation of cases with the verdict "(a medical condition) that cannot be handled/dealt with" (appendix 3), and Analysis of Nasal Anatomical Terminology (appendix 4) have been added as practical references for the reader. Our new translation derives from an advanced linguistic understanding of the text and from its central strong medical orientation culminating in a fluid, logical, medically sound, and contemporary document. The word "surgical" is not used in our translation, as the document deals very little with actual surgery.

The Egyptian physicians' clinical experience led them to record features that were important in formulating their verdicts, and in noting relationships between head or spine injuries and their neurological consequences. Neurological symptoms and findings are not included in the compound (open) severe cranial injuries, but are included in the closed head injuries. This could be related to the numerous possible combinations of neurological

18. Gonzalo M. Sanchez and Alwyn L. Burridge, "Decision Making in Head Injury Management in the Edwin Smith Papyrus," *Neurosurgical Focus* 23/1 (2007): 1–9. Jost J. van Middendorp, Gonzalo M. Sanchez, and Alwyn L. Burridge, "The Edwin Smith Papyrus: A Clinical Reappraisal of the Oldest Known Document on Spinal Injuries," *European Spine Journal* 19/11 (2010): 1815–23. Online: http://www.springerlink.com/content/vk460l07q7028186/fulltext.pdf.

deficits possibly present in the acute stage, depending upon what areas of the brain sustained injury. However, this is most likely related to survivability being more frequent in closed head injuries, allowing for observation and recording of residuals. A similar situation could apply to a complication of the acute head injury, which in fact, constitutes a new entity as in Case #7, First Alternative Course: Infection–*tiꜣ* (Tetanus). Spinal-cord injury neurological deficits are well detailed.

The Edwin Smith Papyrus is of importance to anyone with an interest in medicine and medical history. It is a document that brings us back in time to witness the practice of our profession already as an established "art," not long after the writing of language had begun. It was a time in which terms had to be created for anatomy, for symptoms, and eventually for diseases. This medical didactic text clearly begins with the explanation of the reason for all of us to be in the field: the patient. Case #1, Explanation A, details in ancient terms what it means "to examine a patient." It then follows with a dissertation of the vascular system from which we elucidate the ancient Egyptian physicians' concepts of areas in clinical medicine that we recognize today.

In the Edwin Smith Papyrus we can glean specifics in the following medical fields:

- Anatomy and Physiology:
    - The heart and its relations to the entire body through the pulse
    - Brain convolutions
    - Cerebrospinal fluid
    - The frontal sinus
    - The nasal cavities
    - The anterior fontanelle pulsations

- Anatomical pathology:
    - Craniofacial fractures
    - Bone fragmentation visible inside the ear canal
    - Various soft tissue wounds
    - Various types of bone fractures and joint dislocations
    - Cervical disc tears
    - Cervical compression fracture
    - Cervical burst fracture
    - Infected wounds
    - Necrotic wounds
    - Chest wall injuries to bone and soft tissue;
    - Possible neurofibromatosis
    - Lumbar disc sprain

- Pathogenesis:
    - Traumatic meningismus
    - Systemic infection developing from an open head injury
    - Intracranial tissue damage from external trauma
    - Detection of transmitted brain pulsations in head injuries as being the consequence of cranial vault disruption and comparing this finding to the examination of an infant's open fontanelle
    - A glimpse to their theory about disease spreading through the blood vessels
    - Mechanisms of cervical injuries resulting in spinal cord injury

- Clinical Data:
  - What it means "to study a man"
  - The pulse
  - Tetanus
  - Depressed level of consciousness in head injury
  - Aphasia
  - Epistaxis and otorrhagia in base of the skull fractures
  - Oculomotor paralysis from head injury
  - Spastic hemiparesis
  - Traumatic esophageal cutaneous fistula
  - Spinal cord injury with quadriplegia, urinary incontinence, ileus and priapism
  - Crepitus in comminuted fractures
  - Intercostal pain
  - The meaning of "the period of crisis" after head trauma

- Therapy:
  - "In bed (under observation and support)"—resting a patient in quiet quarters, under observation
  - Use of the sitting position in severe head trauma
  - Auricle of the ear injury surgical repair detail
  - Technique of mandibular dislocation reduction
  - Treatment of wounds by the use of fresh meat and honey
  - Treatment of infected wounds
  - Stitching and applying strips of cloth to wounds
  - Cauterizing an abscess
  - Avoid bandaging in severe head injuries
  - Warning about the presence of large vessels behind the sternoclavicular joints

The Edwin Smith Papyrus is a surviving sample of a comprehensive medical didactic text on trauma, emerging shortly after development of written language, at the birth of scientific medicine. The importance to modern medicine is accurately captured by Goodrich: "The Edwin Smith Papyrus provides modern neurosurgeons with a window in time through which they can wonder at the challenges and insights faced by ancient Egyptian healers at the dawn of the medical profession."[19] Referring to ancient Egyptian medicine, embodied in the "*swnw*" the word for physician, Guido Magno concludes: "If fame is a measure of success, we can only congratulate the *swnu* [sic]. In the Mediterranean world his art was unsurpassed, until it was absorbed by Greek Medicine."[20]

19. J. T. Goodrich, "History in Spine Surgery in the Ancient and Medieval Worlds," *Neurosurgical Focus* 16/1 (2004): 2.
20. Majno, *The Healing Hand*, 140.

Philological Introduction

Edmund S. Meltzer, Ph.D.

I was both delighted and honored when I was invited to join a project to produce a new edition of the Edwin Smith Papyrus including a translation and both Egyptological and medical commentaries.

We devoted a great deal of thought to the grammatical approach to adopt for the translation and decided to proceed according to the Standard Theory, that is, the analysis of the function and syntax of Egyptian verb-forms pioneered and developed by Hans J. Polotsky, elaborated and expanded by other scholars including Mordechai Gilula, John Callender, Paul John Frandsen, Friedrich Junge, Eric Doret, Leo Depuydt, and James Hoch.[21] There are several reasons for this. The primary reason is that I am not convinced by the arguments that have been advanced against it, or the alternatives that some have proposed in its place. I have addressed this in several publications and papers, most recently, "Once Again Initial Adverbials and the Standard Theory," presented at the Annual Meeting of ARCE in Chicago, April 2011. While I am somewhat flexible and open to different approaches, and I do not think that the Standard Theory, at least in its current forms, solves all of the problems of Egyptian grammar, I find the Standard Theory of unmatched heuristic usefulness in working with Egyptian grammar. While working through the cases of Edwin Smith, I found that with very few exceptions (which are discussed in the commentary), the clauses fell very felicitously and elegantly into place and the forms could be identified when a Standard Theory model was applied. While we do not expect the present translation to put to rest different suggested solutions for many passages, I think that it can stand as a cogent and consistent understanding of the text, enhancing the credibility and utility of the Standard Theory while also further enhancing the credibility and validity of the medical content.

As an example of a significant insight resulting from the application of the Standard Theory model, I would draw special attention to the use of the geminating *sḏm.f gmm.k*. There is a very clear reason why the examination description uses the nominal form or Manner Nominalization, and why it should not be taken as a "virtual conditional." The conditional is found in the opening clause or protasis, "If you examine a man" who has a particular type of wound that is specified. Then the examination shows particular findings, "How you find his cranium," "How you find him, etc." (is) in such-and-such a condition. The master physician, that is, the author of the papyrus, knows full well what the student or "intern" will find with that particular type of wound. He is not saying, If you find A you will do A and if you find B you will do B. He is saying, How you will find him is this way. When a particular kind of wound admits two or more possible scenarios or variations that dictate different courses of treatment and he does want to say "If A is happening you will do A and if B is happening you will do B," he uses another marked conditional protasis with *ir gm.k* "If you find," with an explicit conditional, suggesting the inference that in such a case the findings might not be that uniform—but the point is that he uses

21. For orientation see L. Depuydt, "The Standard Theory of the 'Emphatic' Forms in Classical (Middle) Egyptian: A Historical Survey," *Orientalia Lovaniensia Periodica* 14 (1983): 13–54; a valuable overview of Polotsky's work is presented in a review of his *Collected Papers* (Jerusalem: Magnes Press, Hebrew University 1971) by H. S. Smith, P. Johnson and J. Barr, *Journal of Semitic Studies* 18 (1973): 129–44. A teaching grammar with a very accessible account of the Standard Theory is James Hoch's *Middle Egyptian Grammar*. Polotsky's most comprehensive statement is "Les transpositions du verbe en égyptien classique," *Israel Oriental Studies* 6 (1976): 1–50.

a marked or explicit conditional. Otherwise, he is using a form that is not intended as a conditional. The nearly universal tenency to take these *gmm.k* clauses as "virtual conditionals" illustrates the dangers of an approach to Egyptian grammar that takes it as containing a large percentage of "virtual" or unmarked clauses that can be pressed into service almost at the convenience of the translator (a strong tendency of the Gardiner or pre-Standard Theory approach) as compared with an approach in which most clauses are marked for a given grammatical function or identity. The former approach is conducive to producing a translation that largely follows the expectations of the translator; as Junge says, "everybody gets the Egyptian he deserves."[22]

It should be noted that what we and Callender[23] call the Manner Nominalization (a formulation that was also endorsed by R. J. Williams [review of Callender, *Middle Egyptian*, *Journal of Biblical Literature* 98 (1979) 103–4, and on numerous occasions in class discussions]), and Hoch calls the Explicatory Sentence,[24] is also accepted by Borghouts in the recently published English edition of his grammar, *Egyptian: An Introduction to the Writing and Language of the Middle Kingdom* (Leuven: Peeters, 2010), secs. 61–64, in which the form is characterized as "a description of how an action or state unfolds …," "howness," though he explains it as a consequence of imperfective aspect, a connection which we reject. In our view the Manner Nominalization is aspect-neutral, and close attention to the meaning and situation of every adverbial complement reveals incongruities in the attempt to fit them all into a concept of imperfectivity. The adverbial complement or "pivot" can have momentary as well as durative or frequentative meaning (as ibid., sec. 62 ex. 10). Moreover, the multifarious ways in which Borghouts differentiates the concept of imperfectivity make it difficult to draw the line or exclude a proposed example—a situation analogous to the application of the "context of plurality" to geminating participles and relative forms by Schenkel and Allen.[25] In effect, Borghouts' position is a crypto-Gardinerian one. The essential point, though, is that his recent and major synthesis of grammar also utilizes the Manner Nominalization though it departs from our grammatical analysis in some respects.

Conditional protases that themselves contain a Manner Nominalization are discussed by H. Satzinger, "Die Protasis *ir sḏm.f* im älteren Ägyptisch," *Lingua Aegyptia* 3 (1993): 121–35. The identity of the form following *ir* in the simplest or most basic protasis is sometimes the Prospective *sḏm.f* but most typically a form that seems identical with the circumstantial *sḏm.f* and can be identified as the Active *sḏm(w).f* (Hoch, *Middle Egyptian Grammar*, secs. 134, 188; Satzinger, "Die Protasis *ir sḏm.f*," 122–23).

One deceptively simple form that recurs numerous times in Edwin Smith is the favorable verdict or prognosis *iry.i*, for which we have followed Allen (*AM*, 70) in translating "which I will handle/deal with." This seems very felicitously in keeping with the versatility and flexibility of the verb *iri*. I agree with Breasted in identifying this as the Prospective Relative Form, which, when Breasted wrote, had recently been identified by Gunn (Breasted, *Edwin Smith*, 95). This presents a potential problem, however, because as apparent equivalents of "marked" relative clauses with *nty*, relative forms are generally regarded as having *definite* referents or antecedents, an approach that I have not rejected, though "I do not think that participles and attributive adjectives are to be regarded as inherently definite."[26] The prognosis clause seems to involve an indefinite antecedent, "a medical condition," "an ailment," etc. It seems to me that a solution is to be found in the discussion of J. Gwyn Griffiths in his article, "The Relative *Nty* with Generic Reference," *Journal of Egyptian Archaeology* 54 (1968):

22. "How to Study Egyptian Grammar and to What Purpose. A Summary of Sorts," *Lingua Aegyptia* 1 (1991): 401.

23. John B. Callender, *Studies in the Nominal Sentence in Egyptian and Coptic*. Near Eastern Studies 24. Berkeley and Los Angeles: University of California Press, 1984.

24. James E. Hoch, *Middle Egyptian Grammar* (SSEA Publications 15. Mississauga, Ontario: Benben, 1996), sec. 148.

25. See my comments in "Participles, Relative Forms and Gemination in Middle Egyptian: A Working Paper," *Lingua Aegyptia* 1 (*Proceedings of the Second International Conference on Egyptian Grammar (Crossroads II) Los Angeles, October 17–20, 1990* (1991), 232–34.

26. "Problems of Adjectival Constructions in Old and Middle Egyptian" (PhD dissertation, University of Toronto, 1980), II.5.

60–66. Griffiths concludes, "There is still a process of definition involved, but it now relates to a type or class...." In accordance with this analysis, I think that *mḥr iry.i* should be strictly understood as something like "a medical condition of the type that I will handle," or perhaps "the type of medical condition that I will handle," but we shall continue to use the simpler version in our running translation for convenience. (The concept of "specificity" in Egyptian grammar was elaborated in much greater detail by J. B. Callender.[27]

Of the three prognoses or verdicts, *n irw.ny* is the only one that cannot be parsed as a relative form and that should be taken as the true virtual relative, if that is not an oxymoron. Breasted's ingenious explanation as a passive participle + the prepositional adverb *ny*, though impressive, is not feasible because it would not emply the negation with *n* (which observation would also apply to a relative form), nor can there be a question of the archaizing use of *n* for *nn* if, as has become widely accepted, the construction is a form of the *n sḏm.n.f* negation of ability. This prognosis is taken as the variant of the *n sḏm.n.f* with the formative with impersonal subject *ny* by Allen (*ME*, sec. 18.5, pp. 227–28), Westendorf (*GMT*, 177–78, sec. 245) and von Deines and Westendorf in the dictionary of the medical texts.[28] The ending *w* does not find a facile explanation however; Westendorf notes the possibility that it represents the weak radical of the 3ae inf. verb, but acknowledges that this does not have apparent parallels in Smith. I am inclined to accept it nonetheless, in light of the "abnormal" form *dy.n.i* and the writing *iiw.n.i* with the base of the verb *ii*, that is, the reedleaf with legs (Gardiner, *EG*[3], sec. 413). I am open to a clearer and more solidly substantiated identification but have not yet found it. The translation adopted here, "a medical condition) that cannot be handled/dealth with," takes the verb *iri* itself in the same sense as the positive prognosis *iry.i*.

Another principle to which I have tried very hard to adhere in this translation is *lectio dificilior* ("the more difficult reading"). This principle holds that of two or more textual witnesses, the one that presents most difficulty is likely to be the correct or original text because it is more probable that simpler readings have been "dumbed down" or simplified to gloss over difficulties. (This consideration is very pertinent in Egyptian textual studies, where literary texts often survive in schoolboy copies.) Similarly, with only one witness as in Edwin Smith, emendation of a text is considered a last resort and usually a way of evading difficulties rather than trying to explain them. Only under great duress have I departed from this guiding principle of textual study. I have only accepted emendations when they are amply supported by precedents and parallels, whenever possible, forms that occur numerous times in the text, such as *sḏm.<i>n.f* alongside similar passages in which the reedleaf in *sḏm.in.f* is written. This includes arriving at separate readings for two passages that are often emended to bring them in line with each other, when individual viable readings are possible and a sensible meaning can be arrived at for the text as it stands. My teachers, expecially Klaus Baer and Donald Redford, emphasized the importance of *lectio dificilior* and I remember clearly my colleague Jim Sanders at The Claremont Graduate School saying "respect the text, respect the text, respect the text."

In line with this last, it has of course been ever present in our minds throughout this project that the papyrus is written in hieratic, which we transcribe into hieroglyphs as an Egyptological expedient.[29] Hieratic is a more fluid and flexible, and, one might say, spontaneous script than hieroglyphs. Recently I have entered into communication with Dr. Angela McDonald of Glasgow, and she has sent me one conference presentation and two articles prominently featuring the use of hieratic,[30] along with additional reflections and observations.

---

27. *Studies in the Nominal Sentence in Egyptian and Coptic* (Berkeley and Los Angeles: University of Claifornia Press, 1984), 115–203.

28. *Wörterbuch der Medizinischen Texte*. Grundriss der Medizin der alten Ägypter 7/1 (Berlin: Akademie, 1961–62), 94.

29. On the place of hieroglyphs and hieratic in ancient Egyptian literacy and the Egyptological construct of Egyptian language studies, see E. Meltzer, "Hieratic Is Beautiful: Ancient Egyptian Calligraphy Revisited," in *Writing Systems and Cognition* (ed. W. C. Watt; Dordrecht: Kluwer, 1994), 293–301.

30. "Writing as a Weapon in Letters to the Dead," presented at the British Egyptological Conference at the British Museum; "A Metaphor for Troubled Times: The Evolution of the Seth Deity Determinative in the First Intermediate Period," *ZÄS* 134 (2007): 26–39;

I thank Dr. McDonald for her collegiality and generosity. Her work pays detailed attention to the forms of hieratic determinatives that have "automatically" been transcribed a standardized way in most dictionaries and editions of texts, and finds that subtle distinctions and variations relevant to the meaning are present. Thus for instance she writes, "Evidently alongside the giraffe, the cat, the dog, the jackal (in the Coffin Texts only), and the Seth animal may all act as determinatives of *sr*, each perspectivising the meaning of the word in different ways." ("Curiosity of the Cat," 375). Again, "However, the other contexts in which Sethian words are used draw out an additional nuance of their determinative ..." ("A Metaphor for Troubled Times," 30). We think that Dr. McDonald's observations are applicable to the use of hieratic determinatives in P. Edwin Smith, such as the flesh or discharging lips determinative on *wbnw* "wound" and the knife spouting or dripping blood on the word *kft*, although the attempt to translate graphic variants consistently on the basis of the dterminative did not ultimately hold up with sufficient rigor, since for instance the word *wbnw* "wound" referring to the selfsame wound might appear with different determinatives in adjacent or proximate lines of the same case, or in writings of the title of the same ancient medical book that is being cited.

The scribe of the present copy is of course not the author. As all have recognized from the beginning of the truly modern study of this document, the Edwin Smith Papyrus is a copy of an older original. How much older has been debated. We support a date in the range from the end of the Old Kingdom to the early Middle Kingdom, or very roughly ca. 2200–2000 BC. The earlier enthusiastic ascriptions of the work to the Old Kingdom or even to Imhotep himself have been abandoned (though some continue to maintain them; see, e.g., el-Kinawy cited by McDonald in the quote in the following paragraph). There are, however, words and remedies that certainly go back that far, a conspicuous example being *ỉmrw* "Alum(?)," sometimes written with the Old Kingdom value of the *mi* sign as *mr* + the phonetic complement *r*, as was already noted by Breasted. It should be emphasized, though, that not all of the criteria for "archaism" cited by Breasted hold up today. The omission of the preposition *m* is *not* an archaism but rather a Late Egyptianism as described by B. Kroeber.[31]

One statement of McDonald relates to the Seth-animal determinative and the proposed date of a putative *Urtext* or *Vorlage* of the extant papyrus, dovetailing with our own perspective that the original text from which Edwin Smith was copied dates to the First Intermediate Period ("A Metaphor for Troubled Times," 29 n. 14):

> It is generally acknowledged that P. Edwin Smith goes back to an older original manuscript. Breasted's suggestion of an Old Kingdom date (1930, xiii) continues to be cited (e.g., el-Kinawy 2003, 47), and the use of the Seth deity determinative supports a date between the Old Kingdom and early Middle Kingdom.

I concur with the dating of P. Edwin Smith in the Second Intermediate Period or the period covered by the Hyksos and the Theban Seventeenth Dynasty as proposed by Breasted and Allen; Grapow (*Grundriss* 2:88–89) prefers the very end of that range, stating that both Smith and Ebers (which he considers "brother" manuscripts) were written down ca. 1550 BC, and that it is trivial whether, as Breasted opined, Smith is somewhat older than Ebers. Palaeographically, the hand of Smith has many similarities with Ebers, Westcar, and the Rhind Mathematical Papyrus. While there are many broad similarities among hieratic hands of the Twelfth Dynasty through the beginning of the Eighteenth, the preponderance of forms in Smith concentrate in the last part of this continuum. For what it may be worth, I tend to agree with Breasted that Smith is a little earlier than Ebers. It should be noted however that one of the variables in palaeographical dating is the overlapping careers of scribes who wrote at the

"The Curiosity of the Cat in Hieroglyphs," in D. Magee et al., eds., *Sitting Beside Lepsius: Studies in Honour of Jaromir Malek at the Griffith Institute* (Leuven-Paris-Walpole MA: Peeters/Departement Oosterse Studies, 2009), 361–79.

31. Die Neuägyptizismen vor der Amarnazeit (PhD dissertation, Tübingen, 1970), 46–47, citing *GMT*, sec. 340.1 for examples in both Smith and Ebers. For earlier instances of fluctuation and irregularity involving m, see E. Meltzer, "The 'Misplaced Letter to the Dead,' and a Stela, Found Again," paper presented at the annual meeting of the American Research Center in Egypt, Seattle, 2008.

CASE	TITLE	DIAGNOSIS	EXPLANATIONS
1	+		+
2	+		+
3	+	+	+
4	+	+	++
5	+	+	
6	+		++
7	+	++	All
8	+	2nd	All
9	+	+	
10	+	+	+
11	+	+	All
12	+	+	All
13	+	+	
14	+	+	
15	+	+	
16	+	+	
17	+	+	
18	+	+	
19	+	+	+
20	+	+	
21	+	+	
22	+	+	+++
23	+	+	
24	+	+	
25	+	+	
26	+	+	+
27	+	+	
28	+	+	
29	+	+	
30	=	+	+
31	+	+	+
32	+	+	+
33	+	+	++
34	+	+	+
35	+	+	
36	+	+	
37	+	+	++
38	+	+	
39	+	+	+
40	+	+	+
41	+	+	All 5
42	+	+	+
43	+	+	+++
44	+	+	
45	+	+	++
46	+	+	+
47	+	++	+
48	+	+	

Table 1: Rubrications in the Edwin Smith Papyrus signal what the author and/or the scribe considered the most important segments in a given Case. All titles starting in black had a preceding phrase in red color.

same time but were educated earlier or later than their colleagues; thus an older scribe can write an "older" hand while a younger contemporary can write a "later" hand.[32] Therefore this question may not be able to be solved with certainty, though I for one would hesitate to consider it "*unerheblich*" as does Grapow.

One feature of the hieratic hand of P. Edwin Smith, which it shares with other texts of the time continuum referred to above, is the use of a more uncial, if we may use that word, and a more cursive variant of the same sign or group.[33] (I do not designate the forms as more literary and more epistolary or documentary, because the cursive forms occur alongside the less reduced forms in literary texts such as Sinuhe.) Several of the prominent examples of this phenomenon are:

M  and less frequently 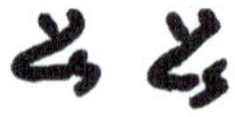

P 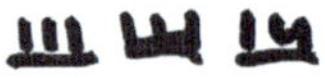, etc., the more cursive , and once the very cursive 

Y (double reedleaf) normally 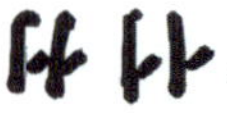, etc., rarely 

Mn with phonetic complement 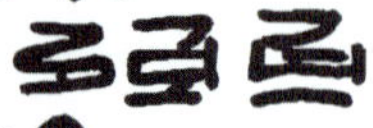 alongside the more cursive 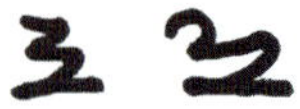

ḥr (face with stroke) 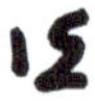 and 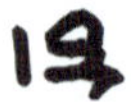

The scribe makes errors that, in a number of cases, he corrects himself, but is, on the whole, an adequately proficient scribe who writes in a good legible hand. There is at least one case in which the scribe seems to confuse a word in taking dictation, writing *iʿi* "wash" instead of **ʿi* "ascend, extend" (Case #40), an error very difficult to explain on the basis of copying a written text.

One last aspect of the scribe's practice needs to be addressed, namely, the use of rubrics or sections in red ink, a feature of many Egyptian papyri. Breasted characterizes this by saying, "the scribe of the Edwin Smith Papyrus employs very plentiful rubrics, so plentiful indeed that his discussion of a case may conclude with a remark in red, obliging the scribe to begin the next case in black in order to secure his desired contrast." He also remarks that when the scribe corrects his own errors, "in almost all cases he has detected these errors and has made his corrections in red ink over black, and in black ink over red" (1:29). Allen parallels Breasted's observation: "Each case begins with a title, usually written in red ink except where the final words in the previous case were in red" (70).

Kilgour made an attempt to define the overall pattern of the scribe's use of rubrics in an article most noteworthy for its extremely negative characterization of Edwin Smith himself (see below).[34] After some remarks on the use of rubrics in other Egyptian texts, Kilgour maintains that the alternation of red and black is a way of "indexing" so as to retrieve information, summarizing that "the use of red ink for titles and diagnoses in surgical cases, aided by a natural and logical arrangement of the cases, facilitated finding information in" the Edwin Smith Papyrus.[35] He states that "the beginning of Case 21 … is out of sequence because the scribe mistakenly wrote the last three-quarters of the treatment in red."[36] We feel that this is very problematic and that, in keeping with the text-critical principle of *lectio dificilior*, we should start with the presumption that the scribe knew what he was doing and had a reason for writing that passage in red, rather than assume that he was in error because

32. See Meltzer, "Misplaced Letter to the Dead"; cf. R. A. Parker, *A Saite Oracle Papyrus from Thebes* (Brown Egyptological Studies 4; Providence: Brown University Press, 1962), 14.

33. See G. Möller, *Hieratische Paläographie* I (Leipzig: Hinrichs, 1927), passim.

34. "Locating Information in an Egyptian Text of the 17th Century B.C.," *Journal of the American Society for Information Science* 44 (1993): 292–97.

35. Ibid., 296.

36. Ibid.

of our own expectations. (In addition, we do not think it is accurate to describe the cases as "surgical cases.") In studying the use of rubrication in the papyrus, we have made a chart that is given here on p. 13 above, showing the occurrence of rubrics (as distinct from corrections of individual signs and words), which we think does much to clarify the overall picture. In our best judgment, the occurrence of rubricized passages indicates the most important segments of a given case, with the proviso that if the end of a case is in red, the title of the next one will be in black. This one adjustment leaves the overall purpose of rubrication intact, that is, the setting off of what were considered the most important segments in red.

The copying of this text in the Second Intermediate/Hyksos period testifies to this period as a time of literary and scribal activity and preservation/proliferation of significant Egyptian cultural documents under Hyksos rule; note the emphasis on Egyptian scribal expertise and literary knowledge by the Hyksos king Apophis described on the scribal palette of Atju.[37] Another prominent example of a period of foreign rule marked by indigenous textual productivity and emphasis on the indigenous textual legacy is the Kassite period in Babylonia.[38]

A vital part of our methodological foundation and of the working method that we have adopted is the relationship between the Egyptological/philological and the medical components of this endeavor. The Egyptological and medical aspects have had a reciprocal and interactive relationship in arriving at the present translation. In each of the forty-eight cases, a preliminary, but in our opinion sound, translation was given to Dr. Sanchez, who interpreted the results clinically and wrote the detailed and comprehensive medical commentaries, and who responded to the translations with queries regarding the clinical corollaries and implications of both lexical and grammatical issues, and the medical consequences of different possible translations of a given passage. In light of all of our work, we can venture a basic reflection. The sophistication of the medical descriptions, diagnoses, prognoses, and prescriptions in this text, explored and explained in great detail by Dr. Sanchez, make us confident in considering the author a "master physician" and "master teacher." The master physician is not intimidated even by very serious symptoms but is guided by a body of precedent as well as experience in assessing the response of different injuries to a wide variety of treatments. The master physician writes in systematic formulations in balanced, elegant, and well-thought-out prose; the master physician is a consummate professional. The master physician cites and quotes earlier medical treatises and explains concepts and phraseology in a manner understandable to his students. This is not some slapdash hastily conceived or executed compilation. This is an impressive display of expertise of which any practitioner could be proud.

In the notes to the translation, we have tried to include those points that indicate why we are translating the text a particular way, and we have tried to convey some of the process of weighing alternatives and the criteria that we have regarded as important in opting for a particular translation. We have included notes that we hope will be helpful to the student who has not previously tackled this type of text. We hope that we have succeeded not only (at least for the most part) in justifying our proposed translations, but in communicating to the Egyptological and non-Egyptological reader alike something of the challenge and excitement and dynamic nature of the translation process as we have experienced it, the interaction with both grammatical structure and medical content, and moreover the interaction with an ancient author who was both a highly skilled and knowledgeable physician and an extremely articulate and intelligent human being.

One point needs to be clarified in the presentation of any new translation of the Edwin Smith Papyrus or indeed any Egyptian text, especially for the non-Egyptological reader. Of course we have undertaken the present work because we think that there are improvements large and small that can be ventured over the work of previous translators and commentators. As already remarked, we are not so overweening as to expect the present

37. D. B. Redford, *Egypt, Canaan, and Israel in Ancient Times* (Princeton: Princeton University Press, 1992), 122; idem, *Pharaonic King Lists, Annals, and Day-Books* (Mississauga: Benben, 1986), 163 and n. 171; H. Goedicke, "The Scribal Palette of Athu (Berlin Inv. Nr. 7798)," *Chronique d'Égypte* 63 (1988): 42–56.

38. See, e.g., Gwendolyn Leick, *The Babylonians: An Introduction* (New York: Routledge 2003), 46, 49–51.

effort to end debate. At the same time, it will be evident and is inevitable that the overlap with the efforts of previous translators is considerable. Egyptian is after all a known language, thanks to generations of pioneering scholars (on whom more below). While there is room for innovation and debate in both grammar and lexicon, the options for translating a given expression are often limited. Most Egyptologists will come up with the same basic text (which is indeed a test of whether a language has been deciphered, and was an early test to confirm the decipherment of Akkadian), as is apparent in comparing the major anthologies of literary and historical texts. Having said that, we reiterate that the potential progress offered by another comprehensive examination of the Edwin Smith Papyrus's medical cases was more than sufficient to justify our undertaking the present work, and we hope that the medical and Egyptological reader will agree.

Edwin Smith and His Contribution

While the Civil War was raging in North America, a conflict in which, with grim irony, unprecedented demands were placed on battlefield surgeons in the treatment of catastrophic wounds, one American, Edwin Smith, who had been living in Egypt since 1858, purchased the papyrus that is the subject of this volume (in January 1862 to be precise). He acquired the document from the well -known dealer and consular agent Mustafa Aga (Ayat), whose name is probably more widely associated with the events surrounding the discovery of the Deir el-Bahri cache of royal mummies. In his edition, Breasted gives a very detailed account of the history of the papyrus, which had to be reconstituted from a composite "papyrus" glued together by the dealer, an extremely patient and painstaking endeavor on Smith's part. Breasted also presents a detailed narrative of many of the events and accomplishments associated with Smith himself, who had studied Egyptology and had what was for his time an expert knowledge of the Egyptian language, and most notably an outstanding proficiency in the hieratic script. Smith was the first to read and communicate to the Egyptological community important hieratic texts including the correct reading of the date of the Ebers Calendar. This leads to one circumstance that has occasioned some confusion, that the larger medical papyrus subsequently acquired by Georg Ebers and known as Papyrus Ebers was in the keeping of Smith before Ebers acquired it, and it had become widely known and referred to by Egyptologists as "Papyrus Smith." This also led to some acrimony and aspersions cast on Smith's reputation, which has come down to our time significantly flawed in the major sources of Egyptological reportage. This is the nature of Barbara Mertz's account, which includes the very backhanded compliment, "Like many of his fellow 'adventurers,' he was no simpleminded crook."[39] Mertz concurs in Breasted's admiration of Smith's linguistic attainments. Her account largely converges with that of John Wilson, who also calls the purchaser of the renowned papyrus an "adventurer."[40] Wilson calls Smith "An equivocal figure," while admitting that "He was a good decipherer of hieratic." Wilson's substantial section on Smith includes shady aspects of his life and career (leaving his family in America, moneylending, involvement with forged antiquities). Wilson further draws attention to idiosyncratic ideas that Smith developed about the analysis of Egyptian words and takes a rather dismissive tone. The ideas may have been wrong, but we should not forget that Egyptian philology was in a more exploratory state at that time. (Also, to the language expertise of Smith's correspondent C. W. Goodwin, Wilson should add Chinese.) While Wilson is critical, presenting Smith "warts and all" as it were, F. G. Kilgour has drawn up what is to all intents and purposes a bill of indictment against Smith in an article ostensibly devoted to the organization and color-coding of information in the Smith Papyrus and other Egyptian texts.[41] In the information structure of the article itself, the biographical section on Smith is more a digression or distraction than anything else and is

39. *Red Land, Black Land: Daily Life in Ancient Egypt* (2nd ed.; New York: Morrow, 2008), 250.
40. *Signs and Wonders upon Pharaoh* (Chicago: University of Chicago, 1964), 52–57, 230.
41. "Locating Information in an Egyptian Text," 292–97.

scarcely relevant to the author's alleged theme. It might have been relevant to point out that Smith succeeded in understanding the sequence and information structure of the papyrus well enough to reconstitute it correctly from the composite collage in which it had been mounted. Kilgour states flatly that "Smith was a born loser"[42] and leaves no stone unturned that would reveal anything discreditable, some of which he seems to narrate with relish. He quotes the last part of Breasted's paragraph, which we cite below, affirming Smith's extraordinary level of understanding of the text, as well as a published reference to Smith's identification of a name on a seal in the Abbott collection with one in a hieratic papyrus[43] and a statement of Deveria that Smith was devoting himself to the translation of the papyrus,[44] but he quotes this all in an *en passant* fashion; he has nothing to add about Smith's scholarly achievements or contributions to Egyptology and essentially glosses over them, seeming to be in a hurry to proceed to the "dirt." He does not seem to entertain the possibility that a person capable of making Smith's contributions to Egyptian studies might not have been such a total loser after all. When at length Kilgour writes that "poor Smith gained his just renown" posthumously with the revelation to the world of the remarkable contents of the papyrus,[45] he does not suggest that Smith himself really did anything to earn that renown and refers only to the work of scholars who studied the papyrus in the twentieth century. To focus on the positive, which we think is substantial enough to justify an appreciative view of Smith's legacy, the letters that he wrote to C. W. Goodwin, mentioned by Breasted, Wilson, and Kilgour, are included in Warren R. Dawson's biography of Goodwin[46] and include Smith's solutions of difficult hieratic forms. Kilgour cites Dawson's work on Goodwin[47] but quotes the letters only insofar as they show Smith in a discreditable light. Also, Breasted's assessment of Smith's surviving notes on the papyrus to which both of them devoted so much labor, already mentioned above, should carry weight (*Edwin Smith*, 21):

> Among Mr. Smith's meager papers handed to me by the New York Historical Society I find a manuscript containing a remarkable attempt by Mr. Smith at a complete translation of the papyrus.... When we recall how scanty was the knowledge of hieratic in the sixties of the last century, when this effort at a translation was written out, not to mention also the very limited knowledge of the Egyptian language itself ..., it is extraordinary how much of the document Mr. Smith has understood.

We are very pleased to be able to announce in this publication that our inquiries have succeeded in locating the elusive Smith manuscript in the files of the New York Historical Society at the Brooklyn Museum, in the form of photostats of thirteen handwritten pages. We tender our grateful thanks to Dr. Edward H. Bleiberg, Curator, Egyptian, Classical, Ancient Near Eastern Art, for cheerfully granting permission to publish it, to Ms. Kathy Zurek-Doule for sending us images of the photostats as well as inverted positive exposures which are far more legible, and to Librarian Sandy Wallace and Graduate Intern Jessica Popkin, all of whom have distinguished themselves by their extremely collegial cooperation and helpfulness. The entire manuscript is illustrated and transcribed with a brief introduction in an appendix to the present work. A truly in-depth understanding will, however, require a far more extensive commentary, which the authors plan to provide in a separate publication. Even at first blush, we are impressed by the accuracy which Smith was able to achieve in some of his translation, the rigorous and methodical nature of his approach and use of terminology, and the striking perceptiveness of his intuitions. Of course his work would have been entirely impossible without his fluency in the reading of hieratic.

42. Ibid., 292.
43. Ibid.
44. Ibid., 292–93.
45. Ibid., 293.
46. *Charles Wycliffe Goodwin, 1817–1878: A Pioneer in Egyptology* (Oxford: Oxford University Press, 1934).
47. "Locating Information in an Egyptian Text," 292–93.

Speaking of the British Egyptologist Samuel Birch, T. G. H. James notes the rudimentary state of the study of hieratic in that era of Egyptology.[48] Muller quotes James:

> One of the most remarkable things about his early work is that he began to study hieratic papyri, notes James … "In 1841, the first hieratic papyri were published with 'very succinct' notes provided by Birch. James notes that 'it was still difficult to decipher these texts, but he made a pretty good shot at determining the nature of their contents.'"

It is remarkable that about twenty years later, Smith was able to do so much more, decades before the availability of any such reference tools as Georg Möller's *Hieratische Paläographie.*

Edwin Smith apparently never published anything in his own lifetime. In this he resembled his fellow pioneer, the far more lauded and lionized Charles Edwin Wilbour (who, it can be remembered, also had a checkered past). The authors think that it is more than a little unfair that Wilbour has a library and a professorship named after him as well as a papyrus and that he is generally regarded as one of the gods or at least patriarchs of early Egyptology, while Edwin Smith only has a papyrus and is remembered, if at all, in very mixed or somewhat negative terms. The full recognition of Edwin Smith's contribution to the study of the papyrus that bears his name, and of his contribution to the progress of Egyptology, is necessary if he is to be restored to his rightful place in the annals of Egyptian philology. As W. H. Auden wrote in his elegy "In Memory of W. B. Yeats,"

> Time that is intolerant
> Of the brave and innocent …
> Worships language and forgives
> Everyone by whom it lives.

Let that be his epitaph, and let this new edition of his papyrus and the long overdue publication of his own manuscript be a tribute to his memory.[49]

48. K. Muller, "Samuel Birch, the Discreet Pioneer Egyptologist," *The Egyptological Seminar News* 3 (1998) 3–4.

49. These lines are part of the original 1939 version but omitted in 1966 and later editions of Auden's shorter collected works: http://www.norton.com/college/english/nap/In_Memory_of_W_Yeats_Auden.htm#poem.

Visual Index

VISUAL INDEX I

Craniofacial Injuries in the Edwin Smith Papyrus

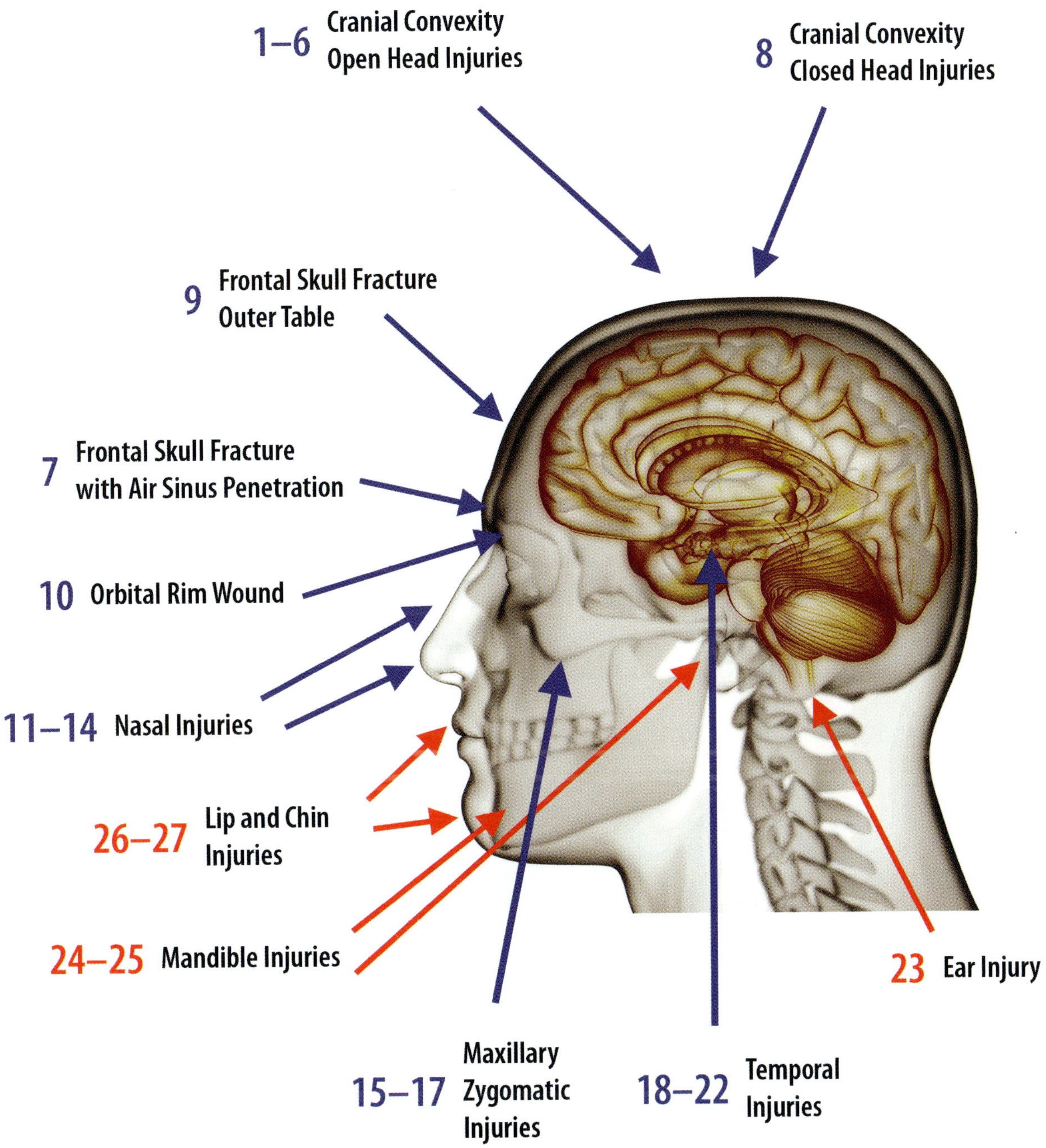

Image courtesy of PHOTO RESEARCHERS, 307 Fifth Ave., New York, NY 10016.

VISUAL INDEX II

Extracranial Injuries in the Edwin Smith Papyrus

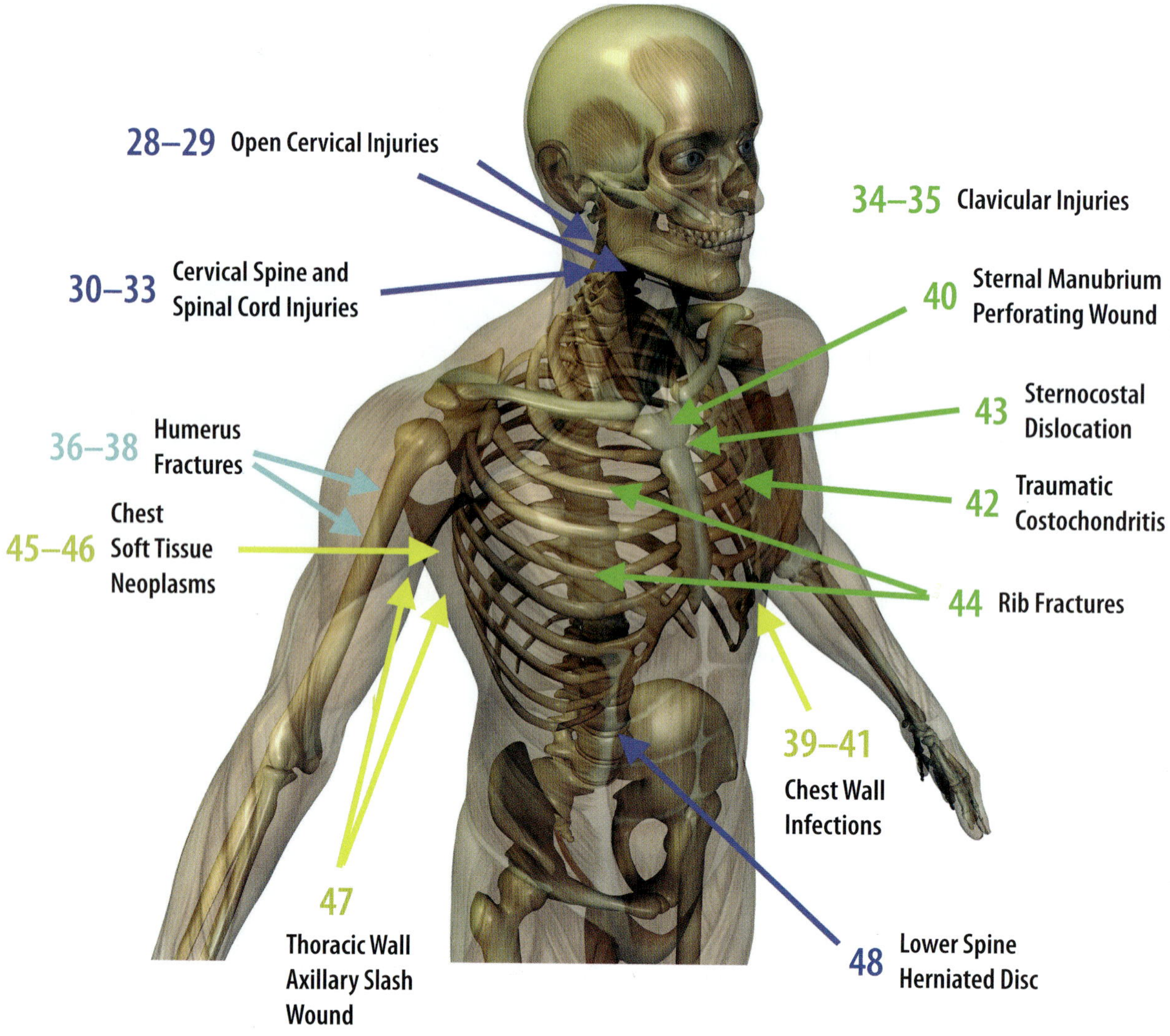

Image courtesy of PHOTO RESEARCHERS, 307 Fifth Ave., New York, NY 10016.

VISUAL INDEX III

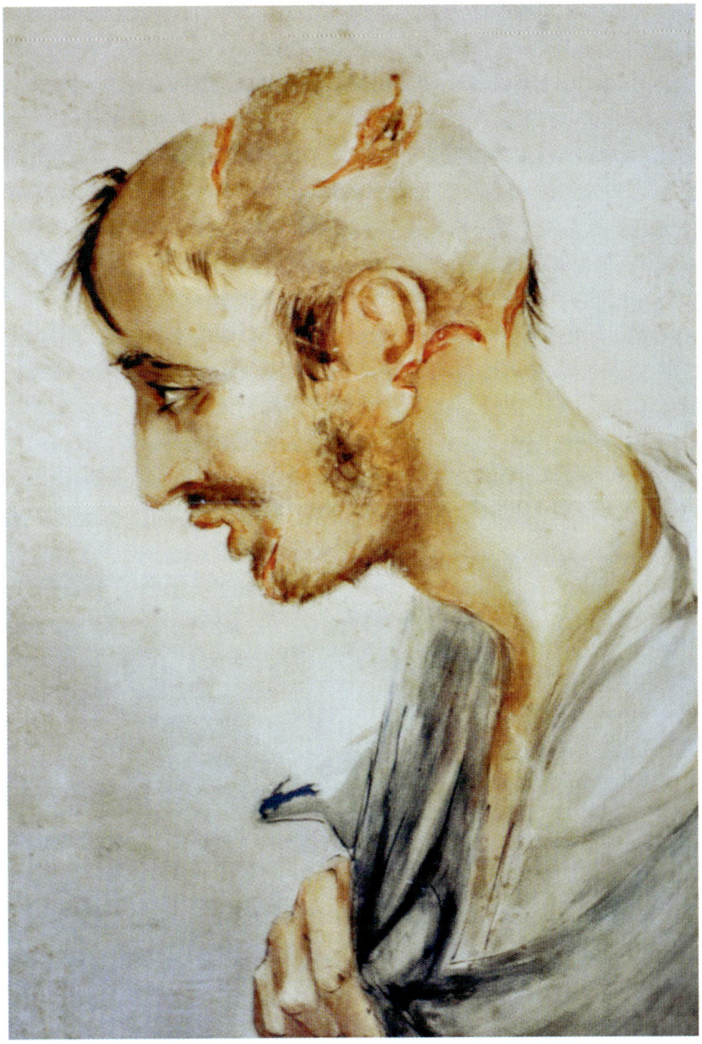

Sir Charles Bell's Trooper 1st Royal Dragoons

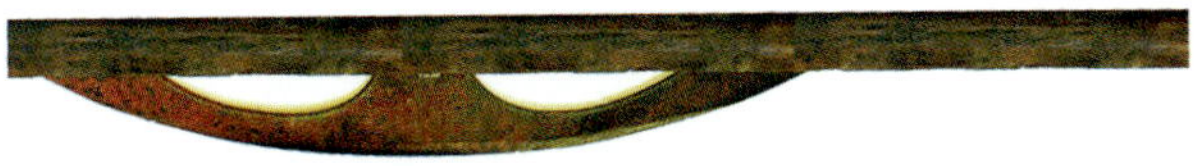

Epsilon Egyptian Battleaxe

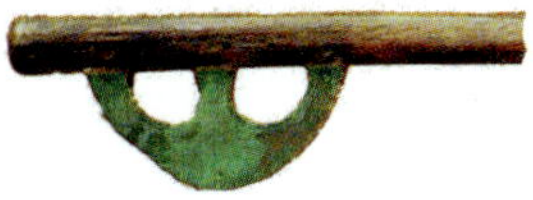

Round Small-Eyed Battleaxe

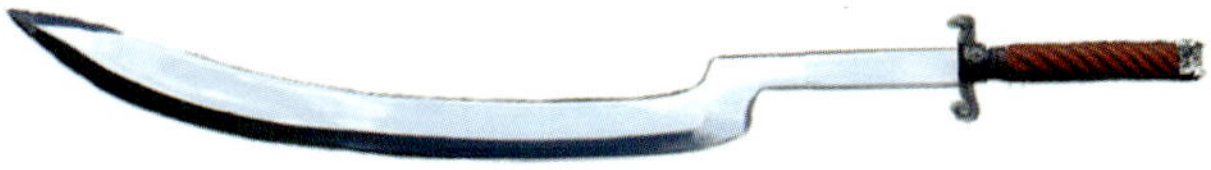

Khopesh Sword (Modern Replica)

VISUAL INDEX IV

Cranial Fractures in the Edwin Smith Papyrus

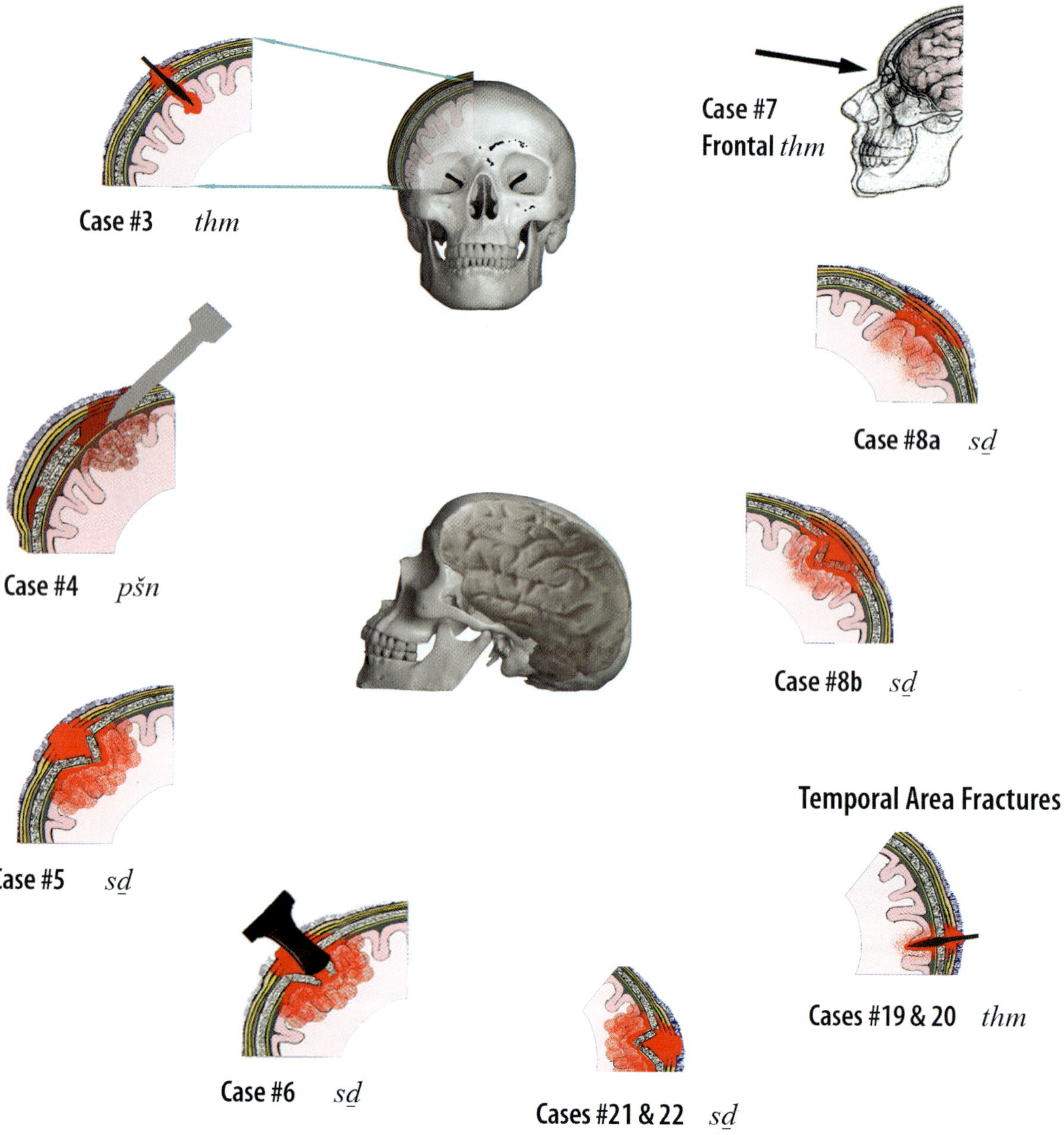

VISUAL INDEX V

CRANIAL INJURIES IN THE EDWIN SMITH PAPYRUS

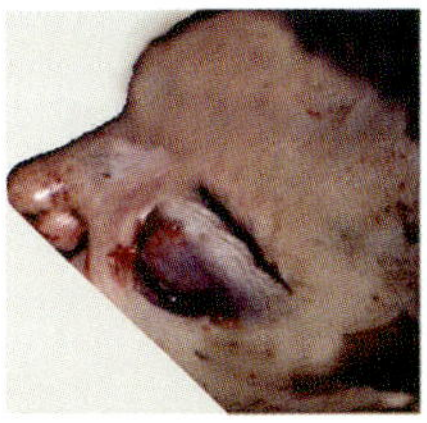

a Periorbital Ecchymosis
from Fractured Orbital Roof(s)

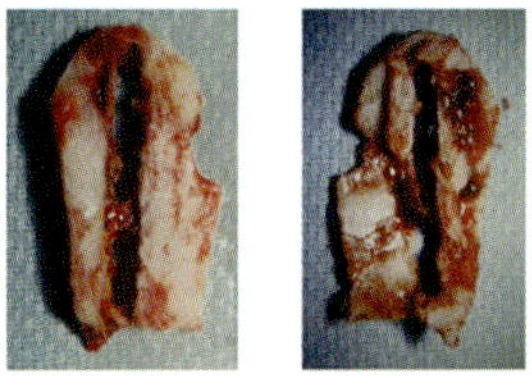

b Penetrating Skull Fracture
by Cutting Weapon

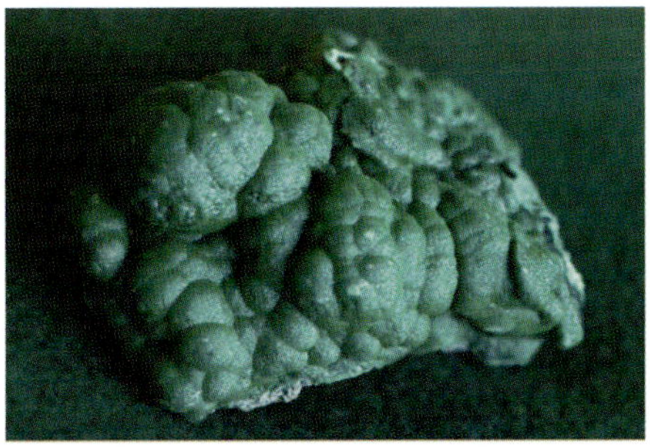

c Botryoidal Malachite $Cu_2(CO_3)(OH_2)$
Naturally occurring copper compound in igneous rocks that have similar appearance to slag produced during copper smelting.
Case #6 Explanation B compares the brain appearance to that of copper slag.

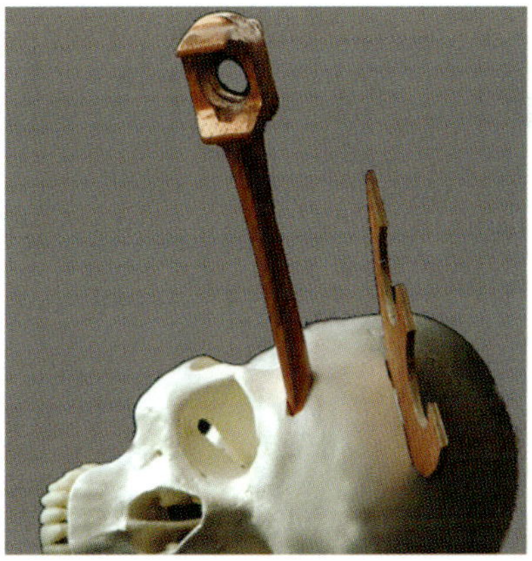

d Syro-Palestinian Axe and Broad-Blade Axe injuries to the right frontal skull as in that of King Seqenenre Tao II.

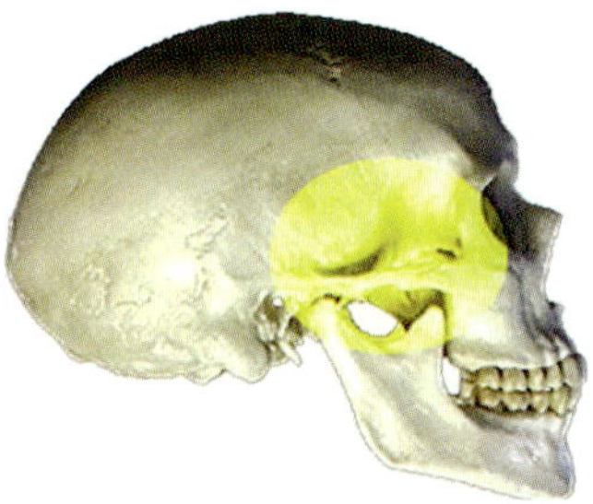

e *gmȝ* Case #18, Explanation B

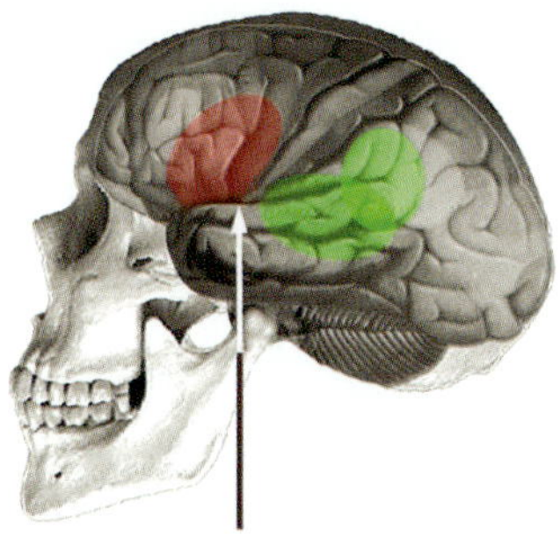

f Speech Areas – Dominant Hemisphere
Broca – Frontal Lobe
Wernicke – Temporal and Parietal Lobes

VISUAL INDEX VI

Case #7: First Alternative Course: Infection (Tetanus)

Frontal cutting wound with compound skull fracture penetrating the frontal air sinus
The patient has developed infection (Tetanus)

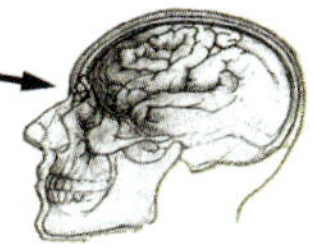

(drawing by Allison Stout)

Necessary knowledge and skills for a slash wound in his head penetrating to the bone and perforating the membranous lined cavities of his braincase.

Signs of Infection

If however you find that man, his flesh having developed heat because of that wound which is in the membranous lined cavities of his braincase.

How you find his forehead (is) clammy with perspiration

his face being flushed

the odor of his braincase being like the excrement of goats.

while that man has developed *ti3* because of that wound

Signs of Tetanus

(Opisthotonus) the ligaments of the back of his neck being taut

(Risus Sardonicus) his teeth, (it) shining

(Trismus) his mouth being immobile / bound

his eyebrows quivering

his face being something like he weeps

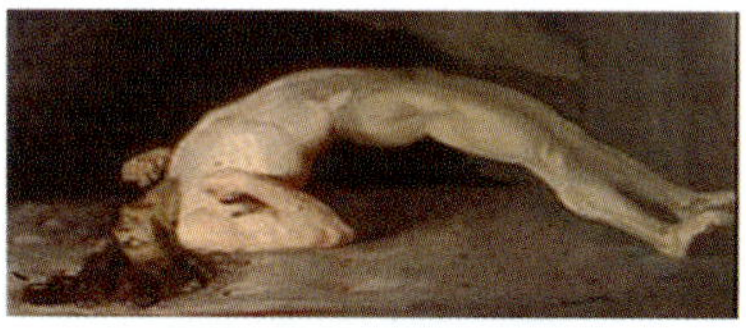

Tetanus following gunshot wounds
Painting by Sir Charles Bell, 1809
(with permission of The Royal College of Surgeons of Edinburgh)

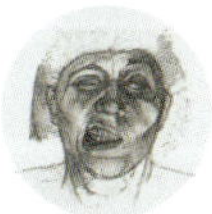

Facial Paralysis in Cephalic Tetanus
(drawing by Allison Stout)

VISUAL INDEX VII

Cerebral Motor Pathways and Hemiparesis

Explanation of Contralateral Weakness in Brain Injury

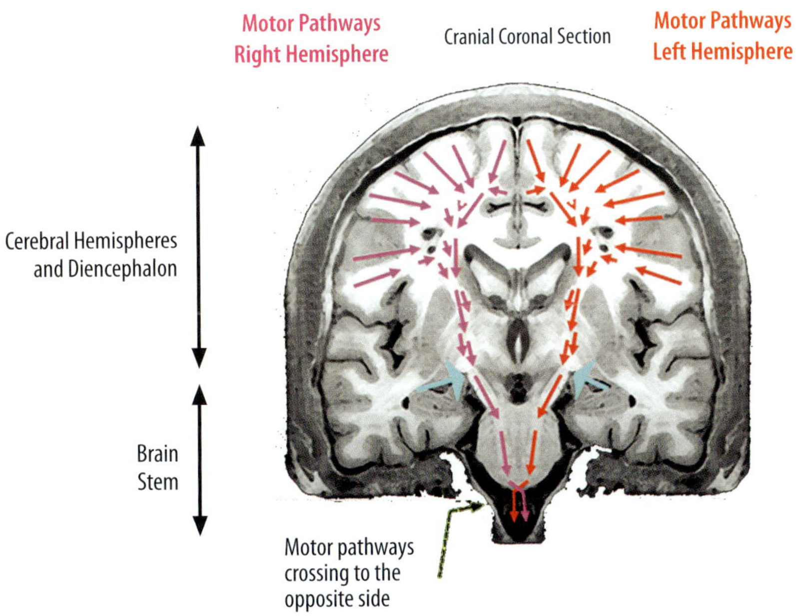

Damage to the motor cerebral cortex or its pathways in the brain will produce weakness to the opposite side of the body, due to their crossing to the other side at the level of the medulla.

The upper brain stem passes through the "tentorial notch," an oval opening formed by the dura mater that separates the cerebellum from the main cerebrum (blue arrows).

Explanation of "Ipsilateral" Weakness in Brain Injury — Case #8

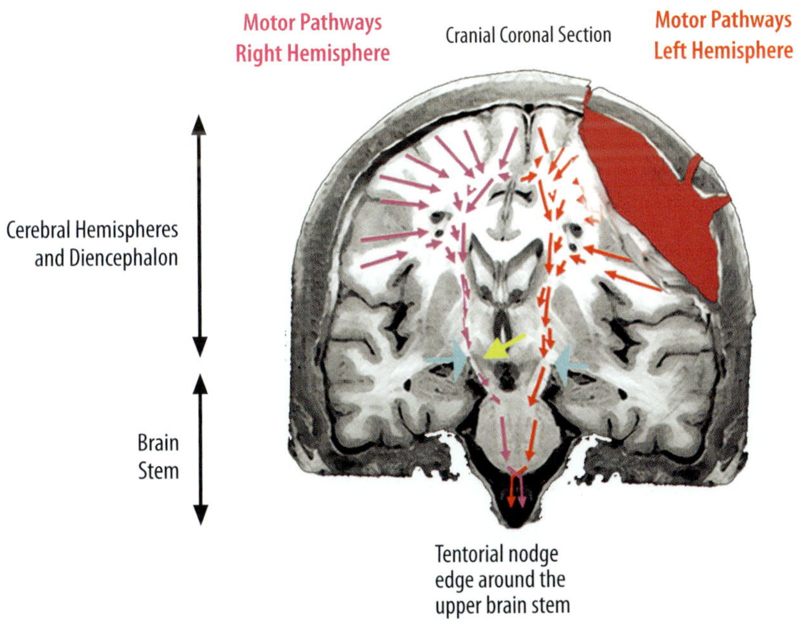

Example of left epidural hematoma producing intracranial mass effect and brain shift from left to right across the midline.

Damage to the left side of the brain would most likely result in weakness of the right side of the body: "contralateral hemiparesis."

The upper brain stem on the right side is being pushed against the tentorial edge, compressing the right motor pathways. This would result in weakness of the left side of the body: "ipsilateral hemiparesis."

VISUAL INDEX VIII

Temporo-Zygomatic Stab Wound

Temporo-Zygomatic Stab Wound

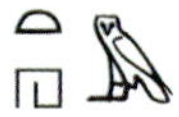

thm

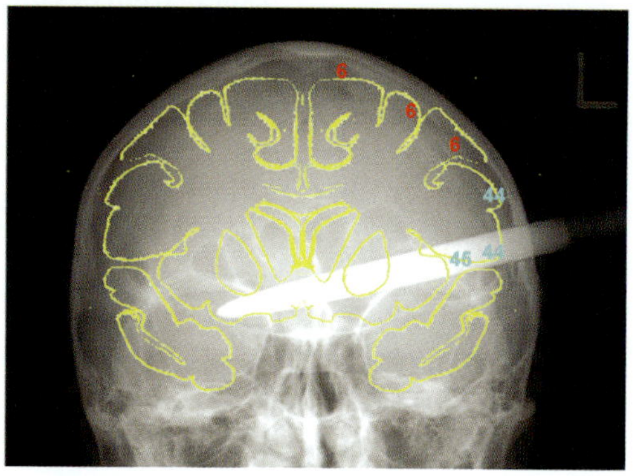

a. Skull X-Ray Simulated Stab Head Injury
Anterior–posterior view with brain overlap. Brodmann cortical areas: 4, 6, 44, 45, 46.

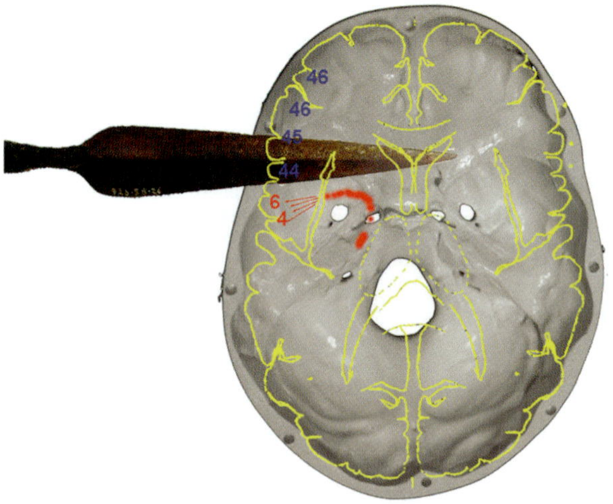

b. Skull Cross Section with Brain Overlay and Simulated Stab Injury to the Left Side of the Head
(Spear reproduction with permission of the ROM.)

Areas in the inferior frontal gyri of the left cerebral hemisphere primarily involved in motor speech functions. Brodmann areas 4, 6, 44, 45, 46.

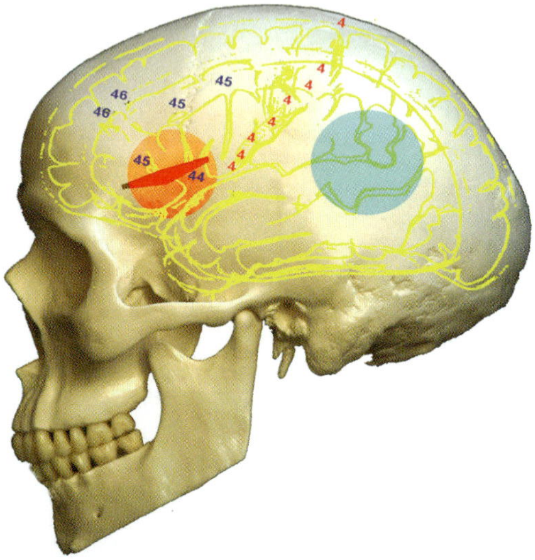

c. Lateral Skull with Brain Overlay and Simulated Stabbing Weapon at the Anterior Temporo-Frontal Areas

Major cerebral cortical speech areas of Broca (orange) and Wernicke (blue) shaded.

Cases on the Main Body of the Papyrus "Recto"

CASE #1:
Scalp Contusion Laceration Penetrating to the Bone
(Reconstructed lost column to Plate I:2–12)

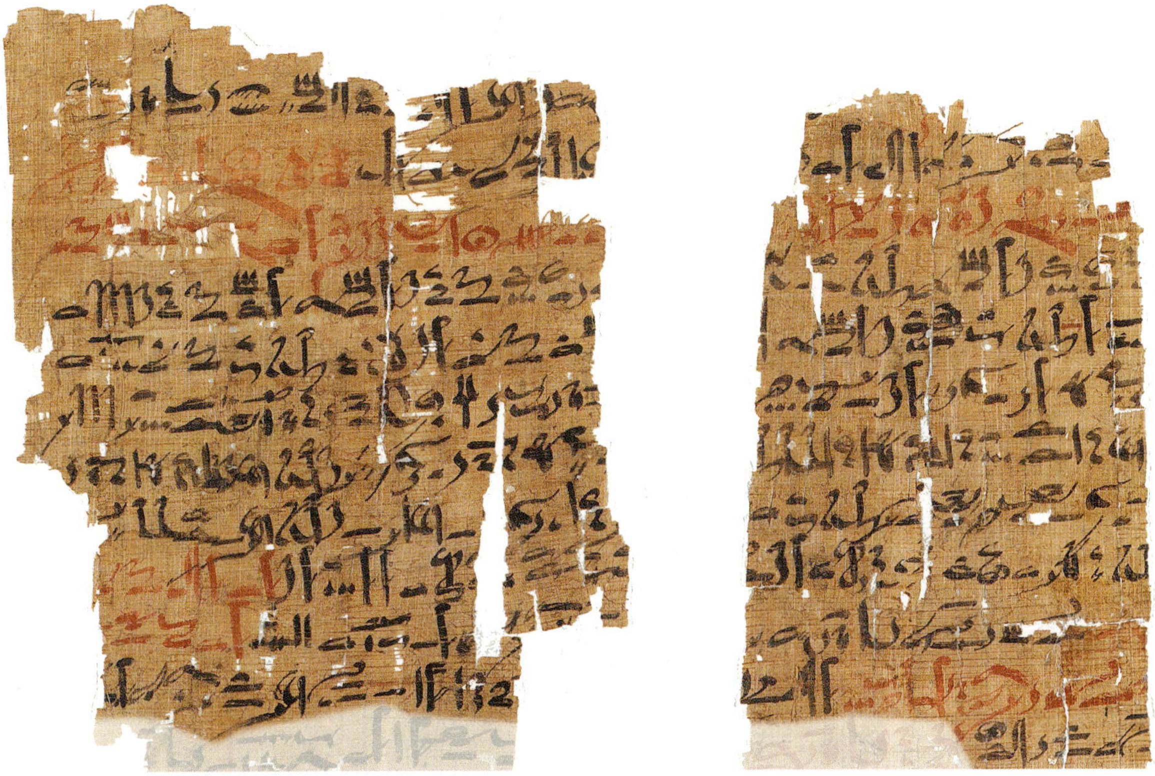

Courtesy New York Academy of Medicine.

2. 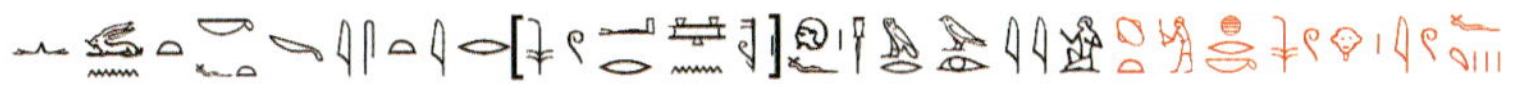
3. 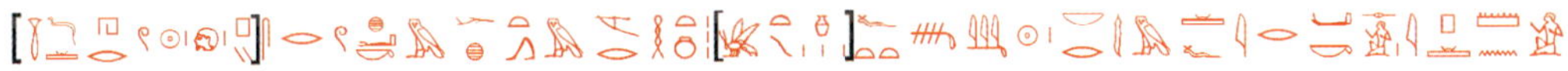
4. 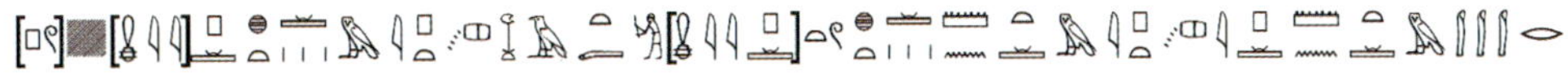
5. 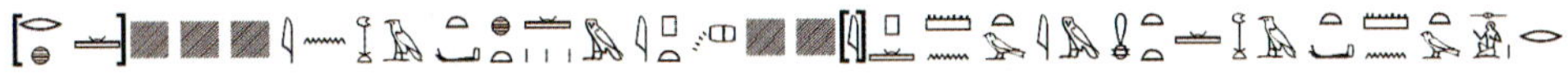
6. 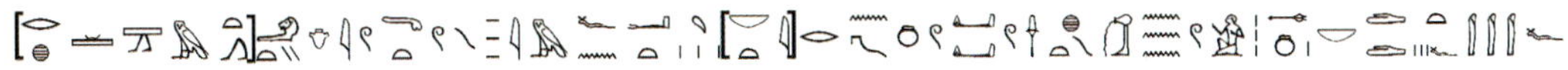
7. 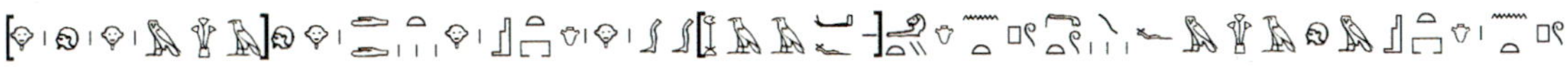
8. 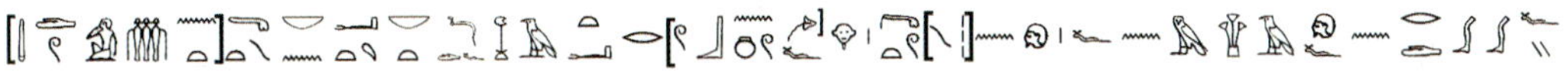
9. 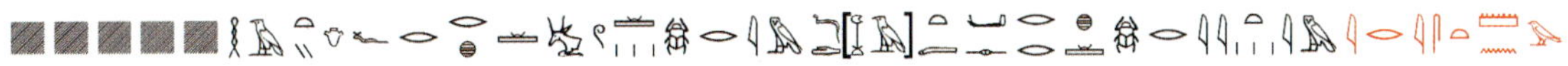
10. 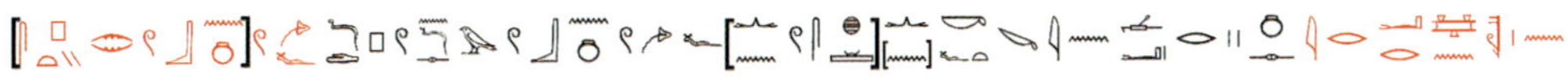

11. 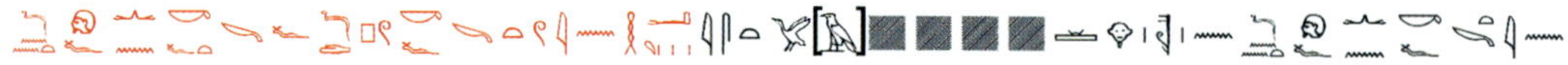

12. 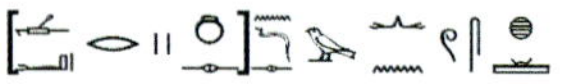

Transliteration

A§ *[šsȝw wbnw m tp.f ʿr n ḳs n ḏnnt.f] [ir ḫȝ.k s n wbnw m tp.f ʿr n ḳs n*

B§ *ḏnnt.f nn kft.f][ḏʿr.ḫr.k wbnw.f wd.ḫr.k ʿ.k ḥr.f] [gmm.k ḏnnt.f wḏȝ.ti*

1§ *n wnt thm pšn sd im.s] [ḏd.in.k r.f ḫry wbnw] m tp.f isṯ [n wnt] spty wbnw.f*

2§ *[…] n wnt kft isṯ ir sw ʿr n ḳs n tp.f mḥr iry.i wt.ḫr.k sw ḥr iwf*

3§ *[wȝḏ hrw tpy] srwḫ.k m-ḫt m mrḥt [bit] ftt rʿ nb r nḏm.f ir ḫȝ.k s ip mn*

4§ *[pw … mi i]pt ḫt m ipt ḥȝt [mi ip].tw ḫt mnt m ḏbʿw r*

5§ *[rḫ …] in ḥȝt ḫt m ip [tw…] [i]p mnt im mitt ḥȝt mnt s r*

6§ *[rḫ šmt] ḥȝty iw mtw im.f n ʿt [nbt] [ir]-nw dd.w wʿbw Sḫmt swnw nb ḏrty.f ḏbʿw.f*

7§ *[ḥr tp ḥr mkḥȝ] ḥr ḏrty ḥr st-ib ḥr wʿrty ḫ[ȝȝ.f] ḥȝty nt-pw mtw.f mkḥȝ m st-ib nt-pw*

8§ *[mdw.f ḫnt] mt nb n ʿt nbt ḏd.f ḥȝt r[dit.f ḏrt].f ḥr mtw n tp.f n mkḥȝ.f n rdwy.fy*

9§ *[…] ḥȝty.f r rḫ šsȝw ḫpr im <m> ḏd [ḥȝ]t s r rḫ ḫpryt im ir isṯ mn*

10§ *[nn (?) spty wbn]w.f ḏd pw nḏs wbnw.f [nn wsḫ] n[n] kft in wʿ-r-snw.s ir ʿr n [ḳs n*

11§ *ḏnnt.f nn kft.]f ḏd pw kft win ḥʿw isṯ p3[?] ḥr ḳs n ḏnnt.f nn kft in*

12§ *[sḳr wbnw.f] nḏs nn wsḫ*

Translation

Title:

[Necessary knowledge and skills for a wound in his head that penetrates to the bone of his braincase:]

Examination:

[If you examine a man for a wound in his head, that penetrates to the bone of his braincase without cutting it, then you must palpate his wound.

You must place your hand upon it.

How you find his braincase (is) intact/uninjured, there not being a bone perforation, split fracture, or smashed-in fracture in it.]

Diagnosis:

[Then shall you say/you are to say concerning him: One who has a woun]d in his head, while his wound does [not] have lips […] there is not/there not being a slash wound, although/while [it penetrates to the bone of] his head—

an injury which I will handle/deal with.

Treatment:

You have to bind it (along) with [fresh] meat [the first day], and you should treat it afterward with oil and [honey], and a dressing every day until he is well.

Explanation A:

As for "you examine a man," [it means] evaluating someone [is similar to] things being counted by a grain measure.

Examining with (a) finger(s) [is similar to] given things being [counted] by a grain measure, counting a given thing with the fingers in order to [know/learn ...] It is measuring things by means of a grain measure which is [in accord(??) therewith(??) ...]

Assessing the injury therein is the same as measuring the injury of a man in order to know the action/movement of the heart.

There are vessels from it to all the body parts.

Now as for one <on> whom the priests of Sekhmet or any physician puts his hands or his fingers—[on the head, on the back] of the head, on the hands, on the seat of the heart, and on the legs—(it is) how he measures the (action of the) heart.

It is a fact that/the case that his vessels of the back of the head and nape are out of the seat of the heart.

It is a fact that/the case that [it speaks from/out of] every vessel of every body part.

He says: "Examining (i.e.) [placing] his [hands] upon the vessels to/of his head, to/of the back of his head and nape, to/of both his legs and [...] his heart, in order to know the necessary knowledge and skills that come to pass/are to be done therein/therefrom,"

<namely>: "[Exam]ining a man by finger in order to know what has happened therein."

Explanation B:

Now as for "a patient/sufferer [whose wound does not have two lips (?)]," it means, "his wound is small, not wide, there being no slash wound, that is/namely, one (side) against the other."

Explanation C:

As for "which penetrates [to the bone of his braincase, there being no slash wound]," that is to say: "It is the knife which has grazed(?) the flesh, while this(?) [ ] on the bone of his braincase, there being no slash wound/cutting by [a blow, his wound] being small, not wide."

Notes

The restorations of the missing portions of the first three cases follow Breasted, *Edwin Smith*, 1:78–139, and 2:xi–xii, plates I–IA, except as pointed out below in the notes.

šsȝw – We pondered for a long time how best to translate this opening word of the title of each case, because we were not entirely satisfied with any of the translations proposed so far: "instructions" (Breasted); "practices," explained more fully as "knowledge gained from practical experience" (Allen, *AM*, 70); "Heilsmittel" (*Grundriss* 7, 2:867); "medical *prescription*" (Faulkner, *CDME*; not with reference to Edwin Smith, but to the Kahun and Ebers papyri, where it is admittedly more accurate). We arrived at "necessary knowledge and skills."

Though we had some trepidation in proposing so long a translation for a single word, and moreover a translation that might seem to be more of a paraphrase, we were increasingly convinced that this translation covers the bases and accounts for the essential aspects of the meaning of the Egyptian better than other definitions; while Allen's extended definition or gloss approaches our meaning most closely, it does not seem to us to have precisely the needed emphasis. An examination of the dictionaries seems to make it inescapable that this word *šsꜣw* is related to *šsꜣ* "be wise, be conversant, be skilled, know; wisdom, skill" (Faulkner, *CDME*, 271). Moreover, it seems clear, as Allen's extended definition also entails, that the root *šsꜣ* does not pertain specifically or exclusively to the domain of medicine but refers to knowledge, wisdom, and skill of a more inclusive nature, used in medical contexts with reference to medicine but not having an intrinsic meaning of that nature. In each case the Master Physician aims to explain the necessary knowledge and skills for dealing with each wound or condition. *Mutatis mutandis*, the prescriptions of Ebers constitute the necessary knowledge and skills for dealing with the conditions enumerated therein. Rather than either curtail or embroider the meaning of the word, we think that we have found a translation that does it justice.

If *gmm.k* is correctly restored, it is a manner nominalization and I am translating accordingly; see philological introduction.

To say "to" someone is normally *n*; *r* would not be preferred.

mḫr – In the present edition we have adopted J. F. Quack's new reading of the word "medical condition, ailment" as *mḫr* rather than *mr* because he raises some reasonable doubt about the traditional reading,[1] but we do so with skepticism and misgivings.[2]

ỉry.ỉ – I accept Breasted's identification as a prospective relative form; see the philological introduction.

r nḏm.f: This is an adjective-verb; "until he is well" is best.

"It is measuring things …." – I restore an emphasizing construction with *Ỉn*, which seems to have been Breasted's understanding. I am suggesting a participial statement and tentatively restoring a verb that starts with *tw*, namely, *twt*, Faulkner, *CDME*, 295–96. Also very conjecturally, the following word could have been the adverb "therewith," *ḥnꜥ* or *ḥnꜥw* (Faulkner, *CDME*, 172). *Ỉn* is not translatable with English "by" in all occurrences.

"all the body parts" – The word "body part" is written as a plural. The modifier "all/every" is not, but that is often the case (Gardiner, *EG*^{3}, sec. 47.1/47).

"one <on> whom …" – In a text of this period, one should take the *w* as a real ending. One would not expect a superfluous *w*. The form *ddw* could not be a geminating *sḏm.f*. Therefore I am taking it as a relative form, which Allen also does but not in exactly the same way. A resumptive <*ḥr.f*> is omitted, but I think the ending on *ddw* is more decisive in establishing the identification of the form.

"how he measures" – *ḫꜣꜣ.f* as manner nominalization.

"speaks from/out of" – See Faulkner, *CDME*, 194 s.v. *ḫnt*.

r rḫ šsꜣw ḫpr ỉm – For the meaning of *šsꜣw* see above. For the possible relevant senses of *ḫpr*, see Faulkner, *CDME*, 189. Allen's translation (*AM*, 73) is somewhat in keeping with ours. The two possible senses are knowledge and skills that should be followed, or knowledge and skills that emerge from working with the case, which is the way Allen takes it.

<*m*> *ḏd* "<namely>" – See Faulkner, *CDME*, 325. <*m*> must be emended; the fact that the preceding word is *ỉm* makes a haplography possible.

"a patient/sufferer [whose wound does not have two lips (?)]" *mn* [*nn spty* (?) *wbn*]*w.f* – The restoration is problematic but I think the likeliest alternative. One expects this explanation to express or paraphrase the idea

1. J. F. Quack, "Zum Lautwert von Gardiner Sign-List U 23," *Lingua Aegyptia* 11 (2003): 113–16.

2. See Gábor Takács, *Etymological Dictionary of Egyptian*, vol. 3: *m-* (Leiden: Brill, 2008), 359–64 for evidence militating in favor of the old reading.

of the wound not having lips. Breasted arrived at that translation for this passage by hypothesizing that the word *mn* "suffer" was written mistakenly for an early occurrence of the Late Egyptian negative existential *mn* (1:115). We cannot follow this as there is no parallel known to us for such an early appearance of the Late Egyptian word, which descends from Middle Egyptian *nn wn*. Allen (*AM*, 73) does not venture a restoration except for completing the word *wbnw* "wound." With some hesitation we are restoring [*nn spty* (?) *wbn*]*w.f.* Breasted (*Edwin Smith*) restores *spty wbnw.f* with no negative, and there seems to be no room for one, but he uses a long writing of *wbnw*. If, however, the scribe employed a short writing, there would be room for *nn* at the beginning of the restoration. Grammatically this would be appropriate, as "a patient/sufferer" is an indefinite antecedent and *nn* often introduces what I call an indefinite or unmarked relative and Gardiner calls a "virtual relative."

"It is the knife. . ." – possibly participial statement without *in* (cf. p. 216 below). For *win* cf. *CDME*, 56.

"that is/namely" – Despite Gardiner's rather misleading heading at sec. 227, *in* is not a free-floating "indeed" and he cites no such examples. The use here is most analogous to Gardiner, *EG*[3], sec. 227.5, defining something more specifically, and I think the passage makes very good sense if this is used. Gilula ("The Stative Form of the Verb *sḏm* 'to hear'," *Journal of the American Research Center in Egypt* 14 [1977]: 37–40) always cautioned against using words such as "indeed" as a "one size fits all" translation for particles. Their syntax is often the key.

Explanation C – I am not venturing a restoration. I think it is smoothest as well as grammatically more precise to translate subordinate clauses "there being no" and "being small," especially since by its position *nḏs* is a stative apparently following a noun. If it is a bare noun (i.e., if we do not have a construction introduced by *iw* or an analogous element), then the normal translation would be subordinate.

Medical Commentary

Type of Injury

Case #1 is a head injury caused by impacting the head with the flat surface of a heavy cutting object, such as a glancing blow from a sword, with enough force to tear the scalp layers, producing a contusion laceration. Explanation "B" provides wound details including that it is a small, open wound with jagged, uneven edges, without clear margins: "now as for 'a patient/sufferer [whose wound does not have two lips (?)],' it means, 'his wound is small, not wide, there being no slash wound, that is/namely, one (side) against the other.'"

The scalp consists of the following layers (fig. 1): skin, usually covered by hair; subcutaneous connective tissue; the galea aponeurotica; loose connective tissue; periosteum. Depending upon location, the thickness of the scalp ranges from 3 to 10 mm in the adult. The scalp is highly vascular and bleeds profusely when lacerated. This layering of tissues allows for considerable cushioning and gliding at the impact site, absorbing 35 percent or more of the energy,[3] protecting the underlying tissues and increasing resistance to skull fracture up to ten times. The presence of hair may afford additional protection.

Explanation C further clarifies that while the scalp was fully penetrated, there are no skull fractures: "As for 'which penetrates [to the bone of his braincase, there being no slash wound],' that is to say: It is the knife which has grazed(?) the flesh, while this(?) [ ] on the bone of his braincase, there being no slash wound/cutting by [a blow, his wound] being small, not wide." It is clear that for the physicians in ancient Egypt that bone violation constituted a more dangerous injury than those situations that only damaged the scalp. This explanation indicates the knife blow to the skull was indirect, the blade of the weapon only glancing/grazing the scalp.

3. E. S. Gurdjian, *Impact Head Injury* (Springfield, IL: Thomas, 1975), 29, 114–35.

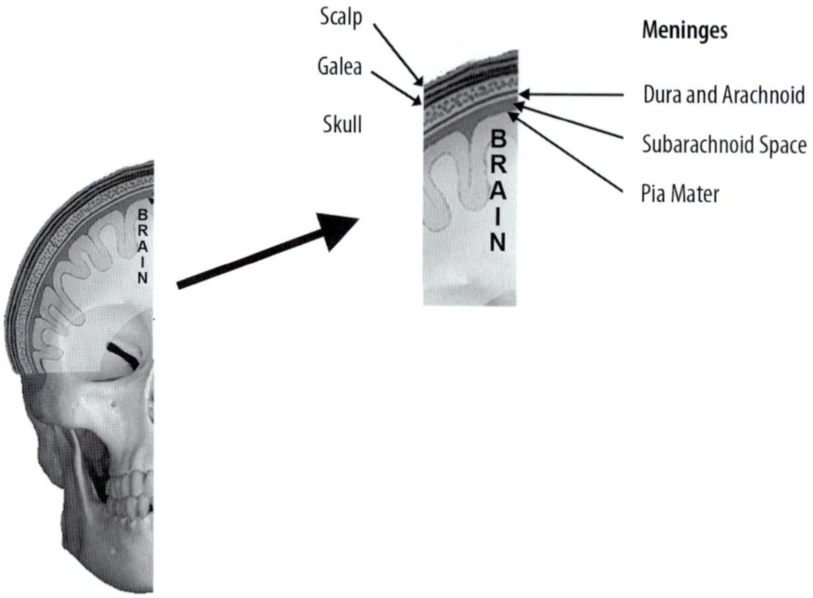

Fig. 1. Layers of the cranium. The cerebrospinal fluid circulates in the subarachnoid space.

In the sequential presentation of injuries in the Edwin Smith Papyrus, Case #1 represents the simplest of the head injuries, one in which there is only a scalp laceration. Modern-day treatment of these injuries requires only cleansing and bandaging.

Many head injuries affect only the superficial tissues and do not produce significant damage to the brain. It is well known that traumatic brain injury (TBI) can occur without skull fracture. Because of frequent devastating effects there is currently intensified attention toward prevention and treatment of traumatic brain injury.

Ancient Medical Methodology and Knowledge

Case # 1 is a minor head injury with a scalp laceration. The text and Explanations B and C adequately describe the extent of the injury and its treatment with emphasis upon the fact that the bone has not been injured. Here the text refers to the types of skull fractures that will be occurring in more severe trauma. The presence of skull fractures undoubtedly weighed heavily in the ancient Egyptian's diagnostic/prognostic assessment of head injuries.

Case #1 contains various anatomical, physiological, clinical, didactic, and wound therapy concepts. In the examination of the patient with a wound of the head, the teacher physician gives the first directive to the student: "You must palpate his wound," and tells him what he is going to find: "How you find his braincase (is) intact/uninjured, there not being a bone perforation, split fracture or smashed-in fracture in it…."

Noted by Meltzer (p. 9 above) is the emphasis in the wording utilized by the master physician, that is, the author of the papyrus: "He knows full well what the student will find in a particular type of wound and he is explicitly instructing him: How you find him is this way." This emphasizes the manner and character of the method of direct knowledge transfer from teacher to pupil that is used throughout the papyrus. The master physician, with the type of injury already clarified, declares that for a patient exhibiting a specific injury, the student will find the patient in a characteristic and defined way. This interpretation of their method of teaching is different from that implied by Breasted's translation as a series of conditional "If you find ..." symptoms, leading to the formulation of a diagnosis.

Wound Dressing

In the treatment of wounds, the Edwin Smith Papyrus does not mention wound washing. The scalp laceration in Case #1 was to be bandaged and fresh meat applied over the wound on the first day, followed by daily applications of dressings with oil and honey, assuring that the wound remained protected and moist.

As for the purpose of applying fresh meat to the wound on the first day of the injury, we can only speculate. But it is safe to say that covering the wound with fresh meat would have maintained tissue moisture, formed a protective barrier and provided some of the coagulating factors, and, it has been suggested also that fresh meat may provide beneficial enzymatic effects (Allen, *AM*, 73). The usefulness of fresh meat relates to the fact that its pH drops to levels of 5.4 to 5.7 at 24 hours after slaughter, but then it begins to rise and starts decomposing when it reaches a pH of 6.5. More recent literature provides examples of the use of large pieces of meat for wound treatment. There is a case cited in the *American Medical and Surgical Journal* in 1831 of a patient having a severely injured hand and forearm from a rattle-snake bite.[4] The application of fresh meat to that patient is reported to have given "comfort to the patient, appeared to reduce swelling in the hand and, by pressure, nearly suppressed the hemorrhage." In the twentieth century, the ancient application of fresh muscle to wounds for controlling hemorrhaging was again found during the performance of modern brain surgery.[5] In the early years of neurosurgery, the problem of hemorrhaging from small vessels during an operation was a serious one. This was due to the consistency of the brain tissue, which made ligature of small vessels impossible. In the years between 1909 and 1911, Victor Horsley in England and Harvey Cushing in the United States, simultaneously studied and used fresh-cut grafts of various tissues for control of venous and capillary vessel bleeding during surgery. They found muscle to be far superior. It became evident that within a few minutes of fresh muscle application to the bleeding surface, platelets and fibrin fibers could be demonstrated microscopically. Muscle adherence to the brain tissue proved strong enough to withstand pressures of 60 to 80 mm Hg. Victor Horsley later found that boiling of the fresh muscle would make it lose its hemostatic properties.[6] So, the use of fresh meat became a critical tool in the early days of modern brain surgery. As a resident physician at the Hospital of the University of Pennsylvania in the 1920s, Dr. Benson Harer Sr., had the opportunity to observe directly one of America's pioneer neurosurgeons, Dr. Charles H. Frazier, apply fresh pigeon flesh to the brain surface for hemostasis.[7] Similarly, Guido Majno relates a conversation he had with an elderly neurosurgeon, telling him that "in his younger days, before safe clotting agents had become available, it was standard practice to check very small hemorrhages on the surface of the brain by applying a tiny bit of muscle taken from the same patient."[8] Using fresh meat for venous and capillary hemostasis served neurosurgery well until the development and implementation of electrocoagulation in 1926. These new technologies and refined instrumentation allowed for consistent control of transoperative hemorrhaging, making neurosurgical cerebral operations safe.

4. Anonymous, "Case of a Bite of a Rattlesnake," *The North American Medical and Surgical Journal* 11 (1831): 227–28.

5. A. Earl Walker, "The Evolution of Neurosurgery," *The Genesis of Neuroscience* (American Association of Neurological Surgeons, 1998), 272.

6. Cited in J. R. Vender et al., "Effect of Hemostasis and Electrosurgery on the Development and Evolution of Brain Turmor Surgery in the Late 19th and Early 20th Centuries," *Neurosurgical Focus* 18/4 (2005): 7. Online http://thejns.org/doi/pdfplus/10.3171/foc.2005.18.4.4.

7. Personal conversations with Dr. W. Benson Harer about his physician father's hospital experiences.

8. Guido Majno, *The Healing Hand: Man and Wound in the Ancient World* (Cambridge, MA: Harvard University Press, 1975), 106.

The addition of oil to bandages would have made them supple and prevented their adhesion to injured tissues. We are not sure if the oil prescribed here was of vegetal or animal origin (grease), since the word *mrḥt* can apply to both. However, extensive use by the ancient Egyptians of various oil-producing plants and the fact that in this papyrus the word *ꜥḏ* is used for animal fat/grease, suggests that *mrḥt* here refers to oils of vegetable origin. Regarding other possible benefits of adding oil to bandages, it has been reported that the administration of antioxidants and free radical scavengers using date-seed oil enhances the healing process.[9] The African oil palm produces two kinds of oil, namely, palm oil and palm kernel oil. Palm oil is rich in beta-carotene, tocopherols, and tocotrienols, well-known antioxidants and oxygen-free radicals. Palm-kernel oil has a high content of saturated fatty acids, similar to coconut oil. One study attributed extensive antimicrobial properties to extracted palm kernel oil,[10] while other investigators have found only minimal inhibition of Escherichia coli using palm kernel oil extract.[11]

The addition of honey would have provided a protective layer with bacteriostatic, antibacterial, and antifungal properties. The beneficial effects of honey are extensively discussed by Majno[12] and additional information of specifics is provided by Bergman et al.[13] and Namias,[14] and Cooper et al.[15] In essence, these bactericidal and fungal effects are due primarily to the high hypertonicity of honey, which draws water away from bacteria, killing them. In addition, honey contains inhibine, an enzyme by which oxygen peroxide is produced. The present use of honey in wounds, burns, and poor healing ulcers, remains a useful therapeutic tool in modern medicine.

Clinical Physiological Implications

The most important aspect of Case #1 is exposed in Explanation A. Here, the teacher-physician approaches the basic principle, the actual focus and purpose of medicine, which is the patient. Very appropriately the teacher begins with his explanation of "What does it mean to examine a man," one of the first steps in the life of every physician from antiquity to our day!

Following the text, this issue is addressed in the following concepts (* = author's clarification):

a) Comparing the process of evaluating a man/a patient as being similar to counting.
b) Counting a given thing with the fingers is measuring things.
c) Measuring things is done in order to know....

9. I. Dammak, F. B. Ben Abdallah, S. Boudaya, L. Keskes, S. Besbes, A. El Gaied, H. Attia, H. Turki, and B. Hentati, "Effects of Date Seed Oil on Normal Human Skin in Vitro," *European Journal of Dermatology* 17/6 (2007): 516–29.

10. O. D. Ekpa and R. U. B. Ebana, "Comparative Studies of Mmanyanga, Palm and Coconut Oils: Anti-Microbial Effects of the Oils and Their Metallic Soaps on Some Bacteria and Fungi," *Global Journal of Pure and Applied Sciences* 1/2 (1996): 155–63.

11. U. N. Ekwenye and C. A. Ijeomah, "Antimicrobial Effects of Palm Kernel Oil and Palm Oil," *KMITL Science Journal* 5/2 (2005): 502–5.

12. Majno, *The Healing Hand*, 115–20.

13. A. Bergman, J. Yanai, J. Weiss, D. Bell, and M. P. David, "Acceleration of Wound Healing by Topical Application of Honey," *The American Journal of Surgery* 145 (1983): 374–76.

14. N. Namias, "Honey in the Management of Infections," *Surgical Infections* 4/2 (2003): 219–26, citing Spencer E. Efem's work ("Clinical Observations on the Wound Healing Properties of Honey," *British Journal of Surgery* 75 [1988]: 679–81) reporting: "Honey was inhibitory against Streptococcus pyogenes, Enterococcus faecalis, Staphylococcus aureus, Escherichia coli, Klebsiella pneumoniae, Proteus mirabilis, Pseudomonas spp., Bacteroides fragilis, Clostridium welchii, Clostridium tetani. Honey was not inhibitory against: Pseudomonas aeruginosa, Clostridium oedematiens." Also citing Elbor Obaseiki, et al. (*Journal of Pharmacy and Pharmacology* 36 [1984] 283–84) about *Candida albicans* having high susceptibility to honey.

15. R. A. Cooper, E. Halas, and P. C. Molan, "The Efficacy of Honey in Inhibiting Strains of Pseudomonas Aureginosa from Infected Burns," *Journal of Burn Care and Rehabilitation* 23/6 (2002): 366–70.

d) Because there are vessels from it (heart) to all the body parts, assessing the injury therein (*the arterial pulse) is the same as measuring the injury of a man.
e) Now as for one <on> whom the priests of Sekhmet or any physician puts his hands or his fingers on the head (*temporal arteries) on the back of the head (*occipital arteries), on the apex of the heart, on the legs (*femoral arteries), it is how he measures the (action of the) heart.
f) Measuring at any of these sites the action of the "heart is in order to know the medical indications occurring therein."
g) Concluding by ourselves repeating a portion of the statement expressed in d: "Assessing the injury therein is the same as measuring the injury of a man."

The above physiopathological concept is itself based upon functional understanding of the direct relationship existing between the physical heart (*ḥ3ty*) and the pulse, which can be palpated at various parts of the body. These are explained in parallel texts in the Edwin Smith Papyrus Case #1 and Ebers Papyrus #854a: "There are vessels from it to all the body parts," and "It is a fact that/the case that [it speaks from/out of] every vessel of every body part." Then the clinical correlation between the information obtained by examining the injured patient's pulse and his state of health is established by the teacher physician.

The Dual Concept of the Heart

The physical heart was recognized by the physicians in ancient Egypt as the center of a system that conveyed needed supplies to all parts of the body through a system of conduits, the *mtw* (canals/vessels).[16] There are two Egyptian words used for heart, *ḥ3ty* and *ib*, both residing in the same physical space. Although there is not full acceptance of the dual concept of the heart,[17] Walker puts forth extensive evidence showing that *ḥ3ty* corresponds mostly to the physical heart,[18] explaining: "the *ḥ3ty* denotes the heart when it is within the human body, the freshly excised heart of an animal at the time of its slaughter and the heart of the deceased left in the mummy to keep him/her alive in the hereafter" (12.3, p. 153).

Referring to *ib*, Walker (12.8; subtitle "*ib* as the psyche or 'self'") explains: "It has been long appreciated that *ib* includes the totality of mental functions within the compass of its meaning. In Freudian terms the *ib* is all the id (basic drives), ego (conscious mentation, will), and superego (conscience, social functioning) of a person. It is the source of one's personality and so it is different in each individual." Furthermore, Walker notes that in the medical texts (12.9) "The *ib* nearly always refers to aspects of the psyche, especially to subjectively experienced symptoms, or to the person him/herself." Walker specifies that in contrast with the *ḥ3ty*, the *ib* is not linked to the *mtw* conduits of the body and does not denote an anatomical entity, the only exception to this concept occurring in the Ebers Papyrus #207.

Alluding to the well-known fact that human anatomical terminology derives mostly from animal butchery, Walker further states: "*ḥ3ty* is cited among the cuts of meat from a butchered animal, whereas *ib* is absent from all but one of the inventories of the cuts of meat from a butchered animal" (12.11; the *ḥ3ty* and the *ib* in the anatomical lists).

16. The term *mtw* is also applied to other elongated structures, like tendons, ligaments, and nerves. Breasted, *Edwin Smith*, 108; Nunn, *Ancient Egyptian Medicine*, 44–49.

17. Robert K. Ritner. "The Cardiovascular System in Ancient Egyptian Thought," *Journal of Near Eastern Studies* 65/2 (2006): 100.

18. James H. Walker, *Studies in Ancient Egyptian Anatomical Terminology* (The Australian Centre for Egyptology Studies 4; Warminster: Aris & Phillips, 1996), 147–86.

Breasted translates *st-ib* as being simply "the pulse," but according to Walker, "the seat of the *ib*" is the apex beat of the heart, which is palpable in the left lower anterior chest. In the Explanation A in Case # 1 of Papyrus Smith, and in Ebers 854a, which gives the anatomical arrangement of arterial pulse sites from head to foot, the *st-ib* is located in the torso between the arms and the legs. This assertion is corroborated in Coffin Text Spell 304.[19] In Explanation A the pulse is sequentially studied on the head, the hands, the *st-ib* and the legs. As mentioned above, the *st-ib* location refers to the pulse on the left anterior chest wall, over the apex of the heart.

Integration of Egyptian functional concepts for the lungs, the heart, and the pulse, are evident from Ebers[20] 855a (99:12–14): "As for the air that enters at the nose, it enters to the heart and lungs, and they convey to the whole body." These means of conveyance are evident in Edwin Smith Case #1, Explanation A.

While avoiding overreading this text and making direct transpositions of these ancient concepts into our current understanding of physiology, we need to be equally cautious not to ignore the expressed understanding of physiological functions and their clinical correlations. Measuring or assessing the pulse gave the physicians in ancient Egypt a direct indication of the heart's condition and of the state of the patient's health by monitoring the various parts of the body. As remarked by Ritner, "The sudden adoption of this standard practice in the later Greek medicine of Alexandria need occasion little surprise."[21]

19. Ibid., 173.

20. For Ebers Papyrus #855a (99:12–14), see Hermann Grapow, *Die Medizinischen Texte in Hieroglyphischer Umschreibung Autographiert* (Berlin: Akademie, 1958), 2. See also Wolfhart Westendorf, "Papyrus Ebers," in *Handbuch der altägyptischen Medizin* (2 vols.; HdO 1.36; Leiden: Brill,1999), 2:692.

21. Ritner, "Cardiovascular System," 100.

CASE #2:
Scalp-Slicing Wound Penetrating to the Bone
(Plate I:12–17)

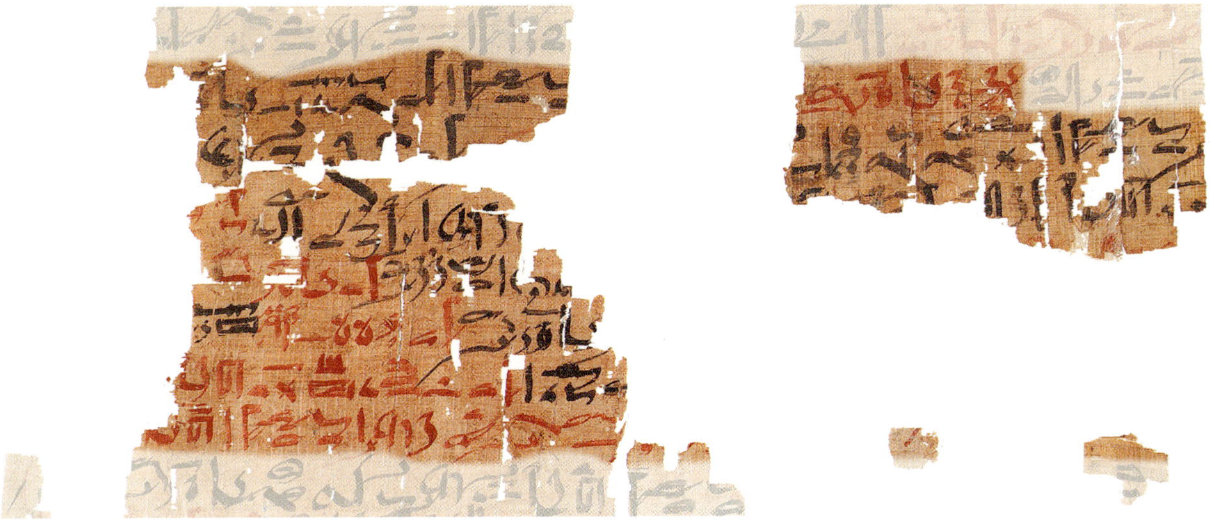

Courtesy New York Academy of Medicine.

Transliteration

12§ *šsꜣw wbnw n [kft m tp.f] ʿr n ḳs ir ḫꜣ.k s n wbn[w-n-*

13§ *kft m tp.f] ʿr n ḳs wd.ḫr.k ʿ.k ḥr.f dʿ[r.ḫr.k wbnw.]f ir gm.k ḏnnt.f [wḏꜣ.ti*

14§ *n w]nt thm im.s d[d].in.k r.f ḫr[y wbnw-n-kft] m tp.f mḥr iry.i wt.ḫr.[k sw ḥr iwf wꜣḏ hrw tpy]*

15§ *[wd.ḫr.k n.f ꜣiwy n ḥbs] [srwḫ.k m-ḫt <m> mrḥt bit ftt] rʿ nb r nḏm.f ir wbnw-n-[kft m tp.f*

16§ *ʿr n ḳs …].f wbnw.f ir ꜣiwy n ḥbsw [sšdwy pw n*

17§ *ḥbsw dd.tw ḥr spty wbnw-n-kft r rdit dmi wʿt] r wʿt ir n wnt pšn thm [sḏ im.s …]*

Translation

Title:

Necessary knowledge and skills for a [slash] wound [in his head] that penetrates to the bone:

Examination:

If you should examine a man for a [slash wound in] his [head], that penetrates to the bone,

you have to lay your hand on it [and you have to palpate] his [wound].

If you find his braincase [sound/uninjured and there is no] bone perforation in it,

Diagnosis:

then you are to say about him, [one who has a slash wound] in his head,

an injury which I will handle/deal with."

Treatment:

You have to bind [it (along) with fresh meat] the first day,

and [you have to apply to him two strips of cloth bandage].

[You should treat him afterward <with> ointment and honey, and dressing] every day until he is well.

Explanation A:

As for "a [slash] wound [on his head, that penetrates to the bone," it means:] … his wound.

Explanation B:

As for "the two binding bandages of cloth," [it means the two bands of cloth which one puts over the lips of the slash wound in order to cause one to join] to the other.

Explanation C:

As for "there is not a split fracture, bone perforation [or smashed in fracture in it," it means …]

Notes

wbnw n kft "slash wound" – It is possible to analyze this as an attributive genitive. For this construction in Middle Egyptian see E. Meltzer, "Problems of Adjectival Constructions in Old and Middle Egyptian" (PhD dissertation, University of Toronto, 1980), ch. IV, sec. 2; Gardiner, *EG*[3], sec. 94 with Observations 1–2; Lefèbvre, *GEC*, sec. 148.

kf – Hannig (*Grosses Handwörterbuch Deutsch–Ägyptisch*. Mainz: von Zabern 2000) "obsidian." Others, however, suggest the translation "flint" (French "silex"); Dimitri Meeks, *Année Lexicographique* 1 (Paris: Impr. de la Margeride, 1980), 397; with query, Sydney H. Aufrère, *L'univers minéral dans la pensée égyptienne* (Cairo: IFAO, 1991), 2:566, 569.

ir gm.k – note the *non*geminating *sḏm.f,* normal after *ir* in the protasis with a 3ae inf. verb (Gardiner, *EG*[3], sec. 444.4). The occurrence of nongeminating *sḏm.f* with 3ae inf, and geminating with 2ae gem. means that in Standard Theory terms it looks at first glance as if the circumstantial *sḏm.f* is used, which would not be expected in a "nominal" slot. This was still "obscure" to Polotsky (*Egyptian Tenses* [Israel Academy of Sciences and

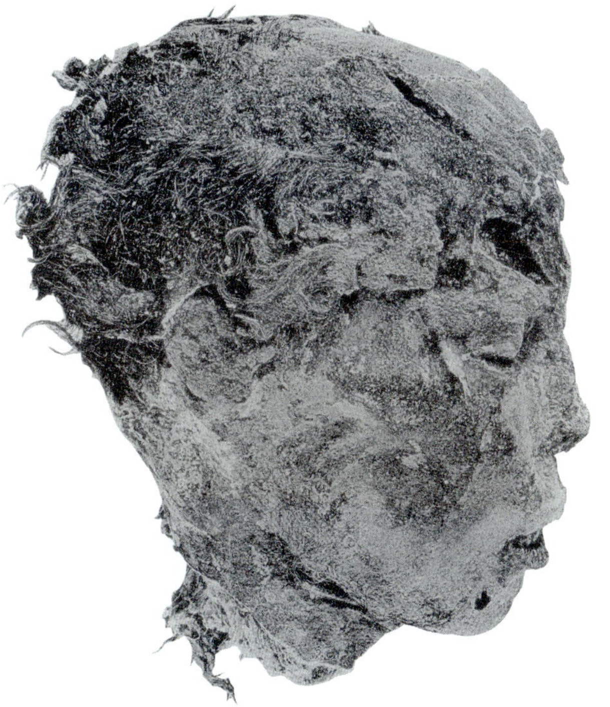

Fig 2. Soldier #14, from Winlock, *Slain Soldiers of Neb-hep-et-Re Mentu-hotpe*, plate VIII A.

Humanities Proceedings 2/5; Jerusalem: Central Press, 1965], sec. 11 with n. 9) but the solution is to be found in the sometimes elusive active *sḏm(w).f.*[22]

wḏ3.ti – stative, accomplished or achieved state.

ḥr – Uses of prepositions are often difficult to categorize. In the case of binding or bandaging a patient's wound *ḥr* oil, meat, etc. we have decided that the great majority of occurrences can be understood as Gardiner's *ḥr* "of addition" (*EG*[3], sec. 165.8), and can be translated "(along) with," similar to the translation "with" employed by both Breasted (*Edwin Smith*) and Allen (*AM*).

mrḥt – The word for "oil/unguent" written with the tall jar as a word sign can be read either *mrḥt* or *mḏt* (Faulkner, *CDME*, 112, 123). I am opting for the reading *mrḥt* because that is the reading indicated whenever the word is spelled out in this papyrus. This was originally Breasted's decision (*Edwin Smith* 1:536).

Medical Commentary

Type of Injury

Following the strict order in the Edwin Smith Papyrus of describing injuries in progression of severity, Case #2 is a full-thickness scalp-cutting wound (fig. 2 and Visual Index III) in which no bone damage has occurred. The *kft* injury is produced by a sharp-edged weapon making a clean cut in the tissues. Weapons of this era likely

22. J. E. Hoch, *Middle Egyptian Grammar* (SSEA Publications 15; Mississauga, Ontario: Benben, 1996), sec. 138, and H. Satzinger, "Die Protasis *jr sḏm.f* im älteren Ägyptisch," *Lingua Aegyptia* 3 (1993): 122–23.

to have produced this type of injury would have been swords, broad axes, arrows, daggers, and spears. The dampening effect of the scalp layers in this sort of trauma is minimal. Due to the great vascularity of the scalp, in these types of injuries there is significant bleeding that needs to be stopped by applying direct pressure and then by approximation of its edges by sutures, staples, or adhesive bandages. Any such injury needs to be inspected visually and by palpation. After being cleansed with soap, water, and antiseptics, wound closure can proceed.

Ancient Medical Methodology and Knowledge

The Egyptian physician clearly addresses the fact that the bone has not been violated, indicating that this trauma was a relatively minor head injury. Again is stressed the importance that the physicians in ancient Egypt attached to bone injury. The cut was to be bandaged and fresh meat applied over the wound on the first day and treated by approximating its edges with two strips of cloth bandage. Their purpose is "to cause one to join to the other." It is likely that these cloth strips had adhesive properties. Guido Majno points out that ancient Egyptian technology included the use of various adhesives, and that adhesive strips are better than stitches in situations in which the treated wound might be infected.[23] The application of fresh meat to the wound on the first injury day would have promoted hemostasis while providing moisture and tissue protection as discussed in Case #1. After the first day, daily applications of dressings with oil and honey followed, assuring that the wound remained protected and moist. Likewise, the bacteriostatic, antibacterial, and antifungal effects of honey produced from its high hypertonicity and by the enzyme inhibine have also been discussed in Case #1.

An example from ancient Egypt of a scalp-cutting wound not penetrating the skull is shown in human remains, and is demonstrated photographically in fig. 2 (Winlock's, *Slain Soldiers of Neb-hep-et-Re Mentu-Hotpe*, #14).[24] This is a warrior showing a right frontal gash measuring 6 by 1 centimeters.

23. Majno, *The Healing Hand*, 94, suggests that gum from acacia trees and various resins could have made bandages adhesive; citing also from A. Lucas, *Ancient Egyptian Materials and Industries* (4th ed. rev. and enl.; London: Arnold, 1962).

24. Herbert E. Winlock, *The Slain Soldiers of Neb-hep-et-Re Mentu-Hotpe* (Mansfield Centre, CT: Martino, 2007), plate VIII A–C.

CASE #3:

Head Injury with Skull Perforation

(Plate I:18–II:2)

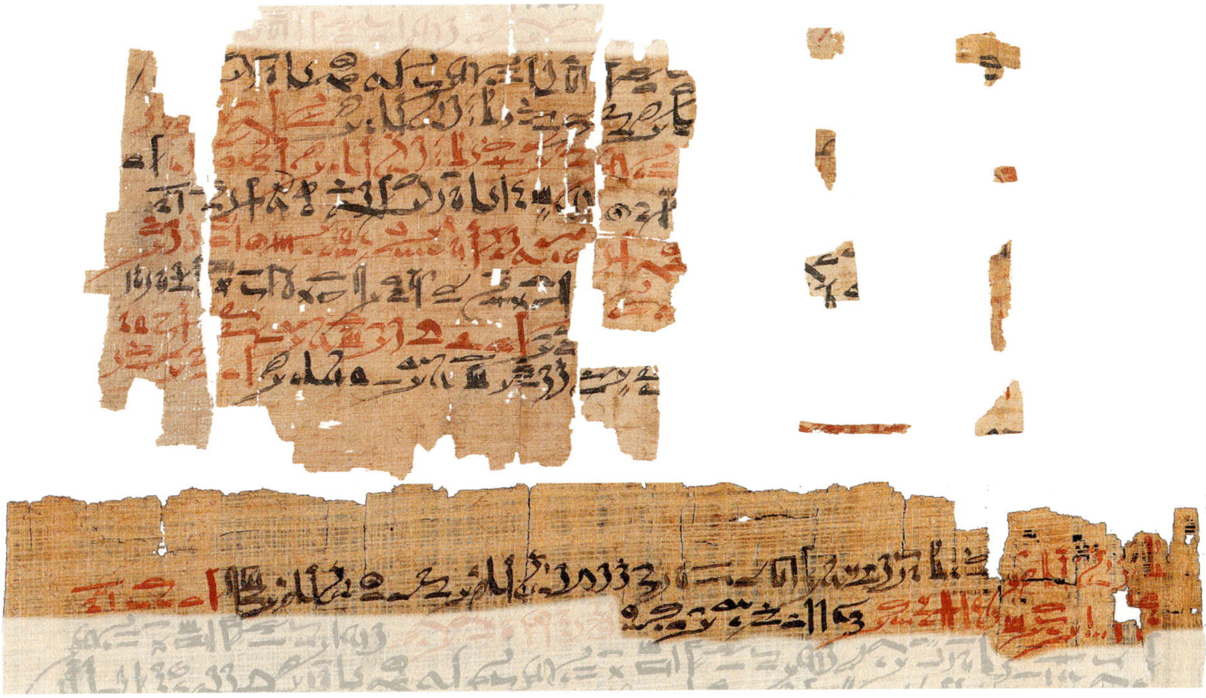

Courtesy New York Academy of Medicine.

18. 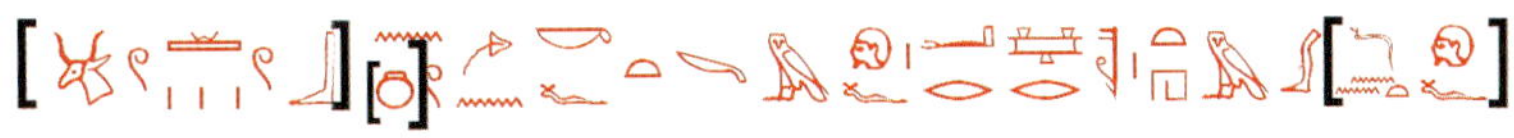

19. 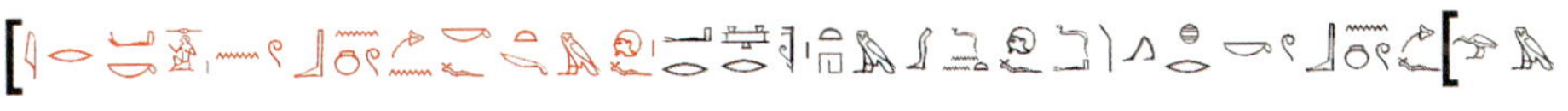

20. 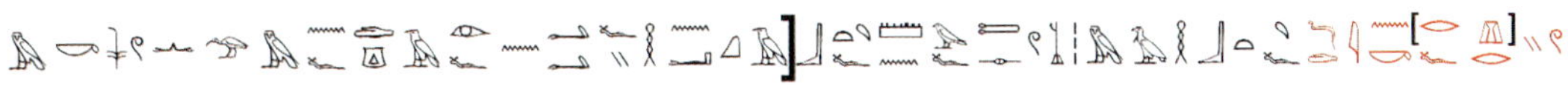

21. 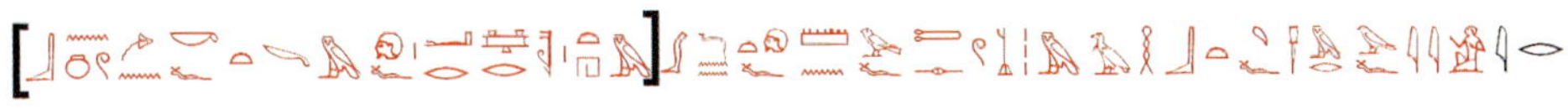

22. 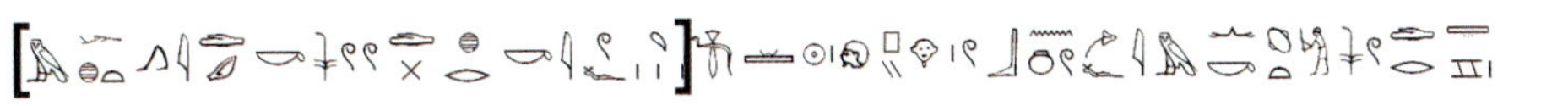

23. 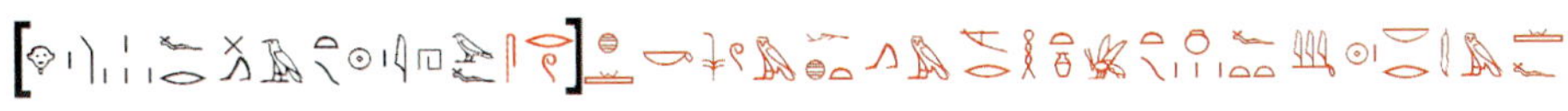

24. 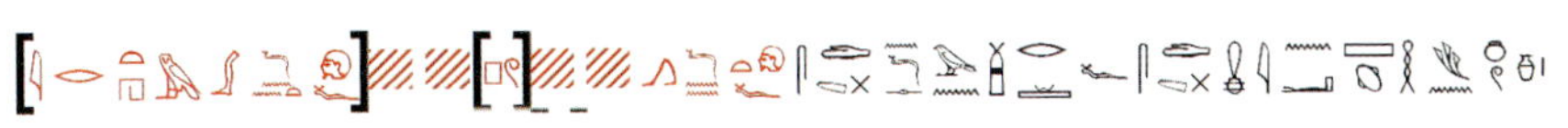

25. 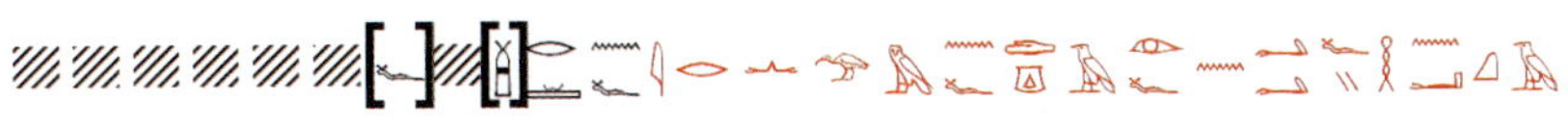

26. 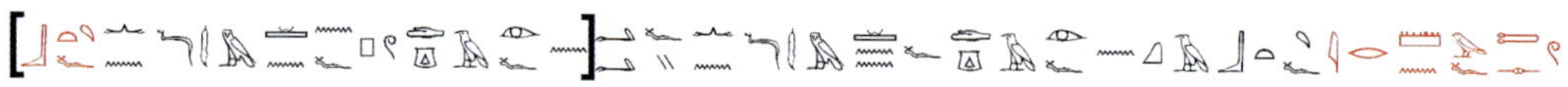

1. 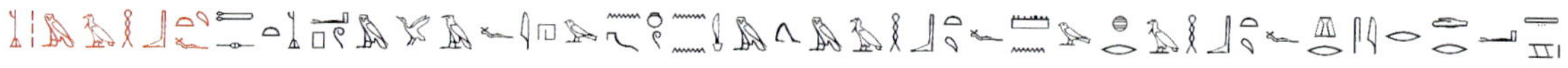

2. 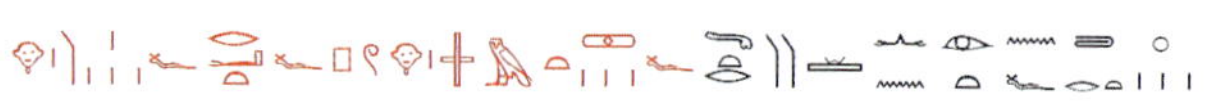

Transliteration

18§ *ḳs thm [ḏnnt.f]*

19§ *[ir ḫꜣ.k s n wbnw-n-kft m] [tp].f ꜥr r ḳs thm ḏnnt.f ḏꜥ.ḫr.k wbnw.f [gmm.k*

20§ *sw n gm.n.f dgꜣ.f n ḳꜥḥwy.fy ḥnꜥ] ḳꜣbt.f mn.f ṯsw m nḥbt.f ḏd.in.k r.f ḫry*

21§ *[wbnw-n-kft m tp.f ꜥr r ḳs thm] ḏnnt.f mn.f ṯsw m nḥbt.f mḫr iry.i ir*

22§ *[m-ḫt id.k sw wd.ḫr.k iwf] wꜣḏ hrw tpy ḥr wbnw.f im.k wt sw d(w?) <sw> r tꜣ*

23§ *[ḥr mniw.f r swꜣ ꜣt ih.f] [srw]ḫ.k sw m-ḫt m mrḥt bit fit rꜥ nb r nḏm.f*

24§ *[ir thm ḏnnt.f … pw … nš] ḏnnt.f sd nḏs n ꜥpr.f sd mi nꜥš ḥnw*

25§ *[… ꜥpr].n.f ir n gm.n.f dgꜣ.f n ḳꜥḥwy.fy ḥnꜥ*

26§ *ḳꜣ[bt.f n nḏm.n n.f pw dgꜣ.f n] ḳꜥḥwy.fy n nḏm.n n.f dgꜣ.f n ḳꜣbt.f ir mn.f ṯsw*

1§ *m nḥbt.f ṯst pw m pꜣ<y>.f ih nw nnm m nḥbt.f mn ḫr nḥbt.f ḫr.s ir d (w) r tꜣ*

2§ *ḥr mniw.f rdit.f pw ḥr imit.f mtr nn irt n.f pḫrt*

Translation

Title:

[Necessary knowledge and skills for a] slash [wound]/knife [wound] in his head, penetrating to the bone and perforating the bone of [his braincase:]

Examination:

[If you examine a man for a slash wound in] his [head], penetrating to the bone and perforating the bone of his braincase, you have to palpate his wound.

[How you] find [him (is) unable to look to his shoulders and] his chest and suffering from rigidity in the back of his neck;

Diagnosis:

then you are to say about him: "One who [has a slash wound in his head, penetrating into the bone (and) perforating] his braincase, while he suffers from rigidity in the back of his neck—an injury which I will handle/deal with."

Treatment:

After [you stitch it, then you should apply] fresh [meat] the first day on his wound.

You should not bind it.

Lay (him) on the ground/Put (him) to the ground [upon his bed under observation and support, until the (critical) period of his injury passes.]

You should treat it afterward with oil and honey and dressing every day until he is well.

Explanation A:

[As for "perforating the bone of his braincase ..." it means ... penetrated(?)] his braincase, a small smash (fracture) because he incurred a smash (bludgeoning), just like the perforation of a jar [...] he has [incurred].

Explanation B:

As for "he is unable to look at his shoulders and his [chest," it means (it is) not comfortable for him to look] to his shoulders, nor comfortable for him to look at his chest.

Explanation C:

As for "he suffers from rigidity in the back of his neck," it means: lifting up from his pain, this which goes astray in/into the back of his neck, so that his neck suffers under it."

Explanation D:

As for "lay (him) down to the ground upon his bed under observation and support," it means, "placing him on his bed." Monitor without administering a prescription to him.

Notes

thm – an active participle.

gmm.k – "Manner nominalization," Callender's understanding of the nominal *sḏm.f.*[25]

mn.f – Circumstantial *sḏm.f*, thus also "while he suffers," below.

ḏ(w?) – The simple *d* writing a verb for "lay, place, etc."need not be an abbreviated writing of *wdi* but can at least as if not more likely be the verb *dw*, frequently written with the *d*, for which see Faulkner, *CDME*, 308, where he cites his note "*dw*, *wdi*, *rdi*," in *Journal of Egyptian Archaeology* 45 (1959): 102. The likelihood of *wdi* is somewhat greater where it follows the pronoun *sw* and a haplography is possible.

[... ?] *ḏnnt.f* – The word *ḏnnt.f* (rubricized) has to go with what precedes, *sd nḏs* with what follows. The question of which verb is to be restored in the lacuna before *ḏnnt.f* cannot be resolved conclusively. The walking-legs determinative is clear. Breasted (*Edwin Smith* 1:136 note a) states that because of the walking legs "we cannot read *thm*." I do not think we can be so categorical; although completely preserved occurrences of *thm* in this papyrus do not show the walking legs (cf. Breasted's glossary, 1:572), the word is attested with the walking legs (Faulkner, *CDME*, 300). Allen's translation "violated" at the end of the lacuna (*AM* 73) suggests that he restores a repetition of *thm* with the different determinative. Another possibility might be *ḏfy* "penetrate" (Faulkner, *CDME*, 322), of which a nominal form *ḏfyt* appears in Case 32 (Breasted, *Edwin Smith*, 1:336, 574). Perhaps another possibility could be *ẖmꜥ*, which is used with the colorful image of a staff penetrating water (Faulkner, *CDME*, 191) and which is attested with the walking legs, though not primarily. Finally, one wonders whether

25. J. B. Callender, *Studies in the Nominal Sentence in Egyptian and Coptic* (Near Eastern Studies 24; Berkeley and Los Angeles: University of California Press, 1984).

ʿḳ "enter" could be considered, since it can be a transitive verb. We are opting for a word meaning "penetrate," though the identity of the word itself remains elusive.

ṯst pw m pꜣ<y>.f ihw… – I take *nw* as a demonstrative pronoun, followed by an active participle, a collocation found in Egyptian. As a demonstrative, *nw* can only be used as a pronoun (as I take it here), or attributively followed by *n*(*y*) + a (normally plural) noun.

ḏ(*w?*) *r tꜣ* – The writing here comprises the same words as above but with one additional sign and a small error. The scribe has written the preposition *r* ligatured with the *d*, before rather than after the determinative, which is the simple arm (not holding anything). Thus when Breasted in his glossary states that the writing of the *d* + simple arm, which he lists under *wdy*, occurs only once in the papyrus, in Case #2, he is overlooking this occurrence, or perhaps he considers it problematic or marginal because of the inversion of the signs just noted.

ḥr mniw.f – This expression recurs in the papyrus. Allen (*AM*, 73–74) simply translates "on his bed," Breasted "at his mooring stakes" (*Edwin Smith*, 1:139, 535) and *Grundriss* 7/1:372 translates "auf seinem Ruhebett," explaining that "the patient is to be kept in a position at rest (sitting or lying down), 'until the time of his affliction has passed.'" We think that the last explanation in this case (D), and a comparison of the passages in which the expression appears, indicate that the authors of *Grundriss* have the right idea and the physician is to keep the patient as stable as possible, while monitoring or "checking" (Allen, *AM*) him. We think however that there is a strong etymological connection with "mooring" (as Breasted, *Edwin Smith*, 1:535, where the word is read *mny.wt*), and that this has the meaning of holding the patient in as stable a situation as possible, as a moored boat stabilized by the mooring post is prevented from drifting away or moving too precipitously. In that sense we think that Breasted's understanding of the word was insightful. *Grundriss* on the other hand connects this writing with *Wb.* 2:75.15–16, referring to a shrine or something similar, perhaps originally a tent and especially the throne hall. Note that the word for "bed" in the Explanation paraphrase is not a repetition of *mniw*.

Medical Commentary

Type of Injury (Visual Index IV)

Case #3 is a stab injury to the head that produced a scalp and skull perforation, an injury we classify as an open or compound skull fracture. The details given in Explanation A of Case #3[26] indicate that the bone penetration was small: "he incurred a smash (bludgeoning)." This skull fracture is compared: "just like the perforation of a jar." In a head injury produced by a sharp object, the scalp tissues are easily penetrated. The pressure required to produce a skull fracture ranges from 435 lbs per square inch to over 900 lbs per square inch, more precisely a

26. There are various opinions about the interpretation of Explanation A, which arise from the uses of the Egyptian word *sḏ* [smash] in the Edwin Smith Papyrus, which could be a verb or a noun (*Grundriss* 4, 1:174 and Westendorf, *Handbuch der altägyptischen Medizin*, 713. Its primary medical applications relate to the mechanism of producing injury by a blow, and to the resulting fracturing effects on bone. These vary in size and extent, depending upon the force and shape of the offending object. Our medical interpretation of "his skull has a small burst fracture because he incurred a smash/bludgeoning, just like the puncture of a jar," is closest to Breasted's and medically agrees with A. Brawanski's ("Die Fälle 1–8 des Papyrus Edwin Smith," *Studien zur altägyptischen Kultur* 29 [2001]: 14–15; Breasted, *Edwin Smith*, 130). It is also our belief that the bone-perforating injury *thm*, produced by a *sḏ* blow in Case #3, refers to a smaller variant of the type of *sḏ* injuries later considered in Cases # 5 and #6, as it is Brawanski's belief. It appears that the division between *thm* bone fractures and *sḏ* smash fractures would depend upon the predominance of multiple bone fragments (an open comminuted fracture) versus a clean punched out bone fracture as in Bregman's illustration, cited by Brawanski. A case in point would be Breasted's inclusion of King Seqenenre's injuries as representative of Case #3, which questionably fall into the "small smash" category. Explanation A gives a simple and as dictated by the times, a "primitive" type of explanation of the cranial injury in contemporary terms, by an excellent illustration of the effects of a blow on a pottery jar by a sharp instrument.

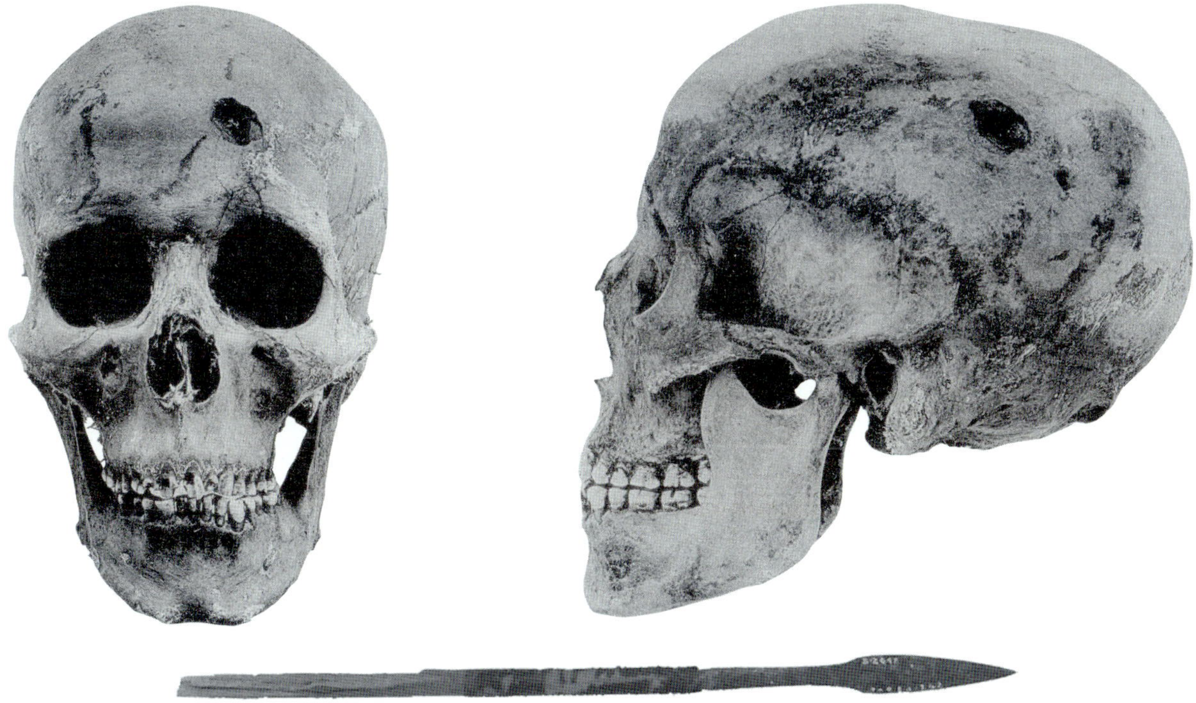

Fig. 3. Left: Soldier #25, left frontal 1-cm-diameter open skull fracture. Right: Soldier #54, left parietal 1-cm-diameter open skull fracture. From Winlock, *Slain Soldiers of Neb-hep-et-Re Mentu-hotpe*, plate IX B and D. Bottom: ancient Egyptian arrow, courtesy of the Royal Ontario Museum.

force of 33.3 to 75 fpds.[27] in terms of transmitted energy. The type of fracture that is produced will depend upon the velocity and the geometry of the offending object or weapon's surface. Most perforating head injuries occur at relatively low velocity and low kinetic energy.[28] The geometry of a pointed object/weapon would cause localized bone failure and perforate the skull with almost no bone deformation at the site of impact. Consequently, the point of skull penetration may not be accompanied by linear fracture lines.[29] If the offending object penetrates intracranially, the meningeal coverings and the brain itself would be damaged leaving tissue destruction, blood, bone fragments, hair, clothing, and so on, in its track. In this case, because of low kinetic energy transmitted by the object, damage is likely restricted to the impacted area.[30] The immediate neurological consequences of such an injury would entirely depend upon the area of brain involved, except for the occasional direct injury to a blood vessel, where brain hemorrhaging would cause more serious brain tissue damage or even death. Most injuries to the brain surface produce some degree of bleeding into and under the covering tissues of the brain, the three meningeal layers: dura, arachnoid, and piamater (fig. 1, Case #1). Bleeding often occurs over or under the dura, respectively causing epidural and/or subdural hemorrhages. Bleeding under the arachnoid layer (subarach-

27. "Foot pound" is a measure of energy (also torque) expended when a force of one pound acts through a distance of one foot in the direction of the force.

28. J. E. Leestma, et al. "Impact Injuries to the Brain and Head," *Forensic Neuropathology* (1988): 190–95. See also, T. W. Trask and R. K. Narayan, "Civilian Penetrating Head Injury," *Neurotrauma* (1996): 868–89 and O. R. O'Neill, G. Gilliland, J. B. Delashaw, and T. J. Purtzer, "Transorbital Penetrating Head Injury with a Hunting Arrow," *Surgical Neurology* 42/6 (1994): 494–97.

29. Leetsma, et al., "Impact Injuries to the Brain and Head," 191.

30. Trask and Narayan, "Civilian Penetrating Head Injury," 882.

noid hemorrhage) occurs in the space where the cerebrospinal fluid circulates, producing meningeal chemical irritation and symptoms of neck rigidity, photophobia, nausea, and vomiting.

Alteration of level of consciousness is a frequent feature of head injury. In a head injury of the type and severity of the one described in Case #3, there is preservation of consciousness in approximately 75 percent of cases. This type of injury would not likely be accompanied by severe neck trauma.

Considering forces of impact produced by various weapons in ancient Egypt, a low velocity *thm*-type of penetrating skull fracture could have been caused by arrows, daggers, narrow chisels, a stone thrown from a sling, or even by a fall on a pointed object. In terms of transmitted energy Gabriel provides specific data on the energy produced by ancient weapons:[31] an impacting arrow would have a force of 47 fpds,[32] a sword/dagger thrust 21 fpds, and spear up to 71 fpds. It is interesting to note that according to Frolich,[33] all thirty-one head injuries recorded by Homer in the *Iliad* were fatal. Data on cranial wounds from arrow warfare from 2000 BC,[34] to the 1990s CE[35] shows these injuries favor the left side of the head on a two to one ratio.[36]

Current management of this kind of injury requires immediate on-site evaluation and transfer to an emergency room where a full neurological evaluation can be done and cranial imaging studies obtained, including skull radiographs and computer tomography. The cervical spine may be also studied if there is clinical evidence, or suspicion of a neck injury. Depending upon clinical neurological findings and the results of x-rays and scans, the patient would likely need to be treated surgically at a neurosurgical facility with cranial and intracranial tissues debridement and repair. The patient would then be closely monitored for several days in a neurological intensive care unit receiving antibiotics and prophylactic anticonvulsive therapy.

Ancient Medical Methodology and Knowledge

The injury in this case has penetrated the scalp and perforated bone. The evaluating physician is directed by the teacher to probe the patient's wound, confirming by touch the nature of the skull perforation. He is then instructed about "How you find him, (is) unable to look to his shoulders and] his chest and suffering from rigidity in the back of his neck…." Furthermore, Explanations C and D provide more clinical details and the reason for neck rigidity in a situation of a cranial penetrating wound. Our modern understanding of the finding of neck rigidity in this case is from traumatic "meningismus," that is, irritation of the meningeal layers covering the brain, secondary to bleeding in the subarachnoid space (traumatic subarachnoid hemorrhage).[37] This space is normally filled with cerebrospinal fluid and surrounds the brain and the spinal cord (fig. 1). The blood spilled intracranially into the spinal fluid creates a great deal of chemical irritation, which transmitted to the neck spinal fluid compartments, results in neck rigidity and pain, both of which are aggravated by neck flexion and rotation.

Accepting that the ancient Egyptian concepts of head trauma were rudimentary in comparison to our current understanding of trauma pathogenesis and its physiopathology, it is remarkable that the ancient Egyptian

31. R. A. Gabriel, "War in the Ancient World 2500 B.C.E.–1453 C.E." *The Great Armies of Antiquity* (Wesport, CT: Praeger, 2002), 24.

32. Fpds: Foot pounds is defined by Webster as a unit of work equal to the work done by a force of one pound acting through a distance of one foot in the direction of the force.

33. Franz Hermann Frölich, *Die Militärmedicin Homers* (Stuttgart: Enke, 1879), 58.

34. Winlock, *Slain Soldiers of Neb-hep-et-Re Mentu-hotpe*, 16–18.

35. G. van Gurp, T. J. Hutchison, and W. A. Alto, "Arrow Wound Management in Papua New Guinea," *Journal of Trauma* 30/2 (1990): 183–88.

36. M. D. du Trevon, and J. R. van Dellen, "Penetrating Stab Wounds to the Brain: The Timing of Angiography in Patients Presenting with the Weapon Already Removed," *Neurosurgery* 13/5 (1992): 905–7.

37. The reader is directed to appendix 2 for a compilation of the neurological symptoms and signs in the Edwin Smith Papyrus.

physicians' notions about the source of neck stiffness in Case #3, parallels our own. They clearly attributed the remote clinical sign of neck rigidity to a traumatic event occurring to the head migrating into the neck: Explanation C: "As for 'he suffers from rigidity in the back of his neck,' it means: lifting up from his injury, this which goes astray in/into the back of his neck, so that his neck suffers under it."

We are not given any symptoms suggesting there was alteration of level of consciousness in Case #3. But we have evidence that the patient is able to understand and to attempt following commands: "He is unable to look to his shoulders and his [chest]."

Having arrived at the diagnosis, the Egyptian physician decided this medical condition to be one he will be able to treat. Treatment included wound care and general supporting measures:

- Stitching is the first measure to be implemented. This would stop bleeding and bring the wound edges together for proper healing.
- Then is the warning against binding the head. No clear reason would currently apply with this kind of injury. It is possible that in antiquity, there would have been concern about masking an infection.
- The general care of this head injury consisted of laying the patient to rest in quiet quarters, until the "critical" period had passed. Such details are given in explanation D: Lay (him) on the ground/Put (him) to the ground [upon his bed under observation and support, until the (critical) period of his injury passes.]
- These treatment measures seem to encompass what we consider to be conservative treatment, bed rest, observation, and supportive care. Not to give the patient a prescription probably refers to keeping him under an order equivalent to our "*nothing by mouth*," which avoids vomiting and airway aspiration in patients in which there is meningismus and/or depressed level of consciousness.
- Once it is clear that the patient will live, the wound is treated with oil and honey dressings, until he recovers.

As with any cavitary injury in antiquity, infection was a major decisive factor with intracranial injuries.

The human remains from ancient Egypt, in Winlock's *Slain Soldiers of Neb-hep-et-Re Mentu-hotpe*, plate IX B reveal head injuries consistent with the *thm* type described in Case #3 (see fig. 3).

CASE #4:
Head Injury with Open, Displaced, Elevated, Skull Fracture
(Plate II:2–11)

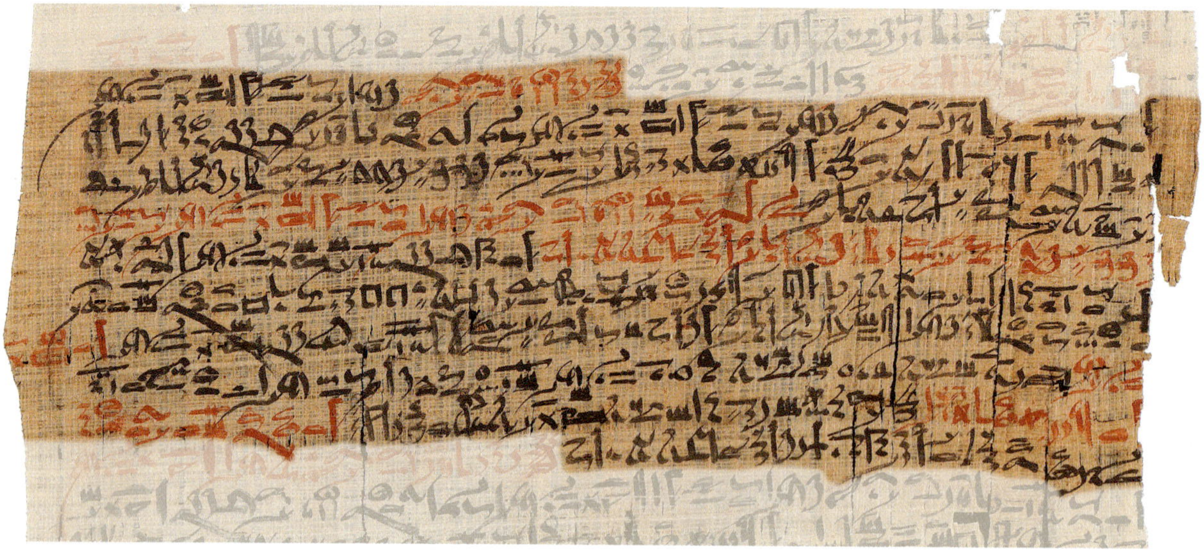

Courtesy New York Academy of Medicine.

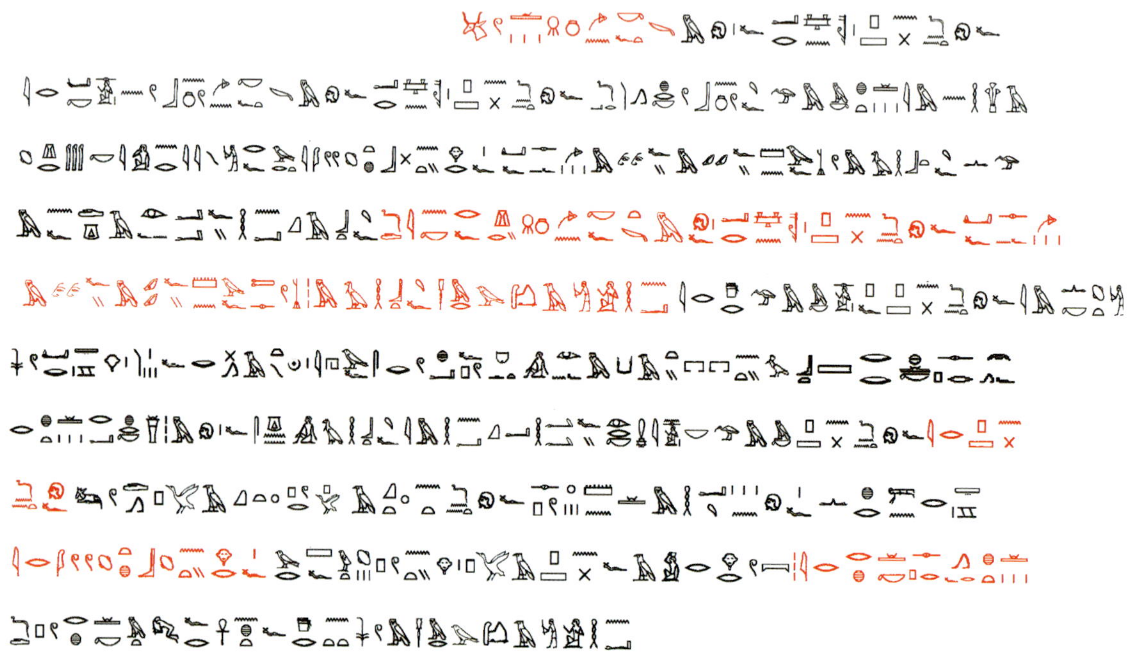

2.
3.
4.
5.
6.
7.
8.
9.
10.
11.

Transliteration

2§ *… šsꜣw wbnw-n-kft m tp.f ꜥr n ḳs pšn ḏnnt.f*

3§ *ꞽr ḫꜣ.k s n wbnw-n-kft m tp.f ꜥr n ḳs pšn ḏnnt.f ḏꜥr.ḫr.k wbnw.f gmm.k ḫt ꞽm nḥꜣ*

4§ *ẖr ḏbꜥw.k ꞽnry r.f wrt i.šw tḫb nty ḥr.f dꞽ.f snf m msdty.fy msḏrwy.fy mn.f ṯsw m nḥbt.f n*

5§ *gm.n.f dgꜣ.f n ḳꜥḥwy.fy ḥnꜥ ḳꜣbt.f ḏd.ꞽn.k r.f ẖry wbnw-n-kft m tp.f ꜥr n ḳs pšn ḏnnt.f dꞽ.f snf*

6§ *m msdty.fy msḏrwy.fy mn.f ṯsw m nḥbt.fmḥr ꜥḥꜣ.i ḥnꜥ ꞽr ḏr gmm.k s pf pšn ḏnnt.f ꞽm.k wt*

7§ *sw dꞽ r tꜣ ḥr mnꞽw.f r swꜣ ꜣt ꞽh.f srwḫ.f pw ḥmst ꞽr n.f mkꜣty nty ḏbt r rḫ.k spr.f*

8§ *r ḫt rdꞽ.ḫr.k mrḥt m tp.f sgnn nḥbt.f ꞽm ḥnꜥ ḳꜥḥwy.fy ꞽrr.k mꞽ n s nb gmm<.w>.k pšn ḏnnt.f ꞽr pšn*

9§ *ḏnnt.f iwd pꜣḳt pw r pꜣḳt nt ḏnnt.f spw mn m ḥꜥw n tp.f n ḫr.n r tꜣ*

10§ *ꞽr šw tḫb nty ḥr.f wr šfwt pw nty ḥr pꜣ pšn fꜣ r-ḥrw ꞽr rḫ.k spr.f r ḫt*

11§ *ḏd pw rḫ.k mt.f r ꜥnḫt.f ḏr-ntt sw m mḥr ꜥḥꜣ.ꞽ ḥnꜥ*

Translation

Title:

Necessary knowledge and skills for a slash wound in his head, that has penetrated to the bone, splitting his braincase:

Examination:

If you should examine a man for a slash wound in his head, that has penetrated to the bone, splitting his braincase, you must palpate his wound.

How you find something therein (is) shaking under your fingers, so that it quakes/so that it shifts from it very much, and how the swelling which is over it protrudes (is) while he bleeds from both his nostrils/nasal cavities and his ears, while he suffers rigidity in the back of his neck, and he is unable to look to both of his shoulder joints and his chest.

Diagnosis:

Then, you are to say about him: "One who has a slash wound in his head that has penetrated to the bone, splitting his braincase, while he bleeds from both his nostrils/nasal cavities and ears and he suffers rigidity in the back of his neck, a medical condition I will fight with."

Treatment:

Since you find that man with his braincase split you should not bandage it.

Put (him) to the ground, upon his bed under observation and support until the (critical) period of his injury passes.

His treatment: it is sitting (upright).

Make for him: two supports of brick until you know he has reached a turning point.

Then, you have to put ointment on his head and soften/massage the area of the back of his neck together with both his shoulders.

How you do (is) likewise for any man whom you find having split his braincase/that his braincase is split.

Explanation A:

As for "splitting his braincase," it means a plate of bone detaches from (another) plate of bone of his braincase, while the pieces stuck fast in the tissue of his head cannot fall (out) to the ground.

Explanation B:

As for "how the swelling which is over it protrudes," it means the tumefaction which is over this split is great and risen upward.

Explanation C:

As for "You know that he arrives at the turning point," that is to say: it means you know whether he will die or he will live since it is a medical condition I will fight with.

Notes

This case is more complicated and presents intricate syntax as well as morphology, so the notes are more extensive.

Connecting *n* as the genitive adjective goes along with the identification of this type of phrase as attributive genitive mentioned above.

ꜥr is an active participle. (The relative form has a separate subject conjugated in the manner of a *sḏm.f* or *sḏm.n.f.*) It is difficult to say whether it should be identified as perfective or imperfective because the verb *ꜥr* belongs to a class that shows no gemination. For the uncertainty surrounding the use of "perfective" and "imperfective," even in verbs that show germination, see E. Meltzer, "Participles, Relative Forms and Gemination in Middle Egyptian: A Working Paper," *Lingua Aegyptia* 1 (1991): 227–40, and L. Depuydt, *Fundamentals of Egyptian Grammar I: Elements* (Norton, MA: Frog, 1999), lxxiii.

gmm.k as manner nominalization: see Hoch, *MEG*, sec. 148 for a similar example, also sec. 138, p. 198.

This set of clauses starting *gmm.k* presents a challenge in arriving at a viable syntactic arrangement that makes satisfying sense and arrives at a coherent understanding of the whole. It would greatly facilitate the flow of these sentences if one could take them confidently with a sense of conditionality, "IF how you find something … and IF how the swelling protrudes …," as other translators have by rendering "should." One might resort to writing "(If)" in parentheses. Sentences receiving this type of translation, beginning with a bare geminating or nongeminating form, sometimes described as "virtual clauses of condition," are cited in grammars (Allen, *ME*, sec. 19.7, 25.11, Gardiner, *EG*^{3}, sec. 216), but in general those sentences can be strictly analyzed as *Wechselsätze* and the present passages cannot. Therefore I am leaving the translation in its present form and following our fundamental understanding of the use of the manner nominalization.

nḥꜣ, properly *nḥꜣ(w)* I take as a stative with the ending omitted as is frequently the case. The meaning "rough" has also been suggested for *nḥꜣ*; see A. B. Lloyd, "Once More Hammamat Inscription 191," *Journal of Egyptian Archaeology* 61 (1975): 54–66. In the same inscription I have taken *nḥꜣ* as "shaking"; see E. Meltzer, "Earthquakes in Ancient Egypt with Emphasis on Upper Egypt," *Earthquake Activity and Dam Stability Evaluations for the Aswan High Dam, Egypt* (USAID Project; Walnut Creek: Woodward-Clyde Consultants, 1985), 257; also idem, "*Nḥꜣ n(y) inr* (Wady Hammamat #191): An Earth Tremor?," paper presented at the annual meeting of the American Research Center in Egypt, New York, 1985.

ꜥḥꜥ.i ḥnꜥ – *ꜥḥꜥ.i* is being taken as a prospective relative form; for the use with an indefinite antecedent corresponding to what Gwyn Griffiths identified as "generic reference," see the discussion of *iry.i* above. *ḥnꜥ* is the prepositional adverb given in Faulkner, *CDME*, 172 (which can also be read *ḥnʿy/ḥnʿw*); see also Elmar Edel, "Die Herkunft des neuägyptisch-koptischen Personalsuffixes der 3. Person Plural *-w*," *Zeitschrift für ägyptische Sprache und Altertumskunde* 84 (1959): 17–38 and idem, *Altägyptische Grammatik* (2 vols.; Analecta Orientalia 34/39; Rome: Pontifico Istituto Biblico, 1955/1964), secs. 750–753; also Meltzer, "Problems of Adjectival Constructions in Old and Middle Egyptian," II.2.

inry also taken here as stative, as this very example is given by Edel, *AG*, sec. 577; Edel lists examples of the *i.* augment and double reedleaf ending for 3ae inf. verbs. If the augment is Frank Kammerzell's adverbial transpositor, that too would fit perfectly (Frank Kammerzell, "Augment, Stamm und Endung. Zur morphologischen Entwicklung der Stativkonjugation," *Lingua Aegyptia* 1 [*Proceedings of the Second International Conference on Egyptian Grammar (Crossroads II) Los Angeles, October 17–20, 1990*] (1991): 389–426; idem, "Norm, Relikt oder Fiktion? Zweifel an der Existenz einer morphologisch-syntaktischen Kategorie 'indikativ-perfektisches *sḏm=f*' im M[ittel]äg[yptischen]," *Göttinger Miszellen* 102 [1988]: 41–57). In this case I take *inry* as a stative of result. Westendorf (*Grundriss* 8, sec. 27) lists this example as prospective *sḏm.f*, which in this passage I think is impossible.

išww has both the augment and repeated *w* both times it occurs. It also has expressed subject and cannot be a stative. I cannot follow Westendorf (*Grundriss* 8, sec. 27, 195.4) in taking it as a prospective *sḏm.f*. The repeated *w* looks on the face of it like gemination. If the second *w* is a *.w* ending, that would suggest the active *sḏm(w).f* form, but in that form the *i.* augment does not co-occur with the *.w* ending (Edel, *AG*, sec, 514). I think it far more likely that *išww* is another nominal *sḏm.f*.

di.f snf, mn.f – Both circumstantial *sḏm.f*.

gmm(w).k "whom you find" is a relative form.

n ḫr.n is the usual negation of ability, like *n gm.n.f*.

mwt.f – If a *t* formative is omitted and we should read *mwt<t>.f*; this could be *sḏmt.f* as the object of a verb, attested in Old Egyptian; Edel, *AG*, sec. 739.

Medical Commentary

Type of Injury (Visual Indexes III and IV)

In following the order of presenting head injuries by increasing severity, Case #4 deals with a fracture that is given the Egyptian term *pšn* (split/elevated fracture). This injury is described in Explanation A as the separation of a plate of skull bone from another plate of bone, with fragments remaining attached to the scalp layers, literally "stuck fast in the tissue of his head cannot fall (out) to the ground."

The skull bones consist of two layers of hard bone with cancellous bone and blood vessels in between. The average thickness of the skull is 0.272 in. Its outer layer is thicker in most areas. Differences in skull thickness influence the stress characteristics of the individual segment of the skull. The vault of the skull is spheroidal in shape, its base is flatter and of irregular surface. A force of 33 fpds or 398 inch-pounds of energy are sufficient to produce a skull fracture. The type of fracture would depend upon the velocity and the shape of the impacting object/weapon.[38]

The fracture in Case #4 is classified by Gurdjian as an "Expressed Fracture" and explained in his "Deformation Studies of the Skull" as currently an uncommon type of fracture.[39] This fracture results in extensive bone failure, undergoing further deformation by secondary impacts and forces. Gurdjian explains that "under these

38. Gurdjian, *Impact Head Injury*, 60.
39. Ibid., 135.

circumstances some bone fragments may turn and extend outward, particularly in places where the radius of the curvature is changing due to the abrupt and sharp curving of the skull." Further damage occurs "as a weapon causing the penetration is under stress because of its attachment to the larger mass which is moving, the skull may be hooked and pulled apart. At times large fragments of the skull may break off and the continuing separation may be influenced by the radius of the curvature of the skull and certain areas of stress concentration present in the bony head."

Based on analysis of two of his personal cases, Ralston[40] classified this type of fracture as an "Open Elevated Fracture of the Skull," and listed the conditions for its production:

- penetration by a long, sharp-edged object
- the force is applied tangentially, so that the penetration is superficial and almost parallel to the surface
- an external component is added, either by a lateral pull on the penetrating object, or by rotation of the head

Breasted (*Edwin Smith*, 140) proposed that the Egyptian long-headed battleaxe was the likely weapon capable of producing this fracture (fig. 4). The energy delivered by a blow with this axe of 70 fpds is more than sufficient to produce a *pšn* skull fracture and would have large scalp and bone contact with variable skull penetration, depending upon the angle of impact. With a 16 cm laceration of the scalp, a 14 cm cut in the bone would be produced. If the impact is perpendicular to the skull, the weapon would penetrate to 2.9 cm or more. Similarly, according to Gabriel,[41] a khopesh sword would deliver 77 fpds of energy. Due to the shallow curve of the weapon, a scalp laceration of 16.2 cm would be produced, accompanied by a depressed skull fracture of 14 cm in length and intracranial penetration of 2.1 cm. The small-eyed axe would deliver 70 fpds, and would produce a scalp laceration of 6.5 cm to impact approximately 5.5 cm of bone. But due to its shape, the axe's intracranial reach would be quite limited. Visual index 5d simulates King Seqenenre Tao II's cranial injuries by various contemporary weapons. On the right is a mid-frontal fracture produced by a small-eyed axe. The shape of the weapon explains a large laceration of scalp and bone, but little intracranial penetration. The penetrating battleaxe would have a smaller contact area on the scalp and bone of 4.3 cm concentrating its full 77 fpds of energy on the skull, with devastating effects. While any of these weapons would be capable of producing the *pšn* skull fracture described in Case #4, the penetrating battleaxe would be most likely to do it, and the khopesh sword, the least.

In addition to the presence of meningismus manifested by neck rigidity and caused by traumatic subarachnoid hemorrhage (see the medical commentary to Case #3) we are given in Case #4 symptoms of bleeding from the ears and nose, which is evidence of associated fractures of the anterior and the middle cranial base[42] (Visual Index Va and fig. 4). Basilar skull fractures are always indicative of a severe head injury. The Egyptian physician called attention to these important indicators of severe head injury, and they undoubtedly influenced his final verdict.

40. B. L. Ralston, "Compound Elevated Fractures of the Skull," *Journal of Neurosurgery* 44 (1976): 77–79; idem, "Medical Reinterpretation of Case Four of the Edwin Smith Surgical Papyrus," *Journal of Egyptian Archaeology* 63 (1977): 116–21. In describing compound elevated fractures of the skull, Ralston accepts that large fragments (plates) could be knocked off the skull by the long Egyptian battle axe. Brawanski disagrees. Ralston's cases were the result of high-speed impacts (one produced by a rotating boat propeller and the other in a motor-vehicle accident) and Brawanski believes them to have been more severe injuries than those that would have been produced by ancient weapons. Brawanski doubts that weapons of Egypt's First Intermediate and Middle Kingdom periods would have the sharpness and the necessary force to cause this type of injury; see Brawanski, "Die Fälle 1–8 des Papyrus Edwin Smith," 19.

41. R. A. Gabriel, "War in the Ancient Word 2500 B.C.E.–1453 C.E.," *The Great Armies of Antiquity* (Wesport, CT: Praeger, 2002), 24.

42. Cranial Base: the skull base is the floor of the cranial cavity separating the brain from the facial structures. The peculiar anatomical landmarks allow for a practical subdivsion into three regions, namely, the anterior, middle, and posterior fossae.

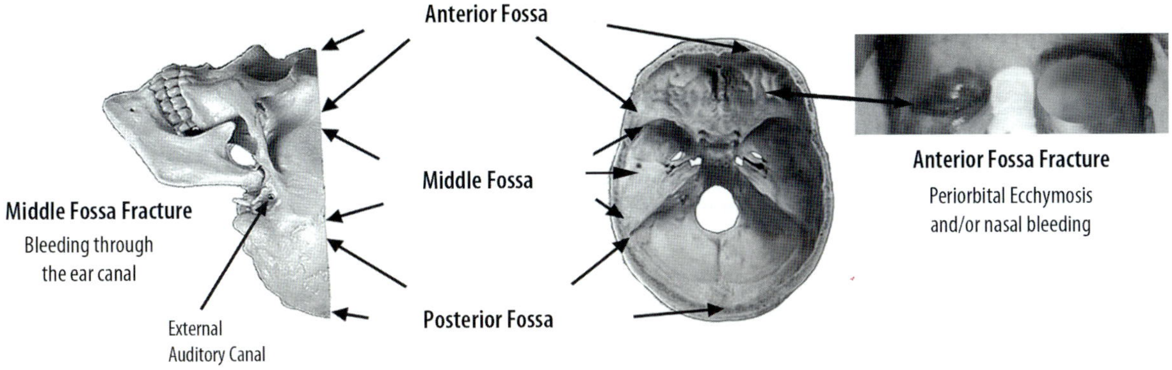

Fig. 4. Skull base. Fractures to the anterior and middle fossae.

The mechanism of injury of an open *pšn* skull fracture resulting in elevation and displacement of large bone skull plates, suggests a tangential blow with a sharp and heavy object. The mechanism of production of the injury in Case #4 implies that some degree of intracranial damage has also occurred with bruising, bleeding, and swelling in the brain, all of which would result in elevation of the intracranial pressure, compounding the original injury. As part of this injury, large plates of fractured bone are elevated by the tangential angle of the blow, potentially providing cranial decompression, benefiting the brain.[43]

Injuries of this kind are now rare, but occasionally seen in boat and airplane propeller accidents.

In regard to the prognosis of this injury for those surviving the initial trauma, infection would play a major role in potential survival. If the dura was not injured, the development of a life-threatening infection would be less likely and the possibility of survival improves.[44]

Current treatment of these injuries begins with prehospital stabilization of the patient's condition including recognition and treatment of rising intracranial pressure. Maintenance of adequate cerebral oxygenation, blood pressure, and cerebral perfusion pressure are essential to avoid secondary brain damage and prevent cerebral herniation.[45] In-hospital management of these and any severe head injury requires full neurosurgical capabilities for evaluation and treatment, from x-ray and imaging studies to neurological intensive care facilities, where all medical, technological, and pharmacological facets of treatment are available. The assistance of a plastic surgeon is often required during the initial and secondary operations.

Ancient Medical Methodology and Knowledge

Examination of the head injury area reveals a large swelling over an open scalp wound. The student physician is told how he will find by palpation of the wound "how you find something therein (is) shaking under your fingers, so that it quakes/so that it shifts from it very much," and that "the swelling which is over it protrudes, (is) while he bleeds from both his nostrils and his ears, while he suffers rigidity in the back of his neck, and he is unable to look to both of his shoulder joints and his chest." The abundant clinical findings to be acquired in

43. Viewing the skull as a closed box, as the injured brain progressively swells, damage wiithin the confined space is exponential.

44. Elisha S. Gurdjian, *Head Injury from Antiquity to the Present with Special Reference to Penetrating Head Wounds* (Springfield, IL: Thomas, 1973), 17.

45. S. I. Stiver and G. T. Manley, "Prehospital Management of Traumatic Brain Injury," *Neurosurgical Focus* 25/4 (2008): 1–11.

a patient suffering from a head injury with a *pšn* skull fracture are summated as: a) a large scalp swelling by a wound in which fractured and displaced irregular large bone fragments are felt inside, shaking under your fingers, so that it quakes/so that it shifts from it very much; b) evidence of bleeding from the ears and nose; c) neck rigidity. This clinical information is sufficient to allow us to form a diagnostic opinion.

These are, indeed, symptoms and signs we use in our neurosurgical practices today in the evaluation of head trauma. The presence of bleeding from the nose and ears in head trauma is most often the reflection of base of skull fractures involving the anterior and the middle cranial fossae. Likewise, the presence of neck rigidity and the patient's inability to "look to both of his shoulder joints and his chest" are evidence of traumatic meningismus.[46] The fact that the patient in Case #4 is able to follow commands ("and he is unable to look to both of his shoulder joints and his chest") indicates that the patient is conscious.

In issuing his verdict, the ancient Egyptian physician indicates that despite the severity of the *pšn* head injury, he still considers it as potentially treatable: "a medical condition I will fight with." This verdict also implies that while giving treatment a try, he realizes he may not succeed.

The recommended treatment is clear and specific, suggesting the existence of an established protocol encompassing various therapeutic measures, which was to be implemented and followed until the patient's condition defined itself. First in Case #4 is the negative and emphatic command, "Since you find that man with his braincase split you should not bandage it." The warning against bandaging the head in this situation is sound. Although there is major skull bone disruption and shifting of the bone plates, the decompression of the intracranial contents provided by such bone motion would afford some relief from the building up of intracranial pressure developing from brain swelling, tissue hemorrhaging, etc. Bandaging of the head would restrict this spontaneous intracranial decompression.

In their treatment plan it followed that the patient must be put to rest, placing him in an upright sitting position within a brick structure that probably would maintain this posture. No explanation is given to us by the physicians of ancient Egypt in this papyrus about their rationale for treating Case #4, and other cases of head injuries, using the sitting position. However, based upon our current understanding of the pathological processes in head injuries, and, clarifying that the ancient Egyptian's concepts and knowledge base were not the same as ours, we still can seek possible explanations for their prescriptions. A key pathophysiological feature of any severe head injury is the presence of elevated intracranial pressure. The higher the intracranial pressure rises, the more brain damage and cell death occurs. Any therapeutic measure that results in controlling or reducing elevated intracranial pressure in severe head injuries is critical to prevent and contain an otherwise irreversible cycle of rising intracranial pressure that ends in death. Placing head-injured patients in the sitting position has been a standard measure in the acute management of elevated intracranial pressure,[47] and only recently has it become clear that the sitting position is not beneficial to every patient.[48] The sitting position helps to decrease intracranial pressure by avoiding intracranial venous overflow caused by head rotation, improves ventilation, and reduces respiratory complications in the semiconscious or comatose patient.

Our understanding is that the sitting position was implemented from the start of treatment, and not after the patient passed the initial "critical period." In this, we have a minor disagreement with Brawanski.[49] In our

46. The reader is directed to appendix 2 for a compilation of the neurological symptoms and signs in the Edwin Smith Papyrus.

47. A. H. Ropper, D. O'Rourke, and S. K. Kennedy, "Head Position, Intracranial Pressure and Compliance," *Neurology* 23 (1982): 1288–91. See also R. M. Chesnut, and L. F. Marshall, "Management of Head Injury: Treatment of Abnormal Intracranial Pressure," *Neurosurgery Clinics of North America* 2/2 (1991): 274.

48. The patient's blood volume needs to be normal if the sitting position is used, or low blood pressure would result in reduction of the necessary arterial intracranial perfusion pressure, further damaging the brain by hypoxia. See M. J. Rosner, et al., "Cerebral Perfusion Pressure, and Head Elevation," *Journal of Neurosurgery* 60 (1986): 636.

49. Brawanski, "Die Fälle 1–8 des Papyrus Edwin Smith," 18.

interpretation, the timing for using the sitting position in the ancient Egyptian's treatment plan was intended to continue "until the critical period of his injury passes." The meaning of "critical period" in Explanation C is explained: "it means you know whether he will die or he will live...."

The treatment plan for Case #4 and other cases of severe injuries in this document unambiguously defines the physician's commitment to his profession and reflects a societal attitude towards the welfare of the injured. The last component statement in Explanation C: "... since it is a medical condition I will have to fight with," follows the above reasoning and appears to be the physician's own justification to go ahead with his treatment, despite the severity of this *pšn* (split) injury. In other words, the physician is stating something to the effect of: "because I decided it is a condition I will have to fight with, I will make the treatment effort for this patient until I know that he lives or he dies."

As for the local wound treatment, it consisted only of comfort measures applied to the head and the back of the neck: "Then, you have to put ointment on his head and soften/massage the area of the back of his neck together with both his shoulders." No direct application of any substance to the wound was specified.

The above form of treatment was also recommended to be used in every *pšn* injury to the skull.

There is limited human remains material from ancient Egypt that can be studied for investigation of major head injuries. One exception is the cache of Winlock's specimens reported in his publication, *Slain Soldiers of Neb-hep-et-Re Mentu-hotpe*. However, because the skulls that could have presented this injury would have been badly fragmented, true *pšn* (split) skull fractures are difficult to identify. In more recent warfare, Sir Charles Bell provides an excellent example of a *pšn* injury in his drawing of a trooper of the First Dragoons wounded in the head by a saber at Waterloo in 1815 (Visual Index III). The injury detached a portion of the back of his skull,[50] producing a *pšn*-type of fracture.

50. Sir Charles Bell (1774–1842) was a Scottish anatomist and surgeon. His drawings of soldiers wounded at Waterloo are conserved at the Royal College of Surgeons, Edinburgh.

CASE #5:
Head Injury with Open, Comminuted, Depressed Skull Fracture
(Plate II:11–17)

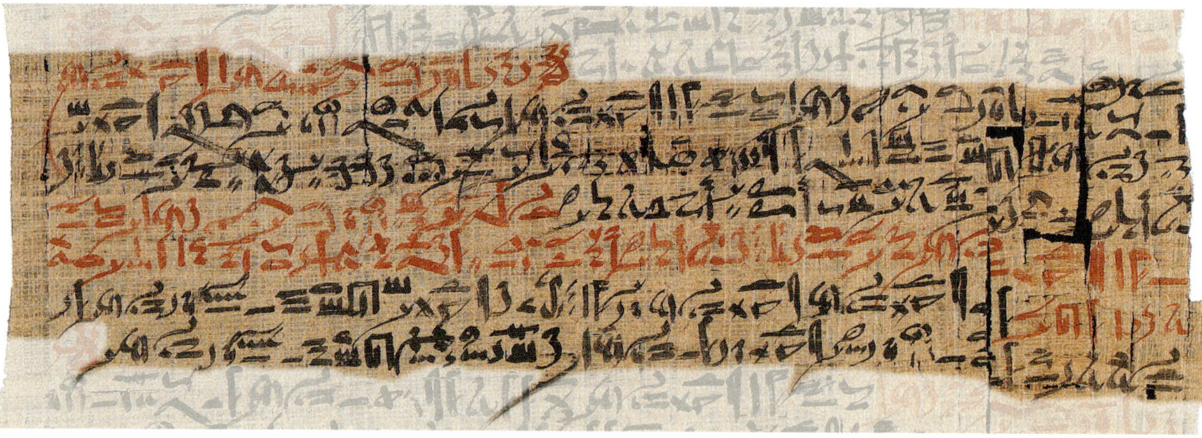

Courtesy New York Academy of Medicine.

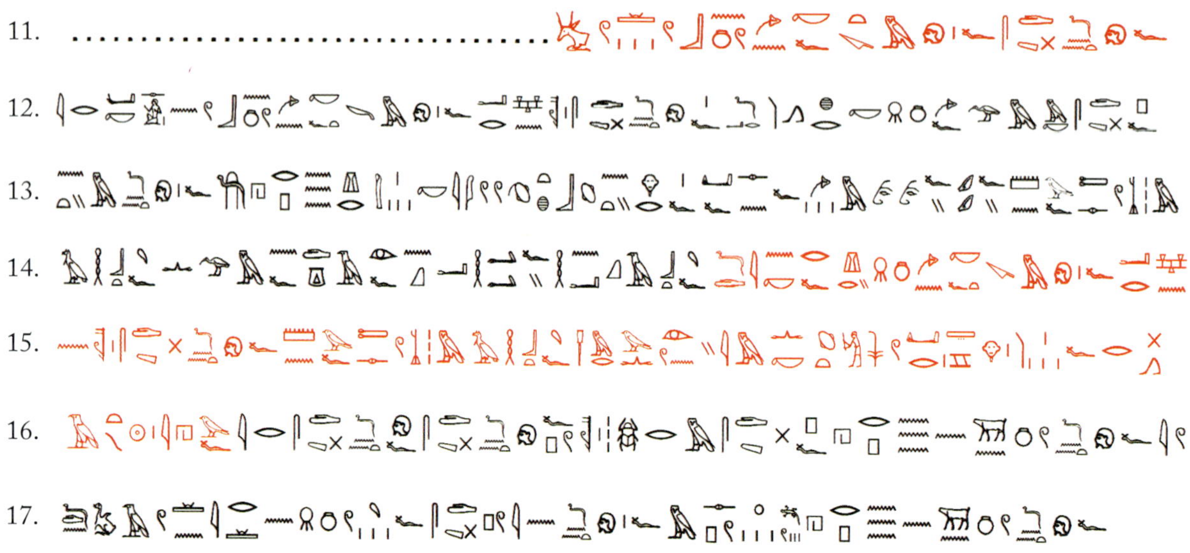

Transliteration

11§ … *šsȝw wbnw-n-kft m tp.f sd ḏnnt.f*

12§ *ỉr ḫȝ.k s n wbnw-n-kft m tp.f ꜥr n ḳs sd ḏnnt.f ḏꜥr.ḫr.k wbnw.f gmm.k sd pf*

13§ *nty m ḏnnt.f mḏ hrp ẖr ḏbꜥw.k i.šw tẖb nty ḥr.f di.f snf m msdty.fy msḏrwy.fy mn.f ṯsw m*

14§ *nḥbt.f n gm.n.f dgꜣ.f n ḳꜥḥwy.fy ḥnꜥ ḳꜣbt.f ḏd.ỉn.k r.f ẖry wbnw-n-kft m tp.f ꜥr n*

15§ *{n} ḳs sd ḏnnt.f mn.f ṯsw m nḥbt.f mḥr n ỉrw.ny ỉm.k wt sw dỉ r tꜣ ḥr mnỉw.f r swꜣ*

16§ *ꜣt ỉh.f ỉr sd ḏnnt.f <m> sd ḏnnt.f pw ḳsw ẖpr m sd pf hrp n ẖnw ḏnnt.f ỉw*

17§ *ḏd.n ṯꜣw n ỉr n wbnw ỉwf sḏ pw ỉn ḏnnt.f m spw ꜥšꜣw hrp n ẖnw ḏnnt.f*

Translation

Title:

Necessary knowledge and skills for a slash wound in his head that has crushed his braincase:

Examination:

If you examine a man for a slash wound in his head, that penetrates to the bone smashing in/burst fracturing his braincase,

you have to palpate his wound.

How you find this crushed fracture that is in his braincase (is) deep and sunken under your fingers, and how the swelling that is over it protrudes (is) while he bleeds from both his nostrils/nasal cavities and his ears

while he suffers rigidity in the back of his neck, and he is unable to look to both of his shoulders and his chest,

Diagnosis:

Then you are to say about him: "One who has a slash wound in his head, that penetrates to the bone, smashing in/burst fracturing his braincase, while he suffers from rigidity in the back of his neck:

a medical condition that cannot be handled/dealt with."

Treatment:

You should not bandage it.

Put (him) to the ground on his bed under observation and support, until the critical period of his injury passes.

Explanation:

As for "smash fracturing his braincase," this means: smash fracturing his braincase, bone fragments which come into being in that smash being depressed into the interior of his braincase.

The "Treatise of What Pertains to His Wounds" states: "It means a smash of his skull into numerous fragments, which sink into the interior of his skull."

The "Compilation of That which Pertains to His(?) Wounds" has said, it means "a smash fracture, that is to say, his braincase being in/consisting of many fragments depressed into the interior of his braincase."

Notes

gmm.k .... mn.f – This section shows the same syntactic structure as Case #4.

n ỉrw.ny – Of the three prognoses or verdicts, this is the only one that cannot be parsed as a relative form and which should be taken as the true virtual relative if that is not an oxymoron. Breasted's ingenious explanation as a passive participle + the prepositional adverb *ny*, though impressive, is not feasible because it would not employ the negation with *n* (which observation would also apply to a relative form), nor can there be a question of the archaizing use of *n* for *nn* if, as has become widely accepted, the construction is a form of the *n sḏm.n.f* negation of ability. This prognosis is taken as the variant of the *n sḏm.n.f* with the formative with impersonal subject *ny* by Allen (*ME*, sec. 18.5, pp. 227–28), Westendorf (*Grundriss* 8, sec. 245, pp. 177–78), and Hildegard von Deines and Wolfhart Westendorf (*Grundriss* 7, 1:94). The ending *w* does not find a facile explanation however; Westendorf notes the possibility that it represents the weak radical of the 3ae inf. verb but acknowledges that this does not have apparent parallels in Smith. I am inclined to accept it nonetheless, in light of the "abnormal" form *dy.n.ỉ* and the writing *ỉỉw.n.ỉ* with the base of the verb *ỉỉ*, that is, the reedleaf with legs (Gardiner, *EG*[3], sec. 413). I am open to a clearer and more solidly substantiated identification but have not yet found it. The translation adopted here, "(a medical condition) that cannot be handled/dealt with," takes the verb *ỉrỉ* itself in the same sense as the positive prognosis *ỉry.ỉ*.

ḫpr – Taken as an active participle of "come into being" rather than a passive participle of "create." The latter (transitive) meaning of *ḫpr* does exist but is rare.

hrp or *hrp*(*w*) – Understood as a stative.

ỉw ḏd.n ... – Typical form for a past statement of fact (Hoch, *MEG*, sec. 31).

ṯꜣw – "Compilation" seems to be the most suitable translation, corresponding to the German *Sammelhandschrift*.

The title of this ancient book presents some challenges and no attempted translation is free of problems. It cannot be simply "Compilation pertaining to," because the Egyptian text gives *ṯꜣw n ỉr*(*y?*) *n* with what would be a redundant or pleonastic construction. Thus, "Compilation of" seems indicated, with *ỉr*(*y*) belonging to what follows. "That which pertains to" seems a natural choice for *ỉr*(*y*), except that in Earlier Egyptian one would expect the feminine form *ỉrt* for the general/abstract designation, and it seems yet another pleonasm that *ỉr*(*y*) is followed by another *n*. This use, however, seems to be paralleled on both counts elsewhere in Smith (*Grundriss* 7, 1:95). Allen's suggestion "Nature" is attractive (*AM*, 75), but *ỉrw* or *ỉr*(*w*) "shape, form, nature" is normally written with the eye hieroglyph (Faulkner, *CDME*, 27). Another appealing possibility is *ỉr*(*y*) "one belonging or pertaining to," referring to a person, as in compounds such as *ỉry-ꜥꜣ* "doorkeeper" and *ỉry-pḏt* "bowman" (Faulkner, *CDME*, 25; *Wb.* 1:104). In this case the compound would refer to the physician who specializes in or is in charge of the treatment of wounds. However, the additional *n* following *ỉr*(*y*) seems to present an obstacle to this interpretation, nor does the word have a person determinative.

It is interesting that the verb "to say" is used to give a quotation from a book, rather than "it is written." Cf. *Wb.* 5:619.

ỉn – The same employment of this particle noted above.

Medical Commentary

Type of Injury (Visual Index IV)

Case #5 is a severe head injury producing an open, comminuted, depressed, skull fracture. The explanation section indicates that in this case, there is a direct shattering blow to the head by a blunt object, driving bone fragments to the interior of the skull. This type of injury is usually produced by a low velocity, high kinetic-energy impact, applied over a small area of the skull vault.[51] If the skull capacity for elastic deformation is exceeded

51. Gurdjian, *Impact Head Injury*, 114–35; Manfred Oehmichen, R. N. Auer, and H. G. König, *Forensic Neuropathology and Associated Neurology* (Berlin: Springer, 2006), 117.

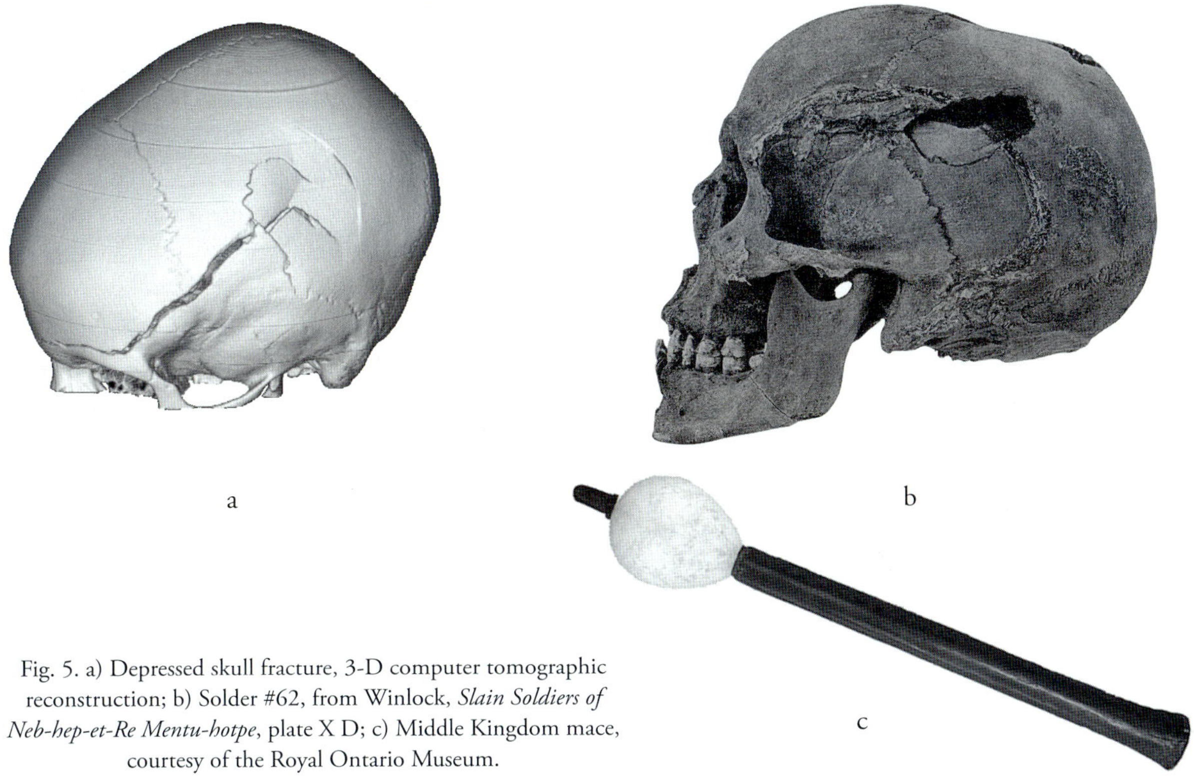

a b c

Fig. 5. a) Depressed skull fracture, 3-D computer tomographic reconstruction; b) Solder #62, from Winlock, *Slain Soldiers of Neb-hep-et-Re Mentu-hotpe*, plate X D; c) Middle Kingdom mace, courtesy of the Royal Ontario Museum.

the outer table of the skull bone bends inward, resulting in an initial "dent" fracture, whose size is directly related to the impacting object. The inner skull table facing the interior of the skull and the brain bends inward and tears. The depressed area of the outer skull table sustains parallel fractures, and its layers collapse. The inner table caves in deeply, resulting in splintering in a reversed-pyramid that projects into the interior of the skull (Visual Index IV and fig. 5a and b). The direction of the radiating fractures and their length depend upon the skull's curvature and the presence of its naturally occurring structural buttresses. Fractures can spread to the skull base. Intracranial tissue damage to the meningeal brain coverings, blood vessels, and underlying brain follows, their consequences related to site of injury in the brain. Hemorrhages result and the brain swells in response to the injury.

The clinical evaluation as described in Case #5 singles out the wound features of a depressed fracture with in-driven fragments. The presence of meningismus and bleeding from the nose and ears are indicative of basilar skull fractures of the anterior and middle cranial base. The importance of the latter two clinical findings has been discussed in Cases #3 and #4. The cranial damage and resulting brain injury are potentially much greater in Case #5 than in previous cases. The verdict issued here reflects the severity of this injury.

As expressed in Case #4, the treatment of severe head injuries today requires prehospital stabilization of the patient's condition including recognition and treatment of rising intracranial pressure. The patient is then transported to a hospital with neurological and neurosurgical capabilities for comprehensive clinical, investigative, surgical, and intensive care management. The treatment of depressed fractures of the skull with in-driven fragments demands the same. Most such resources have only become available and partially effective after the First World War.

In ancient Egypt the injury described in Case #5 would most likely have been caused by blows from maces (fig. 5b and c), the blunt end of axes, large rocks hurled from fortresses upon attackers, and stones launched from slings.[52] In the New Kingdom the extensive incorporation of horses into the Egyptian armies introduced a new source of depressed skull fractures by the hooves or trampling by animals. Multiple examples of these *sḏ* types of injuries are evident in the remains of Montuhotep's soldiers[53] from 2000 BC. Some of these head injuries appear to be primary, while others are "finishing blows," also known as the *coup de grâce*.

Ancient Medical Methodology and Knowledge

The nature of this injury is detailed by its physical characteristics and the confirmation of sunken bone fragments under the examiner's fingers. It is significant that the anatomical pathological substrate of this injury is explained twice by the master physician, who supports his first explanation by referring to another didactic text he calls the "Compilation of That which Pertains to His(?) Wounds."

In addition to describing the findings to be encountered by palpation of a depressed skull fracture with in-driven fragments, the Egyptian physician calls attention to the clinical findings of bleeding from the nose and the ears, and neck rigidity.[54] The patient's level of consciousness is evidently preserved, as the patient attempts to follow commands. There is no specific mention of neurological findings.

In contrast with the previous cases, the verdict in Case #5 is "a medical condition that cannot be handled/dealt with." This conclusion is perfectly understandable as the treatment for severe head injuries with depressed skull fragments during that time. Such medical management requires advanced knowledge of anatomy, physiology, surgical skills, and anesthesia. In short, successful management of depressed skull fractures demands the existence of knowledge and technologies that have only become available in the last one hundred years.

It should be noted that regardless of the dire verdict in Case #5, as in many other cases of severe injuries in this papyrus, the patient was not abandoned; care was provided. Bandaging of the injured head was contraindicated and no other measure prescribed, except for placing him on bed rest and observation, according to what appears to be an established treatment protocol for severe head injuries.

Treatment was given, no matter the "verdict," which was essentially a prediction of the expected success in each case. This is different from today's "triage," which is a process of prioritizing treatment based on severity of the condition and expected outcome based on the treatment that could be given.

Treatment was continued in depressed, compound skull fractures with in-driven bone fragments "until the critical period of his injury passes." This cautious statement implied hope of recovery for some patients, and points to the humanitarian aspects of medical treatment in ancient Egypt.

52. Robert B. Partridge, "Weapons and Military Equipment," *Fighting Pharaohs: Weapons and Warfare in Ancient Egypt* (Manchester, U.K.: Peartree, 2002), 31.

53. Winlock, *Slain Soldiers of Neb-hep-et-Re Mentu-hotpe*, 11–17, plates VIII–X, soldiers ##14, 23, 25, 48, 54, 62, 64, 76, 81 had depressed skull fractures consistent with injuries by stones, maces, and axes.

54. The reader is directed to appendix 2 for a compilation of the neurological symptoms and signs in the Edwin Smith Papyrus.

CASE #6:

Head Injury with Open, Comminuted, Depressed Skull Fracture and Dura Laceration

(Plate II:17–III:1)

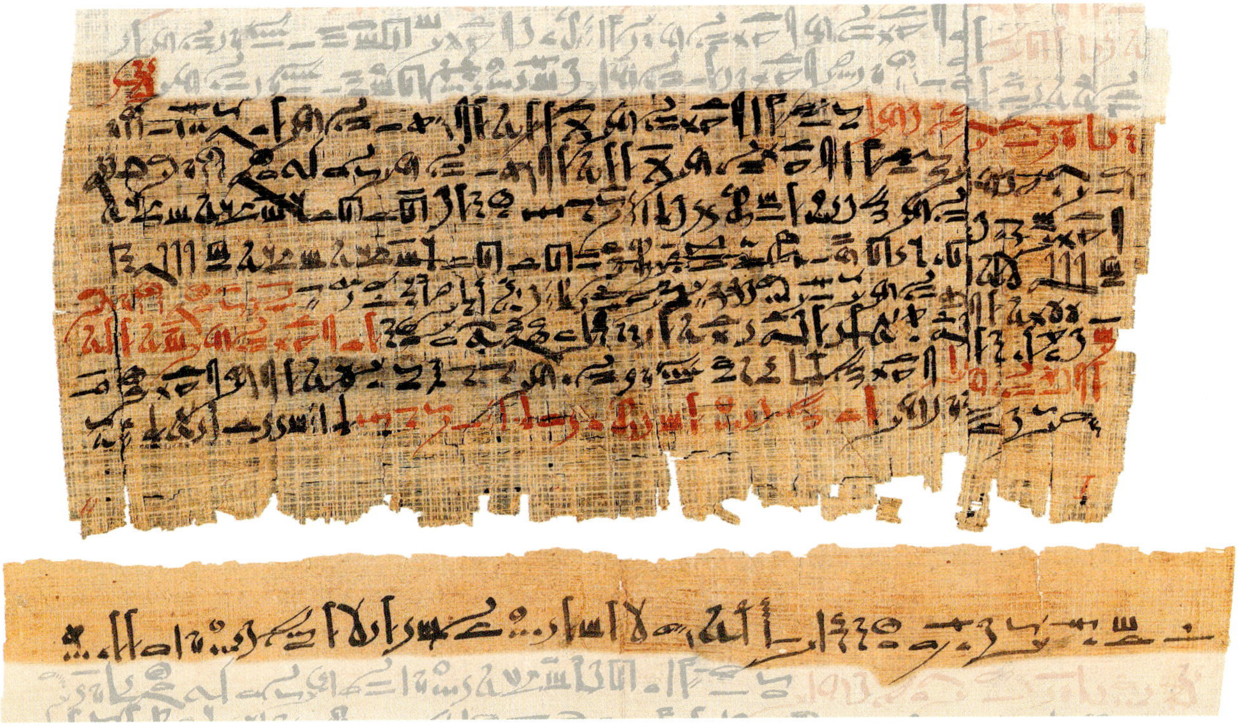

Courtesy New York Academy of Medicine.

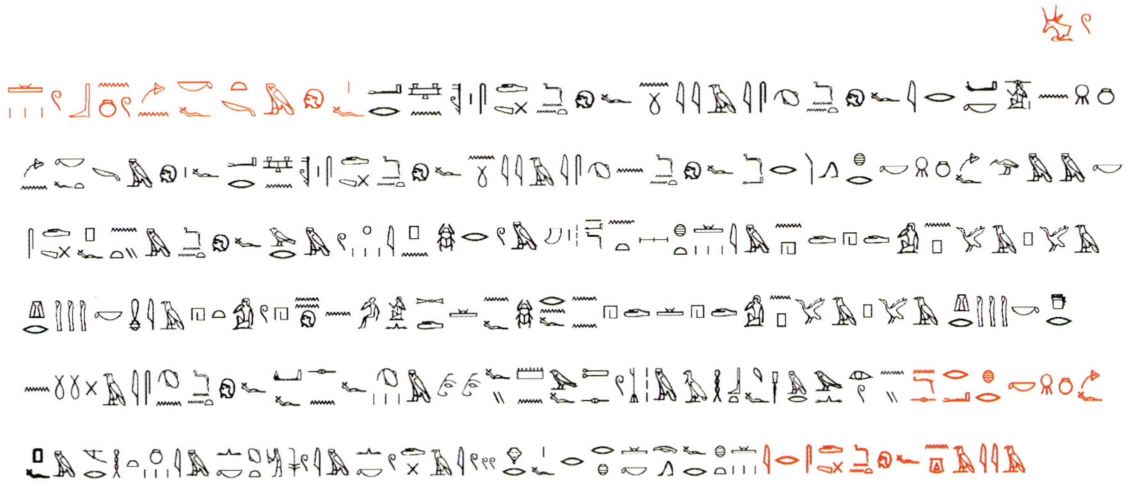

17.

18.

19.

20.

21.

22.

23.

24. 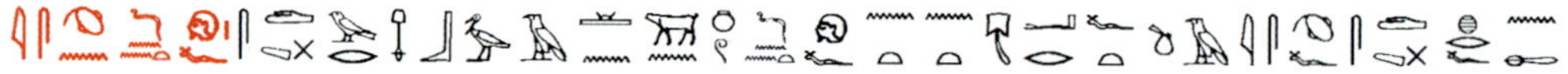

25. 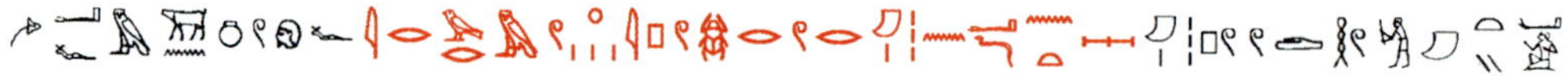

1. 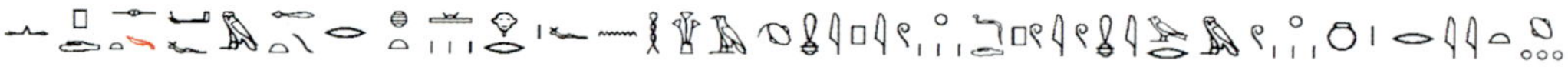

Transliteration

17§ … *šsꜣw*

18§ *wbnw-n-kft m tp.f ꜥr n ḳs sd ḏnnt.f ngy ꜣis n ḏnnt.f ir ẖꜣ.k s n wbnw-*

19§ *n-kft m tp.f ꜥr n ḳs sd ḏnnt.f ngy ꜣis n ḏnnt.f ḏꜥr.ẖr.k wbnw.f gmm.k*

20§ *sḏ pf nty m ḏnnt.f <mi> wrmw ipn ẖpr.w m ḥmt n ꜥnḏt ẖt im nhdhd npꜣpꜣ*

21§ *ẖr ḏbꜥw.k mi ꜣht whnn n ẖrd n ꜥd.n.f ẖpr.n.f n nhdhd npꜣpꜣ ẖr ḏbꜥw.k ḏr*

22§ *ngg ꜣis n ḏnnt.f di.f snf m msdty.fy mn.f ṯsw m nḥbt.f mẖr n irw .ny nsr.ẖr.k wbnw.f*

23§ *pf m mrḥt im.k wt sw im.k wd ꜣiwy ẖr.f r rẖ.k spr.f r ẖt ir sd ḏnnt.f ngy*

24§ *ꜣis n ḏnnt.f sd wr wbꜣ n ẖnw ḏnnt.f ntnt ꜥrft ꜣis.f sd.ẖr.f nẖ*

25§ *.f m-ẖnw ḏꜣḏꜣ.f ir wrmw ipw ẖprw r ḥmt n ꜥḏnt ḥmt pw wdḥw ḥmty*

1§ *n pdst.f m ꜥꜣt r ẖt ḥr.f nẖꜣ mi piw ḏd pw iw mi wrmw nw ryt*

Translation

Title:

Necessary knowledge and skills for a slash wound in his head, that penetrates to the bone, smashing in/bursting in his braincase and exposing the brain of his braincase:

Examination:

If you should examine a man for a slash wound in his head, which penetrates to the bone, smashing in his braincase and exposing the brain of his braincase, you need to palpate his wound.

How you find that fracture which is in his braincase (is) <like> those convolutions that occur in copper of a crucible(?)

and something therein, throbbing and fluttering under your fingers like the weakness of the crown of a child (fontanelle).

He/it cannot be whole/sound.

How it has come to pass/How he has become (is) because of the throbbing and fluttering under your fingers, since the brain of his braincase is exposed/broken open,

while he gives blood from both his nostrils/nasal cavities,

and while he suffers rigidity in the back of his neck—

Diagnosis:

"a medical condition that cannot be handled/dealt with."

Treatment:

You should daub/apply gently that wound of his with oil.

You should not bandage it.

You should not lay the two bandage strips over it until you know he has reached the crisis.

Explanation A:

As for "smashing in of his braincase and exposing/breaking open the brain of his skull," the large smash fracture is open to the inside of his braincase and the dura mater/membrane that envelops his brain has to have ruptured, its fluid being inside his head.

Explanation B:

As for "these convolutions that occur on copper of a crucible(?)," it is "the (molten) copper that a coppersmith pours off before it has been flattened in a stone mold with respect to something upon it that is bumpy, like wrinkles," that is to say, "it is like ripples of discharge."

Notes

Both Breasted (*Edwin Smith* 1: 521) and Faulkner (*CDME*, 51) query the translation "crucible" for *ꜥḏnt*.

nhdhd(*w*) *npꜣpꜣ*(*w*) – statives. For the use of the masculine form after the word *ḫt*, see Gardiner, *EG*[3], sec. 511.2.

n ꜥd.n.f – From this point I change the translation considerably, because I do not think that substantial elements of previous translations can be justified. I do not think that *n ꜥd.n.f* can be taken as a "not yet" or "before" form, for which one would expect the *n sḏmt.f* form, which indeed occurs later in this very case (*n pdst.f*). Allen (*AM*, 75) seems to be thinking of something like an adjective predicate + dative construction, but the adjective predicate would not be negated by *n*, the *sḏm.f* or *sḏm.n.f* of the adjective-verb would, which is actually what we have here (cf. Gardiner, *EG*[3], sec. 144). Thus I take the form as a typical *n sḏm.n.f*, which we have encountered in this text, and I take "he" as referring to the patient, or alternatively "it."

I take *ḫpr.n.f* as a nominal *sḏm.n.f* (manner nominalization). I do not think that *n* in *n nhdhd npꜣpꜣ* works syntactically as a negative, and I take it as the preposition *n*, and *ḏr* as "since."

ꜥrft "that envelops" – active participle.

nḫ.f "its fluid" (Faulkner, *CDME*, 139) – Alternatively it can be taken as a circumstantial *sḏm.f* "since it spews forth."

n pdst.f – *n sḏmt.f* "before" or "not yet" form, noted above.

iw mi wrmw nw ryt – This is a "textbook" case in which *iw* converts a subordinate (adverbial) element, a prepositional phrase, into an independent statement. The locus classicus of this type of sentence is in Sinuhe, *iw mi sḫr nṯr* "It was like the plan of a god." See M. Gilula, "The Stative Form of the Verb *sḏm* 'to hear'," *Journal of the American Research Center in Egypt* 14 (1977): 37–40. Note the analogous example in Case 39 below. It is interesting that the preposition found in the relevant passages in Smith is *mi*, and that this is also the case in *iw mi sḫr nṯr* as well as two other examples in Sinuhe, *iw mi ḫt ꜥꜣ wḥm st* "It is like a great thing, (namely) to repeat it" and *iw mi sšm rswt* "It was like the guidance of a dream" (Gardiner, *EG*[3], sec. 123 n. 2; J. L. Foster, *Thought Couplets in The Tale of Sinuhe* [Münchener Ägyptologische Beiträge 3. Frankfurt: Lang, 1993], 27–28, 56).

Medical Commentary

Type of Injury (Visual Index IV)

Case #6 represents the most severe open-head injury in this papyrus. It is a compound, depressed skull fracture (*sd*) with dura laceration, exposing the brain surface. Its source is an impact from a heavy sharp-bladed weapon. The patient exhibits symptoms and signs of base of skull fracture and post-traumatic meningismus (neck rigidity). Both of these are seen in severe skull fractures and have already been discussed in Cases ##3, 4, and 5. Case #6 describes bleeding from the nose only, a sign associated with anterior basal-skull fracture.

The brain injury in this case is the result of direct trauma by the offending object and from depressed bone fragments. An injury such as this could be caused in modern times by impacts with hammers, pipes, machetes, axes, high speed missiles, and fast moving objects like boat or airplane propellers. Visual index Vb shows the surgically removed portion of a patient's skull, showing a penetrating skull fracture produced by an airplane propeller. When produced by a sharp and heavy or sharp and fast-moving object the scalp wound and the bone penetration are straight and sharp, conforming to the shape of the impacting object. Immediately beneath the point of impact the bone is fractured and driven into the cranial cavity, resulting in depressed fragments and in additional fractures, which radiate outward from both its ends. Intracranial injury includes hematomas (epidural, subdural, intracerebral), and brain edema. Foreign-body material is often introduced by the offending object.

Our management of such wounds today requires full neurological, diagnostic radiological, neurosurgical, and dedicated intensive-care facilities. The current mortality rate by gunshot wounds to the head is 35 percent.[55] The prognosis for life and function are directly dependent upon the site and upon the extent of the brain injury, complications, and the availability of rehabilitation facilities. The biological serum markers S-100 protein and NSE (neuron specific enolase) serial measurements in head injury, respectively measuring astroglial and neuronal damage seem extremely promising in determination of the severity of brain injury and prediction of outcome[56]

Examples of these injuries in antiquity can be seen in the mummy of Egypt's Seventeenth Dynasty king, Seqenenre Tao II, killed in battle (Visual Index Vd and fig. 6, right).[57] Other examples of cranial penetrating injuries are evident in the skulls of Montuhotep's slain soldiers nos. 14 and 62 from the mummy cache from Deir el-Bahari (2000 BC; fig. 6, left and center).[58] Much later, Weber and Czarnetzki[59] studied thirty-three skulls from southwestern Germany, dating to the sixth, seventh, and eighth centuries, in which penetrating injuries produced by swords were evident. They concluded that mortality was directly related to the depth of penetration. The length of the head wounds in lethal cases averaged 8 cm, while the length in healed head wounds averaged only 5 cm. These data are consistent with dura and brain penetration in the lethal cases. If the patient did not die immediately from the brain injury, he would most likely die from infection[60] as dural tears would permit bacteria to enter and produce meningitis, brain abscesses, and cerebritis.

55. F. C. Vinas, et al. "Penetrating Head Trauma." Medscape Reference: http://emedicine.medscape.com/article/247664-overview.

56. Samit S. Mehta, "Biochemical Serum Markers in Head Injury: An Emphaisis on Clinical Utility" *Clinical Neurosurgery* 57 (2010): 134–40.

57. Manfred Bietak and E. Strouhal, "Die Todesumstände des Pharaos Seqenenre (17. Dynastie)," *Annals des Naturhistorischen Museums in Wien* 78 (1974): 45–50. The mummy is presently conserved in the Egyptian Museum, Cairo, Egypt.

58. Winlock, *Slain Soldiers of Neb-hep-et-Re Mentu-hotpe*, 14, 17, plates VIII, X.

59. J. Weber and A. Czarnetzki, "Brief Communication: Neurotraumatological Aspects of Head Injuries Resulting from Sharp and Blunt Force in the Early Medieval Period of Southwestern Germany," *American Journal of Physical Anthropology* 14 (2001): 353–56.

60. Christine F. Salazar, *The Treatment of War Wounds in Graeco-Roman Antiquity* (Studies in Ancient Medicine 21; Leiden: Brill, 2000), 15 –27.

Ancient Medical Methodology and Knowledge

In addition to the explicit and detailed anatomical/pathological description of the injury, with symptoms and signs of base of skull fracture and post-traumatic meningismus[61] (see Cases #3, #4, and #5). Case #6 raises the importance of this document to landmark level in the history of the neurosciences with its descriptions of the following major anatomical and functional concepts:

- The appearance of the brain surface
- Identification of the duramater as a membrane enveloping the brain
- Cerebral pulsatile features in the traumatized patient with widely open/fractured skull
- The existence of cerebrospinal fluid
- The anterior fontanelle in infants

Using common objects and activities of his time, the Egyptian physician compared the appearance of the surface of the brain to the floating supernatant, or slag that forms in bubbles of sulphur dioxide, produced during the process of copper smelting. Metal working was both widespread and common in ancient Egypt, making the bubbled surface of discarded copper slag a familiar sight. The master physician instructs his pupil about how to find this type of wound by palpating the intracranial wound, the brain surface, which would feel "[like] 'these convolutions that occur in copper of a smelter ... bumpy, like wrinkles ... that is to say, it is like ripples of discharge.'" Breasted's translation of *ryt* as "ripples of pus" is not applicable to the description related to copper smelting, but the translation "ripples of discharge" is in complete agreement. This is precisely the material, known as copper slag, which the smith pours off before he forces molten copper into a mold. Although Brawanski has raised doubts about the exact meaning of the material in this case,[62] it appears to us that comparing the floating supernatant in the copper smelting process with the brain surface was an excellent choice. Naturally occurring botryoidal[63] forms of copper compounds formed in igneous and metamorphic rocks[64] are very similar in appearance to the copper slag formed in smelting. We have used illustrations of this copper compound to demonstrate how its surface architecture resembles that of a brain (Visual Index Vc).

In the examination segment, our master physician explains the brain's pulsating motion seen and palpated in the wound of this patient who has a fractured and open skull by comparing it to the pulsating of an infant's soft spot on the crown of his head, what we call the "fontanelle." The fontanelle and its pulsation ceases as the bone sutures close with the child's growth. Further, he explains the pathogenesis of why the examining physician is able to feel head pulsations when palpating the cranial wound in Case #6: "How it has come to pass/How he has become (is) because of the throbbing and fluttering under your fingers, since the brain of his braincase is exposed/broken open."

Reference to the cerebrospinal fluid is made in Explanation A: "As for 'smashing in of his braincase and exposing/breaking open the brain of his skull,' the large smash fracture is open to the inside of his braincase and the dura mater/membrane that envelops his brain has to have ruptured since it spews forth its fluid being inside his head."

In addressing the diagnostic/prognostic segment of this case, the physician's verdict is, "a medical condition that cannot be handled/dealt with." This is an appropriate verdict for the medical and surgical capabilities

61. The reader is directed to appendix 2 for a compilation of the neurological symptoms and signs in the Edwin Smith Papyrus.

62. Brawanski, "Die Fälle 1–8 des Papyrus Edwin Smith," 21–23.

63. "The word is derived from the Greek word for grapes, and means tiny crystals occurring in closely interlocking spherical masses or "bubbles," which can sometimes look like bunches of grapes." Online: http://dave.ucsc.edu/myrtreia/specimens.html.

64. http://www.rocksandminerals.com/rockcycle.htm.

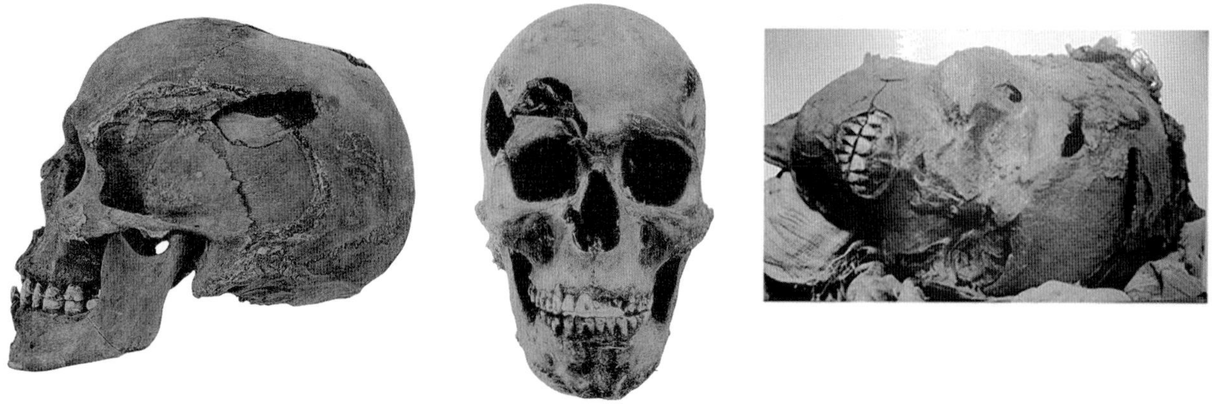

Fig. 6. Left: Soldier #62, plate X D. Center: Soldier #14, plate VIII B. From Winlock, *Slain Soldiers of Neb-hep-et-Re Mentu-hotpe*. Right: King Seqenenre Tao II's head injuries.

existing 3,750 years ago. There were no significant changes in this pessimistic way of the treatment of head injuries until the period between the American Civil War and the end of World War I, when the advent of anesthesia, the understanding of the concept of bacterial infection, and, the implementation of antisepsis and asepsis in the operating room all made possible the development of modern neurosurgery.[65] The mortality from head wounds was reduced from 73.9 percent in the Crimean War (1856) to 35 percent in World War I (1918).[66] The era between the Great World Wars and the end of the Vietnam War produced major improvements in head injury care through the advent of antibiotics, anticonvulsants, neurodiagnostic radiological techniques, formal neurosurgical education, specialized instrumentation, and rapid evacuation and treatment. The mortality rate from head wounds was 14 percent during World War II, dropping to 9.7 percent during the Vietnam War.[67] The current management of head injury continues to improve by widespread use of CT and MRI scanning, cerebral blood flow (CBF) studies, intracranial pressure monitoring and management, and from ongoing advances in our understanding of the biochemical and molecular biology of brain injury.[68]

We have seen in the previous case, despite having received this verdict, a patient with the type of injury considered in Case #6 received some form of treatment. First the warnings "You should not bandage it" and "You should not lay the two bandage strips over it." As in Case #5, the implications are clear for us, they were avoiding any measures that could contribute to elevate the intracranial pressure. The statement "until you know he has reached the crisis" is in accord with our current understanding of the evolution of physiopathological intracranial events after a severe head injury in which the patient's clinical neurological condition either stabilizes (intracranial pressure returns to normal), or deteriorates and the patient does not survive.

Assuming no other systemic injury exists that would produce hypoxia and hypotension, and that no major complications develop (i.e., infection), the "critical period" alluded to in this papyrus refers to the time when the trauma would produce disturbances in cerebral blood flow autoregulation, brain tissue pH changes with reduction in CO_2 reactivity, and when the elevation of intracranial pressure begins to subside, gradually returning to normal. This is, in optimal conditions at the end of two weeks, but, depending on variable complications, it may be much longer or never.

65. T. F. Dagi, "The Management of Head Trauma," *A History of Neurosurgery* (ed. Samuel H Greenblatt; Park Ridge, IL: American Association of Neurological Surgeons, 1997), 289–313.

66. Elisha S. Gurdjian, *Head Injury from Antiquity to the Present with Special Reference to Penetrating Head Wounds* (Springfield, IL: Thomas, 1973), 113.

67. Ibid.

68. Dagi, "Management of Head Trauma."

CASE #7:

Frontal Cutting Wound with Compound Skull Fracture Penetrating the Frontal Air Sinus, Uncomplicated and Infected: Tetanus

(Plate III:2–IV:4)

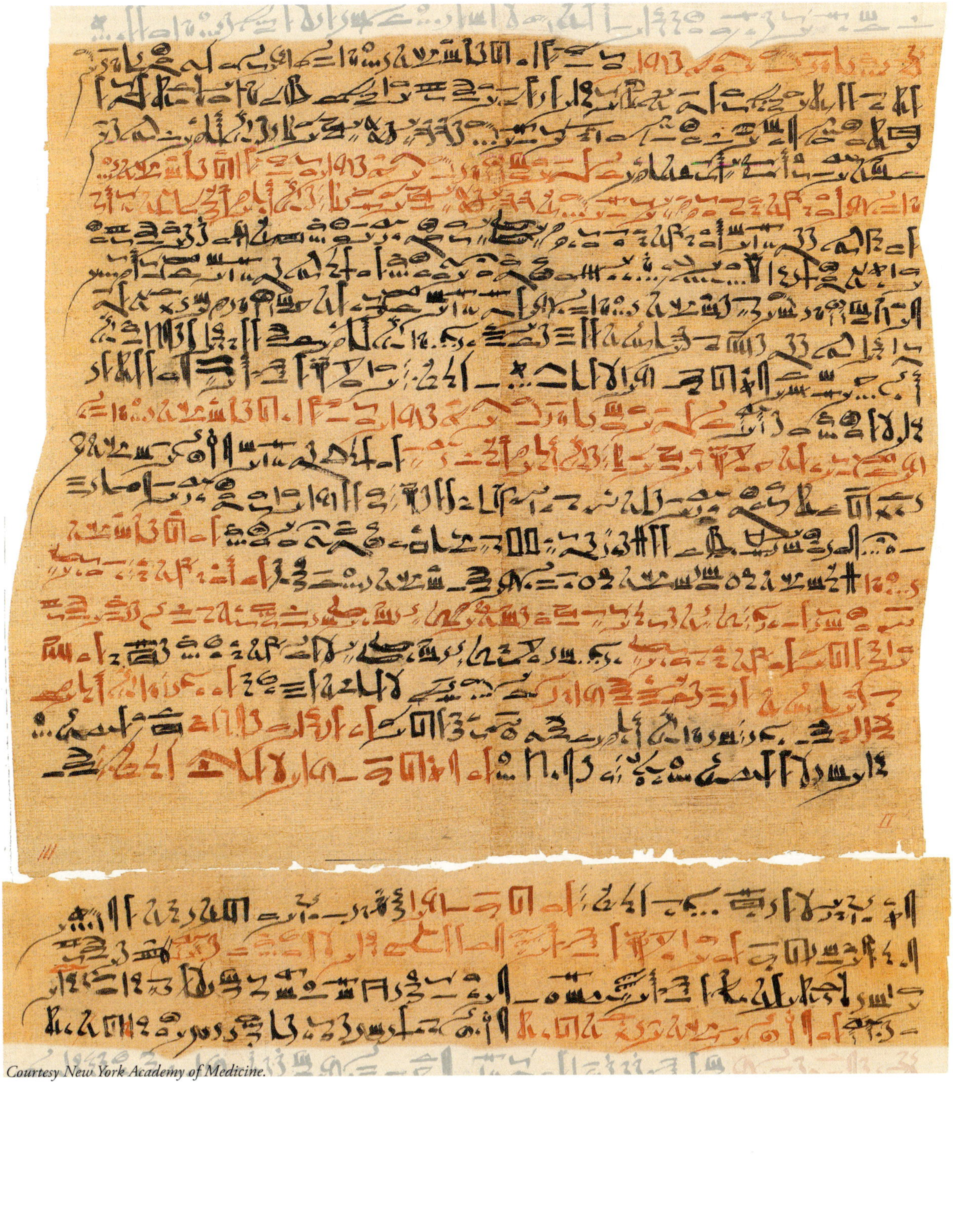

Courtesy New York Academy of Medicine.

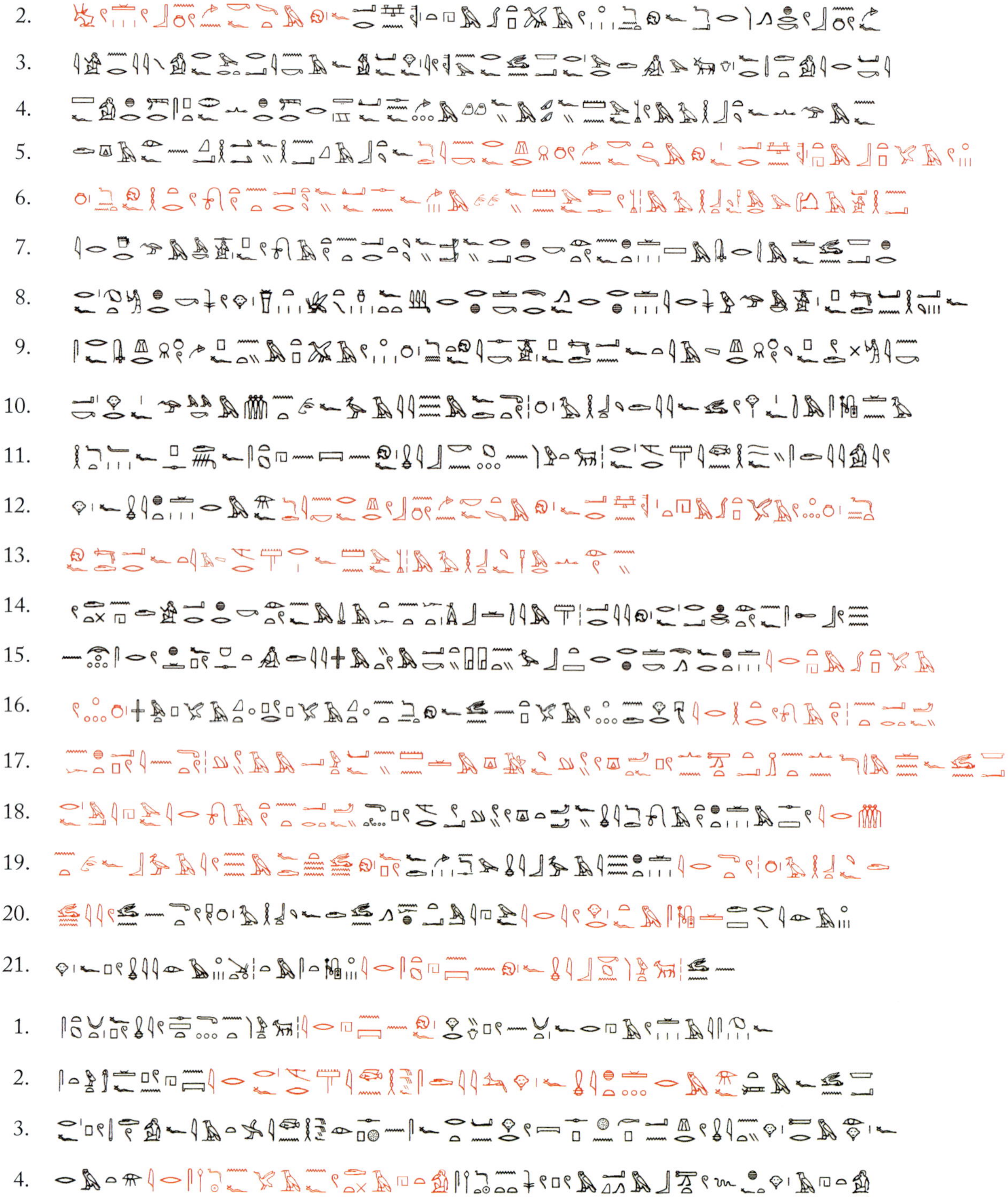
2.
3.
4.
5.
6.
7.
8.
9.
10.
11.
12.
13.
14.
15.
16.
17.
18.
19.
20.
21.
1.
2.
3.
4.

Transliteration

2§ šsꜣw wbnw-n-kft m tp.f ꜥr n ḳs thm tpꜣw nw ḏnnt.f ḏꜥr.ḫr.k wbnw.f

3§ inry r.f wrt rdi.in.k fꜣ.f ḥr.f iw ḳsn r.f wn rꜣ.f wrḏ ib.f r mdt ir ḫꜣ.k

4§ iš.f ḫr r spty.f n ḫr.n r tꜣ di.f snf m msdty.fy msḏrwy.fy mn.f ṯsw m nḥbt.f n gm.n.f

5§ dgꜣ.f n kꜥḥwy.fy ḥnꜥ ḳꜣbt.f ḏd.in.k r.f ḫr<y> wbnw-n-kft m tp.f ꜥr n ḳs thm tpꜣw

6§ nw ḏnnt.f ḥtr wꜣt nt ꜥrt{y}.f{y} di.f snf m msdty.fy msḏrwy.fy mn.f ṯsw m nḥbt.f mḥr ꜥḥꜣ.i ḥnꜥ

7§ ir ḏr gmm.k s pf ḥtr wꜣt nt ꜥrt{y}.f{y} wgyty.fy rdi.ḫr.k ir.tw n.f ḫt šm r nḏm.f wn.ḫr

8§ rꜣ.f wt.ḫr.k sw ḥr mrḥt bit ftt r rḫ.k spr.f r ḫt ir swt gm.k s pf šd.n ḥꜥw.f

9§ srf ḫr wbnw pf nty m tpꜣw ḏnnt.f isk s pf šd.n.f tiꜣ ḫr wbnw pf wd.in.k

10§ ꜥ.k ḥr.f gmm.k mḫnt.f bꜣy m fdt mtw nw nḥbt.f dwn.y ḥr.f tms

11§ nḥdt.f psd.f sty hn n tp.f mi bkn n ꜥwt rꜣ.f mr inḥwy.fy sdy iw

12§ ḥr.f mi ḫt rm.f ḏd.in.k r.f ḫr<y> wbnw-n-kft m tp.f ꜥr n ḳs thm tpꜣw nw

13§ ḏnnt.f šd.n.f tiꜣ mr rꜣ.f mn.f ṯsw m nḥbt.f mḥr n irw.ny

13§ … ir swt gmm.k s pf sḥḏ.n.f pꜣ.n.f

14§ wdt nhd rdi.ḫr.k ir.tw n.f mḏꜣt nt ḫt ḏbꜣ.t m ḥbsw rdy tp <m> rꜣ.f rdi.ḫr.k ir.tw n.f sḫbw

15§ n wꜥḥ srwḫ.f pw ḥmst (w)dy imitw mkꜣty nty <m> ḏbt r rḫ.k spr.f r ḫt ir thm tpꜣw

16§ nw [ḏnnt.f] imitw pꜣkt pw r pꜣḳ nt ḏnnt.f wn tpꜣw n dḥr ir ḥtr wꜣwt nt ꜥrty{y}.fy

17§ nḫt pw in mtw pḥwy ꜣmꜥwt.f ny mn m gmꜣ.f pḥwy wgyt.f pw nn itt-int n nḏm.n n.f wn

18§ rꜣ.f m-ꜥ iḫ.f ir wꜣ nt ꜥrt{y}.fy mtw pw mr pḥwy wgyty.fy mi ḏd wꜣt ḫt šs ir ḫnt.f

19§ bꜣi m fdt wnn tp.f pw fd nḏs mi bꜣi ḫt ir mtw nw nḥbt.f

20§ dwn.y wnn mtw pw nw nḥbt.f dwn nḫt m-ꜥ iḫ.f ir iw ḥr.f ṯms dšr irtyw

21§ ḥr.f pw mi irtyw prt ṯmst ir sty hn n tp.f mi bkn <n> ꜥwt wnn

1§ sty wpt.f pw mi wsš nt ꜥwt ir h n tp.f ḥry-ib pw n wpt.f r-hꜣw ꜣis.f

2§ s-twt.f pw n hn ir rꜣ.f mr inḥwy.fy sdy ḥr.f mi ḫt rm.f tm.f wn

3§ rꜣ.f pw mdw.f iꜣṯ inḥwy.fy ir sp n sfrt n-ḥrw sp n kꜣp n-ḥrw mi nty ḥr ṯrm ḥr.f <ḥr>

4§ rmt ir sḥḏ.n.f pꜣ.n.f wdt ꜣht sḥḏt ntt sw p m ꜥḳ m bṯ ḫft-ḥr ꜣht

Translation

Uncomplicated (Plate III:2–8)

Title:

Necessary knowledge and skills for a slash wound in his head penetrating to the bone, and perforating the membranous lined sinus cavities of his braincase:

Examination:

You need to palpate his wound, it quaking/crepitating (or, that quakes/shifts?) from it very much.

Then you are to make him lift his face, and it is too painful for him to open his mouth, and his heart/mind is too feeble/weary to speak,

and if you observe his spittle hanging down from his lips, unable to fall to the ground, while he bleeds from his nostrils/nasal cavities and his ears, and (while) he suffers rigidity in the back of his neck, and (while) he is unable to look to both of his shoulder joints and his chest,

Diagnosis:

then you are to say about him: "One who has a slash wound in his head, penetrating to the bone, and perforating the membranous lined sinus cavities of his braincase:

the ligament(s) of his lower jaw/mandible being contracted, while he bleeds from both his nostrils/nasal cavities and his two ears, and (while) he suffers rigidity in the back of his neck—

a medical condition I will fight with."

Treatment:

Now since how you find that man (is) with the ligament<s> of his lower jaw{s} and his rami contracted, you have to have something hot made for him, so that he recovers.

His mouth must open.

You must bandage it (along) with ointment and honey and a dressing until you know that he arrives at a turning point.

First Alternative Course

Title: (omitted)

Examination:

If however, you find that man, his flesh having developed heat because of that wound which is in the membranous lined sinus cavities of his braincase while that man has developed *tỉꜣ* because of that wound,

then you should lay your hand on him.

How you find his forehead (is) clammy with perspiration

the ligaments of the back of his neck being taut, his face being flushed,

his teeth, (it) shining, the odor of his braincase being like the excrement of goats, his mouth being immobile/bound, his eyebrows quivering, his face being something like he weeps.

Diagnosis:

Then you are to say about him: "One suffering from a slash wound in his head penetrating to the bone, perforating the membranous lined sinus cavities of his braincase,

He has developed *tỉꜣ,* his mouth being bound while he suffers rigidity in the back of his neck—

a medical condition that cannot be handled/dealt with."

Second Alternative Course

Title: (omitted)

Examination:

But if you should find that man having become white/pale, and he has been lying down weak,

Treatment:

You must cause that one make for him a wedge of wood, padded with cloth, the tip being placed <in> his mouth.

You must cause that one make for him a broth of carob beans (or earth almonds?).

His treatment: it is sitting (upright), laid between two supports, which are <consisting of> brick, until you know that he has passed the crisis.

Explanation A:

As for "perforating the membranous lined sinus cavities of [his head]," it means, "between the bony plate and (another) bony plate of his braincase, there exist membranous lined sinus cavities of tough membrane."

Explanation B:

As for "the cords of his lower jaw/mandible being contracted," it means stiffening by the ligaments of the two ends of his forked bones, which are fastened in his temporal bone. It means: "the ends of his ramus are without movement back and forth and (it) cannot be comfortable for him to open his mouth because of his illness."

Explanation C:

As for "the cord<s> of his lower jaw," it means the ligaments that bind the two ends of his rami are like saying "a cord, a thing consisting of rope."

Explanation D:

As for "his forehead being clammy with perspiration," it means that, "his head is a little sweaty, as if something is damp."

Explanation E:

As for "the ligaments of the back of his neck being taut," it means that the ligaments of the back of his neck are taut and stiff because of his illness.

Explanation F:

As for "his face being flushed," it means his face is red in color like the color of red fruit.

Explanation G:

As for "the odor of the chest/vault of his head being like the excrement of goats," it means, how the odor of the crown of his head is (is) like the urine of goats.

Explanation H:

As for "the chest of his head," (braincase), it is in the middle of his crown in the vicinity of his brain. It is similar to a box.

Explanation I:

As for "his mouth bound; his eyebrows quivering, his face being something like he weeps," it means, he does not open his mouth and his speech is distorted. His two eyebrows maintain a diseased condition because of contorting upward, the condition of drooping downward being like one who is blinking while his face is weeping.

Explanation J:

As for "he having become pale, he has lain down weak and pale," it means that he is entering into an incurable condition in the presence of the debility/weakness.

Notes

ỉnry – Another stative, or alternatively perhaps an active participle.

ỉw ksn r.f wn rꜣ.f – "It is too painful…." Cf. Gardiner, *EG*^{3}, sec. 467; for the "too … to" construction, see also sec. 163.7. These occurrences of *ỉw* + adjectival word are to be analyzed either as *ỉw* + stative of the adjective-verb (Gardiner's preference, especially as suggested by the ending *w* in some examples; cf. Gilula "The stative Form of the Verb *sḏm* 'to hear'") or as *ỉw sḏm.f*, a present statement of fact, Hoch, *MEG*, sec. 31, in such cases employing the *sḏm.f* of the adjective-verb rather than the simple predicate adjective. See also Meltzer, "Problems of Adjectival Constructions," II.6.

wrḏ ib.f r mdt – "too … to" construction, as above.

The description of the symptoms is characterized by series of parallel clauses, most of which we are understanding as circumstantials, either circumstantial *sḏm.f* or stative depending on the syntax. In the case of "his teeth, it shining," I think this fits into the series of circumstantials despite the fronted noun; for a circumstantial *sḏm.f* following a noun in front extraposition, see E. Doret, *The Narrative Verbal System of Old and Middle Egyptian* (Cahiers d'Orientalisme 12, Geneva: Patrick Cramer, 1986), 33–34, or, as he puts it, a noun + *sḏm.f* construction.

ꜥrt{y}.f{y} – The writing of "his lower jaw" as a dual seems to refer to a strong folk concept conceiving the lower jaw as a pair of bones joined in the center at the chin. I do not make a habit of citing Budge, but this spelling is found in the Pyramid Texts and Book of the Dead; E. A. W. Budge, *Osiris: The Egyptian Religion of Resurrection* (New Hyde Park, NY: University Books, 1961), 2:91–93. Budge recounts that the Arab physician Abd el-Latif "spent a good deal of time examining skulls in Egypt, in order to be able to refute by personal observation" the belief that the lower jaw comprised a pair of bones (93). In the case of Edwin Smith, the master physician certainly would have known better, but the scribe might have had a tendency to follow an inaccurate but possibly familiar and widely believed folk tradition and linguistic usage.

rdy tp – Passive *sḏm(w).f*, which is one of Polotsky's (*Egyptian Tenses*) circumstantial or adverbial forms; for the form *rdy*, see Gardiner, *EG*^{3}, sec. 420.

"which are <consisting of> brick" – <*m*> needs to be emended after *nty* because *m* of predication is required.

ntt sw pw m ꜥḳ – *ntt … pw* "this means that," *sw* (depending or leaning on *ntt*) *m ꜥḳ* "he is entering into," pseudo-verbal construction with *m* + infinitive sometimes found when verb involves the meaning of motion (Gardiner, *EG*^{3}, sec. 331), though *ꜥḳ* is not a verb of motion as most strictly defined; it is used intransitively here (*ꜥḳ m* "enter into") and indeed very frequently, but its transitive use is also attested (*Wb.* 1:230–32). Gardiner notes that *m* + infinitive can substitute for *ḥr* + infinitive of the relevant verbs, but *m* + infinitive also has a close relationship with the stative, and in fact the stative or qualitative of some verbs in Coptic is derived not from the earlier stative form but from *m* + infinitive; this was explored by E. F. Wente, "The Syntax of Verbs of Motion in Egyptian" (PhD dissertation, University of Chicago, 1959).

bṯw "incurable condition" – Faulkner, *CDME*, 86.

rdy tp – Passive *sḏm(w).f*, which is one of Polotsky's circumstantial or adverbial forms (Egyptian Tenses); for the form *rdy*, see Gardiner, *EG*^{3}, sec. 420.

This treatment is illustrated in the painting by Robert Thom that illustrates the cover of this volume.

Medical Commentary

Uncomplicated (Plate III:2–8)

Type of Injury (Visual Index IV)

Case #7 discusses a head injury with a compound skull fracture that has penetrated the cranial cavity.[69] Because perforation (*thm*) has occurred into "there exist membranous lined sinus cavities of tough membrane," anatomically located "between the bony plate and (another) bony plate of his braincase," Chapman suggested that these cavities are the frontal air sinus.[70] Although Chapman's term of "membranous lined sinus cavities of his braincase" is adequate, the Egyptian master physician has further identified the *tpꜣw* anatomical location in Explanations G and H. These explanations are given in relation to the second alternative course, where an infection has developed in the area of the frontal air sinus in the patient described in the first alternative course. The infection has produced a foul odor from the injured site, "the chest of his head." This structure is "similar to a box" and located "in the vicinity of his brain" and "in the middle of his crown." The Egyptian word *wpt* refers to horns, crown of the head, vertex, and apex. James Walker[71] disagreed with Chapman, interpreting *wpt* as the brow, proposing instead it referred to the two parietal bones and their joining sagittal suture in the midline of the skull. But Walker also cites two funerary texts that allude to the ureaus serpent arising from the top of the king's forehead, namely, Coffin Text Spell 817 and Pyramid Text Spell 396. Both texts lend support to the brow interpretation of *wpt*. Using a different approach in the study of the word *wpt*, it is certain that many of the Egyptian anatomical terms applied to humans derived from butchery practice and it is of anatomical interest that the origin of the cow horns is from the frontal bone and that the horn cavities themselves interconnect with the frontal air sinuses.[72] In this context, *wpt* could very well apply to the anatomical location of "the chest of his head." On human anatomy, a midline sagittal section of the skull helps identify the shape, location, and relationships of the frontal air sinus in concordance with those features attributed to the "chest of his head" (Visual Indexes I and IV).

The possibility of this injury penetrating the main cranial cavity has also been considered, but in addition to the wealth of information about "the chest of the head's" location, the specific word for the duramater: 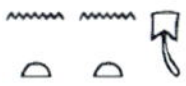 *ntnt* is not used to describe the lining of these cavities. Instead, the word *dḥr* "hide" is used.

The Clinical Picture

Objective analysis of the provided data indicates that upon examination of the patient:

69. Walker, *Studies in Ancient Egyptian Anatomical Terminology*, 62.

70. P. H. Chapman, "Case Seven of the Smith Surgical Papyrus: The Meaning of *tpꜣw*," *Journal of the American Research Center in Egypt* 29 (1992): 35–42.

71. Walker, *Studies in Ancient Egyptian Anatomical Terminology*, 62, 63.

72. Klaus-Dieter Budras and Robert E. Habel, *Bovine Anatomy* (Hannover: Schlütersche, 2003), 34, 35.

- On palpation of the head wound there is crepitation, indicating comminuted bone fractures.
- Upon command, the patient is asked to lift his face. This implies the patient is not unconscious and he is able to understand and to follow commands.
- Level of consciousness is described as depressed, as it is noted: 1) "his heart/mind is too feeble/weary to speak." As this is a head injury case the authors interpret "*ib*" as "mind," related to the effect on speech, not as heart or *ḥ3ty* in this instance (see Case #1 under "The Dual Concept of the Heart"). Indeed, heart arrhythmias and failure can occur in severe head injuries, but these are usually terminal events developing in a patient in whom brain damage has affected the lower brain stem, a very different situation to the one portrayed in the first alternative course of Case 7. Shock can also be a cause of feeble pulse, but that does not appear to be the situation in the first alternative course as we lack evidence for major hemorrhaging or extensive body damage. 2) "you observe his spittle hanging down from his lips, unable to fall to the ground." In a drowsy patient, normal reflexive swallowing is depressed and along with dehydration would produce thick saliva.
- It is too painful for him to open his mouth and the ligament(s) of his lower jaw/mandible being contracted. The physician's treatment recommendations at this stage indicate that he attributes the mouth symptoms to local oral causes (Breasted, *Edwin Smith*, 179). Explanation B clearly identifies the Masseter muscles as those being contracted, that is "trismus."
- There is evidence of basal skull fractures: "while he bleeds from his nostrils and his ears."
- There is evidence of traumatic meningismus[73] from subarachnoid hemorrhage:
  1) "and he suffers rigidity in the back of his neck,"
  2) "and he is unable to look to both of his shoulder joints and his chest."

The current evaluation and treatment of this type of injury today would require initial clinical assessment, as was performed by the physician in ancient Egypt, complemented by systemic evaluation and tetanus shots. Once radiological and scanning studies of the head and neck are completed, surgical wound exploration, culturing, debridement, and repair would proceed. Follow up management would be in a neurological/neurosurgical intensive care unit with appropriate antibiotic coverage.

In regard to the presence of "trismus" in Case 7, all we can say for certain is that in absence of known facial-mandibular injuries to account for a local source of trismus, the possibility of early tetanus infection exists.[74] However, the physician's treatment recommendations suggest that, at the moment, he attributes the mouth symptoms to local (oral) causes. We presume that Case #7 is the Egyptian physician's first encounter with this newly injured patient. If so, it is unlikely that he would be already in the presence of tetanus infection, since it requires a period of incubation.

Ancient Medical Methodology and Knowledge

Because sufficient and clear clinical facts are provided in the text from the ancient Egyptian physician's findings in the Examination, we are able to understand the nature/extent of the head injury in the first alternative course. The same applies to the clinical objectivity displayed in the physician's diagnostic conclusions. The verdict regarding treatability of this injury is defined as "a medical condition I will fight with." Treatment is given, but there is uncertainty about its success. The only measures are local treatment to the contracted oral muscles with something hot: "His mouth must open." Then honey, ointment, and dressings were to be applied "until

73. The reader is directed to appendix 2 for a compilation of the neurological symptoms and signs in the Edwin Smith Papyrus.

74. Breasted, *Edwin Smith*, 49; A. P. Leca, "Maladies Infectieuses, épidémies," *La Médicine Ėgyptienne au Temps des Pharaons* (Paris: R. Dacosta, 1971), 208. Leca considers that in Case 7, three stages of tetanus are successively described.

you know that he arrives at a turning point." Examples from Egyptian antiquity of penetrating head injuries to the frontal sinus area shown in Soldiers #14 and 23 from Winlock's *Slain Soldiers of Neb-hep-et-Re Mentu-hotpe* (fig. 7).

First Alternative Course: Infection–*tiꜣ* (Tetanus 75; plates III:8–13, 16–21; IV:2–4)

Type of Injury (Visual Index VI)

Presented in the first alternative course is the same head injury patient described in the initial injury: a head injury with a compound, comminuted skull fracture, penetrating the cranial cavity in the area of the frontal air sinus. But now the patient has developed an infectious complication.

By separating this section as "first alternative course," the authors signal its significance as a new clinical entity. While Breasted considered this portion of Case #7 as a "Second Examination," we have elected, due to its importance in the history of medicine, to study it under the subtitle "First Alternative Course: Infection." The text begins: "If however, you find that man [referring here to the initial injury described at the start of the case as a patient with 'a slash wound in his head penetrating to the bone, and perforating the leathery cavities of his braincase'], his flesh having developed heat because of that wound which is in the membranous lined sinus cavities of his braincase, while that man has developed *tiꜣ* because of that wound."

The new examination findings in the first alternative course are given under two words: *srf* = heat from inflammation/infection and *tiꜣ*, a word left untranslated by Breasted and which has been the subject of intense interest ever since. Both of these entities have developed because of the wound. Each of these have symptoms and signs expressed in the texts of examination, diagnosis, and Explanations "B" through "I."

Those associated with *srf* = heat from inflammation/infection are:

- "his forehead being clammy with perspiration" (see Explanation D),
- "his face being flushed"[76] (reddish discoloration, see Explanation F),
- "the odor of the chest/vault of his head being like the excrement of goats" (this statement refers to the smell of an infected intracranial wound;[77] see Explanation G).

Those associated with *tiꜣ* are:

- "the ligaments of the back of his neck being taut" (see Explanation E)
- "his teeth, it shining" (see Examination)
- "his mouth being immobile/bound" (see Examination, First Alternative Course, and Explanation I)
- "his eyebrows quivering" (see Explanation I)
- "his face being something like he weeps" (see Explanation I)

75. Tetanus in the authors' opinion. See the rest of the medical commentary of the first alternative course.

76. W. Schenkel, "Die Farben in ägyptischer Kunst und Sprache," *Zeitschrift für ägyptische Sprache und Altertumskunde* 88 (1963): 140–41, notes the word *tms* most likely refers to a particular shade of red.

77. The smell of wounds is caused by a mixture of short chain organic acids produced by anaerobic bacteria, and a mixture of amines and diamines like cadaverine and putrescine, the product of other proteolytic bacteria. C. W. Moss, et al. "Gas Chromatography of Bacterial Fatty Acids with a Fused Silica Capillary Column," *Journal of Clinical Microbiology* 28 (1974): 80–85. Frequently isolated bacteria from these wounds are anaerobes Bacteroides and Clostridium species, and aerobes Proteus, Pseudomonas species and Klebsiella. A. D. Parry, P. R. Chadwick, D. Simon, B. Oppenheim, and C. N. McCollum, "Leg Ulcer Odour Detection Identifies Beta-Haemolytic Strepto-coccal Infection," *Journal of Wound Care* 4/9 (1995): 404–5.

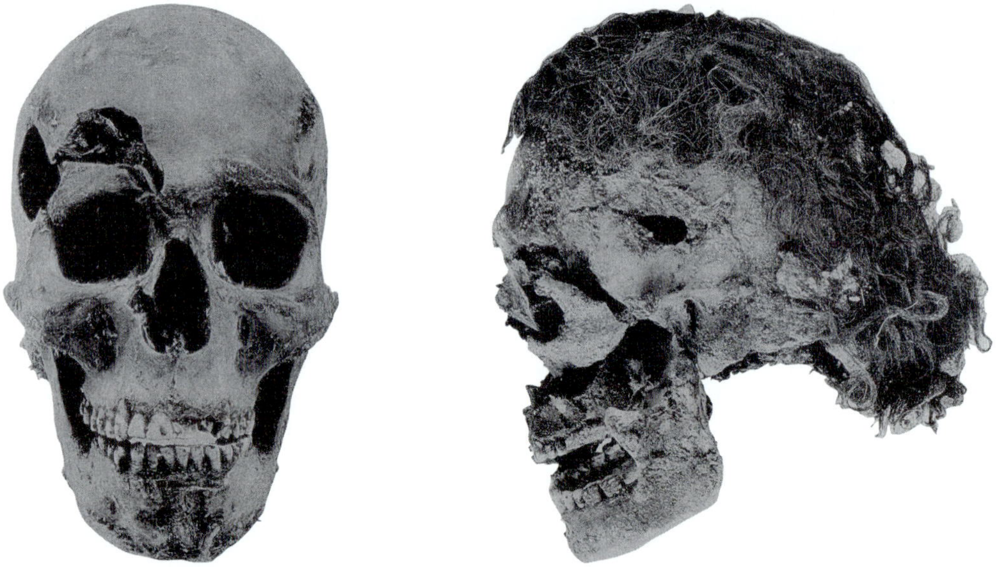

Fig. 7. Left: Soldier #14, plate VIII B. Right: Soldier #23, plate IX A, showing penetrating wounds to the frontal air sinus areas. From Winlock, *Slain Soldiers of Neb-hep-et-Re Mentu-hotpe*.

While both sets of symptoms developed because of the head wound, there are differences in the hieroglyphic determinatives of the word "wound." The developing of heat from inflammation/infection is attributed to: "that wound which is in the membranous lined sinus cavities of his braincase." But the development of *tiꜣ* is "because of that wound." That this data complex was intended to be singled out as a clinical entity is further supported by the structure of the Diagnosis in Case #7b (Breasted's Second Diagnosis). Typically in the Edwin Smith papyrus the Diagnosis includes repetition of the "Title," to which the new diagnosis is added and a new verdict is attached:

- The full title of what we labeled as Case #7 First Alternative Course would have been: "Then you are to say about him, one having a knife slash in his head penetrating to the bone, and perforating the membranous lined sinus cavities of his braincase."
- The new diagnosis "he has developed *tiꜣ*, his mouth being bound while he suffers rigidity in the back of his neck."
- New verdict: "a medical condition that cannot be handled/dealt with."

Breasted suspected tetanus in this case: "The ancient surgeon was perhaps indicating that the patient is suffering from Tetanus." But he could not go further to prove it: "the only new conclusion unfortunately contains an unintelligible term." It is apparent that the word *tiꜣ* holds the key to elucidate what this infectious complication is.

The Meaning of *tiꜣ*

Without a specific explanation in Breasted's translation for *tiꜣ,* it has remained subject to speculation. Its various interpretations, including the *Grundriss*'s (7, 2:937) *tiꜣ* as a verb translated as "to have illness of the teeth," and *tiꜣw* as, "the illness of the teeth" prove unsatisfactory.[78] Based on his findings in nonmedical literature that several words with the *tiꜣ* common radical were related to actions taking place with the jaws contracted (like snarling, grinning, and humming), Bardinet proposed similar interpretations for *tiꜣ*, and *tiꜣw*, to be applied in the Medical Papyri.[79] The word *tiꜣ* would signify "to tighten the jaws/teeth," and *tiꜣw* would signify "contraction of the jaw musculature, or trismus." Applied in this context, these words would be used for conditions associated with the pathological contraction of the jaws, the symptom we call "trismus."[80]

The appearance and development into the clinical picture of the word *tiꜣ* in the first alternative course needs to be analyzed:

- *tiꜣ* appears in two locations:
    1. in our proposed first alternative course, describing a complication of the initial head injury.
    2. in the first alternative course in the examination section as a new symptom complex along with fever.
- *tiꜣ* signals a delayed complication of the head injury in which a penetrating skull fracture has occurred.
- *tiꜣ* and fever are directly attributed by the Egyptian physician to the head wound.
- *tiꜣ* as such is not included as a "symptom" in the first alternative course examination, but as a "syndrome," including four various symptoms:
    1. "the ligaments of the back of his neck being taut" (neck muscle rigidity, see Explanation E).
    2. "his mouth being immobile/ bound: ... He does not open his mouth and his speech is distorted" (see Explanation I).
    3. "his teeth (it) shining" is convincingly explained by Bardinet[81] as akin to "snarling," and consistent with "*risus sardonicus*."
    4. "his face being something like he weeps" is defined in Explanation I.
- *tiꜣ* as a syndrome appears in the first alternative course's diagnosis with a specific name: "*tiꜣ*."
- The "*tiꜣ*" medical complex is recognized as the infectious complication arising from the open-head injury described in the initial injury.
- Fever is not mentioned in the diagnosis section of the first alternative course, but *tiꜣ* seems to have absorbed most of the symptoms listed in the examination section, including those symptoms related to fever.
- It is the presence of *tiꜣ* in the diagnosis section of the first alternative course that transforms Case #7 into an intractable and hopeless case.
- The specific location for the word *tiꜣ* singles it out as the identifying characteristic of, and/or, the name for the new ailment "and he has developed *tiꜣ*."

---

78. An "illness of the teeth" is unlikely in this case where we are dealing with a deteriorating clinical condition in a severely injured individual. A toothache would have been the least of his problems, or his complaints.

79. It is necessary to review here other medically related information about the word *tiꜣ* in the medical papyri. We follow Bardinet in his excellent review of appearances of these cases: Papyrus Kahun #5, #23, #24, and #33, Papyrus Berlin 75, and Papyrus Deir el Medineh (J. Černý, *Papyrus hiératiques de Deir el-Médineh*, Tome I, pl. 10, 1. Catalogue complété et édité par G. Posener, [Le Caire, 1978] = Documents de fouilles, 85). See Thierry Bardinet, *Dents et mâchoires dans les représentations religieuses en la pratique médicale en Égypte ancienne* (Studia Pohl, Series Maior 15; Rome: Pontifico Istituto Biblico, 1990), 166–87.

80. Westendorf, *Handbuch der altägyptischen Medizin*, 2:718.

81. We agree with Bardinet's adoption of the word *psḏ* "shining" as descriptive of the patient's teeth signifying that the patient's canine teeth are visible enough to the observer to "shine," like other white objects. This is an oblique way of saying that the patient's mouth is open wide enough to expose his teeth to view. The clinical portrayal of *risus sardonicus* fits the image very well. However, Bardinet's reconstruction to a stative verbal form *nḥḏwt.f psḏ<ty>*, meaning "to be in a state of shining" does not comply with the text as written (*nḥḏwt.f psḏ.f*) and ignores the suffix pronoun *f*. No reconstructions are necessary since the text as written reads "his teeth, it shines" with the singular "it" referring back to "his teeth." Bardinet, *Dents et mâchoires*. 170–71.

- The term *tiꜣ* is then described by multiple symptoms/examination findings consistent with, and distinctively characteristic of tetanus infection (Visual Index VI).

The simple substitution of the word *tiꜣ* in the first alternative course, for the symptom of "trismus" would be unsatisfactory. The diagnosis would read "and he has developed trismus," followed immediately by "his mouth being bound." This sentence also describes trismus (Explanation I). This would be an unlikely repetition, unless the physician was referring to a unique form of "trismus." "He has developed "*tiꜣ*" (the "trismus of tetanus"), his mouth being bound."

As the possibility of Tetanus infection is strongly considered in this case, it is necessary for the benefit of the nonmedical reader to review information about this disease.

Tetanus Infection[82]

Tetanus is an infectious disease caused by the anaerobic bacilli "clostridium tetani." These bacilli normally participate in the breakdown of organic matter and survive in inanimate matter, soil in particular. Its main reservoirs are heavily manured soil,[83] but it is also found in the intestinal tract and feces of animals and man, in conditions that are neutral or alkaline. Clostridium tetani is introduced into the injured tissue in its spore form. In the presence of dead tissue, impaired circulation, and the absence of oxygen, the spores develop into their vegetative form, producing a powerful toxin known as tetanospasmin or neurotoxin. This substance attacks the nervous system by blocking inhibitory impulses to the muscles, resulting in the generalized muscular contractions/spasms, which are the hallmark of tetanic infection.

Without treatment the disease is almost invariably lethal. Today, there are globally about one million cases of tetanus reported annually,[84] with a mortality rate between 40 and 78 percent.[85]

Tetanus infection is diagnosed by clinical means.[86] There usually is a history of a wound or of a traumatic occurrence in which contamination occurs, including obstetric-gynecologic, neo-natal, and dental events. The period of the development of the symptoms varies from twenty-four hours to one month. The usual incubation period is between seven and fourteen days. The symptoms of tetanus begin with nonspecific irritability and headaches. This is followed by muscular rigidity and spasms characteristic of tetanus, which begin in specific muscle groups:

- "Trismus," the contraction of masticatory muscles, is often the first symptom and produces difficulties with opening the mouth and chewing.
- "*risus sardonicus*" is produced by rigidity and spasms of the facial muscles, and produces distortion of the face, giving the false impression of a forced grin.
- Muscular rigidity in the neck muscles affects initially the back of the neck, similar to what is seen in meningitis.

82. M. V. Solbrig, "Tetanus," *Neurology in Clinical Practice* 2 (2000): 1340–42. See also R. Veronesi and R. Focaccia, "The Clinical Picture," *Tetanus: Important New Concepts* (Amsterdam: Excerpta Medica; 1981), 190–95. J. Sanford, "Tetanus - Forgotten But Not Gone," *New England Journal of Medicine* 332 (1995): 812–13.

83. B. Bytchenko, "Microbiology of Tetanus," *Tetanus: Important New Concepts* (ed. R. Veronesi; Amsterdam: Excerpta medica, 1981), 28–29. See also K. Todar, "The Genus Clostridium," Todar's Online Textbook of Bacteriology, University of Wisconsin Department of Bacteriology. Online: http://www.textbookofbacteriology.net/Bacillus.html.

84. T. P. Bleck, "Clostridium Tetani (Tetanus)," *Principles and Practice of Infectious Diseases* (5th edition; ed. Gerald L. Mandell, John E. Bennett, and Raphael Dolin; Philadelphia: Churchill Livingstone, 2000), 2:2537.

85. K. Todar, "The Genus Clostridium."

86. R. J. T. Joy, "Tetanus," *The Cambridge World History of Human Disease* (ed. Kenneth F. Kiple; Cambridge: Cambridge University Press, 1993), 1043–46.

- Spasms spread to the entire back, producing a backward arching posture, a symptom known since Hippocratic times as "opisthotonos." There is also significant rigidity of the abdominal muscles.

The generalized, painful, and violent muscular spasms are triggered by the slightest stimulation of the patient; his condition is more tragic by the fact that his mind remains clear. In fact, it is not until spasms of the throat muscles produce breathing difficulties that hypoxia[87] and loss of consciousness develop. At first, the patient will awaken once the spasm subsides, but as these episodes increase in frequency and severity prolonged hypoxia leads to death.

Signs of infection and respiratory complications become evident with high fever and profuse sweating from the disease itself. Later, as the infection progresses, complicating pneumonia becomes another source of fever. Without specific treatment, tetanus usually progresses to death.[88]

A clinical variant called cephalic tetanus is a form of the disease that develops shortly after an injury from contamination of head wounds.[89] The period of tetanus incubation in facial injuries is short. A case of initial cephalic tetanus will likely be followed by the generalized disease.[90] In addition to the classic symptoms of tetanus (trismus, *risus sardonicus*, and swallowing and breathing difficulties), there is paralysis of the facial nerve on the same side as the wound. This is manifested in sagging of the facial muscles and inability to close the eye or to "purse" the lips.

Recognition of Tetanus in Antiquity

Tetanus is a disease as old as mankind,[91] and it is reasonable to posit that it existed in ancient Egypt.[92] No direct proof of tetanus has yet been obtained from skeletons or mummified tissues,[93] but data from Case #7 of the Edwin Smith Papyrus and from the Kahun Medical Papyri indicate that the symptoms of tetanus were recognized in ancient Egypt.

The diagnosis of tetanus is clinical[94] and it is a disease with few differential diagnoses.[95] Tetanus was recognized in the Hippocratic book of Epidemics VII[96] dating to the fourth century BC, describing a case that originated from a wound infection, and a case of a woman whose clinical picture is very similar to that described in the Kahun Gynecological Papyrus, Case #5 (1:15–20).[97]

---

87. Poor oxygenation, from poor breathing and secondary pulmonary infections.

88. Veronesi and Focaccia, "The Clinical Picture," 190–95.

89. Ibid., 190.

90. Sanford, "Tetanus - Forgotten But Not Gone," 812–13.

91. B. L. Gordon, *Medicine through Antiquity* (Philadelphia: Davis, 1949), 105.

92. Egypt's geography, the ancient Egyptians agricultural and husbandry practices, their exposure to war and occupational injuries, and their obstetric practices, all provided the ideal conditions for tetanus to thrive.

93. A. T. Sandison, "Evidence of Infective Disease," *Journal of Human Evolution* 1 (1972): 213–24.

94. Joy, "Tetanus," 1043.

95. Bleck, "Clostridium Tetani (Tetanus)," 2537.

96. Mirko D. Grmek, *Diseases in the Ancient Greek World* (Baltimore: Johns Hopkins University Press, 1989), 342. Grmek writes, "In the commander of the large ship, whose right forefinger, bone and all, had been crushed by the anchor, an inflammation appeared, a dry gangrene, and some fever. He was mildly purged on the fifth day. The bouts of fever subsided then as well as the pain. A part of the finger fell off. After the seventh day, an ikhor (a sero-purulent discharge from a wound) came out properly. Afterward, he said that with his tongue he wasn't succeeding in explaining everything. Prediction: the backward spasm is on its way. The jaws began clenching, then it went to the nape of his neck; on the third day, he was totally convulsed backward, with sweating; on the sixth day after prediction, he died."

97. Hermann Grapow, "Papyrus Kahun #5 (1:15–20)," in *Grundriss* 5:459. The last words in this case indicate that if the muscle contractions have spread from the buttocks to the collar bones in a woman affected with *tiꜣ = r-mn ḫpdw.s b[ṯt]w pw* = It is an incurable disease. For discussion see Westendorf, *Handbuch der altägyptischen Medizin*, 1:84–85.

Conclusion

Interpreting data from Case #7 first alternative course under current concepts of tetanus, we recognize that all of the necessary elements to arrive at its diagnosis are present in this case. Breasted's hypothesis regarding tetanus and Case #7 was not initially accepted. Although many authors suspected it,[98] Bardinet's work in 1990 first made firm the conclusion of tetanus in Case #7.[99] More recently, Alexander Brawanski disagreed, arguing that the symptoms in Case #7 could be those of meningitis, or a brain abscess, or seizures.[100] Taking each of these symptoms separately, they could correspond to these entities and their alternative origins can be explained by the head injury and by bacterial infections other than tetanus. In fact, it is common to have multiple bacteria present in wound contamination. However, it is the combination of the characteristic findings specific to tetanus with the word *tiꜣ* used in ancient Egyptian for trismus that makes it so unlikely that the infectious complication developing in Case #7's initial injury, as the first alternative course, could be anything but tetanus (Visual Index VI).

Ancient Medical Methodology and Knowledge

It is important to stress the didactic nature of this ancient text and to emphasize the master physician's instructions to his pupil toward reaching the specific diagnosis he is looking for in his examination "If however you find that man…." Then is the rich and detailed description of a syndrome. In this infectious complication of a compound head injury we are given a major insight into the development of objective and rational medicine. The Egyptian teacher is transitioning from the understanding of the ill effects of trauma, a visible cause, into the acceptance of the ill effects of an invisible complication, a systemic infection. He is attributing the invisible complication to a wound, and giving a name to that complication. The recognition by ancient Egyptians of a cluster of characteristic symptoms served them as somatic "indicators" of what we now label "Tetanus." It is also evident that they recognized that this complication could have originated elsewhere. The first alternative course indicates the presence of a complex of symptoms affecting various parts of the body, as arising from a forehead wound: "while that man has developed *tiꜣ* because of that wound" (Plate III, l. 9), "He has developed *tiꜣ* his mouth being bound while he suffers rigidity in the back of his neck" (Tetanus; Plate III, l. 13). Another instance of this infectious complication appears in the Kahun Medical Papyrus Case #5 (1:15–20)[101] describing what appears to be a case of post-partum tetanus: "it is *tiꜣw* caused by the uterus."

The Egyptian physicians also realized that the presence of *tiꜣ*/trismus as a "local symptom" in itself may have no serious consequences, as was described in the Kahun Medical Papyrus Case #33 (3:25–26).[102] However, the form of *tiꜣ*/tetanus that bound the mouth and produced rigidity in the back of the neck in a patient with a compound skull fracture that had penetrated the frontal air sinus, and in which the physician recognizes a complex of symptoms, was seen as that which could portend grave implications for the patient's health and his chances of survival.

---

98. C. B. Courville, "Injuries to the Skull and Brain in Ancient Egypt," *Bulletin of the Los Angeles Neurological Society* 14/2 (1949): 53–82. Gustave Lefèbvre, *Essai sur la médecine égyptienne de l'époque pharaonique* (Paris: Presses universitaires de France, 1956). Paul Ghalioungui, *Magic and Medical Science in Ancient Egypt* (Amsterdam: Israël, 1963), 62. A. P. Leca, "Maladies Infectieuses, épidémies," *La Médicine Égyptienne au Temps des Pharaons* (Paris: R. Dacosta, 1971), 207. P. H. Chapman, "Case Seven of the Smith Surgical Papyrus: The Meaning of *tpꜣw*," *Journal of the American Research Center in Egypt* 29 (1992): 35–42. John F. Nunn, *Ancient Egyptian Medicine*, 181–82. R. L. Miller, "Tetanus after Cranial Trauma in Ancient Egypt," *Journal of Neurology, Neurosurgery and Psychiatry* 63/6 (1997): 758. Bleck, "Clostridium Tetani (Tetanus)," 2537. Nabil I. Ebeid, *Egyptian Medicine in the Days of the Pharaohs* (Cairo: General Egyptian Book Organization, 1999), 211. He considers that Tetanus is present in Case #7 from the onset. This is a concept with which the authors do not agree.

99. Bardinet *Dents et Machoires*, 162–87.

100. Brawanski, "Die Fälle 1-8 des Papyrus Edwin Smith," 16–39.

101. Hermann Grapow, "Papyrus Kahun #5 (1:15–20)," *Grundriss* 5:459.

102. For Papyrus Kahun #33 (3:25–26), see ibid., 494. Also see the comments by Bardinet, *Dents et Machoires*, 183.

Whether the Egyptian physician's recognition of this complication they called "*tiꜣ*" advanced to the status of true conceptualization as a disease is uncertain. However, it is suggested by their formulation of data in, and around, the word *tiꜣ*.

Grmek characterized primitive thought in the ontological conceptualization of disease as not clearly distinguishing "between the cause of the phenomenon and the phenomenon itself."[103] Commenting upon observable pathological events, Grmek points out the confusion between symptoms and diseases: "a confusion that is easy to understand—and even justified—in a medical system that defines nosological entities by their primitive symptoms or through a syndrome varying in makeup." The diagnosis of Case #7, first alternative course, "He has developed *tiꜣ*, his mouth being bound, while he suffers rigidity in the back of his neck," follows Grmek's pattern. The English used the term "lockjaw" for tetanus, following the same trend.

Second Alternative Case Head Injury Subacute Stage (Plate III:13–15)

Type of Injury

Once the acute stage of a head injury is over, there is still the need to bring the patient back to health, to avoid complications and to rehabilitate him. Step-down care facilities and rehabilitation wards would be the next phase in the care of these patients today. The patient's condition has evolved from the acute head injury with penetration of the skull cavity now, passing onto a subacute stage. He has become stable but he is weak and requires support and nourishment.

Ancient Medical Methodology and Knowledge

It is clear that supportive measures to restore this patient to health required the ability to feed him using high calorie content fluids. The recommendation to insert this padded wedge into the patient's mouth was intended to hold open his jaws since he was unable to open his mouth on his own, thus facilitating both his breathing and the administration of fluids and nutrients, like the prescribed broth of carob beans (or earth almonds?). The patient is treated in the sitting position, which provides the advantages for his airway alluded to in Case #4.

103. Mirko D. Grmek, ed., *Western Medical Thought from Antiquity to the Middle Ages* (trans. Antony Shugaar. Cambridge, MA: Harvard University Press, 1998), 253.

CASE #8:
Closed Head Injuries with Comminuted Skull Fracture
(Plate IV:5–18)

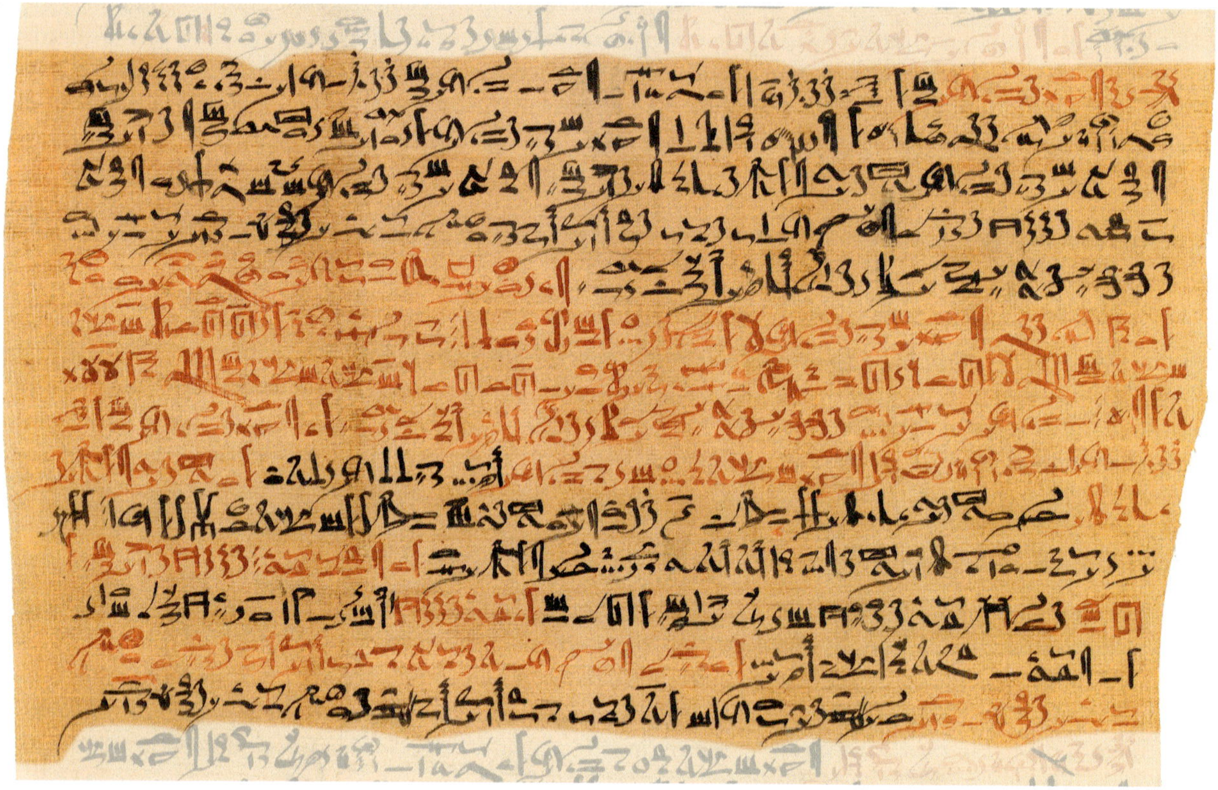

Courtesy New York Academy of Medicine.

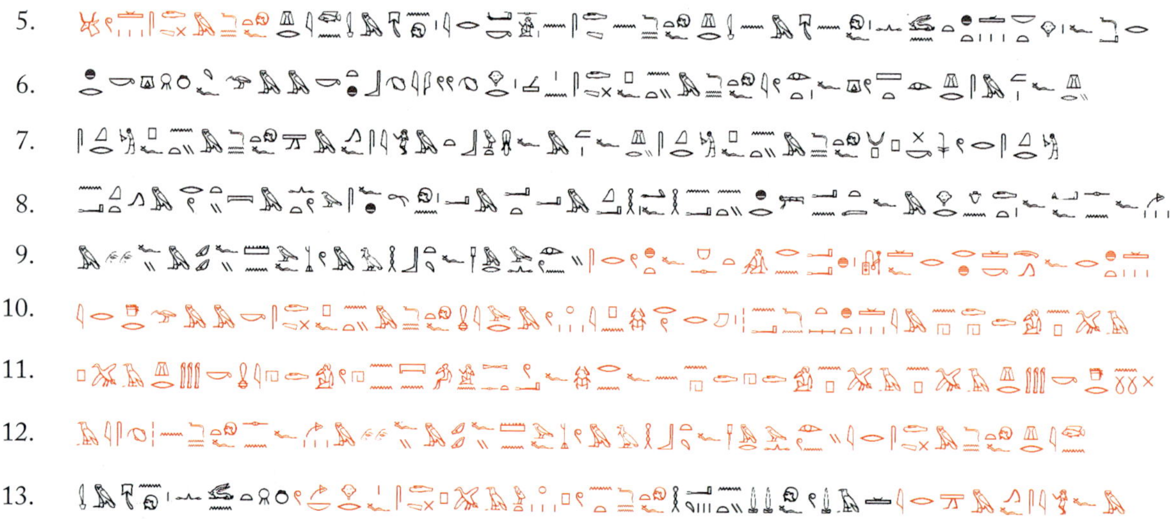

14. 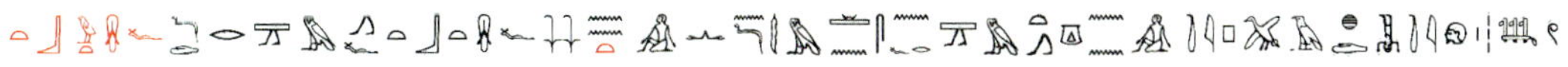

15. 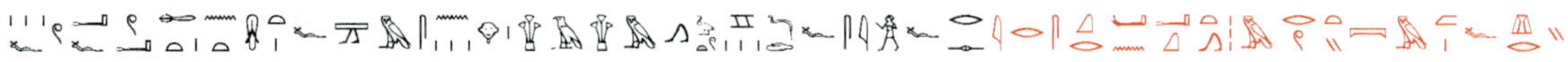

16. 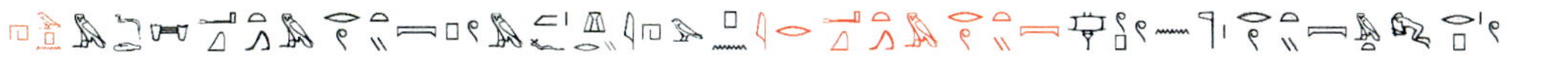

17. 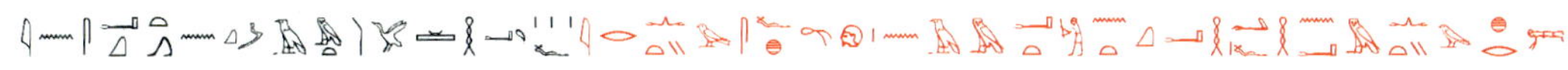

18. 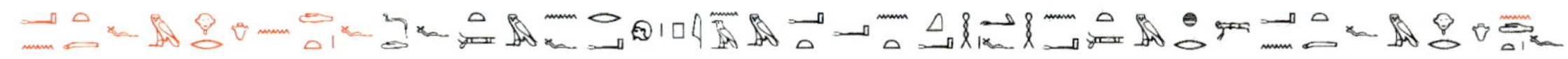

Transliteration

5§ *šs3w sd m dnnt.f hr inm n tp ir h3.k s n sd dnnt.f hr inm n tp.f n wnt ht nbt hr.f*

6§ *dʿr.hr.k wbnw.f gmm.k thb išww hr-s3 n sd pf nty m dnnt.f iw irt.f gwš.t(i) hr.s m gs.f hry*

7§ *skr pf nty m dnnt.f šm.f sy m tbt.f m gs.f hry skr pf nt m dnnt.f wpp.k sw r skr n*

8§ *ʿkt m rwty m iwt<y>w sfh tp n 3mʿt m kʿh.f hnʿ nty hr ʿnt.f m hry-ib n drt.f di.f snf m*

9§ *msdty.fy msdr.wy.fy mn.f tsw m nhbt.f mhr n irw.ny srwh.f hmst r nʿʿ.f r rh.k spr.f r ht*

10§ *ir dr gmm.k sd pf nty m dnnt.f, mi wrmw ipn hpr.w r hmt n ʿndt t im nhdhd np3p3*

11§ *hr dbʿw.k mi hd whnn n hrd n tst.f hpr.n.f n nhdhd np3p3 hr dbʿw.k dr ngg*

12§ *3is n dnnt.f di.f snf m msdty.fy m msdrwy.fy mn.f tsw m nhbt.f mhr n irw. ny ir sd m dnnt.f hr inm*

13§ *n tp.f n wnt wbnw nb hr.f sd p3kwt pw nt dnnt.f hʿw nty d3d3.f wd3 ir šm.f si.f m*

14§ *tbt.f dd.f r šm.f tbt.f nnt n ndm.n.s n.f r šmt gnn.t p3hd.ti tp.w s3hw.f*

15§ *wʿf n ht nt tbt.f šm.sn hr h3h3 s3tw dd.f si.f r.s ir skr n ʿk.tw m rwty m gs.f hry*

16§ *ih pn mdd ʿkt m rwty pw m gs.f hr ih pn ir ʿkt m rwty t3w pw n ntr n rwty mt.(t) r3-pw*

17§ *in s-ʿkt n km3t hʿw.f ir iwty sfh tp n 3mʿt nt kʿh.f hnʿ m iwty hr.n*

18§ *ʿnt.f m hry-ib n drt.f dd.f tm nft r tp p(w) in 3mʿt nt kʿh.f hnʿ tm hr ʿnt.f m hry-ib n drt.f*

Translation

Case #8a

Title:

Necessary knowledge and skills for a crushed fracture in his braincase, under the skin of the head:

Examination:

If you should examine a man for a smashed in/burst fracture of his skull under the skin of his head, there not being anything on it, you must palpate his wound.

How you find the swelling (is) distended on the outside of that crushed fracture which is in his braincase.

His eye is askew under it, on his side which is under that blow which is in his braincase, while he walks shuffling with his foot on his side which is under that blow which is in his braincase.

Diagnosis:

How you should distinguish him from one whom something which enters from outside has stricken (is): being one who cannot loosen the end of the forked bone in his shoulder joint, and one whose thumbnail/fingernail bends down into the middle of his hand, while he bleeds from his nostrils/nasal cavities and from his ears, and he suffers rigidity in the back of his neck—

a medical condition that cannot be handled/dealt with.

Treatment:

His treatment is sitting (upright) until he regains color and until you know he has reached a turning point.

Case #8b

Examination:

Now since how you find that crushed fracture which is in his skull (is) like those convolutions that happen in copper of a crucible(?), and something within, yielding and fluttering under your fingers like the weak spot of the crown of a child (fontanelle) before it has joined,

how it has come to pass/how he has become (is) because of the yielding and fluttering under your fingers, since the brain in his braincase breaks open,

while he bleeds from his nostrils/nasal cavities and his ears,

and he suffers rigidity in the back of his neck—

Diagnosis:

"a medical condition that cannot be handled/dealt with."

Explanation A:

As for "a crushed fracture in his skull under the skin of his head and there is not any wound on it," it means while the bony plates of his skull burst fractured, the skin that is <on> his braincase is intact.

Explanation B:

As for "when he walks, he shuffles with his foot," say concerning him when he walks with his foot dragging, "It cannot be comfortable for him to walk, it (i.e., the foot) being weak, and hanging down, the tips of his toes contracting/curled up towards his instep, so that they go stumbling along the ground." He says/it means, "he limps because of it."

Explanation C:

As for "one whom something that enters from outside has smitten," in his side which has this injury: it means, "one whom that which enters from outside presses/strikes in his side which has this injury."

Explanation D:

As for "that which enters from outside," it means the breath of a god from outside, or a dead man, that is to say, that which what his flesh produces has caused to enter.

Explanation E:

As for "one who cannot loosen the end of the forked bone of his shoulder joint, and being one whose fingernails cannot bend down into the middle of his hand," he says/it means, "one for whom the head of the bone by the fork of his shoulder fails to loosen, and one whose fingernail(s) cannot bend down into the middle of his hand."

Notes

The notes to Case #8 are somewhat detailed because some of the syntax is quite intricate and I want to explain the justification for the translation clearly for the reader.

išww – Here taken as a stative.

iw irt.f gwš.t(i) – All translators render "since"or "while." However, in Middle Egyptian *iw* + noun + adverbial (including stative) is normally independent whereas it is bare noun + adverbial that is circumstantial (cf. Hoch, *MEG*, sec. 16). In Late Egyptian or texts showing marked Late Egyptian characteristics, *iw* becomes the circumstantial converter and the translators' understanding of this sentence would not raise an eyebrow. (No pun intended.) This text seems to operate consistently according to Classical or Middle or Earlier Egyptian norms and it seems difficult to justify the circumstantial translation of this clause. I have to infer that although it seems to break the flow of the clauses, this is deliberate on the part of the author, because the behavior of the eye is important enough for a demarcated independent statement, where we might say, "NB: His eye is askew," or something like that.

gs.f cannot refer to "its side," namely, "of his eye," because the word for eye (*irt*) is feminine, and is moreover followed by an agreeing feminine stative form *gwš.t(i)*. Analogously, *gs.f* cannot mean "its side,"referring to his foot (*tbwt.f*), because *tbwt* is also feminine. Moreover, *ẖry* is a nisbe adjective, not a stative or an adverbial form. Therefore in both cases as far as I can make out it has to be "his side which is under that blow which is in his braincase," and in this case Breasted and Allen are right.

šm.f – Circumstantial *sḏm.f*.

wpp.k sw … – This is a difficult and ambiguous passage that presents dilemmas both lexically and syntactically. The meaning "distinguish A from B" for the collocation *wpi … r …*" is well-enough supported that I do not think it can be ignored in this passage (*Wb*. 1:298; *Grundriss* 7, 1:182–83), although it results in what can be seen as a roundabout and rather awkward description, interposing what the patient is not and then transitioning back to what he is. I further take *sḳr.n …* as a relative form and *ꜥḳt* as an active participle. As for the syntax of the sentence itself, there is an initial temptation to place the nexus after *wpp.k sw* "How you distinguish him (is)," but then the latter part of the sentence becomes unwieldy and an assortment of apples and oranges. Following the understanding of "emphatic" sentences developed by Junge, emphasis and sentential meaning (though I am still uncertain about some of his conclusions), the *r* segment would not be on the other side of the nexus but the following series of adverbials/circumstantials would. It is perhaps worth noting that if we are understanding it correctly, *wpi … r …* "to distinguish … from …" seems to express a concept of what we refer to as "differential diagnosis." (The Greek word "diagnosis," if I understand it correctly, conveys the meaning of knowing between or among different alternatives.)

The segment "and one whose thumbnail" is incorporated in the series of adverbials by being introduced with the preposition *ḥnꜥ*.

n ṯst.f – This is the "before" or "not-yet" form *n sḏmt.f*, and we translate accordingly. This differs from the somewhat parallel passage in Case #6.

ngg – Nominal *sḏm.f* after preposition *ḏr*.

gnn.ti pꜣẖd.ti – Statives, which must depend on *tbwt.f* "his foot," because *ṯbwt* is feminine.

mḏd ꜥḳt m rwty... – Taking *mḏd* or *mḏd(w)* as a relative form.

in – The same use of the particle in that we have encountered earlier.

sꜥḳt.n ḳmꜣt ḥꜥw.f – *ꜣ sḏm(w).n.f* relative form with the subject or actor expression *ḳmꜣt ḥꜥw.f*, which is another relative form, the whole being analyzed as "That which WHAT HIS FLESH PRODUCES (the second relative form) has caused to enter." By the upper case I do not imply emphasis, I only try to show clearly what the subject of the relative form (the second relative form) is.

iwty ḫr.n ꜥnt.f – "one whose fingernail cannot fall," a relativization with *iwty* of the typical negation of ability *n sḏm.n.f.* There is clearly an *n*, which Breasted transcribes above the hand sign in *ḏrt* at the end of the line below, but it obviously belongs with the verb form above. Gardiner (*EG*[3], sec. 203.6) states that *iwty + sḏm.n.f* is "not very common" and gives an example that may be an unusual case of the inclusion of a past *sḏm.n.f* as translated by Gardiner, but which can also be interpreted as the negation of ability, *iwt(y) sḏr.n rmṯ špt r.f* "one on account of whom no one CAN SPEND the night disappointed."

tm n.f rdi(w) – A relative form negated with *tm*; the *n.f* is not part of the verbal complex, but a pronominal dative "for him," yielding the finished translation "for whom." *rdi(w)* is the negatival complement.

tm ḫr(w) – Another relative form negated with *tm. ḫr(w)* is the negatival complement.

Medical Commentary to Case #8a

Type of Injury (Visual Index IV and VII)

Case #8a is a closed head injury with skull fracture (*sḏ*) (figs. 8a and b) that is presented with specific clinical neurological findings, including cranial nerve deficit—"His eye is askew"—and hemiparesis. Both of these sets of clinical findings are localized to the same side of the body as the head injury.

The oculomotor cranial nerve complex includes cranial nerves III, IV, and VI. In head trauma the most frequently injured is the "abducens nerve," cranial nerve VI. The function of this nerve is outward motion of the eye; its paralysis results in medial deviation of the eye, towards the nose.

Neurological symptoms and findings consistent with hemiparesis are given (fig. 8c). First is leg weakness affecting the patient's gait "shuffling his foot." We are in agreement with Walker's[104] interpretation, Explanation B providing an exquisite description of spastic paretic gait: "'when he walks, he shuffles with his foot,' say concerning him when he walks with his foot dragging, 'It cannot be comfortable for him to walk, it (i.e., the foot) being weak, and hanging down, the tips of his toes contracting/curled up towards his instep, so that they go stumbling along the ground.'" He says/it means, 'he limps because of it.'" Second is the description of upper extremity spastic paresis: "being one who cannot loosen the end of the forked bone in his shoulder joint, and one whose thumbnail/fingernail bends down into the middle of his hand." It is our impression that the upper extremity symptoms are consistent with spastic hemiparesis (Explanation E) and that attributing these to the patient in Case #8a would make clinical sense.

The shoulder joint is immobile, by spasticity keeping the extremity close to the body, the hand and fingers in paralytic contraction, so that the patient is unable to make a fist (fig. 8c).

Contralateral hemiparesis is by far more common in head injuries, than paralysis of the limbs on the same side as the injury. Brawanski points out that the Edwin Smith papyrus, being a teaching text, should be presenting common "case types" and considers "confusing sides" to be a scribal mistake.[105] However, since in Case #8a the affected leg and arm are clearly identified as being on the same side of the body as the head injury, we need

104. Walker, *Studies in Ancient Egyptian Anatomical Terminology*, 83–87.

105. Brawanski. "Die Fälle 1–8 des Papyrus Edwin Smith," 30–33.

to stay with the text as is and consider the less common ipsilateral leg paresis in Case #8a. The motor pathways originate in the brain and stay on the same side of the skull until crossing at the level of the lower brain stem to the opposite side, descending in the spinal cord (Visual Index VII).

Ipsilateral hemiparesis can result from:

- Major damage occurring to the brain on the opposite side of the head injury, from violent shifting, impacting against the opposite side of the cranium, also called "contre-coup" injury. This possibility for Case #8a originated with Breasted (*Edwin Smith*, 205) and has been challenged by Alexander Brawanski[106] raising additional questions: Are the upper extremity findings consistent with a spastic paresis from brain injury? Are they related to brachial plexus injury? Do they belong to the patient in Case 8a?[107]
- Injury to the opposite side of the descending brain stem as it is compressed against the tentorial notch. This occurs from shifting of the intracranial contents from the side of the injury towards the intracranial midline, from brain edema and hemorrhaging (Visual Index VII).

Completing the clinical picture in Case #8a, the patient is also showing signs of base of skull fractures of the anterior and middle fossae and of traumatic meningismus: "while he bleeds from his nostrils and from his ears, and he suffers rigidity in the back of his neck."[108]

Today the management of closed head injuries requires immediate neurological and systemic assessment and support. As expressed in the medical commentary to Case #4, the treatment of severe head injuries today requires prehospital stabilization of the patient's condition including recognition and treatment of rising intracranial pressure. Imaging studies and the clinical course will dictate the need for intracranial pressure monitoring, craniotomy, or conservative treatment in Neurological Intensive Care. First order of issue is to control elevated intracranial pressure and cerebral perfusion pressure with clinical and imaging follow-up as required. The closed head injury described in Case 8a corresponds to a moderate to severe head injury. The annual mortality per 100,000 patients with closed head injuries are 7 percent for moderate and 36 percent for severe. Residual neurological deficits are severe with permanent disability ranging from 10 to 100 percent.[109]

Ancient Medical Methodology and Knowledge

A clear description of a large swelling under intact scalp is given along with those findings of fractured bone plates felt through the skin. The observed neurological findings in the eye and the lower extremity are directly associated to the head injury. Making these connections undoubtedly led them to objective and rational understanding of body functions.

In this section is the important interjection of the diagnostic statement: "How you should distinguish him from one whom something which enters from outside has stricken (is)," (see Explanations C and D) intended to call attention to clinical differentiation to be made in Case #8a. Introducing early clinical pathogenetic concepts, the physician states regarding this patient with a closed head injury, in whom there are major symptoms of weakness despite the absence of an open wound: "one whom something that enters from outside has smitten …

106. Ibid.

107. Author's (Meltzer) note: Purely on the basis of syntax it seems to me that all of the bulleted points after the colon are most likely presented as the symptoms of the patient in Case #8a, and the symptoms of the patient whom something from outside has stricken (as in a patient who had a spontaneous stroke) are not specified.

108. The reader is directed to appendix 2 for a compilation of the neurological symptoms and signs in the Edwin Smith Papyrus.

109. Leonardo Rangel-Castilla and Jaime Gasco, "Closed Head Trauma." Medscape Reference: http://emedicine.medscape.com/article/251834-overview.

presses/strikes in his side which has this injury." Furthermore, the physician indicates that this patient may not be clinically much different from another individual who has suffered a spontaneous intracranial event: "that which what his flesh produces. . . ." Today, an example of such would be a stroke,[110] but for the ancient Egyptians it would be explained as caused by some evil that has entered the head (". . . presses/strikes in his side which has this injury." This extraordinary concept in Case #8 indicates the ancient physician's understanding of causation of intracranial injury without an open wound, beyond the damaging effect produced by demonic forces.

The final mechanism of the neurological injury in closed head trauma was difficult for the Egyptian physician to comprehend; however, he/she was unequivocal in stating that it was the strike on the outside of the head that produced the symptoms/signs, and, thus, differentiated from a patient who may have similar symptoms from a spontaneous event occurring inside the head, such as a stroke (by breath of a God or a dead man, or demonic causation), attaching a rational cause to Case #8a.

The verdict in Case #8a: "a medical condition that cannot be handled/dealt with," points to the reality of a fixed neurological deficit, for which nothing can objectively be done. This verdict does not necessarily reflect a lethal situation as suggested by Breasted (Breasted, *Edwin Smith*, 1:206). In spite of this verdict, the patient was cared for by those measures for head injuries applied in treating other cases of severe head injuries in the Edwin Smith papyrus with a sitting position and supportive measures, continued until the crisis passed.

Examples of severe closed head injuries with major fractures are evident in Soldier #14 from Winlock, *The Slain Soldiers of Neb-hep-et-Re Mentu-hotpe*, plate VIII A–C (see fig. 8d).

Medical Commentary to Case #8b

Type of Injury

In accordance with the Edwin Smith Papyrus methodology of arranging trauma according to their increasing severity,[111] we believe Case #8b represents a closed head injury in which greater damage has occurred from that described in Case #8a. The skull has been sufficiently fractured (*sd*) and comminuted to allow palpation of tissues and brain pulsations through the unbroken scalp. The text here is almost the same as in Case #6, which deals with an open head injury with the brain exposed. This entry has created a great deal of discussion, including whether it may have been a scribal error, or whether this text is out of place, or both.[112]

---

110. Attributed to Dr. Joachim Stephan by Westendorf, *Handbuch der altägyptischen Medizin*, 718–19.

111. The injuries in Papyrus Smith are generally arranged according to increasing severity. This order is maintained in the several closed-head injuries, Cases ##11–12, 16–17, 21–22.

112. "The observation of the pulsations in the brain, beneath a fracture which has been accompanied by no visible injury or rupture of the soft tissues over the fracture, would of course be impossible unless the surgeon operated and laid back a flap of skin covering the fracture"; Breasted, *Edwin Smith*, 208.

Westendorf assumes there is a breach under the intact scalp in Case #8: "Dieser Abschnitt vom aufgebrochenen Gehirn mit fast wörtlicher Parallele zu Fall 6 kann nicht hierher gehören, da von einem Bruch unter der unverletzten Kopfhaut die Rede ist. Wahrscheinlich fehlen wesentliche Teile (Splitterbruch mit ähnlichen Symptomen und aufgebrochenem Gehirn)" ("This section about the broken-open brain with nearly verbatim parallel to Case 6 cannot belong here, since it is a question of a fracture under the intact (unwounded) scalp. Apparently essential parts are missing (splinter fracture and similar symptoms and broken-open brain"; Westendorf, *Handbuch der altägyptischen Medizin*, 719 (translation by Meltzer).

Brawanski comments, "Hier fehlt wahrscheinlich ein ganzes Stück des Textes, wenn man von dem Aufbau der anderen Fälle ausgeht. Westendorf hat diesen ergänzt. Da dieser Teil aber nichts Neues gibt, sondem nur eine Wiederholung der eingangs in dem Fall genannten klinischen Befunde, habe ich diesen hier nicht ergänzt" and "Mit Westendorf nehme ich an, daß die Passage bezüglich der Schrumpeln aus Metall und dem Flattern im Wundbereich ein Versehen des Schreibers ist und mit dem hier geschilderten Krankheitsbild nichts zu tun hat" ("Die Fälle 1–8 des Papyrus Edwin Smith," 32). ("Here apparently an entire piece of the text is missing, if one proceeds from the construction of the other cases. Westendorf has completed this. Since, however, this part does not give anything new, but only a repetition

It is certain that skull fractures can occur in the absence of a wound. This issue has specifically been addressed in regard to Case #8 by Courville, Ralston, and Chapman.[113] It is also possible to feel pulsations transmitted to the examiner's palpating fingers through the intact scalp. While accepting this fact, Courville still questions how the ancient physician could see the brain "corrugations" in a closed wound. In response, we must refer to the fact that the text of Edwin Smith Papyrus in Case #8b speaks only of palpating, not of seeing: "and something within, yielding and fluttering under your fingers." This clearly is a tactile sensation not a visual one. The same can apply in a massive closed head injury with bone fragmentation such as in Case #8b, in describing feeling: "like those convolutions that happen in copper of a crucible(?)." Palpation through the scalp of broken bone, brain tissue, blood clots, and swollen scalp would feel mushy and possibly pulsatile, making it uncertain for the examining physician to know exactly what he was feeling. For all practical purposes, these tactile sensations to the finger would not have felt much different to him from those he experienced palpating an open cranial wound, as the one described in Case #6.

Current experience with head trauma in emergency rooms indicates an occurrence of major skull bone disruption in closed head injuries up to 25 percent. During the examination of post-craniotomy surgery cases, particularly post severe trauma, it is possible to feel transmitted brain pulsations through the intact scalp at the site of a large bone defect. The same can be found on occasion in closed head injuries with major skull bone disruption.

The clinical picture in Case #8b includes the common findings seen on the examination of a patient with a severe skull fracture: meningismus, and bleeding through the nose and the ears. In contrast with Case #6, which contains almost the same text referring to the pulsations and appearance of the brain, Case #8b includes evidence of basal skull fracture from both the anterior and the middle fossa whereas, Case #6 has only bleeding through the nose indicative of a fracture to the anterior base of the skull (fig. 4). The skull fractures in Case #8b consist of extensive comminution of the braincase with significant damage to the brain. There are no other neurological signs or details given as to this patient's condition. The patient's outlook is poor.

Ancient Medical Methodology and Knowledge

It is important to note that the entire text in Case #8b is rubricated.[114] This signals the specific importance given to it by the Egyptian physicians as a separate clinical entity. Being a closed head injury, the instructions from the master physician need to be taken also under the premise of palpation: "how to find that smashed in/

of the clinical findings (diagnoses) named at the outset of the case, I have not completed this here. With Westendorf, I assume that the passage relating to the wrinkles out of metal and the fluttering in the region of the wound is a blunder of the scribe and has nothing to do with the image of the illness (clinical picture) portrayed here.")

113. C. B. Courville commenting on Case #8 of the Edwin Smith Papyrus, says, "It is also obvious in the second part of the case report that the pulsations of the brain were transmitted to the examiner's palpating fingers. But how he could see the 'corrugations' of the brain in a closed wound is problematical" ("Injuries to the Skull and Brain in Ancient Egypt," *Bulletin of the Los Angeles Neurological Society* 14/2 [1949]: 66). As Breasted (*Edwin Smith*, 208) points out, there may have been a subsequent surgical incision, but if so, no mention is made of it.

B. L. Ralston: "Smith Case #8 is rendered: Compound Comminuted Fracture of the Skull Displaying no Visible External Injury. As a compound fracture is one which communicates with the exterior through a laceration of overlying soft tissues and skin, the title is self-contradicting … As described in Smith Case #8, comminuted depressed fractures may occur in the absence of a wound …" ("Medical Reinterpretation of Case Four of the Edwin Smith Surgical Papyrus," *Journal of Egyptian Archaeology* 63 [1977]: 116).

P. H. Chapman: "Case #8 describes an extensive fracture beneath the intact scalp. Such injury might not be recognized unless it were in the forehead, where there is no hair and the frontal bone is remarkable for its pronounced, symmetrical convexity" ("Case Seven of the Smith Surgical Papyrus: The Meaning of *tp3w*," *Journal of the American Research Center in Egypt* 29 [1992]: 39).

114. "Rubricated" meaning that particularly important sections of the text are written in red ink. See table 1 (p. 13) and discussion on pp. 14–15.

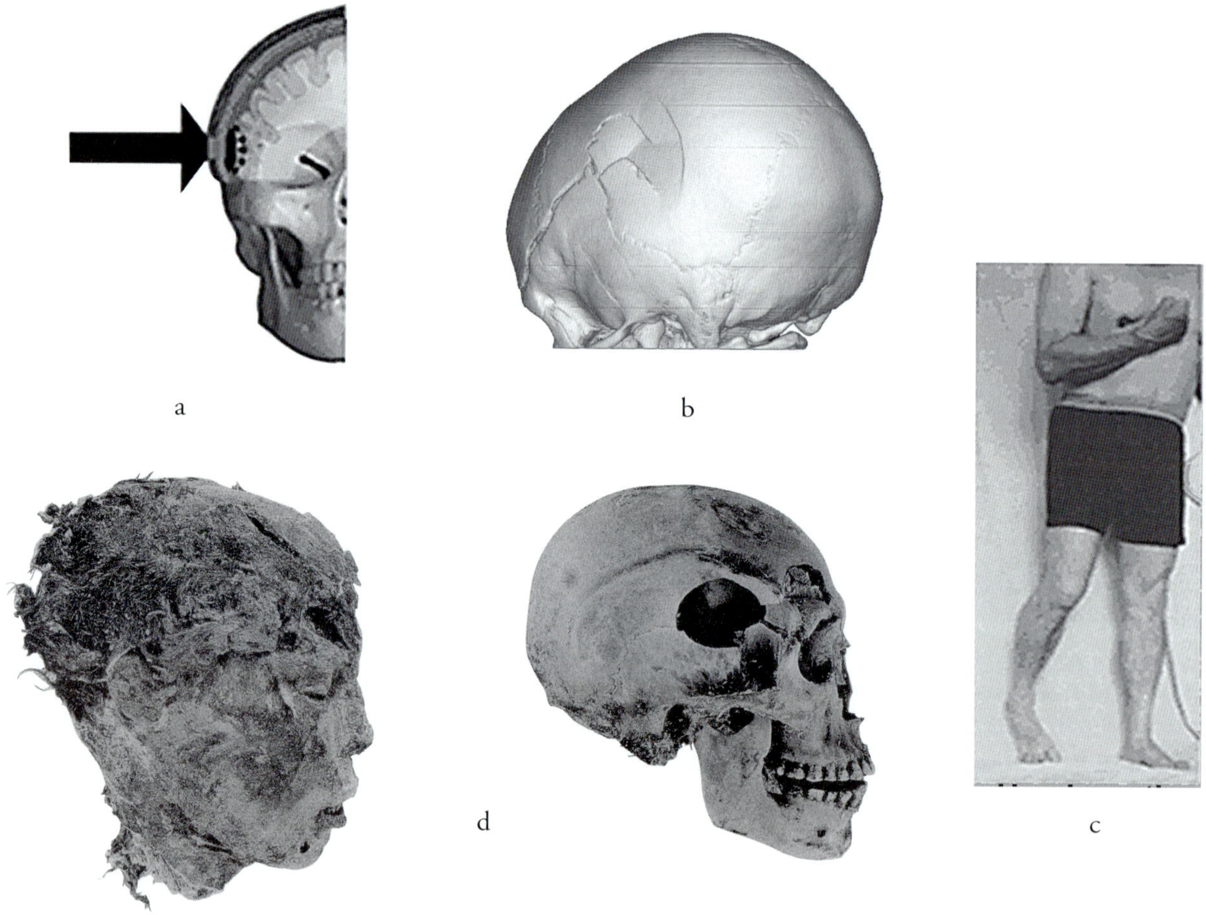

Fig. 8. a) Closed head injury force transmitted to the brain; b) Closed depressed skull fracture, 3-D CT scan; c) Hemiparetic posture and gait; d) Soldier #14, from Winlock, *Slain Soldiers of Neb-hep-et-Re Mentu-hotpe*, plate VIII A and C.

burst fracture which is in his skull (is) like those convolutions that happen in copper through smelting, and something within, yielding and fluttering under your fingers." The physical findings of major bone and intracranial contents disruption are described by the examining physician ("like the weak spot of the crown of a child (fontanelle) before it has joined," "since the brain in his cranium breaks open") and repeats the findings of Case #6 (the most severe of the open head injuries), namely, the skull is severely fragmented and the dura lacerated, allowing intracranial pulsations and the brain surface to be palpated. But Case #8b being a severe closed, comminuted skull fracture, the tissue disruption is palpated through unbroken scalp.

As expected, the verdict in Case #8b is "a medical condition that cannot be handled/dealt with." No treatment was offered.

CASE #9: Wound in the Forehead, Fracturing the Outer Table of the Frontal Bone

(Plate IV:19–V:5)

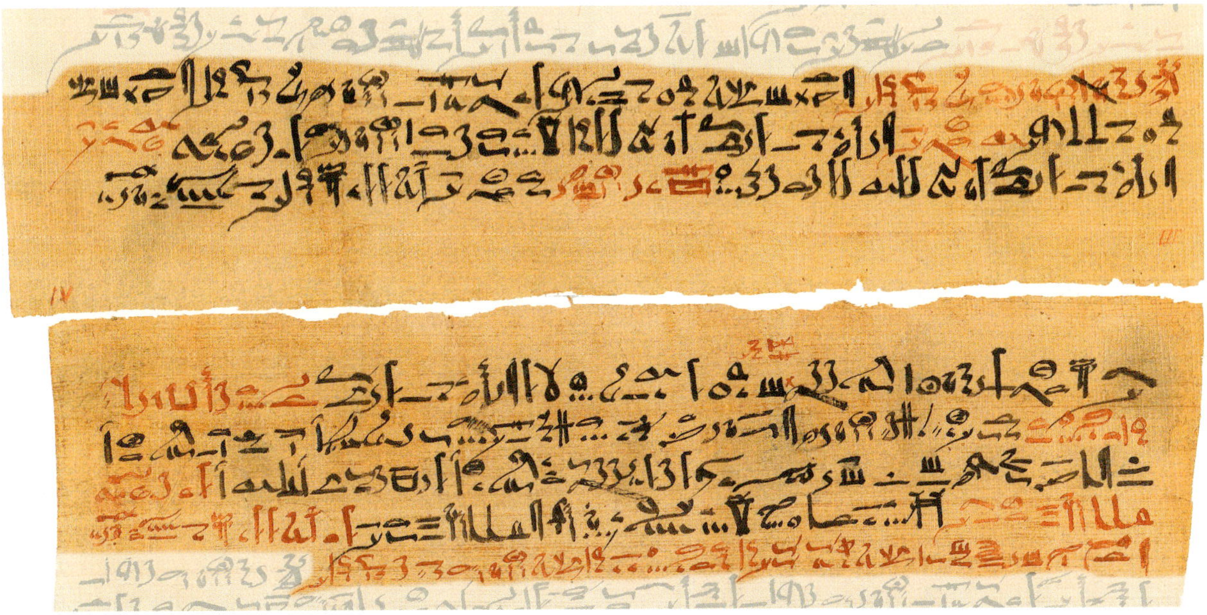

Courtesy New York Academy of Medicine.

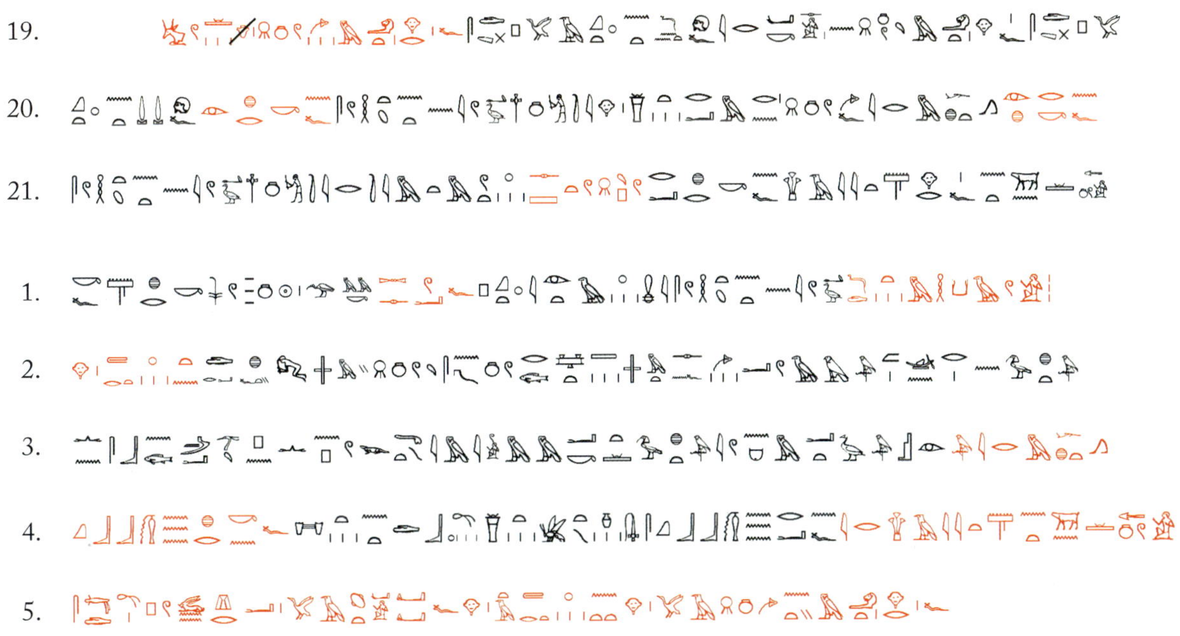

Transliteration

19§ *šsꜣw wbnw m ḥꜣt-ḥr.f sḏ pꜣḳt nt ḏnnt.f ir ḫꜣ.k s n wbnw m ḥꜣt-ḥr.f sḏ*

20§ *pꜣḳt nt ḏꜣḏꜣ.f ir.ḫr.k n.f swḥt nt niw nḏ.ti ḥr mrḥt rdi m rꜣ n wbnw.f ir m-ḫt ir.ḫr.k n.f*

21§ *swḥt nt niw nḏ.ti ir.ti m tmtw sš(w).t(w)(?) wbnw pw rdi.ḫr.k n.f ḥꜣyt ḥbs ḥr.f nt ẖn-swnw*

1§ *kfꜣ.ḫr.k sw ẖmt-nw hrw gmm.k ṯs.f pꜣḳt irtyw mi swḥt nt niw dd.t m ḥkꜣw*

2§ *ḥr pẖrt tn dr ḫfty imy wbnw snwr wꜣt imyt snfꜥwꜣ.ti ḥr gs-dpt n r n ꜣḫt*

3§ *nn sbn mꜣꜥ pn n npw mt<w> im iw.i m mkt ꜣḫt iw nḥm.t(w) sꜣ Wsir ir m-ḫt*

4§ *ḳbb.ḫr.k n.f mḏt nt d<ꜣ>bw mrḥt bit ps sḳbb rd n.f ir ḥꜣyt ḥbs nt ẖn-swnw*

5§ *sšd pw wnn ḫr ꜥ pꜣ wt dd.f ḥr tꜣ pẖrt ntt ḥr pꜣ wbnw nty m ḥꜣt-ḥr.f*

Translation

Title:

Necessary knowledge and skills for a wound in his forehead, smashing in/burst fracturing the bony plate of his braincase:

Examination:

If you examine a man for a wound in his forehead, smashing in/burst fracturing the bony plate of his braincase,

Treatment:

you must prepare for it/him: the egg(shell) of an ostrich, ground with ointment and placed in the mouth of his wound.

Now after, you must apply to it/him the ground egg(shell) of an ostrich ground so that it is made into powder.

That is how the wound is dried/that is what dries the wound.

You must apply to it/him the cloth bandage of a physician's medical kit over it.

You must uncover it the third day.

How you find (is): How it joins/knits together the bony plate of the braincase (is) with the condition similar to the egg(shell) of the ostrich.

What is said as Ritual Power over this prescription:

"Driving out the enemy within the wound (and) causing the hostile force that is within the blood, a robber of Horus, to tremble.

The protection of the utterance of The Beneficial/Effective Goddess (Isis):

This temple will not collapse.

The blood vessel(s) therein have not sickened(?), for I am in the Beneficial /Effective Goddess's protection.

The son of Osiris is saved!"

Afterward, you have to cool for him a compress of figs and ointment and honey, cooked, cooled, and applied to him.

Explanation:

As for "the bandage of cloth belonging to a physician's medical kit," it is "a head binding which is under the charge of this bandager, which he ought to place over this medication that is on that wound that is in his forehead."

Notes

sd – Active participle

rdi(*w*) – For the stative form without the feminine ending, see Gardiner, *EG*[3], sec. 309, though the noun is not plural here.

nḏ.ti ir.ti m tmtw – Both statives, the second being taken as a stative of result.

sš(*w*)*t*(*?*) or *sš*(*w*)*.t*(*w*)(*?*) *wbnw pw* – understanding either "that which dries" (active participle) or "How … is dried" (passive *sḏm.tw.f* as manner nominalization in a nominal sentence with *pw*). There are two roots referring to dryness, *sšr* (< *swšr*) (Faulkner, *CDME*, 262; *Grundriss* 7, 2:733, 734, 802) and *šw* (Faulkner, *CDME*, 263; *Grundriss* 7, 2:841). For the morphophonological process by which the *w* of *wšr* is so frequently omitted in the causative, see, for example, *ssẖ* < *wsẖ* and *mrḥt* < *wrḥ*. (I am indebted to the late Prof. Klaus Baer for introducing this phenomenon in his classes many years ago.) Words from both of these roots are used in medical contexts. Although the writing in the present passage does not have the feather of *šw*, and although *sšr* is spelled out in Case 46, I am inclined (with query) to read the present example as *sš*(*w*) because it seems to be the simpler error and entails the least elaborate presumption of what was omitted.

gmm.k ṯs.f – Both manner nominalizations. *ṯs* is a biliteral not 3ae inf. verb and does not geminate.

ḥkꜣw, ḥkꜣ – For a discussion of "magic" as a "loaded" and culturally pejorative term and the choice of "ritual power" as a more objective and value-free designation, see Meltzer, "Introduction to Old Coptic Texts of Ritual Power," *Ancient Christian Magic: Coptic Texts of Ritual Power* (ed. M. W. Meyer and R. Smith; San Francisco: HarperSanFrancisco, 1994), 13–20. It is ironic that the publisher insisted on the use of the word "magic" in the title because of its mystique. This approach to the terminology of "magic" is not agreed upon by all authorities (so that for instance Robert K. Ritner, Terence DuQuesne, Geraldine Pinch and other major authors continue to use the word "magic"), but in all of my scholarly work I have maintained it consistently for close to twenty years. Breasted's own extremely pejorative dismissal of "magic" is made very clear in his characterization of this case as "a grotesque product of superstition and belief in magic, accompanied indeed by a magical charm" (*Edwin Smith* 217); one can almost hear a scandalized exclamation, "Oh horrors!" and "a curious hodge-podge of superstitions" (220). This is understandable (though it cannot be condoned) from a scholar who, although forward-looking and even visionary in significant ways, was deeply attached to "Judeo-Christian" monotheism (thus lionizing Akhenaten) and saw Egyptian religious ideas and practice in the later periods as degenerating into "magic" (*The Development of Religion and Thought in Ancient Egypt*, New York: Scribner, 1912, repr. New York: Harper & Row, 1959; *The Dawn of Conscience*, New York: Scribner, 1933), going so far as to say that "the general reliance on such devices … must have seriously poisoned the life of the people" (*Development of Religion and Thought*, 309). In the process of his judgmental discussion of the "magical" element of this case, Breasted leaves entirely unexplored the therapeutic rationale and benefits of the treatment mandated in this case, which Dr. Sanchez discusses at length below in the medical commentary.

wꜣt – Since "malignancy" has a specific medical meaning in English and the text is not talking about anything that can be identified as cancerous, I think it should be avoided. *Grundriss* 7, 1:161 defines it as

"Something evil(?) Something bad(?)," referring to *Wb.* 1:244, 249. I would also add *Wb.* 1:246 *wꜣ* "curse." My suggested translation, also somewhat makeshift, would be "hostile force."

ꜥwꜣ(y) "robber" – For this word as one of many designations of hostile beings who can attack an individual and have to be counteracted or guarded against, see J. R. Ogdon, *Sharing New Ideas on the Phenomenon of Possession in Ancient Egypt* (Estudios del C.E.A.E. 1/A. Buenos Aires: Centro de Estudios del Antiguo Egipto, 1997), 28.

Taking *n* as genitival adjective "of," not suffix-pronoun "our" (for which three strokes would have to be emended).

ꜣḫt – This word describes Isis as first and foremost "effective" in her ritual power and healing ministrations. She healed Horus's scorpion stings. For the meaning of *ꜣḫ*, see F. D. Friedman, "The Root Meaning of *ꜣḫ*: Effectiveness or Luminosity," *Serapis* 8 (1985) 39–46.

npw is a verb (*Wb.* 2:248, cf. the comment in *Grundriss* 7, 1:457) having to do with diseased condition though its meaning cannot be pinpointed precisely. The negative is *n* as written in the *n sḏm.f* past negation, and *n<n>* is not to be emended.

wnn – active participle.

It is perhaps possible that the greater frequency of the demonstrative *pꜣ* in this Explanation suggests that it belongs to a more colloquial or informal register of language than the text which it is annotating. For registers of language in an Egyptian context, and different registers appearing in the same text, cf. O. Goldwasser, "On Dynamic Canonicity in Late-Egyptian: The Literary Letter and the Personal Prayer," *Lingua Aegyptia* 1 (1991): 129–41. The point is not chronological priority or lateness, because the *pꜣ*-series is solidly attested in the Hekanakhte Letters in the late Eleventh or early Twelfth Dynasty.

Medical Commentary

Type of Injury

Case #9 deals with a comminuted fracture (*sd*) of the outer table of the frontal bone.[115] Brawanski considers it to be at any place within the skull vault,[116] but actually the frontal area is clearly specified in the text. Following a systematic pattern in the Edwin Smith Papyrus of dealing with case presentation in an anatomical orderly manner, from medial to lateral and top to bottom, and, because only the outer skull plate is involved, the skull injury of Case #9 must be located over the frontal squama, the area above the frontal air sinus (Case #7) and the eyebrow (Case # 10). Soldier #25 (fig. 9a) from Winlock, *Slain Soldiers of Neb-hep-et-Re Mentu-hotpe*, plate IX B, displays frontal bone injuries on both sides. The right frontal fracture appears to involve only its outer table, whereas his left frontal fracture is a penetrating fracture (*thm*) as discussed in Case #3.

Today, treatment of this type of injury would require debridement of the soft tissues and the fragmented skull outer table under general anesthesia, as well as control of bone hemorrhaging and repair of the skull defect to be done at the time of surgery if the wound is not contaminated, or electively at a later time. Bone bleeding is controlled today by the use of bone wax, which is made of 88 percent refined beeswax and 12 percent isopropyl palmitate, or by using clumps of dry microfibrillar collagen hemostat material (Avitene) applied to the bleeding bone and held temporarily under light pressure with dry cotton pads. Bone reconstitution is cosmetically important and it has been one of the fields in which plastic and reconstructive surgery has been interested in using bone

115. The skull is formed by external and internal compact bone layers, with a spongy/cancellous bone layer (diploe) in between. The diploe is highly vascular.

116. A. Brawanski, "Mittelgesichtsverletzungen im Pap. Smith (Fälle 9–14)," *Studien zur altägyptischen Kultur* 35 (2006): 45.

substitutes that can easily be molded and can integrate into native bone. One such material is Hydroxyapatite cement, a product of research into biomaterials and methodologies made of calcium phosphate salts that has osteoconductive physical characteristic serving as a scaffold allowing for the ingrowth of new vasculature and infiltration of osteogenic precursor cells into the graft site. The scalp would also need repair with cosmetic closure.

Ancient Methodology and Knowledge

The two aspects of treatment in Case #9 are a) physical treatment of the wound with the main purposes of "drying" it and reconstitution of the integrity of the skull surface, and b) the implementation of "ritual power" over the wound. Our retrospective analysis is necessarily incomplete, as we cannot fully immerse in the past and always find rationale for their every treatment. When we do find rationale for their specific treatments and successes, it is tempting to imagine the ancient Egyptian medical practitioners having the same basis as we now have. This is of course impossible, the simple reality being that the ancient Egyptian treatment prescriptions in Case #9 were taught and passed on based on experience of successful results, not scientific data as we enjoy.

The First Treatment Component: Wound Care

To treat the compound comminuted outer skull plate fracture of the frontal bone, the ancient physician applied ground ostrich eggshell with oil into the mouth of the wound, followed by application of powdered ostrich egg shell with the stated purpose being to dry the wound. The mixture of oil and ground ostrich egg shell would likely have been made to the consistency of putty that could easily be pushed into the bleeding diploe layer of the skull bone. The addition of powdered ostrich egg shell would further cover the surface irregularities and small cracks in the surrounding skull plate. Next, the head wound was covered with "the cloth bandage of physician's medical kit." This particular statement was further clarified by "it is a head binding which is under the charge of this bandager," indicating that the head binding should be of the kind an embalmer would use, a head wrapping, as we currently apply to all of our craniotomy patients. A compress of figs and honey ointment, cooked and cooled, was applied for the purpose of cooling, or soothing the wounded area, covered by the head bandage.

Three days later the bandage was removed and the master physician tells the pupil, "How you find (is): How it joins/knits together the bony plate of the braincase (is) with the condition similar to the egg(shell) of the ostrich." In other words, the skin is probably still open allowing visualizing the underlying skull, which now appears as if the bony plate of the skull is joined/knit together, the formerly fractured skull plate now looking like the ostrich egg shell. Even if the skull defect would eventually heal, it would not be in two or three days, but its appearance at this early stage is as if it has healed. In modern terms this is called "mimicry," and for all practical purposes the appearance of their bone repair at this stage would look no different than our cranioplasties (using modern materials) at the time of wound closure.

Could this type of treatment of a compound, comminuted, skull fracture of the outer table of the frontal bone have had any somatically based experience? Could it have been effective? The first stated aim of the ancient physician was to dry the wound. The source bleeding from such a wound is from the scalp and bone. Scalp bleeding is controlled by direct pressure of the soft tissues. Bone bleeding originates from the honey-combed diploe layer of the skull, located between the inner and the outer plates or tables. Bone wax used today for control of bone bleeding is made, as indicated above, of 88 percent refined beeswax and 12 percent isopropyl palmitate. Hemostasis is achieved by physically plugging the honeycombed trabecular structure of the cancellous bone under the hard outer skull plate and also into small linear fractures radiating from the main fracture site. The Isopropyl palmitate component in bone wax is a palm-oil-based emollient, moisturizer, and thickening agent.

The ancient Egyptians used ground ostrich egg shell with oil and dry powdered ostrich egg shell over it for the same purpose: "that is what dries the wound." Ostrich shell is 2 mm thick and strong enough to stand a force of 55 kg. Its mineral matrix constitutes 97 percent of its weight and is formed by calcium carbonate (97.4%), magnesium phosphate (1.9%), and tricalcium phosphate (0.7%).[117] The coarse granularity of the ground ostrich egg shell with oil could have been made to the consistency necessary to plug bleeding cancellous bone. The additional application of powdered egg shell on top of it would have further sealed the covered surface, and, smoothed out, would appear in a short time as healed skull bone "with the condition similar to the egg (shell) of the ostrich."

"Mimicry" is now an extensive area of biomedical research for materials capable of mimicking living tissues particularly to replace and mimic bone. These biomimetic materials are substances able to stimulate the tissues for eliciting specific responses at the interface with bone, to create a continuous transition from tissue to implant material. Among the biogenic minerals, calcium figures prominently. Two major compounds found in nature are calcium carbonate and calcium phosphate. Calcium carbonate is found mainly in shells of marine creatures and eggshells and calcium phosphate in bone and dentin of vertebrates.[118] The most successful materials found so far are the synthetic calcium phosphates or "apatites." These substances are able to replicate the structure and composition of bone mineral-hydroxylapatite (HA) and have biocompatible behavior with most of the cell types such as osteoblasts, osteoclasts, and fibroblasts. These properties of apatites favor the formation of bone on their surfaces by attachment, migration, proliferation, and differentiation of bone-forming cells.[119] Lakshminarayan et al.[120] have isolated and purified ansocalcin from goose eggshell matrix. In *in vivo* experiments, this substance nucleates polycrystalline aggregates of calcite crystals. Investigating the possibilities of using ostrich eggshell as a bone substitute, L. Dupoirieux[121] conducted research in rats and rabbits with cranial defects, applying a paste of powdered ostrich egg as interpositional graft to fill a complete bone defect and as onlay graft to fill partial defects. They were also used as onlay grafts in rabbit mandibles. Bone healing without integration of the grafted material occurred in the interpositional grafted animals. In the onlay model, the grafts were partly osteointegrated. No further studies using ostrich egg shell for this purpose have been reported. It is known that in the osteogenic process of bone cells the topography and roughness of the surface are important: "pore diameters between 15 and 50 µm I stimulate fibrovascular growth, between 50 and 150 µm stimulate osteoid formation and in the range of 150–500 µm lead directly to mineralized bone." One potential advantage of using ostrich egg shell is their large pore diameter, averaging 785 µm.[122] However, the ideal pore size and their surface distribution that would maximize bone growth in a graft, are unknown.[123]

Certainly, the ancient Egyptian physical treatment measures employed in Case #9 for a compound comminuted skull fracture of the frontal squama outer skull table could have been effective in terms of containing bone bleeding and obtaining acceptable cosmetic bone repair. (Author GMS covered a cortical bone defect in a

117. L. Dupoirieux, L. "Ostrich Eggshell as a Bone Substitute: A Preliminary Report of Its Biological Behaviour in Animals – A Possibility in Facial Reconstructive Surgery," *British Journal of Oral and Maxillofacial Surgery* 37/6 (1999): 467.

118. A. L. Olivera, J. F. Mano, and R. L. Reis, "Nature-Inspired Calcium Phosphate Coatings: Present Status and Novel Advances in the Science of Mimicry," *Science Direct. Current Opinion in Solid State & Materials Science* 7 (2003): 310.

119. Ibid., 312, 316; Rodríguez I. Zubillaga, G. Sánchez Aniceto, J. J. Montalvo Moreno, "Anterior Subcranial Approach: Discussion and Historical Review of the Surgical Technique," *Revista Española de Cirugía Oral y Maxilofacial* 31/1 (2009): 5–6. Online: http://scielo.isciii.es/scielo.php?pid=S1130-05582009000100001&script=sci_arttext&tlng=en.

120. R. Lakshminarayanan, R. Manjunatha Kini, and S. Valiyaveettil. "Investigation of the Role of Ansocalcin in the Biomemineralization in Goose Eggshell Matrix," *Proceedings of the National Academy of Sciences* 99/8 (2002): 5155–59. Online: http://www.pnas.org/content/99/8/5155.full.

121. Dupoirieux, "Ostrich Eggshell as a Bone Substitute, 467–71.

122. M. H. Abbaspour-Fard, B. Emadi, and M. H. Aghkhani, "Fertility Recognition of Ostrich Egg Using Physical Properties," *Journal of Applied Sciences* 10 (2010): 1405–12. Online: http://scialert.net/fulltext/?doi=jas.2010.1405.1412&org=11.

123. Olivera, Mano, and Reis, "Nature-Inspired Calcium Phosphate Coatings," 312.

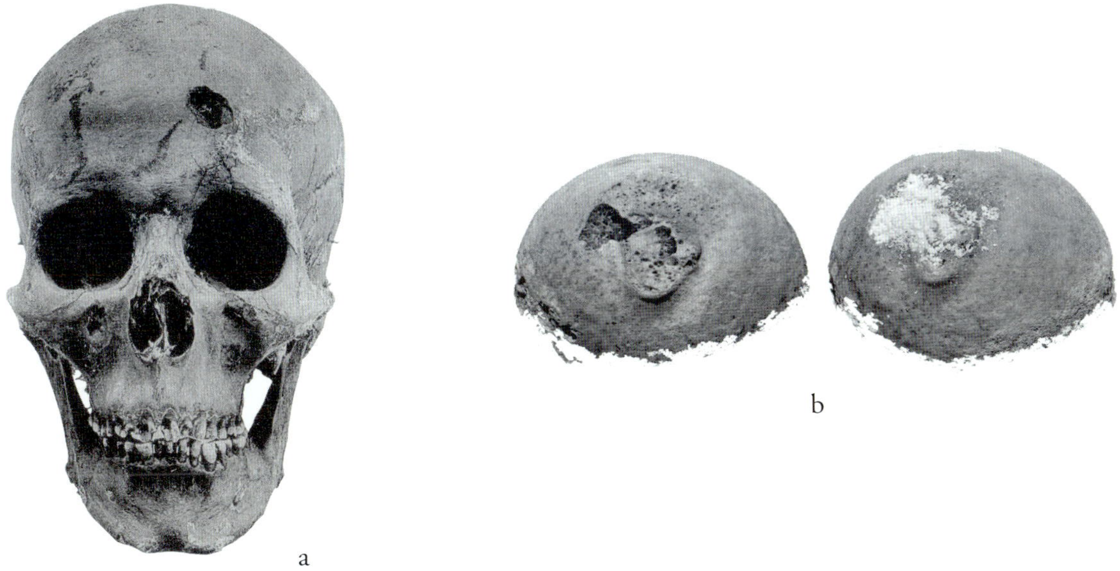

Fig. 9. a) Soldier #25, from Winlock, *Slain Soldiers of Neb-hep-et-Re Mentu-hotpe*, plate IX B; b) Cadaver femoral head with diploe bone defect (left), filled with a paste of ostrich egg shell and vegetable oil by G. M. Sanchez; sealed appearance after six months (right).

dry cadaver femoral head with a paste of ground ostrich egg shell and oil. The cancellous bone covered defect had the smooth appearance of cortical bone as it dried and remained unchanged after six months' observation, fig. 9b). The external application of honey to the wound would likely have prevented infection.

The Second Treatment Component: Implementation of Ritual Power

Ritualistic Implementation

Preferring the use of "ritual power" instead of "magic," we refer to Meltzer's work in "Old Coptic Texts of Ritual Power." The treatment in Case #9 was complemented by the use of a ritual power recitation said over the wound. This part of the treatment caused Breasted to dismiss Case #9 as one with no place in the Edwin Smith Papyrus:[124] "This case represents our surgeon's sole relapse into the superstition of his age, of which he has elsewhere so surprisingly divested himself." Breasted's unfortunate conclusion is an example of what Meltzer describes as a problem with the "evaluative connotation of 'magic' as false, deceptive, discredited, or morally tainted, contrasted with both science (a correct, enlightened understanding of natural law and causation) and religion (a correct, enlightened understanding of the divine and spirituality)." Contrary to Breasted's opinion, the empirical, religious, and ritual power dimensions were all concurrent and complementary within medical care in ancient Egypt.[125] According to Ritner, boundaries between ancient Egyptian magic, religion, and medicine were not

124. Breasted, *Edwin Smith*, 217, 220: "This treatment is a curious hodgepodge of superstitions, without a suggestion of the scientific attitude of mind which is so prominent in the ancient surgeon's discussion of the other cases."

125. Bruno Halioua, *La médecine au temps des pharaons* (Paris: Liana Levi, 2002), 38–41.

strictly observed.[126] The Egyptian perceptions about the supernatural causation of illnesses meant that prayer and magic spells and rituals played a vital role in therapeutics and the practice of the healing arts was intimately linked to religious beliefs and practices.[127] Further elaborating on the subject, Meltzer explains the nature, medical applicability and implementation of ritual power: "These texts and practices answered the needs of the people who employed them in times of crisis, hurt, or loss, or in the continual difficulties of everyday life. Thus, the bottom line in these texts is empowerment, and the texts themselves are appropriately described as texts of ritual power." "Ritual power figures prominently not only in texts (which are, after all, texts dealing with ritual power in a specific context), other 'religious' texts, 'medical' texts, and stories. The texts are not abstract or disembodied entities. The rituals in which they figure are by no means limited to mere recitation but involve a wide range of practices often mentioned or described explicitly by the texts."[128]

The medical, magical, and funerary texts are full of allusions to the curing of Horus, particularly through the magic of his mother Isis. According to Walker,[129] Horus the son of Osiris "was a passive archetypal victim/sufferer/patient for the earlier part of Egyptian history, any ordinary Egyptian was readily able to identify himself with this Horus."

Borghouts describes the role of the person implementing ritual power: "The ritual specialist expresses the will of supernatural powers by impersonating them, hence, elsewhere, the frequent initial presentative clause 'I am god X'."[130] Meltzer further clarifies: "this an example of the ritual specialist playing the role of, and being for that duration and purpose an embodiment of, the divine being or power."[131]

We see these elements of the ritual-power specialist in the three segments from Case #9 delineated below:

1) What is said as ritual power over this prescription:
   - "Driving out the enemy within the wound (and) causing the hostile force that is within the blood, a robber of Horus, to tremble.
2) The protection of the utterance of The Beneficial/Effective Goddess (Isis):
   - This temple will not collapse.
3) The blood vessel(s) therein have not sickened(?), for I am in the Beneficial /Effective Goddess's protection.
   - The son of Osiris is saved!"

While the ultimate goal is to save Horus, and to prevent collapse of "this Temple," the ritual power directly alludes to specific actions locating and driving out the enemy within the wound and within blood vessels (1). Its beneficial action completed, the ritual specialist, playing the role of the divine being, declares the ultimate results: "The blood vessels therein have not sickened (3), the son of Osiris (Horus) is saved! (3)." This portion of the ritual power brings us to the realization that it is a vocalized version of Egyptian early concepts of pathogenesis involving their terms *mtw* and *wḫdw*.

Ritual Power Recitation: Expression of an Early Concept of Pathogenesis?

For the Egyptian physician, trauma and its resulting wounds were understood and treated by somatically based means. In contrast, internal medical problems had unknown and invisible causes that they generally

126. Ritner, *Mechanics of Ancient Egyptian Magical Practice*, 4–5.
127. James H. Walker, "Egyptian Medicine and the Gods," *The Bulletin of the Australian Centre for Egyptology* 4 (1993): 83–101.
128. Meltzer "Old Coptic Texts of Ritual Power," 14.
129. Walker, "Egyptian Medicine and the Gods," 83–101.
130. J. F. Borghouts, *Ancient Egyptian Magical Texts* (Leiden: Brill, 1978), X.
131. Meltzer "Old Coptic Texts of Ritual Power," 17.

believed to be produced by malevolent external powers, including living and dead persons, gods and goddesses.[132] But it is also evident that the ancient Egyptian physicians suspected that disease could also have other origins, which they explained using the anatomical and pathophysiological Egyptian concepts of *mtw* and *wẖdw*. The word *mtw*[133] was used for various elongated anatomical structures, including blood vessels, tendons, and nerves. The word *wẖdw*[134] is more difficult to define because of its multiple attributes and pathogenic capabilities. It signified a morbid principle, or a "pain material" associated with putrefaction in the bowel. It functioned as the exact opposite to that of life-giving blood.[135] The *wẖdw* could be manifest on the surface as *wḥꜣw*[136] or in any part of the body[137] causing disease by spreading via the *mtw*. The *wẖdw* could also appear in a wound,[138] produce "accumulations"[139] and inflammation.[140] But the *wẖdw* could also be killed. Majno[141] summarizes the *wẖdw* properties: "In essence, what bacteria can do, it (*wẖdw*) could do." Westendorf,[142] calls attention to the fact that *wẖdw* is always written with the general illness determinative , but there is no inference of demonic character in the word, even in those few occasions when it appears associated with these.[143]

132. Unknown and invisible causes of disease have been with man for millennia, until discovery of the microscope and pathogenic bacteria in the nineteenth century.

133. Cases #1 (plate I:6,7,8); #7 (plate III:10,17,18,19,20); #9 (plate V:3); and #34 (plate XII:1)

134. Bardinet, *Les Papyrus Medicaux*, 128–38; Westendorf, *Handbuch der altägyptischen Medizin*, 329; Nunn, *Ancient Egyptian Medicine*, 61–63; Majno, *The Healing Hand*, 129. Although *wẖdw* does not occur in the Edwin Smith Papyrus, it is important to acknowledge its role in the ancient Egyptian understanding of disease processes.

135. Bardinet, *Les Papyrus Medicaux*, 128–38. Blood gives life; the *wẖdw* attacks the blood.

136. Ibid., 266, as a rash (Ebers Papyrus #114, #116); 267, internal (Ebers Papyrus #118); 267, in the mouth (Ebers Papyrus #122); 268, in the leg (Ebers Papyrus #128).

137. Ibid., 267, internal (Ebers Papyrus #118); 267, in the mouth (Ebers Papyrus #122); 268, in the leg (Ebers Papyrus #128).

138. Ibid., 268 (Ebers Papyrus #130).

139. Ibid. (Ebers Papyrus ##126, 127).

140. Ibid., 266–67 (Ebers Papyrus ##115, 119).

141. Majno, *The Healing Hand*, 129.

142. Westendorf, *Handbuch der altägyptischen Medizin*, 329

143. Bardinet, *Les Papyrus Medicaux*, 50 (Ebers Papyrus #131); 308–9 (Ebers Papyrus #385).

CASE #10:

Eyebrow Laceration Penetrating to the Bone

(Plate V:5–9)

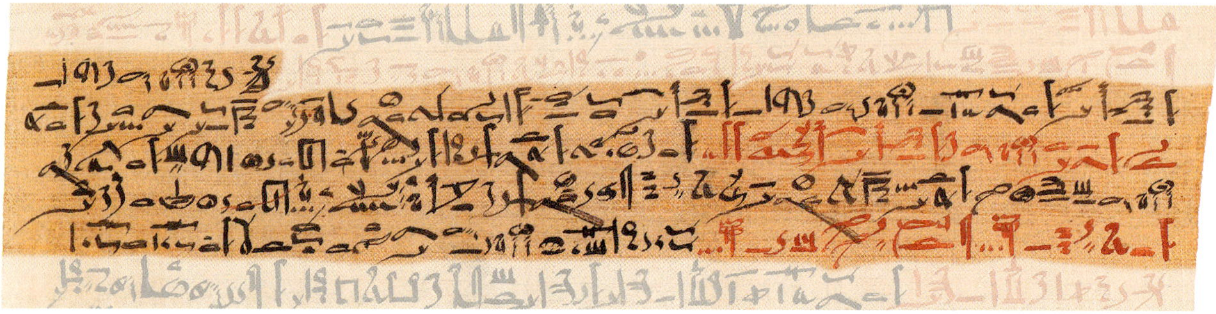

Courtesy New York Academy of Medicine.

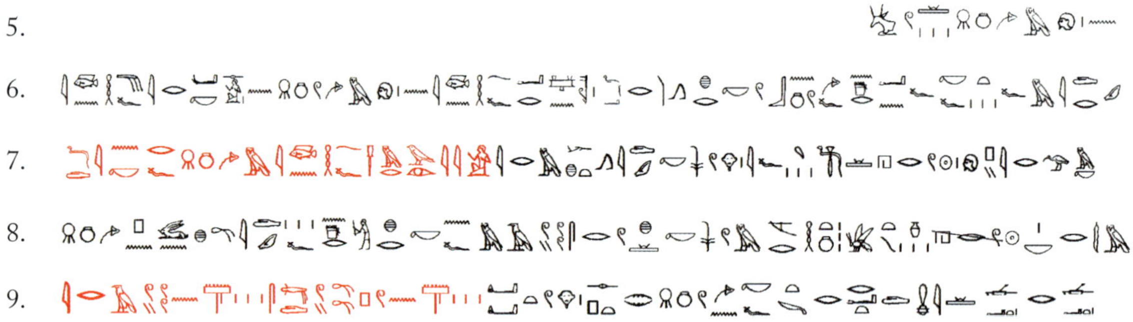

Transliteration

[5§] … *šsꜣw wbnw m tp n*

[6§] *inḫ.f ḏꜥr.ḫr.k wbnw.f nḏr n.f kft.f m idr*

[7§] *ḏd.in.k r.f wbnw m inḫ.f mḫr iry.i* *ir m-ḫt id.k sw ir gm.k*

[8§] *wbnw pn wnḫ idrw.f nḏr.ḫr.k n.f m ꜣiwy srwḫ.k sw m mrḥt bit hrw nb r nḏm.f*

[9§] *ir ꜣiwy n ḥbsw sšdwy pw n ḥbsw* *dd.tw ḥr spty wbnw n kft r rdit dmi wꜥt r wꜥt*

Translation

Title:

Necessary knowledge and skills for a wound in the top of his eyebrow:

Examination:

If you examine a man for a wound in the top of his eyebrow, penetrating to the bone, then you must palpate his wound.

Hold fast for him his slash wound with thread.

Diagnosis:

Then you are to say about it/him: "A wound in his eyebrow, a medical condition which I will handle/deal with."

Treatment:

After you stitch it, <then you must bind it> (along) with fresh meat the first day.

If you find this wound shifted (with respect to) its stitches/(with) its stitches shifting, then you must hold (it) fast for him with two bandages.

You need to treat it with oil and honey every day, until it/he is well.

Explanation:

As for "two cloth bandages," it means "two bandages of cloth, that one places/are placed over the lips of the slash wound, in order to make one join to the other."

Notes

wbnw pn wnḫ idrw.f – There are two possible analyses yielding very similar translations. Either *wnḫ* can be a stative *wnḫ*(*w*) followed by a qualifying noun, "(it) being shifted with respect to its stitches," or a circumstantial *sḏm.f* with *idrw.f* as the subject, "its stitches shifting." For the syntactic questions surrounding such examples, see Meltzer, "Problems of Adjectival Constructions in Old and Middle Egyptian," II.6 and III.

dd.tw – Relative form "that one places," or "that are placed." The author could have used a passive participle *dd*(*w*) for the meaning "that are placed," and the reason for the choice of construction in this passage is not clear.

Medical Commentary

Type of Injury

This injury is located at the orbital rim/eyebrow level. Following the orderly topographic organization of injuries in the Edwin Smith papyrus this wound is placed inferior to that of Case #9 and lateral to Case #7. It is a full-thickness scalp cut reaching the bone without fracturing it. There is no description of associated injuries to neighboring structures. Treatment of such an injury requires thorough irrigation and debridement. Cosmetic closure is indicated, as meticulously described by Trott,[144] placing 5-0 nonabsorbable monofilament alignment sutures first at the superior and inferior margins of the brow hair. If deep (dermal) sutures are necessary to approximate the superficial fascia, 5-0 absorbable suture material can be applied next. The remainder of the skin laceration is closed with nonabsorbable sutures. No dressing is necessary, but antibacterial ointment is applied daily. Sutures are removed in three to five days.

Case #10 describes sometime after the first day, the possibility of finding the sutures becoming loose. Such an occurrence could be secondary to an inordinate amount of soft tissue swelling at the time of suturing, or to the presence of jagged skin edges that did not approximate well from the start. In such a situation, the wound could be reinforced with adhesive strips, or resutured.

144. Alexander T. Trott, *Wounds and Lacerations: Emergency Care and Closure* (3rd ed.; Philadelphia: Mosby, 2005), 162.

Ancient Medical Methodology and Knowledge

It should be noted that wound suturing was effected immediately after examination of the patient's wound. This would have promptly stopped bleeding and would favor proper healing. It is clear that suture material and instruments of the time were relatively coarse, not the ideal for an area of the anatomy requiring fine cosmetic surgery. The application of fresh meat over the wound on the first day was appropriate in line with their established practices. Daily dressings with honey and oil would continue until the wound healed. In the event that sutures became loosened, the wound margins were held fast with "two bandages of cloth, that one places/are placed over the lips of the slash wound, in order to make one join to the other." This form of treatment of secondary wound approximation in Case #10 utilizes the wound closure technique described for Case #2, a scalp laceration. As in that case, the cloth bands probably had adhesive properties, functioning as our current "steri-strips," "butterfly strips," and other variants of sutureless wound closure materials and techniques.

CASE #11:

Fracture of the Nasal Septum

(Plate V:10–15)

Courtesy New York Academy of Medicine.

10. 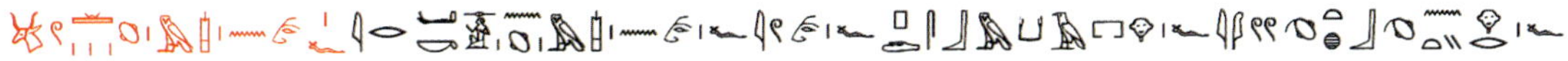

11. 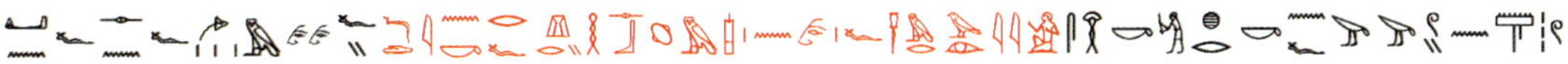

12. 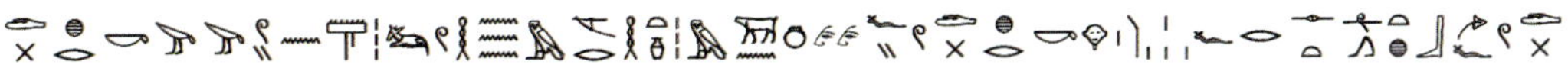

13. 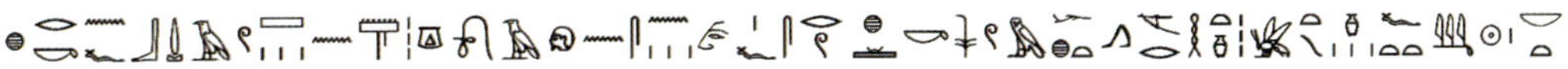

14. 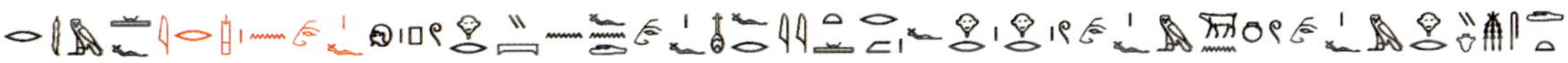

15. 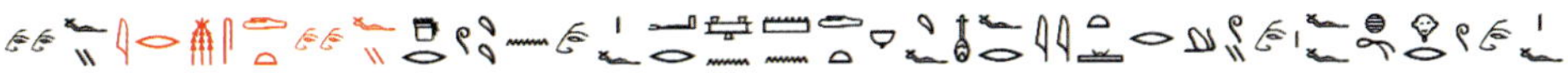

Transliteration

10§ *šsꜣw ḥsb m iwn n fnd.f ir ḫꜣ.k s n ḥsb m iwn n fnd.f iw fnd.f pds mkꜣ ḥr.f i.šw ṯḫb nty ḥr.f*
11§ *di.n.f snf m msdty.fy ḏd.in.k r.f ḫry ḥsb m iwn n fnd.f mḥr iry.i sk.ḥr.k n.f <m> sšmwy n ḥbsw*
12§ *wd.ḫr.k sšmwy n ḥbsw iwḥ m mrḥt m-ẖnw msdty.fy wd.ḫr.k <sw> ḥr mniw.f r stꜣ ṯḫb.f*
13§ *wd.ḫr.k n.f bḏꜣw n ḥbsw gwꜣ.n.sn fnd.f srwḫ.k sw m-ḫt <m> mrḥt bit ftt rꜥ nb{.t}*
14§ *r nḏm.f ir iwn n fnd.f tp pw ḥry n fnd.f nfryt r gs.f ḥr ḥrw fnd.f m ẖnw fnd.f m ḥry-ib msdty*
15§ *.fy ir msdty.fy ḏrwy n fnd.f ꜥr n mndt.f nfryt r pḥwy fnd.f fḫ ḥrw fnd.f*

Translation

Title:

Necessary knowledge and skills for a fracture in the pillar of his nose:

Examination:

If you examine a man for a fracture in the pillar of his nose, and his nose is flattened, his face having been leveled, and (how) the swelling which is upon it protrudes (is) when he has bled from both his nostrils/nasal cavities,

Diagnosis:

then you are to say about him: "One who has a break/fracture in the pillar of his nose: a medical condition which I will handle/deal with."

Treatment:

Then you must clean/wipe out for him two swabs of cloth.

Then you must place two swabs of cloth, saturated with oil, within both his nostrils/nasal cavities.

Then you must put upon his mooring post/bed in order to reduce his swelling.

Then you must place for him stiff rolls of cloth, they having restricted (sic) his nose (or, whose nose they have restricted??).

You should treat it afterwards <with> oil and honey and dressing every day until it/he is well.

Explanation A:

As for "the pillar of his nose," it is the upper top of his nose/top of his nose which is above down to its side and on the upper part of his nose within his nose in the midst of his two nostrils/nasal cavities.

Explanation B:

As for "his two nostrils/nasal cavities," (these are) the two sides of his nose reaching/penetrating to his cheek, down to the back of his nose, leaving the upper part of his nose.

Notes

ỉw fnd.f pds(*w*) – Independent clause.

mkꜣ cannot be an infinitive because bare infinitive cannot be a circumstantial "leveling." *ḥr* + infinitive would be required. Bare infinitive does appear as a "narrative infinitive," frequently in a series of actions, but that does not fit in this context and it is not the equivalent of a circumstantial or adverbial form. Therefore I suggest a passive *sḏm*(*w*)*.f* form, which is one of the adverbial forms identified by Polotsky (*Egyptian Tenses*, 2–6), but that normally gives an anterior or prior rather than simultaneous circumstance (Doret, *Narrative Verbal System*, 93–94 and Table 13). Passive participle + noun in an adjective predicate pattern. "His face is flattened" is also possible (Gardiner, *EG*^{3}, sec. 374), but is a less usual construction.

ỉšww as nominal *sḏm.f* (manner nominalization).

dỉ.n.f – Circumstantial *sḏm.n.f* (anterior or prior circumstance)

sk.ḫr.k n.f … – In idiomatic English we would have to say "clean/wipe out (his nostrils/nasal cavities) for him (with) two swabs of cloth." I am refraining from emending words here because of the possibility that it might come under the heading of Gardiner's additional paragraph in his 3rd edition, sec. 84 A, 423: "Direct object after verbs of apparently intransitive or passive sense," in which he includes *wrḥ* "be anointed," and one that occurs throughout our text, *mn* "suffer." We have never proposed an emendation with the latter, but it must be admitted that Gardiner's listing highlights a gray area or factor of uncertainty regarding some cases in which we, and Breasted, typically emend <*m*>. (One of Gardiner's examples is *ḥtp* "rest on," which calls to mind the ambivalence of the Hebrew verb *škn* "dwell," which can be found followed both by a direct complement and by the preposition *b*-.)

bḏ3w – "stiff rolls" (Faulkner, *CDME*, 86), which I think makes excellent sense.

gw3.n.sn – This does not work as a nominal *sḏm.n.f* (for some grammarians categorized as a type of relative form, "abstract relative form" or "personal substantival form"). The meaning in that case would be "how they have restricted his nose," which as far as I can see does not seem to connect with anything syntactically, and I do not think that an independent or self-standing nominal form fits in the present passage. As an ordinary relative form it would have to mean "whose nose they have restricted," that is, the *sn* has to be the actor of the verb and the *n* segment in *n.sn* marks it for the past, broadly defined. "*They are what restricts his nose/holds his nose firmly," would be expressed quite differently, by a participial statement, **ntsn gw3 fnd.f.* I think that a likelier choice for this passage is circumstantial *sḏm.n.f*, even though that yields an anterior or prior circumstance, "they having restricted his nose," which is incongruous because the stiff rolls have only just been applied. Because of the principle of *lectio dificilior* I am reluctant to emend it by deleting the *n*.

tp ḥry n fnd.f "the upper top of his nose" or "top of his nose which is above" – I think Allen's (*AM*) understanding as the bridge of his nose makes sense.

ʿr, fḫ – active participles. For *fḫ* "leave," see Faulkner, *CDME*, 98; this is analogous to Allen's (*AM*) translation. Though the phraseology seems somewhat circuitous, when translated this way I think that it yields a comprehensible description of the anatomy of the nostrils/nasal cavities.

nfryt r – Understood in the sense of "all the way to the end of," not "down to" in a literally downward direction.

Medical Commentary

Type of Injury

Identification of the nasal injuries described in Cases 11–14 requires a brief review of the specific anatomical features and the most common mechanisms of injury to the specific area considered in each case.

The nasal structures are formed externally by the nose (fig. 10) and internally by the nose cavity and its walls. The nasal cavity connects exteriorly through the nostrils and internally with the main respiratory tract at the nasopharynx. The main nasal cavity has accessory chambers, the frontal, maxillary, sphenoid, and ethmoid air sinuses, located in the surrounding cranial bones.

The nose consists of bony and cartilaginous structures, which are attached to the internal nasal structures in the facial bones and cranial base. The nasal skeleton is formed by paired nasal bones joining in the midline with each other, superiorly to the frontal bone, laterally to the lacrimal bones and the frontal process of the maxilla (fig. 10b). The nasal bones are joined in the midline, posteriorly, by the bony septum, which is formed by the perpendicular plate of the ethmoid bone. The sphenoid plate attaches to the vomer bone inferiorly and posteriorly. In turn, the vomer attaches inferiorly to the maxilla and palatine bones, at the nasal floor (fig. 11). The cartilagenous components of the nose form the lower two thirds of the nose. These are the upper lateral cartilages and the alar cartilages (fig. 10). The lateral cartilages attach superiorly to the nasal bones and receive the septal quadrangular cartilage from inside the nose, at the midline. The quadrangular cartilage also attaches to

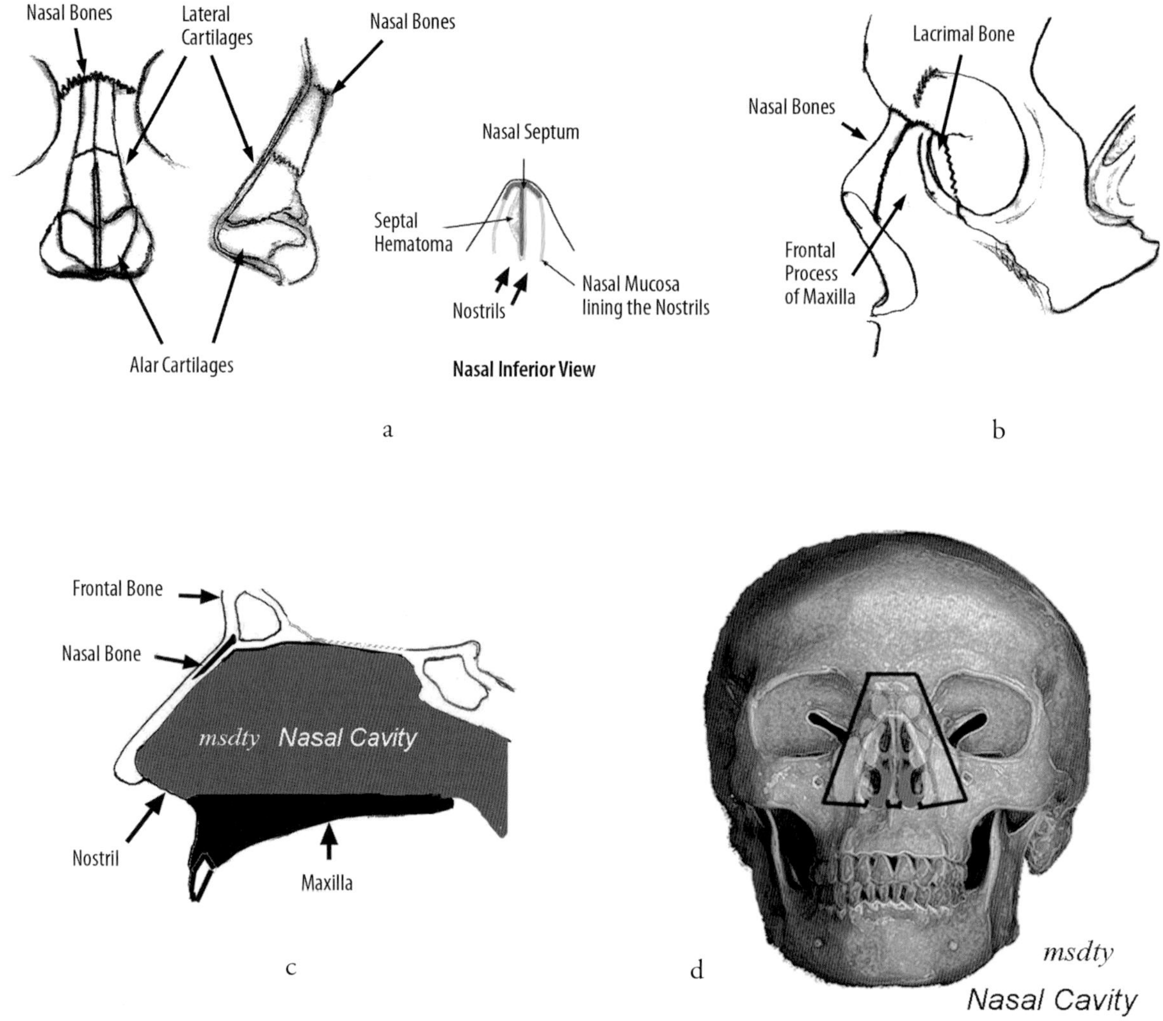

Fig. 10. Anatomy of the nose. a) external bone and cartilages of the nose ; b) external nasal bone structures; c) schematic off-the-midline sagittal section; d) nasal cavity boundaries.

the bony septum, to the quadrangular plate of the ethmoid above, the vomer posteriorly and to the nasal floor (maxilla) below (fig. 11).

It is of interest that another meaning for the Egyptian word for nose *fnḏ* is "beak," which helps us visualize their description of the various parts of the nose. It seems these descriptions refer to beak, or pyramidal shape, which would be observed in a person reclining on his back and face up. In this manner, "top of his nose," would correspond to the tip of the nose. Under this point of view the structural injury described in this case explanation A is easier to follow. It identifies the anatomical boundaries of *iwn fnd* = "the pillar of the nose" as:

- "it is the upper top of his nose/top of his nose which is above...." At the uppermost part of the nose, the nasal ridge is formed by the lateral and the alar cartilages.
- "down to its side." The lateral sloping of the nasal cartilages from the midline.

- "and on the upper part of his nose within his nose in the midst of his two nostrils/nasal cavities." This describes the septal quadrangular cartilage joining the lateral cartilages from inside, in the midline, descending between the two nostrils.

Explanation B refers to the nasal anatomical details of the nasal cavities, including the maxillary air sinus extensions (fig. 10d). Understanding of the text can be facilitated with the patient in the supine brow-up position (fig. 11 right).

- As for "'his two nostrils/nasal cavities,' (these are) the two sides of his nose reaching/penetrating to his cheek," seems to refer to the maxillary sinuses.
- "down to the back of his nose" would be the nasopharynx.
- "leaving the upper part of his nose" would be the nostrils.

In agreement with Breasted, the injury in Case #11 corresponds to the anterior and inferior part of the nose, the cartilaginous portion of the nose and its vertical supporting column (fig 12), a point elegantly discussed by Brawanski in his combined analysis of Cases #11 and #12.[145] The naturally weak areas are in the cartilaginous structures and their junctions with the nasal bones and the septum at the maxillary crest. Whether this "fracture" has occurred at the cartilaginous/nasal bone junction, and corresponding septum, or if it has also involved the inferior and thinner portion of the nasal bones, it is impossible to tell.

The direction of force to the nose during injury determines the pattern of the fracture. In Case #11 it is likely this fracture resulted from a direct frontal, or a superiorly directed blow which involved the nasal septum in a transverse direction, as do the majority of septum fractures[146] (fig. 12). Statistically speaking, nasal fractures are the most common type of facial fractures. In our day, most nasal bone fractures are caused by fights (34%), accidents (28%), and sports (23%).

Presenting symptoms and findings in this type of injury are:

- Change in nasal appearance with a flattened out nose, local swelling, deformity and tenderness.
- Bleeding from the nose (epistaxis) resulting from mucosal disruption.
- Nasal airway obstruction is possible.
- Infraorbital ecchymosis, a common sign in nasal fractures.

Routine radiographs are not necessary in most cases, but computer tomography often is helpful for management decisions.

Recommended treatment measures begin with elevation of the head and use of cold compresses in the periorbital and nasal region, while waiting for edema to subside. The current experience with nasal fractures involving the septum suggests that prompt identification and reduction of the fracture before significant edema has developed are important to avoid potential complications. Necrosis of the nasal septum by unrelieved pressure from a hematoma, or infection in the hematoma itself could occur.

145. Brawanski, "Mittelgesichtsverletzungen im Pap. Smith (Fälle 9–14)," 48–53.

146. It is a horizontal or axial plane that theoretically divides the body in a superior and an inferior portion.

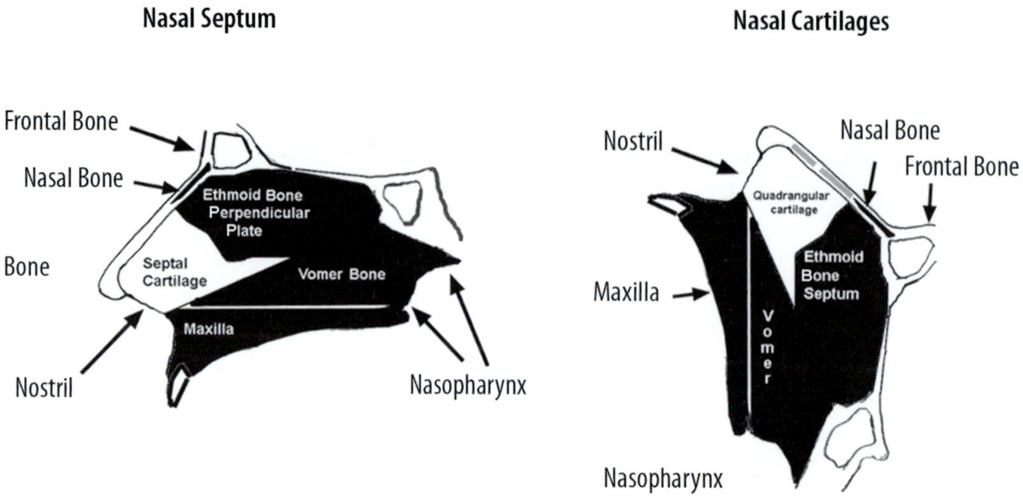

Fig. 11. Author's rendition of Egyptian nasal perspective. Left: Nasal lateral midline view. Right: Nasal anatomy in the brow-up position.

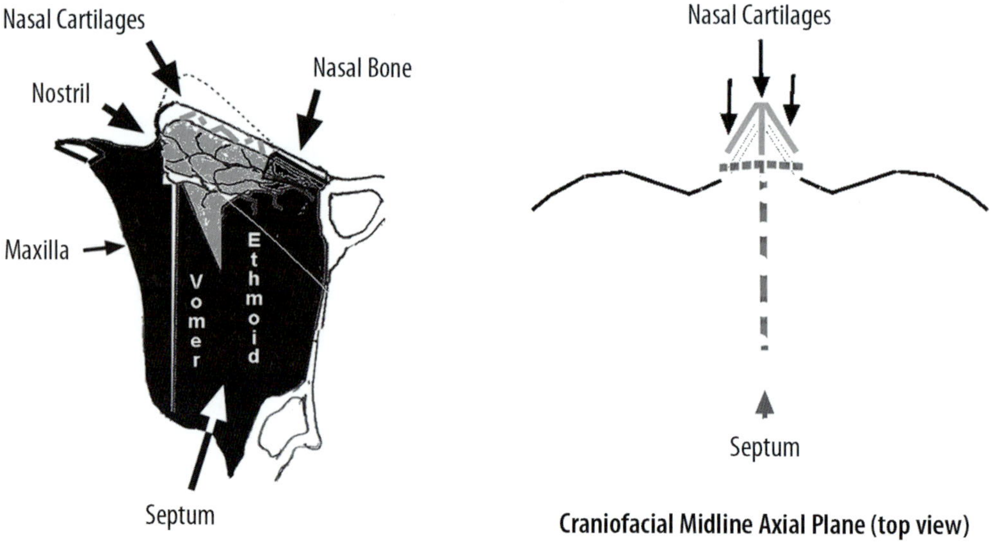

Fig. 12. "Pillar of the Nose" failure. Nasal cartilaginous fracture. Right: Nasal anatomy in the brow-up position.

Ross and Becker[147] summarize the various treatments of these injuries and Mayorga and Higgins[148] provide closed reduction guidelines. Closed reduction is done in cases of simple fractures of the nasal septal complex, whereas open reduction is needed in extensive fracture dislocations of the nasal septum, open septal fractures and septal hematomas. The optimal timing for reduction in patients with minimal swelling is within three hours,

147. A. T. Ross, and D. J. Becker, "Nasal and Septal Fractures." Medscape Reference: http://emedicine.medscape.com/article/878595-overview.

148. Oliver Majorga and Natalie P. Higgins, "Nasal Fracture Reduction: Treatment & Medication." Medscape Reference: http://emedicine.medscape.com/article/82831-treatment.

but when there is significant edema, reduction needs to be delayed from three to ten days, when the edema has resolved. Close reductions are done under local anesthesia with or without sedation. Antibiotic prophylaxis is mandatory prior to intranasal packing. Once fracture reduction has been achieved, lubricated internal packing is necessary to stabilize it, coupled with an external splint. The internal packing is removed in five days and the external splint in seven days.

Ancient Medical Methodology and Knowledge

This is a *ḥsb* type of fracture, which today we would consider a simple linear fracture as compared to a comminuted fracture. The anatomical identification of this nasal injury is provided by the ancient Egyptian's detailed description of *iwn fnd* = "the pillar of the nose" in explanation A, supported by the clinical features ("his nose is flattened, his face having been leveled, and (how) the swelling which is upon it protrudes (is) when he has bled from both his nostrils/nasal cavities) and by the specifics of their treatment measures:

- Cleaning of the injured area.
- Packing the interior of the nose with two swabs of cloth, saturated with oil within both his nostrils/nasal cavities, to reshape the injured area.
- Placing the patient in bed under observation and support in order to reduce his swelling. No clear prescription was issued for keeping the patient in the sitting position, but it is likely that it was, or at least the head of the bed must have been elevated, if their stated purpose for the patient being put to his bed was for the specific purpose of reducing his swelling.
- Placing for him stiff rolls of cloth in order to restrict/support the nose (externally).
- Fracture stabilization by internal and external splints advocated by the Egyptian physician in Case #11 is the same as employed today.
- Daily dressings with oil and honey were prescribed. These were probably awkward to use initially (over the external splints).

Our conservative form of treatment for this particular injury by closed reduction is practically unchanged from that presented in Case #11.

CASE #12:
Nasal Comminuted Depressed Fracture
(Plate V:16–VI:3)

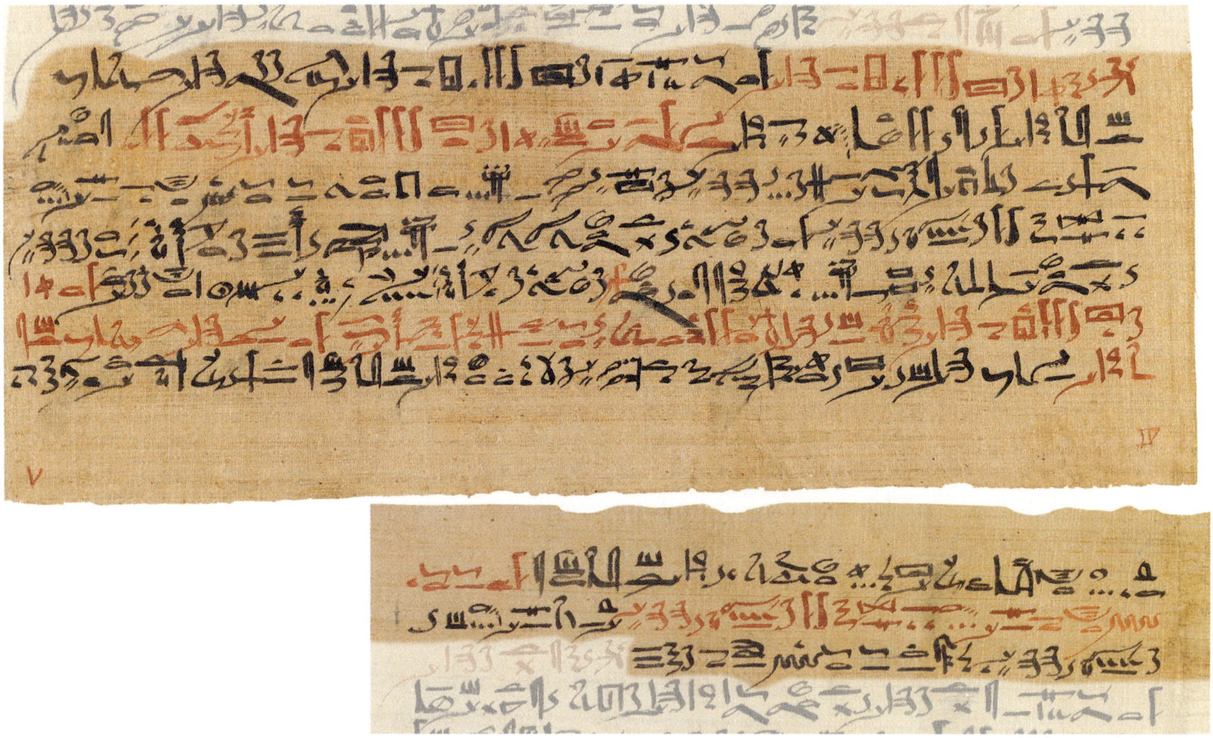

Courtesy New York Academy of Medicine.

16.
17.
18.
19.
20.
21.
22.

1. 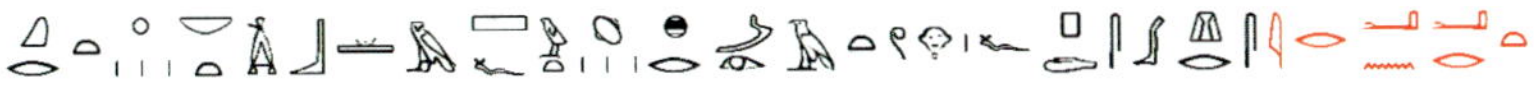

2. 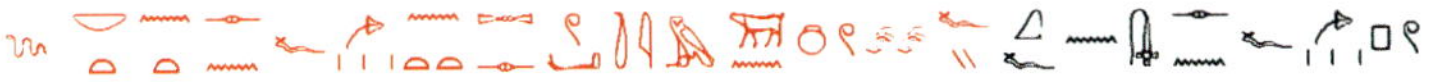

3. 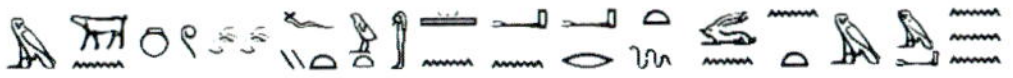

Transliteration

16§ *šsȝw ḥsb m štyt nt fnd.f ir ḫȝ.k s n ḥsb m štyt nt fnd.f gmm.k fnd.f ḫȝb*

17§ *pds ḥr.f iw i.šwy tẖb nty ḥr.f ḏd.in.k r.f ẖry ḥsb m štyt nt fnd.f mḥr iry.i sẖr.<i>*

18§ *n.k sw <w>d m st.f sk n.f imyw msdty.fy m sšwy n ḥbsw r pr.t ꜥnꜥrt nbt nt snf*

19§ *ntt ṯs.ti m-ẖnw msdty.fy ir m-ḫt wd.ḥr.k sšmwy n ḥbsw iwḥ m mrḥt rdi(w) m msdty.fy*

20§ *wd.ḥr.k n.f bḏȝwy n ḥbsw wt ḥr.s srwḫ.k sw m-ḫt m mrḥt bit ftt rꜥ nb r nḏm.f ir ḥsb*

21§ *m štyt nt fnd.f ḥry-ib pw n fnd.f nfryt r pḥwy ꜥr n imytw inḥwy.fy ir fnd.f ḫȝb pds*

22§ *ḥr.f dnb fnd.f pw šf.w r ḏr.f wr mndty.fy m mitt ḫr ḥr.f pds ḫr.s nn sw m ḳd.f mty m-ꜥ ntt*

1§ *ḳrwt nbt ḏbȝ m šfwt ḫr mȝ.tw ḥr.f pds ḫr-s ir ꜥnꜥrt*

2§ *nbt nt snf ntt ṯs.ti m-ẖnw msdty.fy ḳfn snf pw*

3§ *m-ẖnw msdty.fy twt n ꜥnꜥrt wnnt m m-ꜥ mw*

Translation

Title:

Necessary knowledge and skills for a fracture in the chamber/vault of his nose:

Examination:

If you examine a man for a fracture in the chamber/vault of his nose how you find his nose (is) crooked, his face having been flattened, (and) the swelling which is over it is protruding,

Diagnosis:

then you are to say about him: "One who has a fracture in the chamber/vault of his nose, a medical condition which I will handle/deal with."

Treatment:

<Then> you <should> cause it to fall in, it being put in its place (or, so that it is put in its place).

Swab for him the insides of both his nostrils with two swabs of cloth, until every eel of blood (all the clotted blood), which has knotted/coagulated inside both of his nostrils/nasal cavities, comes out.

Afterwards, you must place two plugs of cloth saturated with oil, and placed/so that they are placed in both his nostrils

You have to apply to him two stiff rolls of cloth, bandaged over it.

You should treat him afterwards with oil and honey, and dressing every day until he is well.

Explanation A:

As for "a fracture in the chamber/vault of his nose," it is in the middle of his nose, down to the back, and extending to between his two eyebrows.

Explanation B:

As for "his nose is crooked, his face having been flattened," it means his nose is bent and very swollen in its entirety, both of his cheeks (being) likewise, so that his face is flattened because of it; it is not in its proper shape seeing that all the hollows of his face are blocked up with tumefaction, so that his face looks flattened because of it.

Explanation C:

As for "every eel of blood which has knotted/coagulated inside both of his nostrils/nasal cavities," it means that the clotted blood inside both of his nostrils/nasal cavities is like the eel that exists in water.

Notes

ỉr... gmm.k – In my understanding, the nominal *sḏm.f* or manner nominalization does not continue the "if" protasis; see above.

pds ḥr.f – taking this form as most likely a passive *sḏm(w).f*, as above.

ỉw šwy – The statement of fact *ỉw sḏm.f* does contain the circumstantial *sḏm.f* but it does not operate as a circumstantial clause. It operates according to what I characterized during my years of teaching as Polotsky's "equation" *ỉw* + circumstantial = indicative or *ỉw* + adverbial = statement. The *ỉw*-clause will be circumstantial in Later Egyptian. It can be noted that, unlike *ỉw* + noun + adverbial, *ỉw* + suffix-pronoun + adverbial is neutral or bivalent in Middle Egyptian with respect to independence/dependence.

sḫr.<ỉ>n.k – I am accepting the emendation of the *sḏm.in.f* form.

<w>d m st.f – The *d* by itself is an attested writing (see above), but it is very easy to see this passage as haplography omitting one of the two curl *w*'s in the sequence *sw wd*. I think the verb is most likely a stative of result, "so that it is put."

r prr.f (sic) – The emendation of *r pr<t>.f*, an *r sḏmt.f* construction, is very tempting but not necessary. If one takes the text as it stands, one has the nominal *sḏm.f* after a preposition, which also works syntactically; for *r* + *sḏm.f* with the meaning "until," see Gardiner, *EG*^{3}, sec. 163.11. Cf. *r nḏm.f* "until he is well," which occurs frequently in this text.

ṯs.ti – stative.

rdi(w) – Taking as likely stative of result.

mndty.fy m mitt – noun + adverbial, a subordinate clause which goes with the preceding, not a new sentence.

ḫr ḥr.f pds(w) – The particle *ḫr* seems to reinforce the meaning of the stative of result. For the construction, see Gardiner, *EG*^{3}, sec. 239, n. 4.

ḏbꜣ(w) as stative after feminine plural noun; see above.

Medical Commentary

Type of Injury

The location of the nasal *ḥsb* fracture (linear fracture) in Case #12 is over the upper third of the nose, the area called the chamber or vault of his nose: "it is in the middle of his nose, down to the back, and extending to between his two eyebrows," an explanation that, as in the previous case, is easier to understand visualizing the individual lying down in the brow-up position. A vault is an architectural form designed to provide a space with a ceiling. The arch formed by the nasal bones medially, joining the frontal process of the Maxilla, provide a bony ceiling for the antero-superior part of the nose. The upper nasal septum is formed by the perpendicular plate of the ethmoid bone. The quadrangular cartilage inferiorly adds vertical support (fig. 10). The thickness of the nasal bones decreases inferiorly, consequently, most fractures occur in their lower half.

The nasal bones and underlying cartilage are susceptible to fractures because of the prominence of the nose in the center of the face, and its vulnerability to breaking. The type of fracture in Case #12 is produced by a lateral force, involving the lower half of the nasal bone, the nasal process of the maxillary bone, the perpendicular plate of the ethmoid, probably involving the rest of the septum. A strong force in any direction can cause comminution of the nasal bones, resulting in a C-shaped deformity of the nasal septum. The failure begins under the dorsum (bridge) of the nose, extending posteriorly and downward through the perpendicular plate of the ethmoid and the cartilaginous septum[149] (fig. 13a). Most commonly, as previously noted, nasal bone fractures are sustained in fights (34%), accidents (28%), and sports injuries (23%).

Patients usually present with swelling over the nasal bridge and a difference in the appearance or shape of the nose. These lateral impact injuries typically cause a depression of one nasal bone and may result in a lateral displacement of the contralateral nasal bone (fig. 13b).

The physical examination would reveal swelling over the nasal bridge, gross deviation of the nasal bones, and, frequently, periorbital ecchymosis.

The elevation of the head and use of cold compresses in the periorbital and nasal region can be helpful while waiting for edema to subside. The potential for optimal results lies in the reduction of the fracture within the first several hours following the injury before significant edema has appeared. If this window has passed, subsequent reassessment of the injury is advisable, with correction planned between four and seven days following the injury. The reduction of nasal fractures may be performed using an open or a closed technique, but, most nasal fractures may be reduced successfully with closed reduction.[150]

Whenever a septal hematoma is identified, it should be aspirated immediately.

Not all nasal fracture reductions require internal packing with antibiotic-impregnated gauze in each nostril for one to five days, depending primarily on whether the septum needed reduction and whether fractured segments are mobile to gentle palpation. An external rigid splint is applied over a layer of surgical tape.[151]

Nasal fractures usually heal in six weeks.

149. Majorga and Higgins, "Nasal Fracture Reduction."

150. V. R. Dev, et al., "Nasal Fracture Surgery Treatment & Management." Medscape Reference: http://emedicine.medscape.com/article/1283709-treatment.

151. Ibid.

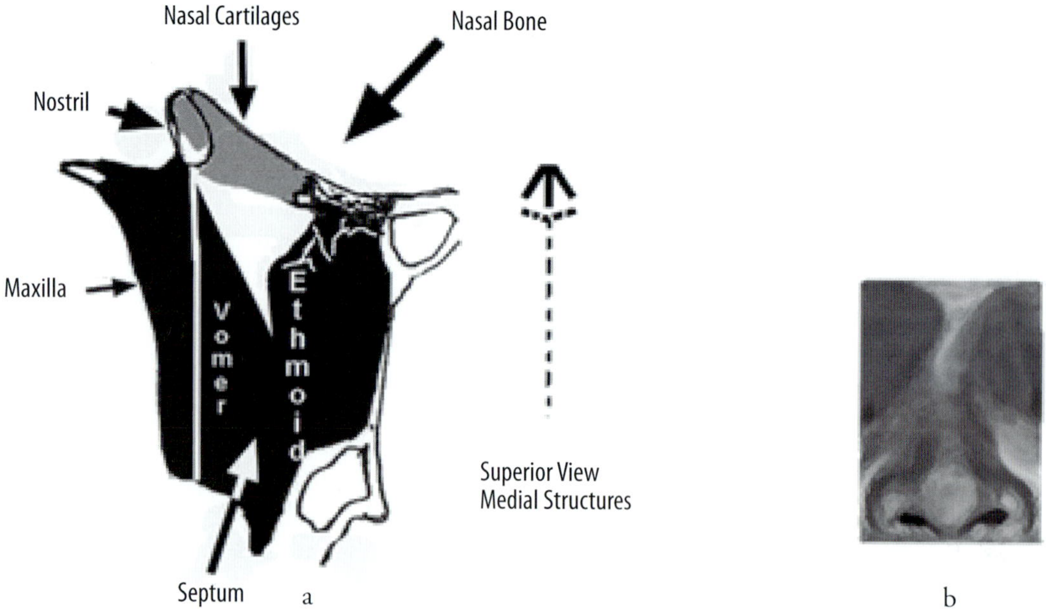

Fig. 13. a) Skeletal nasal vault failure; b) Lateral displacement.

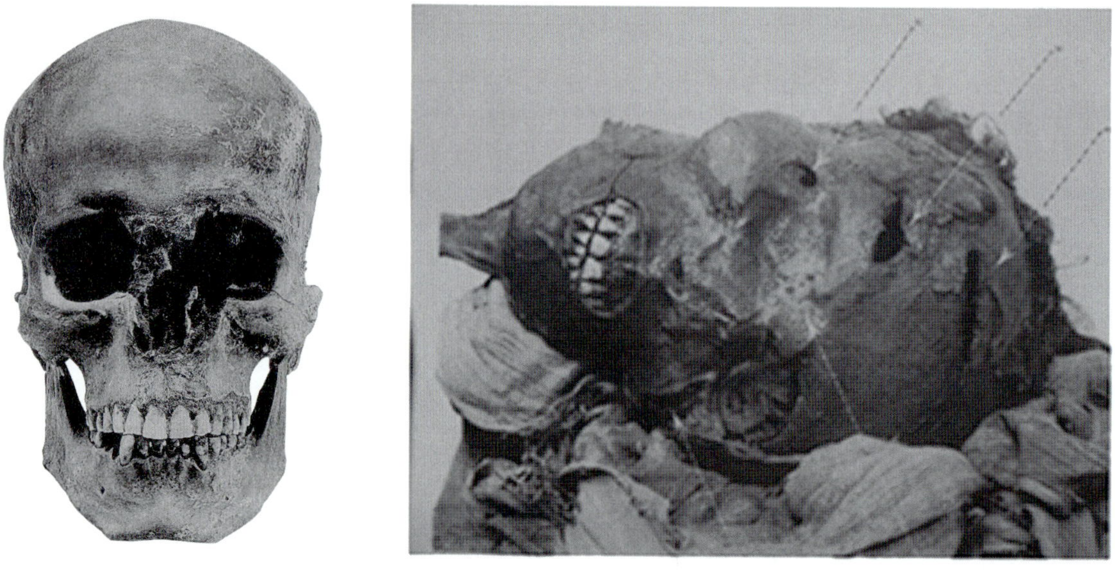

Fig. 14. Nasal fractures in human remains. Left: Soldier #58, from Winlock, *Slain Soldiers of Neb-hep-et-Re Mentu-hotpe*, plate X C. Right: King Seqenenre mummy.

Ancient Medical Methodology and Knowledge

Case #12 is rich in anatomical, clinical, and therapeutic information. Explanation A provides an excellent anatomical description of the area of the nasal bone, joining the frontal process of the maxillary bone, ethmoid perpendicular plate and frontal bone "down and back" (in the brow-up position; fig. 11). Explanation B details the external facial deformities of clinical importance and their causation: "As for 'his nose is crooked, his face having been flattened,' it means his nose is bent and very swollen in its entirety, both of his cheeks (being) likewise, so that his face is flattened because of it; it is not in its proper shape seeing that all the hollows of his face are blocked up with tumefaction, so that his face looks flattened because of it" (fig. 13b). Explanation C describes blood clots formed inside the nose as further explanation of the importance of removing "every eel of blood which has knotted/coagulated inside both of his nostrils/nasal cavities" (fig. 10a and d). The comparison of the stringy blood clots found inside the nasal cavities are compared with the appearance of eels that live in water.

The treatment of these unstable nasal structures consisted of:

- Prompt manual reduction of the fracture: "<Then> you <should> cause it to fall in, it being put in its place (or, so that it is put in its place)."
- Thorough cleansing of intranasal clots: "Swab for him the insides of both his nostrils with two swabs of cloth, until every eel of blood (all the clotted blood), which has knotted/coagulated inside both of his nasal cavities, comes out."
- Lubricated internal nasal packing: "Afterwards, you must place two plugs of cloth saturated with oil, and placed/so that they are placed in both his nostrils."
- External nasal splinting: "You have to apply to him two stiff rolls of cloth, bandaged over it."
- Followed by local dressings with oil and honey.

The treatment principles implemented by the Egyptian physician for this type of fracture are the same as those we employ now with closed reduction. Modern therapeutics has added the use of antibiotics, anesthesia, and surgery, but the underlying principles for the care of a broken nose remain the same.

Examples of trauma to this area from ancient Egyptian human remains can be seen in soldier #58 from Winlock, *Slain Soldiers of Neb-hep-et-Re Mentu-hotpe*, fig. 14 left, and in King Seqenenre Tao II's mummy, fig. 14 right.

CASE #13:
Closed, Comminuted Nasal Fracture with Basilar Skull Fracture and Cerebral Contusion
(Plate VI:3–7)

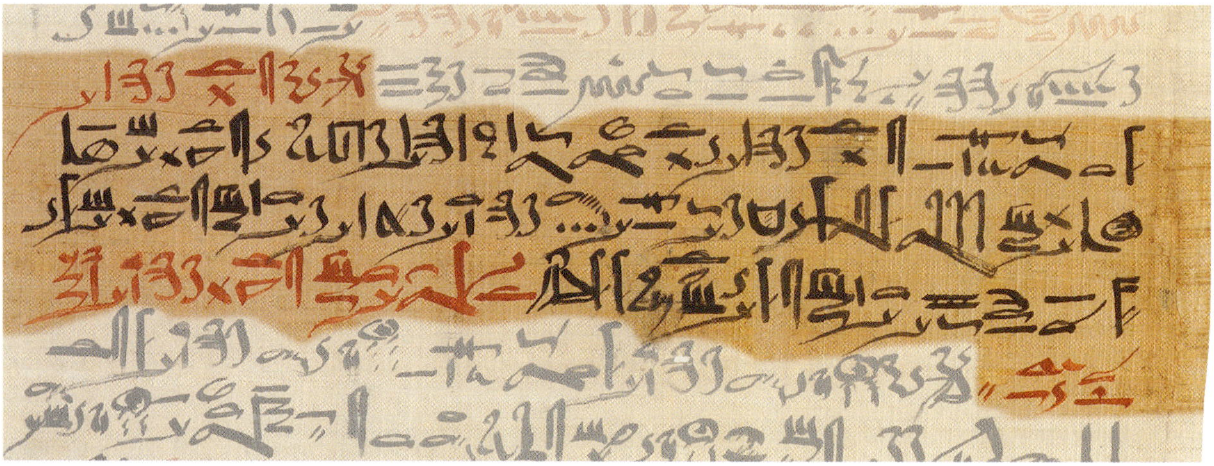

Courtesy New York Academy of Medicine.

3. 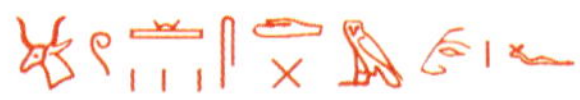

4. 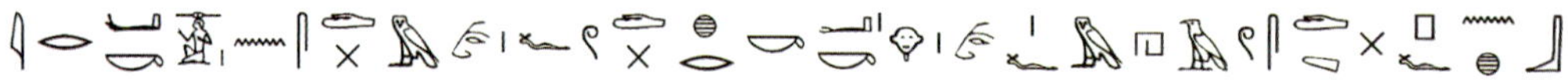

5. 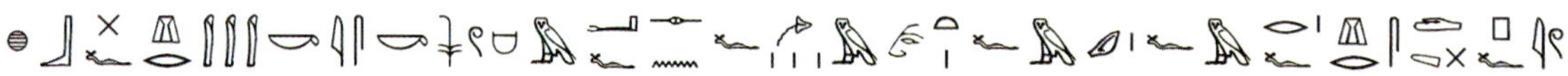

6. 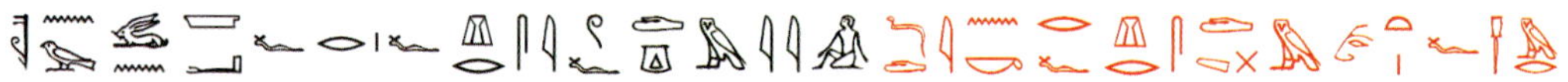

7. 

Transliteration

3§ *šs3w sd m fnd.f*

4§ *ir h3.k s n sd m fnd.f wd.hr.k ʿ.k ḥr fnd.f m-h3w sd pf nḫbḫb.f*

5§ *ẖr ḏbʿw.k isk sw ḥm di.f snf m šrt.f m msḏr.f m r3.f ẖr sd pf jw*

6§ *ḳsn wn.f r3.f ẖr.s iw.f dgmy ḏd.in.k r.f ẖr<y> sḏ m šrt.f mḥr*

7§ *n irw.ny*

Translation

Title:

Necessary knowledge and skills for a crushed fracture in his nose:

Examination:

If you examine a man for a crushed fracture in his nose, you must place your hand on his nose on the area of that smash/burst fracture while (or, so that??) it shifts under your fingers,

and while assuredly, he bleeds from his nasal walls, from his ear and from his mouth because of that crushed fracture,

and it is painful when he opens his mouth because of it, and he is torpid.

Diagnosis:

Then you are to say about him: "One who has a smash/burst fracture in his nasal walls, a medical condition that cannot be handled/dealt with."

Notes

nḫbḫb.f – "while it shifts" (circumstantial *sḏm.f*), or possibly "so that it shifts" (prospective *sḏm.f*)? A medical question that presents itself is, would the palpation be a "testing of the water" in which the physician had to see, very carefully, with hands sensitive to movement and nuances, whether and how much it would shift?

isk sw ḥm di.f – Non-enclitic or initial particle *isk* (cf., Depuydt, *Fundamentals of Egyptian Grammar*, 1:258; Doret, *Narrative Verbal System*, 25) + dependent pronoun subject + enclitic or noninitial particle *ḥm* (Gardiner, *EG*[3], sec. 253, Hoch, *MEG*, sec. 186.3) + circumstantial *sḏm.f* (Doret, *Narrative Verbal System*, 31, 213, index, s.v. *sk/sṯ*). The clause of concomitant circumstance conveys the meaning "at the same time," the particle *ḥm* does not but emphasizes that the patient surely or assuredly bleeds.

iw ḳsn(w) – *iw* + impersonal stative as a statement, see above.

wn.f – Circumstantial *sḏm.f*

šrt.f – See excursus below.

Medical Commentary

Based on the information contained in this papyrus regarding nasal anatomical terminology, we have decided to interpret *fnḏ* as nose; *msdty.fy* as nasal cavities/nostrils and *šrt* as the nasal walls. Discussion about these interpretations can be reviewed in appendix 4.

Type of Injury

Case #13 is a closed comminuted nasal area fracture (*sd*) and is not a simple injury to the nose as the title of this case or Breasted's "Compound Comminuted Fracture in the Side of the Nose" may imply. In the modern classification of cranio-facial fractures, Case #13 is a major craniofacial injury that qualifies as a comminuted

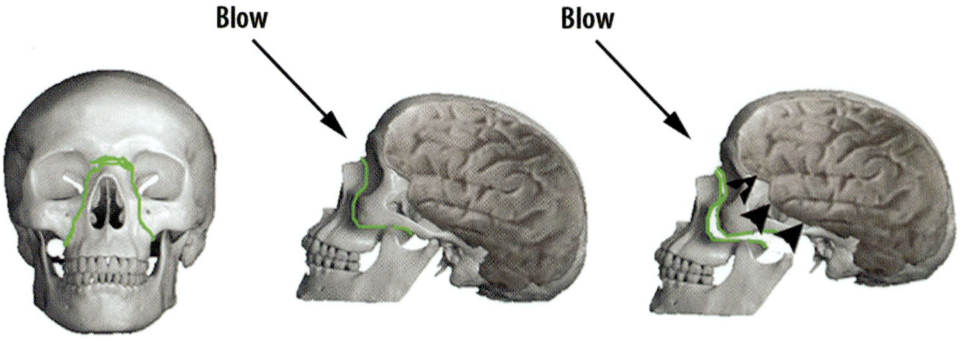

Fig. 15. Le Fort Fracture II.

skull fracture, variant of the Le Fort II cranio-facial disruption,[152] also called "Pyramidal Fracture." The pure Le Fort patterns of craniofacial fractures seldom occur, but mixed variants are common (fig. 15). The type and mechanism of injury necessary to produce a Le Fort II fracture in Case #13 has also produced trauma to the frontal and temporal lobes of the brain by transmitted force from the impact site.

These injuries are today considered under the category of "smash fractures" and named for the primary area of facial involvement.[153] Case #13, under current subclassification, would be considered as a Naso-Frontal, Facial Smash Syndrome. It is also described as a "smash fracture" of the nose in the Edwin Smith Papyrus. The impact producing this type of fracture is a downward blow to the nasal area. The disruption of the skull base is asymmetric in this case with bleeding from his nasal cavity, his ear and his mouth (fig. 4). Nasal bleeding can originate from the direct nasal trauma that produced the compound nasal fracture and could also arise from the anterior skull base. Bleeding from the one ear most likely indicates a unilateral basilar skull fracture in the middle fossa. The source of bleeding from the mouth in Case #13 can be arising from the disrupted nasal structures, or from temporal petrous bone fractures and the roof of the mouth itself, as this type of complex cranio-facial separation tears basal areas of the skull.

Even today with extensive resources available to us to evaluate, monitor, and treat these kind of trauma, we still have significant limitations. The management of cerebral contusion remains indirect, consisting mostly of controlling brain swelling, optimizing cerebral circulation, perfusion pressure, and oxygenation.

Possible complications of basilar skull fractures, such as infection and cerebrospinal fluid leaks are treated today with antibiotics. Persistent leaks require surgical intervention.

---

152. M. J. Noffze, and R. S. Tubbs, "René Le Fort 1869–1951" *Clinical Anatomy* 24 (2011): 278–81. By producing experimental facial fractures in cadavers in 1901, René Le Fort, ("Étude expérimental sur les fractures de la machoire supérieure," *Revue de Chirurgie* 23 (1901): 208–27) observed that these fractures followed the lines of least resistance in the facial bones. He described three main patterns of facial and skull disconnection:

i) Le Fort I a separation of the palate from the maxilla at the level of the piriform rim.

ii) Le Fort II separation of the maxilla from the face. Involve the nasofrontal junction, the frontal process of the maxilla, the anterior maxilla and the medial inferior orbital rim.

iii) Le Fort III separation of the face from the cranium.

153. Additional information on facial fractures can be found in Jesse E. Smith and Carlos L. Perez, "Nasal Fracture Imaging." Medscape Reference: http://www.emedicine.com/radio/topic468.htm#section-introduction#section-introduction. For further reading and discussion of the terms *fnd*, *šrt*, and *msdt*, see our Medical Commentary in Case #14 and Alexander Brawanski's analysis in "Mittelgesichtsverletzungen im Pap. Smith (Fälle 9–14)," 54–56.

Although highly sophisticated surgical reconstruction techniques are now routine, there remain to date, limitations to facial bone reconstruction.

Ancient Medical Methodology and Knowledge

Case #13 is a *sd* (smashed) unilateral injury to the midline facial region. It represents the most severe of the closed comminuted fractures of the nasal area and it is placed in its proper ascending order of severity, characteristic of the Edwin Smith Papyrus. While the blow was to the nasal area, the internal damage to underlying structures was far-reaching. The essential clinical features in this case appear deceptively minor. These are shifting of the fractured nose under the examiner's hand, and hemorrhaging from the nose, ears, and mouth. But there is accompanying evidence of brain injury manifested by "and he is torpid." Alteration of consciousness in Case #13 is identified by the word *dgmy* 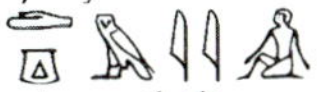, which, in our opinion is most consistent with "torpor," an altered level of consciousness/response/sensibility and motor activity. All of these symptoms and clinical findings are indicative of the degree of craniofacial disruption and cerebral contusion.[154]

The complexity of the skull and neurological injury placed Case #13 beyond any practical treatment capabilities in ancient Egypt, explaining the unfavorable verdict, "a medical condition that cannot be handled/dealt with."

154. The reader is directed to appendix 2 for a compilation of the neurological symptoms and signs in the Edwin Smith Papyrus.

CASE #14:
Perforating Wound to the Interior of the Nasal Walls
(Plate VI:7–14)

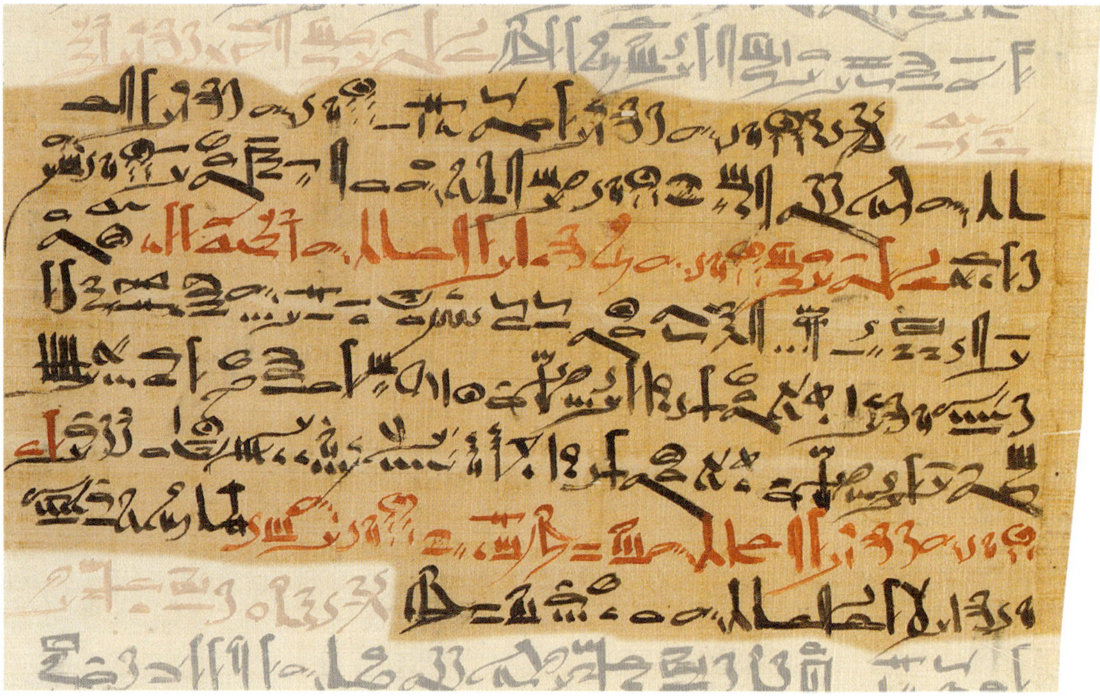

Courtesy New York Academy of Medicine.

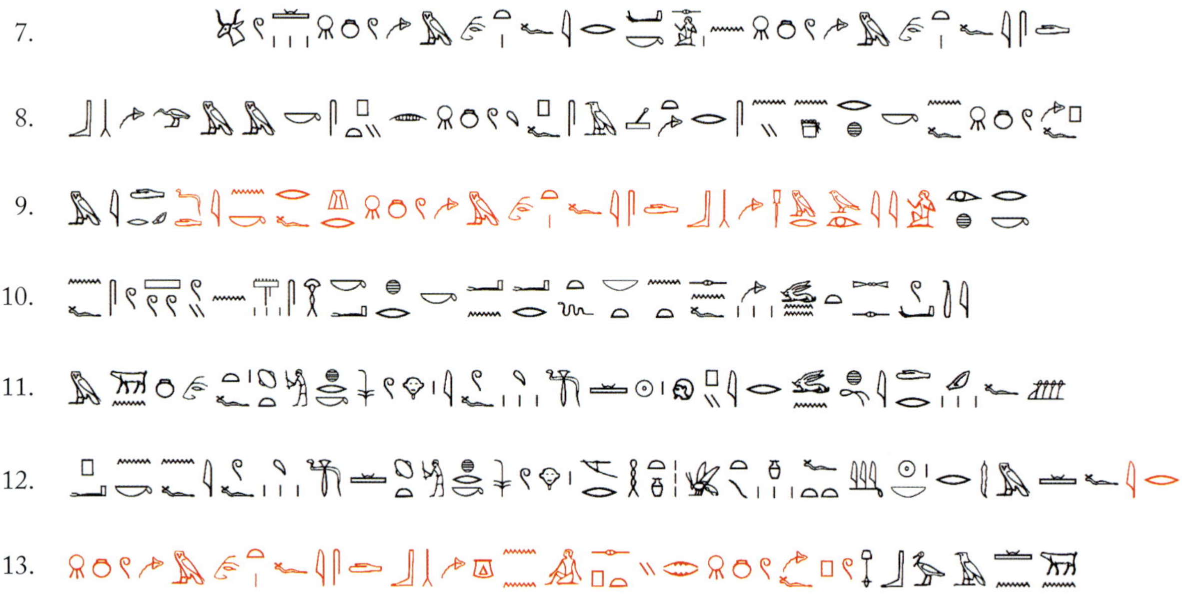

16. 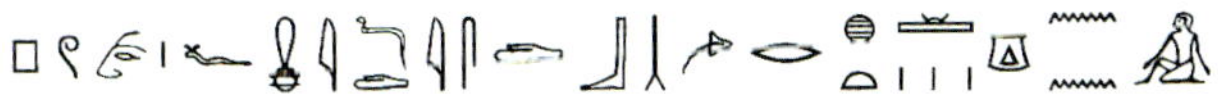

Transliteration

7§ *... šsꜣw wbnw m šrt.f ir ḫꜣ.k s n wbnw m šrt.f isdb*

8§ *gmm.k spty wbnw pf sꜣ.t<i> r sny nḏr.ḫr.k n.f wbnw pf*

9§ *m idr dd.in.k r.f ḫr<y > wbnw m šrt.f isdb mḥr iry.i ir.ḫr.k*

10§ *n.f sšwy n ḥbsw sk.ḫr.k ʿnʿrt nbt nt snf wnnt ṯs.ti*

11§ *m-ḫnw šrt.f wt.ḫr.k sw ḥr iwf wꜣḏ hrw tpy ir wnḫ idrw.f*

12§ *šsp.<i>n.k n.f iwf wꜣḏ wt.ḫr.k sw ḥr mrḥt bit ftt rʿ nb r nḏm.f ir*

13§ *wbnw m šrt.f i.sdb gnn spty wbnw.f pw wbꜣ n ḫnw*

14§ *fnḏ.f mi ḏd sdb r ḫt gnn*

Translation

Title:

Necessary knowledge and skills for a wound into his nasal walls:

Examination:

If you should examine a man for a wound in his nasal walls pierced and collapsed, how you find both lips of that wound (is) shifted one from the another. Then you must draw together/approximate that wound for him with thread/stitching.

Diagnosis:

Then you are to say about him: "One who has a wound in his nasal walls, pierced and collapsed, a medical condition which I will handle/deal with."

Treatment:

You must make for him two swabs of cloth.

You must clean out every eel of blood that exists, coagulated inside his nasal walls.

You must bandage it (along) with fresh meat the first day.

If his stitches shift /loosen, then you are to take (off) the fresh meat for him, and you must bandage it (along) with oil and honey, and a dressing every day until it/he is well.

Explanation:

As for "a wound in his nasal walls, pierced and collapsed," it means, "when the lips of his wound are pulpy/soft and open to the inside of his nose," according as "penetrated/punctured" is said concerning things that are soft.

Notes

isdb – stative (*Grundriss* 8, sec. 164)

šsp.<i>n.k – Agreeing with the emendation to *sḏm.in.f* form.

gnn spty… – This is a 2ae gem. not a 3ae inf. verb (Faulkner, *CDME*, 290), and in this case it is a circumstantial not nominal *sḏm.f.*

sdb – Regarding the possible difference in meaning between *isdb* and *sdb*, it should be noted that there is a parallel passage in Case #26 reading *ḏd.f isdb r ẖt gn* (cf., *Grundriss* 7, 2:826). stative is still morphologically possible without the *i*-augment (and von Deines and Westendorf take this example as a stative also; *Grundriss* 8, 119 with n. 1). Examining all of the occurrences of this root, we have decided that the best understanding is "pierced and collapsed," which also involves the sense of being obstructed.

ẖt modified by form without *t* ending; see above.

Medical Commentary

Based on the information contained in this papyrus regarding nasal anatomical terminology, we have decided to interpret *fnḏ* as nose; *msdty.fy* as nostrils - nasal cavities and *šrt* as the nasal walls. Discussion about these interpretations can be reviewed in appendix 4.

Type of Injury

Case #14 is an open injury piercing the nasal wall, causing tissue to collapse and infold into the nasal cavity. This injury is one of three classified in the Edwin Smith Papyrus as an *isdb* wound, which can be understood as a piercing injury of tissue not supported by bone, whose soft lacerated, and now, disorganized tissue layers, infold (Case #14, Case #26), or outfold (Case #37), obstructing the wound itself.

Regarding technical issues in the treatment of these injuries, it needs to be stressed that the anatomical constitution of tissues in the nose is variable, including, at various points, skin, muscle, independent cartilages, bone, fibro-fatty tissue, and an inner layer of mucosa. A perforation of these tissues by a piercing weapon could easily produce the shifting of layers and their infolding into the nasal cavity.

The current treatment of these injuries requires inspection of the wound and nasal cavity with removal of blood clots, and with particular attention to the possibility of septal hematomas and their drainage. Wound debridement and repair follows as well as mandatory antibiotic coverage. Today repair is best left to the plastic surgeon as it demands precise technical rules to be followed due to the unique nature of these tissues. The mucosal layer needs to be closed with 5–0 or 6–0 absorbable sutures (0.1 mm to 0.07 mm diameter, equivalent to American wire gauge 35–38, 38–40). Cartilage needs not to be sutured, but must be completely covered. The skin of the nose is inflexible and has little redundancy and tears easily with percutaneous stitching. Meticulous skin closure needs to be accomplished using 6–0 nonabsorbable material (0.07 mm diameter American wire gauge 38–40).

Ancient Medical Methodology and Knowledge

As discussed above, the Egyptian physician was detailed in his description of the injury as it penetrated soft and unsupported nasal wall tissue and the shifting of layers of wound margins. These were important in the need, without delay, to correct and carefully restore the margins of these types of wounds. However, given the technology of the day, it was a difficult task. Clearing the nasal cavity from blood clots followed wound closure. Fresh meat was applied over the wound the first day. The master physician calls attention to inspecting the wound for proper healing in that first day, recommending to discontinue the application of fresh meat if the stitches "shifted," meaning the tissue margins were not properly joined. This could have been due to edema or to skin maceration compromising the effectiveness of suturing. As Brawanski points out,[155] wound closure could fail if its edges are not well apposed, or from factors related to the suturing material itself, made of linen or flax. In Case #14 there is no prescription to apply "two linen strips" (adhesive?) to the wound margins, as in other cases in this papyrus where the stitches are found to become loose. Instead, the wound received daily applications of oil and honey dressings, and their protective and antibacterial properties have been discussed above (p. 38).

155. Brawanski, "Mittelgesichtsverletzungen im Pap. Smith (Fälle 9–14)," 55–57.

CASE #15:

Necrotic Maxillary Stab Wound

(Plate VI:14–17)

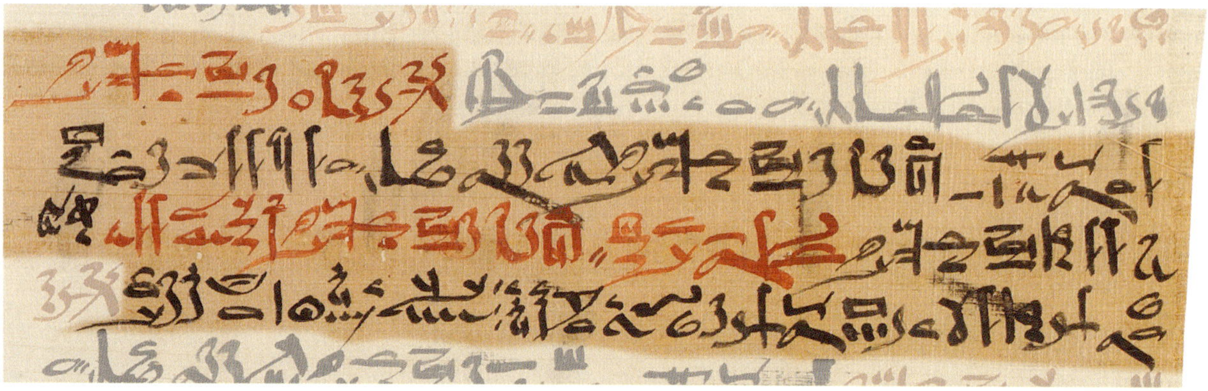

Courtesy New York Academy of Medicine.

14. 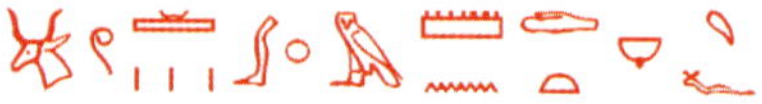

15. 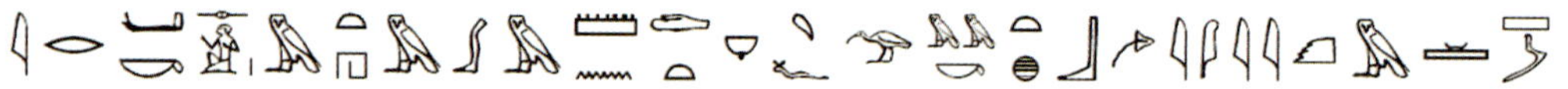

16. 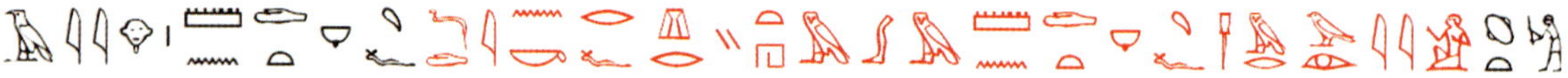

17. 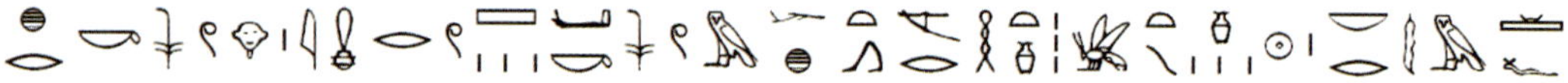

Transliteration

14§ *šsꜣw thm m mndt.f*

15§ *ỉr ḫꜣ.k s n thm m mndt.f gmm.k ṯḥb i.šw.y km šmꜣ.y*

16§ *ḥr mndt.f ḏd.in.k r.f ḫry thm m mndt.f mḥr iry.i wt*

17§ *ḫr.k sw ḥr imrw ḫꜣ.k sw m-ḫt <m> mrḥt bit rꜥ nb r nḏm.f*

Translation

Title:

Necessary knowledge and skills for a perforation in his cheek:

Examination:

If you should examine a man for a perforation in his cheek, how you find the swelling (is) protruding, black, and necrotic/abnormal upon his cheek.

Diagnosis:

then you should say about him: "One who has a perforation in his cheek, a medical condition which I will handle/deal with."

Treatment:

You must bandage it (along) with alum (or, a bandage with alum[?] shavings?) and you should treat it thereafter <with> oil and honey every day until it/he is well.

Notes

išwy km(w) šmꜣy – statives.

šmꜣy is apparently related to *šmꜣw* "disease-demons, disease-bringing entities" (Faulkner, *CDME*, 266; *Wb.* 4:471). This is in turn considered to be related to *šmꜣw* "foreigners, wanderers" (Faulkner, *CDME*, 266; *Wb.* 4:470). For thematic connections between disease and foreigners, and disease as a result of the presence of foreigners, see D. B. Redford, *Pharaonic King-lists, Annals and Day-books* (Mississauga, Ont.: Benben, 1986), 276–96. Returning to the word *šmꜣy* itself, in line with the apparent meaning of infection or inflammation, it is perhaps tempting, though quite tentative, to wonder if it could possibly be connected to *šmm* "be hot, have fever, become feverish," *šmmt* "fever, inflammation" (Faulkner, *CDME*, 267, *Wb.* 4:468–69 s.v. *šm*). One wonders whether they might share a biliteral root *šm*. There is an extensive literature devoted to biliteral roots in Egyptian as well as Semitic and elsewhere in Afroasiatic.[156] Even if an etymological connection is not valid, one wonders if a punning association between *šmꜣy* etc. and *šmm* could have reinforced the idea of fever in connection with *šmꜣy*.

imrw – *Grundriss* 6, 33 considers it "an unknown mineral(?)." *imrw* surprisingly does not seem to be referred to in Aufrère's *L'univers minéral dans la pensée égyptienne*. The spelling *imirw* (sic) is at first glance suggestive of a "mixed spelling," the Egyptian way of indicating phonetic change while keeping at least some of the original spelling intact, and seems to indicate a phonetic change from *imrw* to **imiw* (cf. Gardiner, *EG*^{3}, sec. 279; Hoch, *MEG*, sec. 7). More specifically I think it very likely that the writing *i* + *mi* + *r* + *w* is a holdover from an Old Kingdom writing in which the original phonetic value *mr* of what we think of in Middle Egyptian as the *mi* sign was used, with *r* as the original phonetic complement; see Edel, *AG*, sec. 762. Old Kingdom texts feature writings with the phonetic complement *r* and some with the complement *i* in which the change has already taken place (Edel, *AG*, sec. 30). The word *ibnw* referred to by Nunn (*Ancient Egyptian Medicine*), is given in *Grundriss* 6, 22–23, where it is defined as "alum" on the basis of the Coptic derivative ⲱⲃⲉⲛ. Thus also Aufrère, *L'univers minéral dans la pensée égyptienne*, 2:605–6. I am grateful to Dr. Gonzalo Sanchez for sending me the article on Edwin Smith by Brawanski ("Die Wirbelsäulenverletzungen des Papyrus Edwin Smith (Fälle 29–33)," *Studien*

156. See, e.g., Giovanni Conti, *Studi sul bilitterismo in semitico e in egiziano* (Quaderni de semitistica 9; Florence: Istituto di linguistica e di lingue orientali, Università di Firenze, 1980); Edel, *AG*, sec. 427–28 with *Nachträge*, sec. 427; C. T. Hodge, "Afroasiatic S-Causative," *Language Sciences* 15 (1971): 41–43; A. S. Kaye, "The Nature of the Root in Semitic and Egyptian," *Festschrift in Honor of the Twenty-Fifth Anniversary of California State University, Fullerton* (ed. J. Kalir; Fullerton, CA: California State University, 1984), 93–111; Meltzer, review of Jürgen Osing, *Die Nominalbildung des Ägyptischen*, *Journal of the American Research Center in Egypt* 15 (1978): 142–45; William A. Ward, *The Four Egyptian Homographic Roots B-3: Etymological and Egypto-Semitic Studies* (Studia Pohl, Series Maior 6; Rome: Pontifico Istituto Biblico, 1978).

zur altägyptischen Kultur 32 [2004]: 59–80). Brawanski discusses the word *imrw* (65–66). He writes that the understanding as a bandage can be justified because the determinative is ambiguous and could represent either a stone or a piece of bandage, and he suggests a rendering that includes both elements: "astringent bandage (with metal shavings)." He notes that if used with care, analogies can be made with the Coptic medical Papyrus Chassinat from the ninth to tenth centuries AD, which refers to the addition of metal shavings to a salve medium. Brawanski does not refer to the work of Aufrère on minerals and the identification of alum referred to earlier. Thus, the suggested parenthetical translation follows the translation and discussion of Brawanski, "Wirbelsäulenverletzungen des Papyrus Edwin Smith (Fälle 29–33)," 65–66, but with query because of what I think are the uncertainties that remain.

Medical Commentary

Type of Injury

This is a stab wound to the maxillary-zygomatic area. This appears to be a soft tissue perforation of the maxillary area, which is elevated by underlying hemorrhage and swelling with necrotic tissue visible on its surface. The facial soft tissues over the maxilla are very thin and bone injury would have very likely simultaneously occurred. Under these circumstances gangrene results from tissue devascularization at the injury site and could also arise from infection. Even though infection would have been an ever-present complication with such a wound, Case #15 gives no evidence suggesting that infection has developed. Injuries such as this can be encountered in our day from motor vehicle and construction accidents, recreational wilderness sports, and are common in warfare by explosives.

Today's evaluation of zygomatic/cheek-penetrating lacerations must include examination of the parotid gland and the facial nerve branches. Examining the facial nerve function requires testing motor function in each of its branches: temporal, zygomatic, nasal, buccal, mandibular, and cervical. Treatment of simple cheek lacerations is done under local anesthesia with thorough wound cleansing. Along with damaged and necrotic tissue debridement, removal of foreign bodies is mandatory. Suturing is done with 6-0 monofilament (0.07 mm diameter, equivalent to American wire gauge 38-40) taking special care in reconstruction of skin creases. Deep lacerations may require parotid gland or nerve repair, which should be done at the time. Should the wound have signs of a deep necrotizing infection (a complication produced by beta-hemolytic streptococcus or clostridia), aggressive medical and surgical treatment would be necessary to avert potentially lethal complications of toxic syndrome or gas gangrene.[157]

Ancient Medical Methodology and Knowledge

Perforating facial injuries such as the one described in Case #15 would have been frequent in warfare with injuries produced by arrows, daggers, or small missiles. The prominent position of the malar/zygomatic area in the face makes it quite vulnerable. The injured tissues are described in detail as being swollen, black, and necrotic. The word *šmꜣy* as used here conveys the sense of diseased tissue that is not evolving towards normal healing. In Case #15 the problem appears to be tissue necrosis more than an infection. In Case #41 we will see that the same word, *šmꜣy*, indicates sepsis probably associated with tissue necrosis. *šmꜣy* is apparently related to *šmꜣw* "disease-demons, disease-bringing entities."

157. Trott, *Wounds and Lacerations*, 162–64, 271–72.

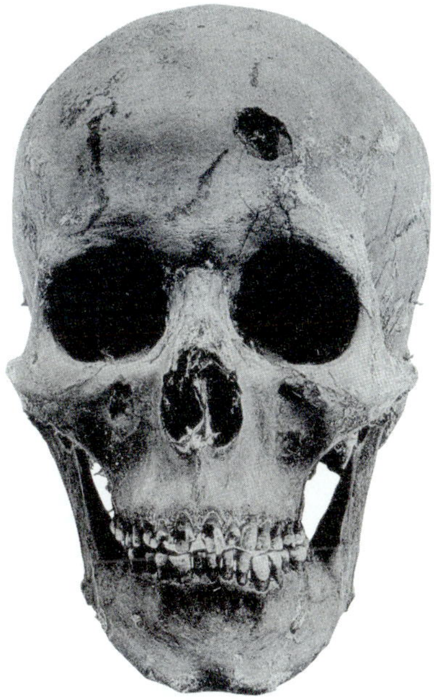

Fig. 16. Right maxillary fracture and left frontal penetrating fracture.
Soldier #25, from Winlock, *Slain Soldiers of Neb-hep-et-Re Mentu-hotpe*, plate IX B.

The initial wound treatment was bandaging it with alum.[158] Our assumption is that alum would be acting as an astringent, favoring soft tissue contraction and reducing inflammation. Afterward oil and honey bandages are advocated. As discussed above, these substances would have provided wound protection and bactericidal effects. The patient was expected to do well.

From the human remains material available for study from ancient Egypt, the mummy of King Seqenenre Tao II[159] exhibits a left cheek injury with malar bone fracture produced by a Syro-Palestinian penetrating battle-axe. The king's injury is much more severe than the one described in Case #15. The king received other head injuries, four of which were lethal (figs. 6, 14, and Visual Index V). Soldier # 25 of Winlock's *Slain Soldiers of Neb-hep-et-Re Mentu- hotpe* (fig. 16) shows a right maxillary penetrating injury and other craniofacial fractures.

158. J. W. Estes, *The Medical Skills of Ancient Egypt* (Canton, MA: Science History Publications, 1993), 139.

159. M. Bietak and E. Strouhal, "Die Todesumstände des Pharaos Seqenenre (17. Dynastie)," *Ann Naturhistor Mus Wein* 78 (1974): table 6.

CASE #16:
Closed, Displaced Maxillary-Zygomatic Fracture
(Plate VI:17–21)

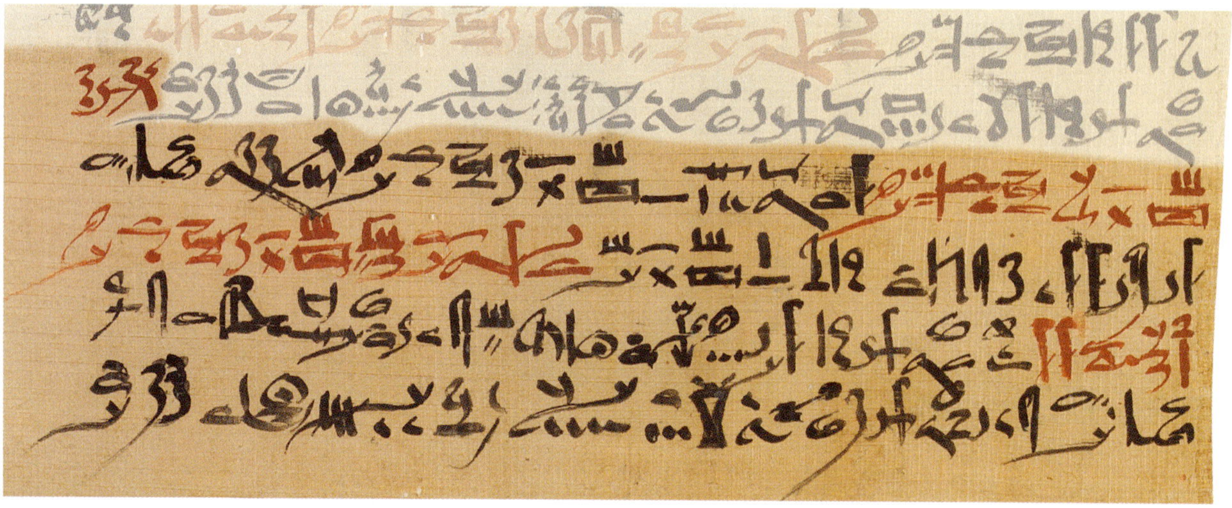

Courtesy New York Academy of Medicine.

17. 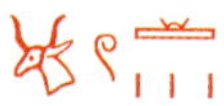

18. 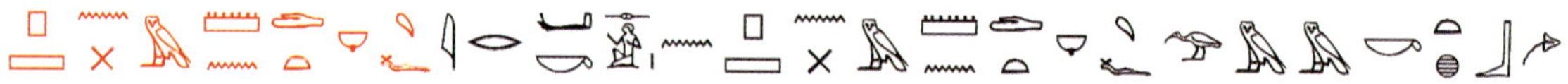

19. 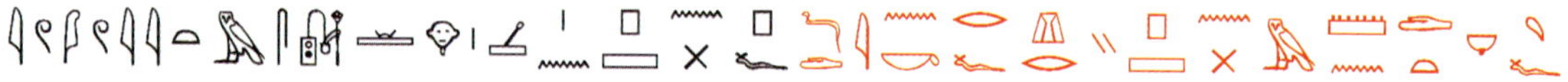

20. 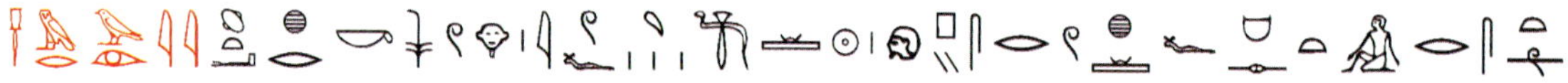

21. 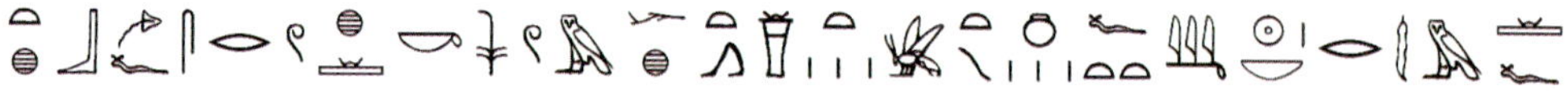

Transliteration

17§ … *šsꜣw*

18§ *pšn m mndt.f ir ḫꜣ.k s n pšn m mndt.f gmm.k tḥb*

19§ *iw šwy ṯms ḥr-sꜣ n pšn pf ḏd.in.k r.f ḫry pšn m mndt.f*

20§ *mḥr iry.<i> wt.ḫr.k sw ḥr iwf wꜣḏ hrw tpy srwḫ.f ḥmst r sṯꜣ*

21§ *tḫb.f srwḫ.k sw m-ḫt mrḥt bit ftt rꜥ nb r nḏm.f*

Translation

Title:

Necessary knowledge and skills for a split fracture in his cheek:

Examination:

If you should examine a man for a split fracture in his cheek, how you find the swelling (is): it is(?) protruding/ swollen and red on the outside of that split/fracture,

Diagnosis:

then you are to say about him: "One who has a split fracture in his cheek, a medical condition which <I> will handle/deal with."

Treatment:

Then you have to bandage it (along) with fresh meat the first day.

His treatment is: sitting (upright), in order to reduce his swelling.

You should treat it afterwards with ointment and honey and a dressing every day until it/he is well.

Notes:

iw šwy (sic?) – The precise identification of the form is difficult and the syntax seems to be unusual, though the general meaning is clear. *Grundriss* 7, 2:841–42 seems a bit uncertain or inconsistent in handling this form, or this type of writing (whether or not it always represents the same form). Von Deines and Westendorf (840) list a writing *iwšwy* in Case 12 as *sḏm.f* without dividing it into *iw* + *šwy*, as we did (we took it as a statement of fact with *iw sḏm.f*). In the present passage, von Deines and Westendorf (842) read *gmm.k tẖb šwy tms ḥr sꜣ n pšn pf*, which at least implies that they are emending the text to delete the *iw* or are otherwise disregarding it. It cannot be a *iw sḏm.f* construction here. I also cannot justify taking *iw* as a writing of the prothetic reedleaf at this time period, though in later periods it would not raise an eyebrow, nor do I think an emendation meets the standard of textual criticism to which we are attempting to adhere. Somewhat provisionally I am taking it as *iw* + impersonal stative, with the *iw* governing two statives, both *šwy* and *tms*(*w*); see Gilula, "The stative Form of the Verb *sḏm* 'to hear'," 38–39. The grammatical phenomenon is "gapping"; cf. Doret, "La forme *sḏm.n.f* Narrative," 13–22. The syntax of the passage is unexpected, because most frequently the complement to a manner nominalization such as *gmm.k tẖb* is a circumstantial or adverbial element, not a statement. Nor is the passage beginning with *gmm.k* a *Wechselsatz*, because that formation overwhelmingly comprises a pair of "balanced" or "correlative" or "reciprocal" nominal forms or manner nominalizations (Hoch, *MEG*, sec. 152). The one type of exception admitted by Polotsky is the type of sentence in which an affirmative first member is followed by a negative second member using the *n sḏm.n.f* negation, whereas in other cases the expected construction with *tm* is used; see H. J. Polotsky, "Ägyptische Verbalformen und ihre Vokalisation," *Orientalia* 33 (1964): 282. I am leaving a question mark in both the transliteration and translation because of the various uncertainties surrounding this form.

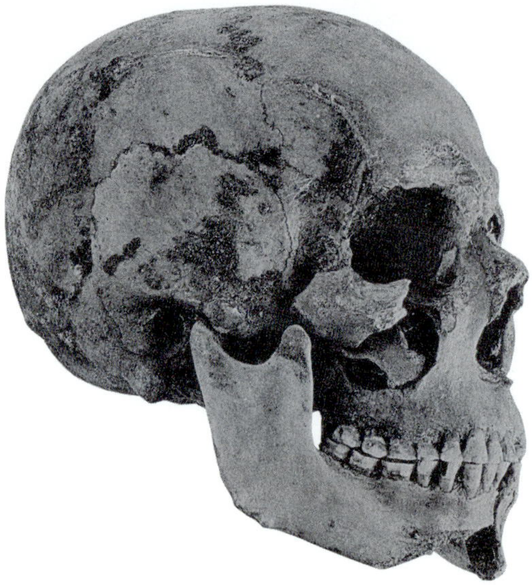

Fig. 17. Displaced maxillary-zygomatic fracture. Soldier #29, from Winlock, *Slain Soldiers of Neb-hep-et-Re Mentu-hotpe*, plate X B.

Medical Commentary

Type of Injury

The injury in Case #16 is a *pšn* fracture, a closed, split-type fracture of the malar/zygomatic bone on the face. By its prominent position in the face the cheek area is, second to the nose, vulnerable to injury. The word *pšn* is used consistently in this papyrus for injuries in which bone fragmentation involves bone plate separation and displacement produced by tangential blows. Production of such fracture requires an impact of 100 g or more.

Common symptoms in such injuries are pain, edema, and local ecchymosis of the cheek and eyelids. Traumatic trismus and orbital floor disruption are not uncommon.[160] Although no specific neurological symptoms are noted here, in this type of trauma a significant degree of force is transmitted to the orbit and the brain.

Ancient Medical Methodology and Knowledge

The appearance of the wound indicates significant swelling but not an open wound. There is no evidence of alteration of level of consciousness, speech impairment, or eye injury. Local treatment is implemented by initial covering of the traumatized area with fresh meat for the first day, then by oil and honey dressings until the wound heals. Keeping the patient in the sitting position is recommended to reduce the patient's facial swelling.

In the human remains material from ancient Egypt, a *pšn* [split/elevated fracture] injury over the right maxilla is evident in soldier no. 29 of Winlock's Deir el-Bahari cache (fig. 17).

160. J. L. Burns and S. J. Blackwell, "Plastic Surgery," *Sabiston Textbook of Surgery* (18th ed.; ed. Beauchamp Townsend and Mattox Evers; Philadelphia: Elsevier, 2008), 2142; T. T. Tollefson and E. B. Strong, "Zygomaticomaxillary Complex Fractures." Medscape Reference: http://emedicine.medscape.com/article/867687-overview.

CASE #17:
Cranio-Facial Injury with Comminuted Maxillary-Zygomatic Fractures and Basilar Skull Fractures of the Anterior and Middle Fossae
(Plate VII:1–7)

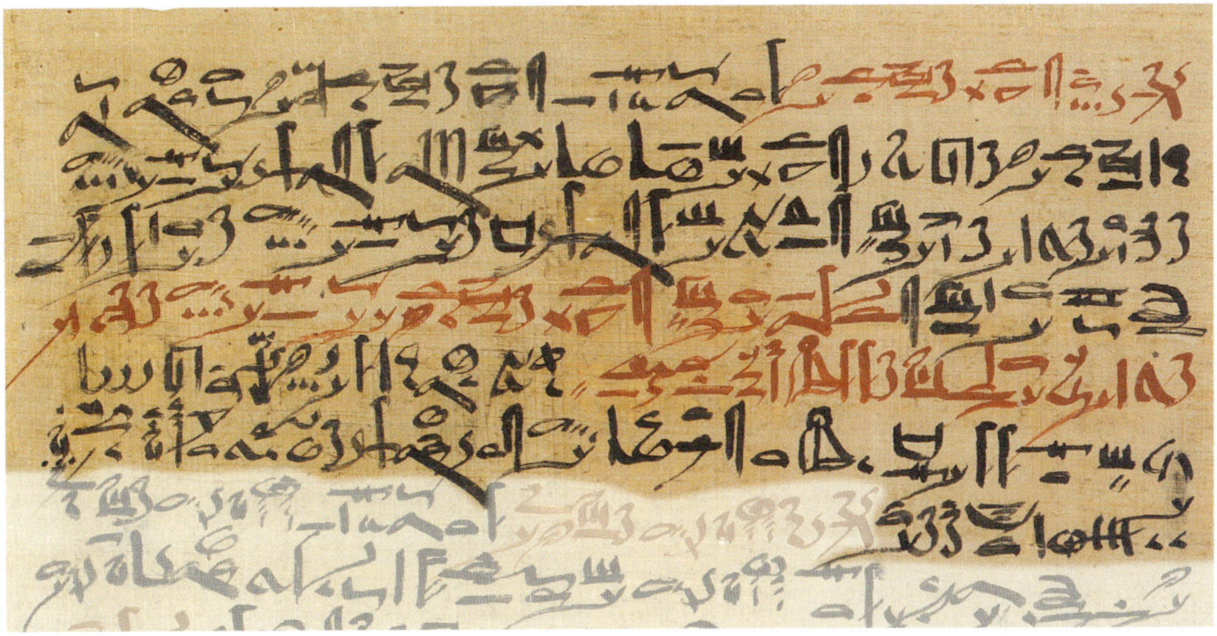

Courtesy New York Academy of Medicine.

1. 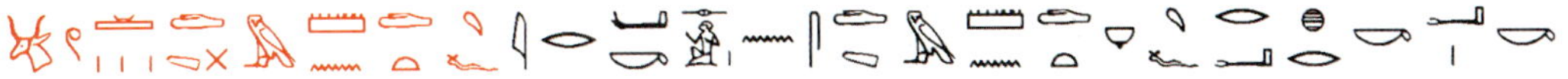

2. 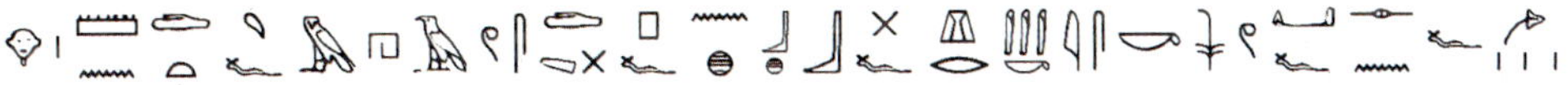

3. 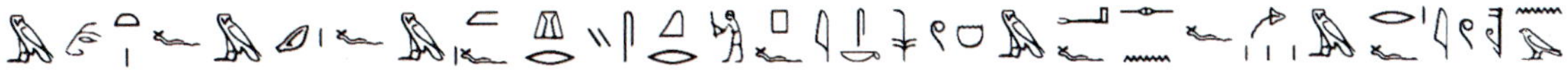

4. 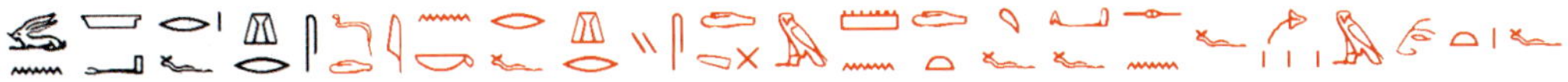

5. 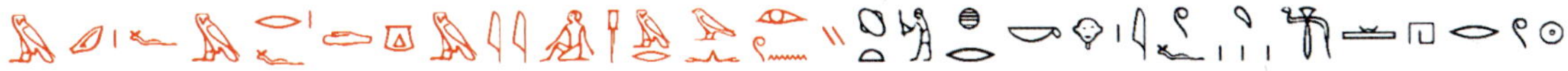

6. 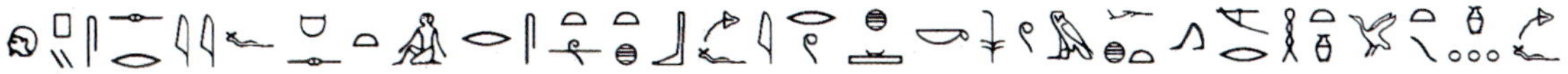

7. 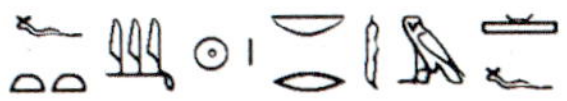

Transliteration

1§ *šsꜣw sḏ m mndt.f i͗r ḫꜣ.k s n sd m mndt.f rdi͗.ḫr.k ꜥ.k*

2§ *ḥr mndt.f m-hꜣw sd pf nḫbḫb.f ẖr ḏbꜥw.k. i͗sk sw di͗.f snf*

3§ *m šrt.f m msḏr.f m gs.f ẖry sḳr pf i͗sk sw ḥm dj.f snf m rꜣ.f i͗w ḳsn*

4§ *wn rꜣ.f ẖr-s ḏd.i͗n.k r.f ẖry sd m mndt.f di͗.f snf m šrt.f*

5§ *m msḏr.f m rꜣ.f dgm.y mḥr n i͗rw.ny wt.ḫr.k <sw> ḥr i͗w.f wꜣḏ hrw*

6§ *tpy sry.f ḥmst r sṯꜣ tḫb.f srwḫ.k sw m-ḫt mrḥt bi͗t*

7§ *ftt rꜥ nb r nḏm.f*

Translation

Title:

Necessary knowledge and skills concerning a crushed fracture in his cheek:

Examination:

If you should examine a man for a crushed fracture in his cheek, you must put your hand on his cheek in the environs of that crushed fracture, that it might shift/crepitate under your fingers, while he is bleeding from his nasal walls and from his ear on his side that has that injury from a blow/strike wound, while at the same time assuredly he bleeds from his mouth, and opening his mouth is painful/it is painful when his mouth has been opened(?) because of it,

Diagnosis:

then you are to say about him: "One who has a crushed fracture in his cheek, while he bleeds from his nasal walls, from his ear, and from his mouth and is torpid, a medical condition that cannot be handled/dealt with."

Treatment:

You must bandage <it> (along) with fresh meat the first day.

His treatment protocol(?) is sitting (upright), in order to reduce his swelling.

You should treat it afterward with oil and honey, and dressing every day until he/it is well.

Notes

hꜣw – Faulkner, *CDME*, 157.

nḫbḫb.f – Prospective *sḏm.f*. Because of the intervening *sḏm.ḫr.f* form, it is not feasible to take *nḫbḫb.f* as a continuation of the *i͗r sḏm.f* protasis.

i͗w ḳsn(w) wn rꜣ.f – *i͗w* + circumstantial *sḏm.f* as statement of fact, or possibly *i͗w* + stative + passive *sḏm(w).f*, though I think that is the less likely rendering. This is not identical to the passage in Case 13, *i͗w ḳsn(w) wn.f rꜣ.f*, which I understand as *i͗w* + stative + circumstantial *sḏm.f*.

sry.f – This word is a lexicographical challenge; Dr. Sanchez has summed up the result of our discussions as follows: *Grundriss* 7, 2:773 gives *sri* the translation "lagern (?)." If we consider that Case #17 falls into the category of severe head injuries—an impact to the cheek in which there have also been fractures to the base of the skull (bleeding from the nose, the ear, and the mouth) and the patient is torpid—in these cases it makes sense to treat this patient under observation/isolation/encampment/stored, deposited, etc. As previously discussed, the sitting position helps to reduce intracranial pressure and facilitate breathing. If "lagern" applies, it can be referring to the actual "observation/isolation/encampment." The purpose of such a setting is to allow the patient to be under quiet observation. "*Lagern*" could also apply to supporting the patient, literally, in the sitting position.

The word "protocol" makes sense in the sense that it encompasses measures to be implemented automatically in an emergency room or an Intensive care unit in specific situations, such as burns, or head injuries, or heart attacks. This word also applies to the treatment of Case #20 (head injury) and Case #32 (neck injury but without neurological spinal cord involvement, and head injury also).

Wb. 4:190 gives another verb *sr* with walking legs determinative, which it does not define. Meeks, *Année Lexicographique* 1, 332, defines it as "to show, to introduce," citing *Koptisches Handwörterbuch* (Heidelberg: Winter, 1965–77), 537 where it is compared with Coptic ⲥⲱⲓ. It probably has nothing to do with the present word.

Medical Commentary

Type of Injury

This case is the most severe trauma to the malar/zygomatic bone area in the papyrus, and is a comminuted "smash/*sd*" type of closed fracture of the malar/zygomatic bone caused by focused blunt trauma. The clinical information indicates that this probably is a craniofacial injury. As with Case #13, pure Le Fort patterns of craniofacial fractures seldom occur, but mixed variants are common. Case #17 likely represents a Le Fort type III[161] cranial fracture from a blow to the upper maxilla or nasal bridge, or a Le Fort type II variant of cranial fracture from a blow to the lower or mid-maxilla (fig. 18a).

The cheekbones are formed by the zygomatic-maxillary complex (ZMC), which is composed of the zygomatic bone articulating with the frontal bone, the maxilla, the greater wing of the sphenoid, and the temporal bone. During impact, this bone complex is pushed backwards and out, with downward rotation (fig. 18a). Crepitus was found during examination of the fracture site, and profuse bleeding was present from the mouth. In this kind of injury, bleeding from the mouth could originate from disruption at the base of the skull, the jaw and/or the maxilla. Bleeding is also described occurring from the nostril and the ear on the side of the injury, a pattern of hemorrhaging consistent with ipsilateral basilar skull fractures of the anterior and the middle fossa of the skull.[162]

The clinical features in Case #17 are similar to those in Case #13. While both are consistent with craniofacial disruption and extensive damage to the face and to the entire cranium, the difference is the site of impact. A common feature to both these injuries is their severity, with evidence of traumatic brain injury manifested by alteration of the level of consciousness and listlessness. This symptom is expressed by the word *dgmy* 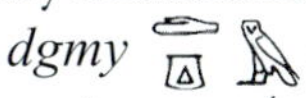, which, in our opinion, is most consistent with "torpor," defined as an altered level of consciousness/response/sensibility and reduced motor activity. The latter feature is emphasized by use of the  determinative.

For further discussion of the term *dgmy* please refer to the medical commentary in Case #22.

Today management of this kind of injury requires, prior to addressing treatment of the fractures, stabilization of the patient's general condition with proper ventilation and circulation, neurological evaluation, and

161. Burns and Blackwell, "Plastic Surgery," 2142; Kris S. Moe, Patrick Byrne, David W. Kim, and Adele R. Tawfilis. "Maxillary and Le Fort Fractures." Medscape Reference: http://emedicine.medscape.com/article/1283568-overview.

162. The reader is directed to appendix 2 for a compilation of the neurological symptoms and signs in the Edwin Smith Papyrus.

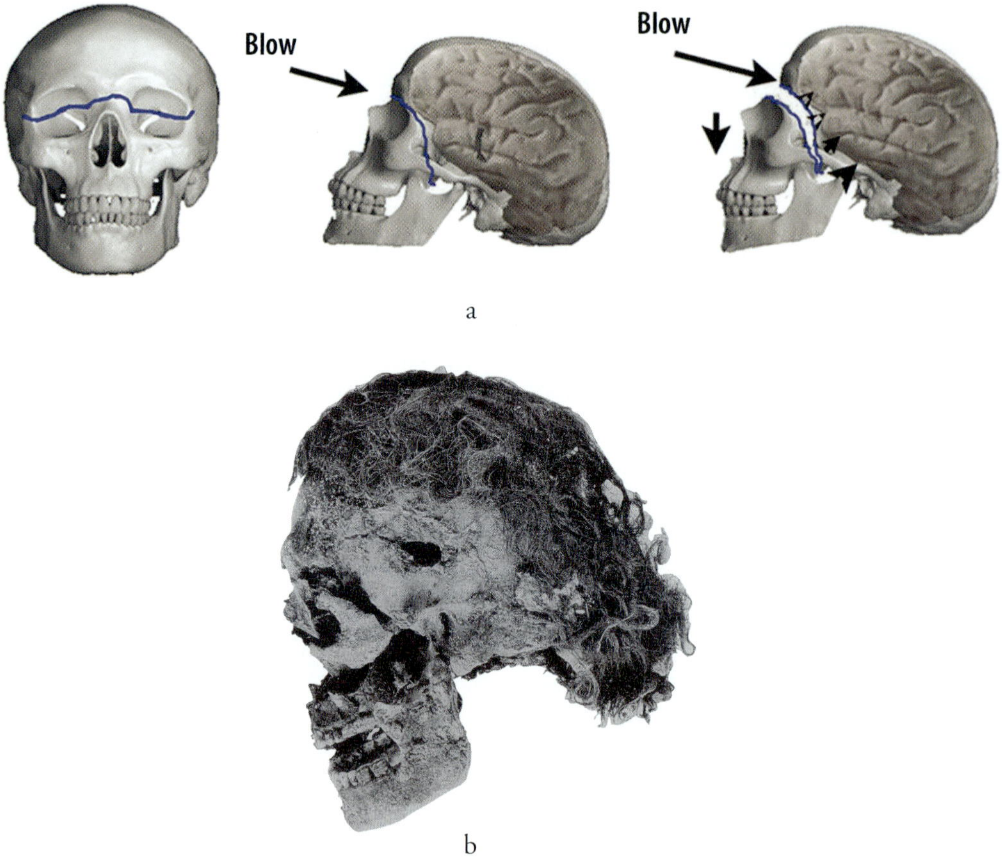

Fig. 18. a) Le Fort Fracture III; b) Soldier #23, from Winlock, *Slain Soldiers of Neb-hep-et-Re Mentu-hotpe*, plate IX A, with Le Fort III fracture.

assessment of the cervical spine. The surgical treatment is complex exposure, decompression, reconstruction and fixation, requiring surgeons in the maxillofacial, ear, nose, and throat specialties.

Ancient Medical Methodology and Knowledge

Instructions are for examination of the fractured area for bone shifting, crepitus, and difficulty opening of the patient's mouth. As in the other case of major craniofacial injury, Case #13, the verdict is, "a medical condition that cannot be handled/dealt with." This verdict conveys the fact that there was not expectation of correcting the problem by the treatment measures available at that time. However, the patient is not abandoned, and wound treatment and supportive care in the sitting position are implemented. With the patient's level of consciousness being depressed (torpid), it is likely that some sort of physical support to keep him in the sitting position was necessary, that being perhaps the meaning of the word "*sry*," which was interpreted by Allen, "He should be forced to sit" (*AM*, 85). Local trauma measures and support were all that the ancients could do for these complex injuries.

Soldier #23 of Winlock's Deir el-Bahari cache shows evidence of a Le Fort type III fracture (fig. 18b).

CASE #18:

Temporo-Zygomatic Laceration

(Plate VII:7–14)

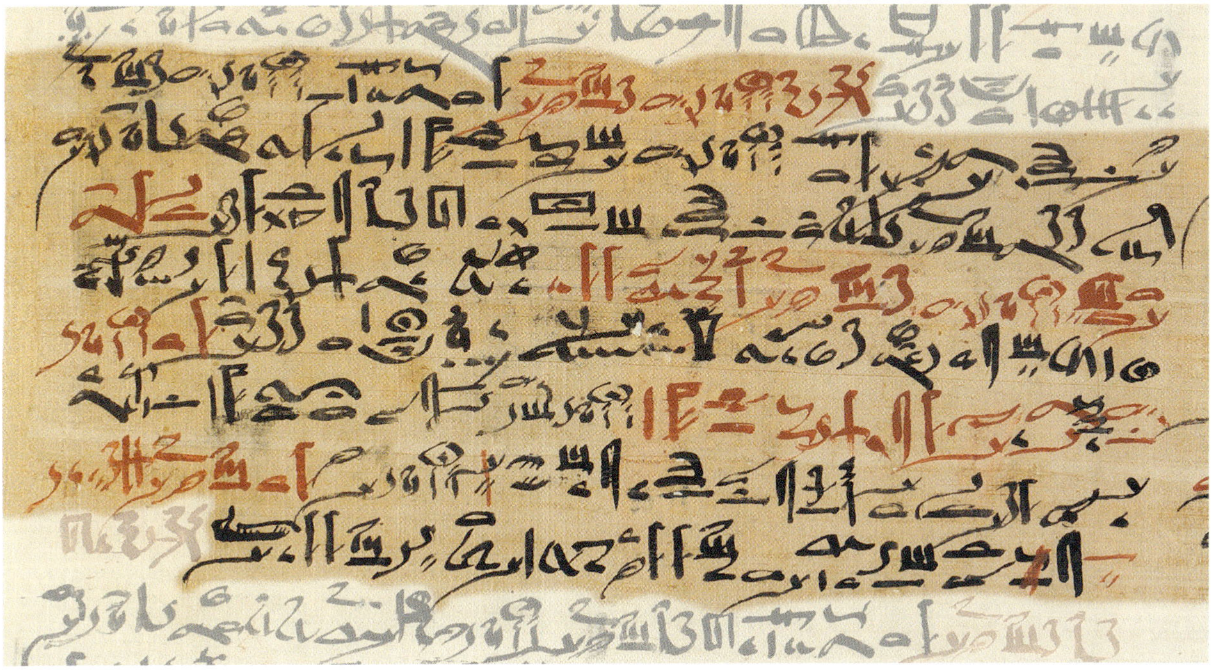

Courtesy New York Academy of Medicine.

7. 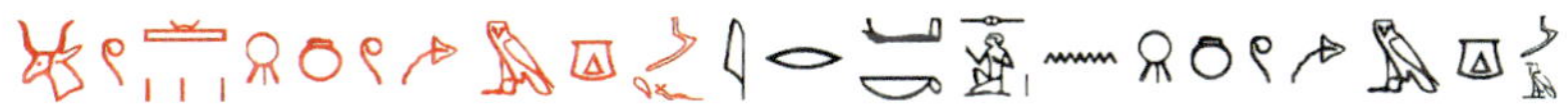

8. 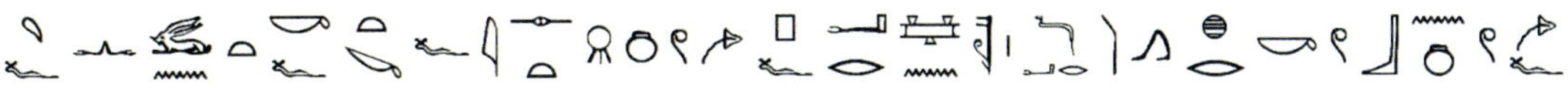

9. 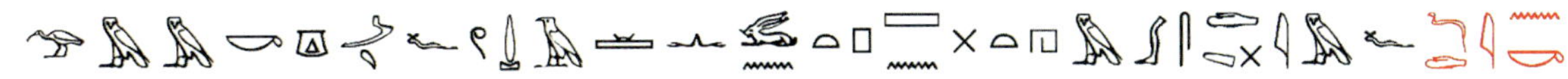

10. 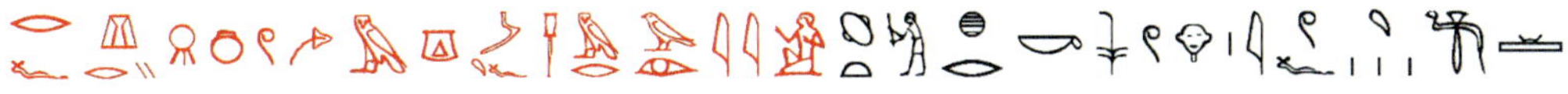

11. 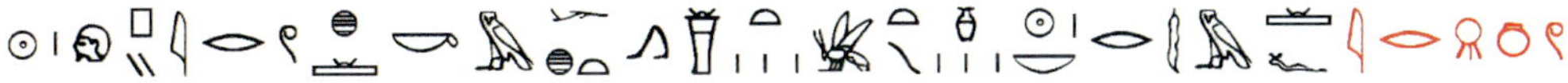

12. 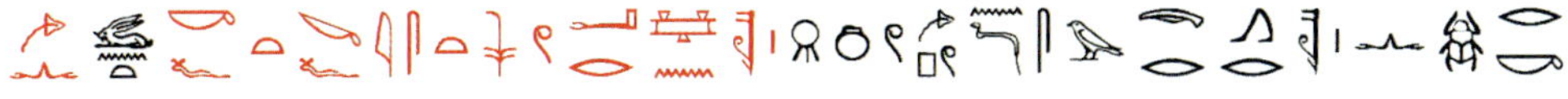

13. 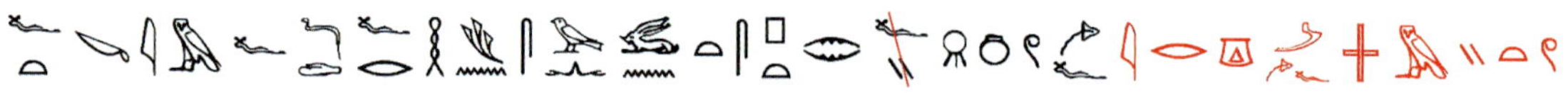

14. 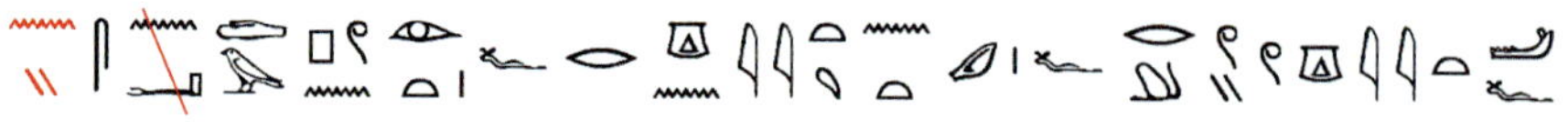

Transliteration

7§ … *šsꜣw wbnw m gmꜣ.f ỉr ḫꜣ.k s n wbnw m gmꜣ.f*
8§ *nj wnt kft.{f} ỉsṯ wbnw pf ꜥr n ḳs ḏꜥr.ḫr.k wbnw.f*
9§ *gmm.k gmꜣ.f wḏꜣ n wnt pšn thm sḏ ỉm.f ḏd.jn.k*
10§ *r.f ḫry wbnw m gmꜣ.f mḥr ỉry.i wt.ḫr.k sw ḥr ỉwf wꜣḏ*
11§ *hrw tpy srwḫ.k m-ḫt mrḥt bỉt rꜥ nb r nḏm.f ỉr wbnw*
12§ *n wnt kft.{f} ỉsṯ sw ꜥr n ḳs wbnw pw nḏs spr r ḳs n ḫpr*
13§ *kft ỉm.f ḏd.f r ḥns n wnt spty{.fy} wbnw.f ỉr gmꜣ.f jmytw-*
14§ *ny sꜥnd pw n ỉrt.f r gnyt nt msḏr.f r pḥwy wgyt.f*

Translation

Title:

Necessary knowledge and skills for a wound in his temple/zygomatic region:

Examination:

If you should examine a man for a wound in his temple/zygomatic region and there is no slash wound although that wound has penetrated to the bone, you must palpate his wound. How you find his temple/zygomatic region (is): intact, there being no split fracture, perforation, or crushed fracture in it.

Diagnosis:

Then you are to say about him: "One who has a wound in his temple/zygomatic region, a medical condition which I will handle/deal with."

Treatment:

Then you must bandage it (along) with fresh meat the first day

and you should treat afterwards with ointment and honey every day until it/he is well.

Explanation A:

As for: "a wound: there is no slash wound although it has penetrated to the bone," it means: that wound is small, reaching to the bone, and no slash wound has occurred in it.

He speaks about/refers to "narrowness" since there are no lips of his wound.

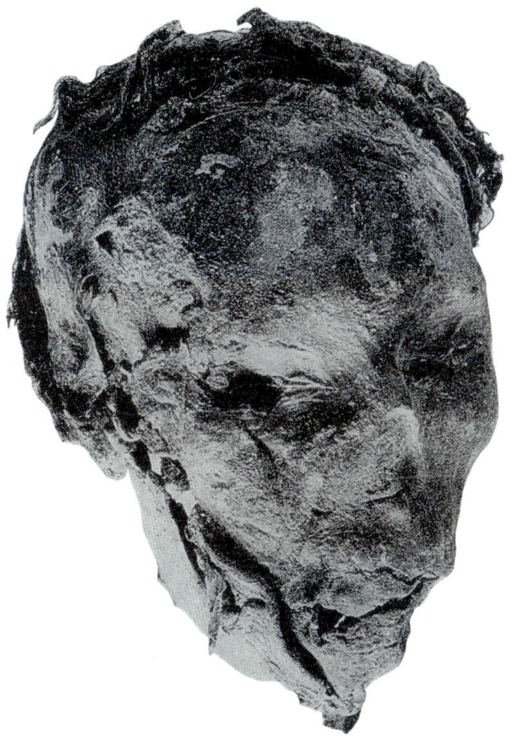

Fig. 19. Soldier #29, from Winlock, *Slain Soldiers of Neb-hep-et-Re Mentu-hotpe*, plate X A, displaying injury to the temporo-zygomatic area.

Explanation B:

As for: "his temple/zygomatic region," it means the area between the corner of his eye, to the auricle of his ear, at the end of his ramus.

Notes

ʿr or *ʿr*(*w*) – stative.

wḏꜣ(*w*) *n wnt pšn thm sd im.f*, also *n wnt sprty.{fy}* – *n wnt* used here as circumstantial, in the first example parallel with the stative as a complement of the nominal form/manner nominalization. In the second example, the translation "since there are no lips" conveys the circumstantiality. For *n wnt* attested as subordinate (circumstantial, used as so-called virtual, or better, unmarked or indefinite relative), see Gardiner, *EG*³, sec. 109, though Gardiner did not understand the role of circumstantiality.

n wnt kft.{f} – Though the scribe was apparently uncertain about or uncomfortable with this writing, it is actually a valid possessive variant or parallel to the existential *n wnt* + noun with no suffix-pronoun, literally, "its slash wound does not exist/not existing," that is, "it has/having no slash wound"; Gardiner, *EG*³, sec. 115. See also Meltzer, "*Iw wn/nn wn* + Indefinite Noun in Old and Middle Egyptian," though that paper deals with examples using *nn wn*.

n wnt spty.{fy} wbnw.f – although the scribe has crossed out the *.fy*, it can be noted that as originally written this could be taken as an example of a rare construction that has been labeled "prolepse of the genitive" (W.

Golenischeff, unpublished manuscript pages shown to me by Keith Seele); see Meltzer, "Problems of Adjectival Constructions in Old and Middle Egyptian," 201–4. This construction is also present in Elizabethan English and Mishnaic Hebrew.

Medical Commentary

Type of Injury

As a contusion laceration of the soft tissues of the temporo-zygomatic region, the area defined by the ancient Egyptians as *gmꜣ*. Case #18 represents the simplest of the group of injuries to this area in the papyrus. It is a wound without a defined cut.

Modern management of these wounds requires a thorough examination, if necessary under local anesthesia. Cleansing with removal of foreign material is followed by protective bandaging. If necessary, a tetanus immunization is given. As with any head injury, it is necessary to perform a thorough neurological evaluation of these patients with follow up as required by the individual case.

Ancient Medical Methodology and Knowledge

In its didactic exposition of head trauma the Edwin Smith Papyrus moves to the side of the head to describe injuries to the temporal region. Case #18 is a laceration of the scalp and temporalis muscle, reaching, but not penetrating bone. Its importance lies in the fact that it accurately describes the characteristics of the wound and determines that the only required treatment consists of topical measures. There is no need for suturing. Explanation B in Case #18 defines precisely the anatomical boundaries of the zygomatic arch, the *gmꜣ*: "it means the area between the corner of his eye, to the auricle of his ear, at the end of his ramus" (Visual Index Ve).

An example of such injury from antiquity is seen in fig. 19 (soldier #29, from Winlock's *Slain Soldiers of Neb-hep-et-Re Mentu-hotpe*, plate X A).

CASE #19:

Temporal-Zygomatic Intracranial Stab Wound

(Plate VII:14–22)

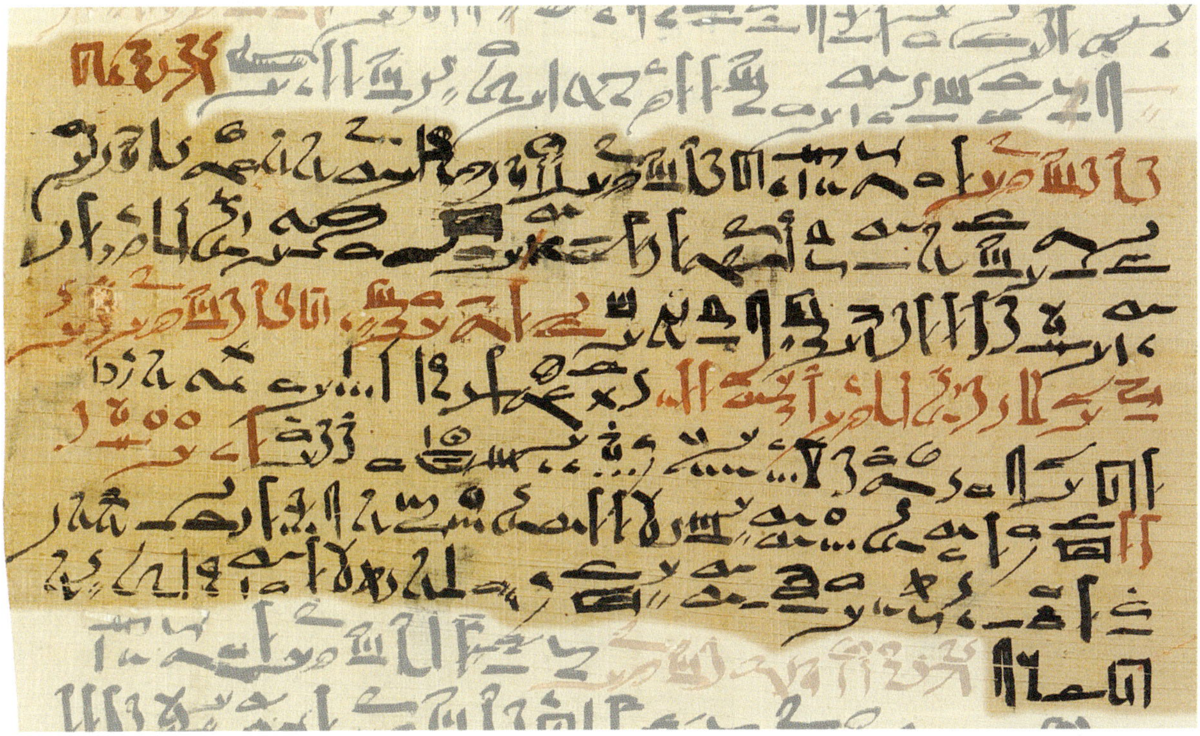

Courtesy New York Academy of Medicine.

14. 

15. 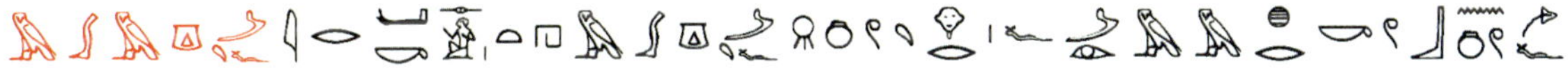

16. 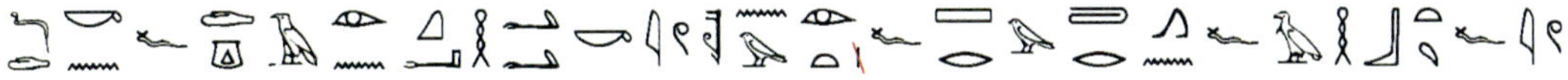

17. 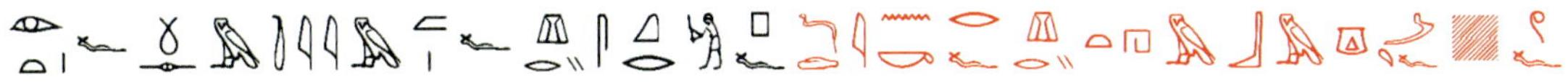

18. 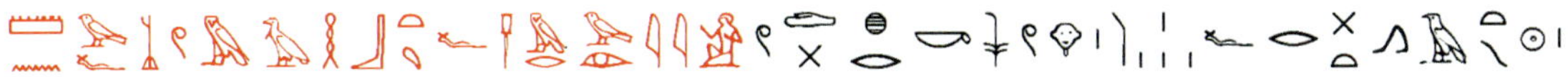

19. 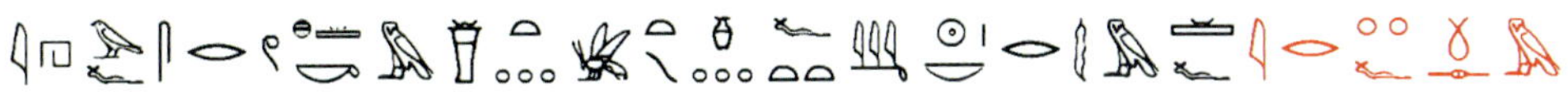

20. 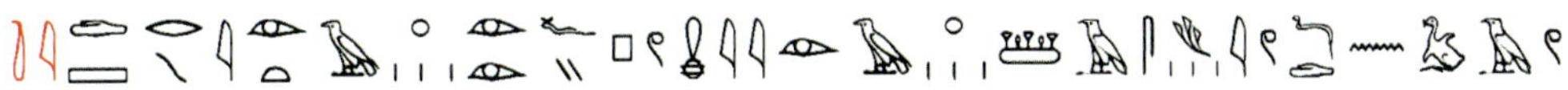

21. 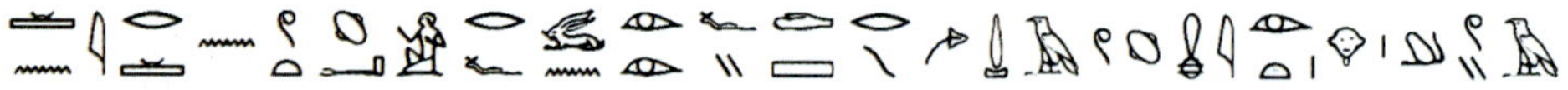

22. 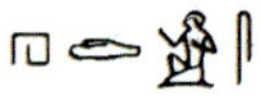

Transliteration

14§ *... šsꜣw thm*

15§ *m gmꜣ.f ir ḫꜣ.k s <n> thm <m> gmꜣ.f wbnw ḥr.f mꜣꜣ.ḫr.k wbnw.f*

16§ *ḏd.k n.f dgꜣ n ḳꜥḥwy.k iw ḳsn irt.f šrr pẖr.n.f nḥbt.f iw*

17§ *irt.f šsm.ti im gs.f ẖry sḳr pf ḏd.in.k r.f ẖry thm m gmꜣ.f [i]w.f*

18§ *mn.f ṯsw m nḥbt.f mḥr iry.i wd.ḫr.k sw ḥr mntw.f r swꜣt ꜣt*

19§ *iḥ.f srwḫ.k m mrḥt bit ftt rꜥ nb r nḏm.f ir irty.f šsm.ti*

20§ *dšr irtyw irty.fy pw mi irtyw šꜣs iw ḏd.n ṯꜣw*

21§ *n ir n wt r.f wnn irty.fy dšr ḏꜣw mi irt ḥr pḥwy*

22§ *ꜣhd.s*

Translation

Title:

Necessary knowledge and skills concerning a bone perforation in his temple/zygomatic area:

Examination:

If you should examine a man <for> perforation <in> his temple/zygomatic area, with a wound on it, then you have to look at his wound.

You should say to him: "Look to both of your shoulders." His doing so is painful so that how he has turned his neck is (only a) little, and his eye is bloodshot in his side that has that injury from a blow.

Diagnosis:

Then you are to say about him: One who has perforation in his temple/zygomatic area, [and] he [is] suffering from rigidity in the back of his neck, a medical condition which I will handle/deal with."

Treatment:

You must position him upon his mooring post/bed, until the (critical) period of his injury has passed.

You should treat with ointment and honey, and a dressing every day until it/he is well.

Explanation:

As for "both his eye(ball?)s are bloodshot and red," it means the color of both his eyes is like the color of coriander berries.

The "Compilation of That Which Pertains to the Bandager/Embalmer" has said about it: "How both his eyes are (is) red (with blood?) and diseased like an eye at the end of its exhaustion."

Notes

iw ḳsn and *iw irt.f šsm.ti* should both be taken as present tense in this passage.

sšm.ty – In my view we should clearly take the preposition as *m* and the stative form as *šsm.ty* with double reedleaf, although the subject seems to be singular (*irt*). The parallel passage in the explanation suggests that the scribe may well have been thinking about two eyes rather than one eye (though one must note that in the explanation there is no double reedleaf).

šri pẖr.n.f nḥbt.f – I think the form should probably be taken as the prospective *sḏm.f* of the adjective-verb. Moreover, I think that *pẖr.n.f* (the only element in this sequence which is explicitly past) is not a circumstantial but a nominal *sḏm.n.f* or manner nominalization (which in this text we have so far generally seen in the *sḏm.f*).

[*i*]*w.f mn.f* – Restoring this with considerable probability as a *iw.f sḏm.f* statement of fact (Hoch, *MEG*, sec. 37). This construction does actually contain the circumstantial *sḏm.f*, and is an example of what I call the Polotsky "equation," *iw* + circumstantial = indicative. Thus, as a statement of fact it does *not* mean "while he suffers," but it would if it were a bare circumstantial *sḏm.f*. I have tried to show the effect of the restoration with brackets.

The group used for the first writing of "his eyes," two circles + *.f*, probably has to be read as a writing *irty.fy*, thus *Grundriss* 7, 1:68, where the circle occurs in several writings including ones with *-t*, because of the grammatical agreement of the stative ending *.ti*, but on the basis of orthography it would be extremely tempting to take it as a writing of *b3*(*3*)*.f* (= later *br.f*) (!) "his eyes," or better, "his eyeballs," a logographic writing of the word *br* found in Walker (*Studies in Ancient Egyptian Anatomical Terminology*, 268), defined there as "the eyes." This word, the ancestor of Coptic ⲃⲁⲗ "eye," is listed in *Wb.* 1:465, where it is attributed to the Ptolemaic period. It does, however, have a much earlier history, which is discussed by J. F. Borghouts ("The Evil Eye of Apopis," *Journal of Egyptian Archaeology* 59 [1973]: 115–16), going back to a word *b3*(*3*) in the Coffin Texts, defined by Borghouts as "pupil (of the eye)," and also apparently the same as a component of reduplicated verbal roots in the Pyramid Texts. It would not make much sense for the pupils of the eyes to be bloodshot. An apparent solution can be found in William A. Ward, *The Four Egyptian Homographic Roots B-3: Etymological and Egypto-Semitic Studies* (Studia Pohl, Series Maior 6; Rome: Pontifico Istituto Biblico, 1978), 47 and 141–46, which corrects the definition to "eyeball" and cites a passage in a Middle Kingdom "magical" papyrus published by Roccati, in which *irt* and *b33* are parallel, and "eyeball" gives a much more satisfactory sense than "pupil" for *b33*. Ward considers the varied relationships among Egyptian words in the semantic field "eye" and "see," as well as words in Semitic languages. (It also seems to me that in class in Toronto, Prof. R. J. Williams mentioned that the Egyptian ancestor of Coptic ⲃⲁⲗ actually meant "eyeball," and the class, which included Ron Leprohon and myself, proceeded to make puns on "eye"–"ball/ⲃⲁⲗ." In the present passage it would have made excellent sense for the "eyeballs" to be bloodshot as a parallel with the simple word for "eyes." However, as noted above, we would have to emend and delete a clearly written *.ti* ending, and in accordance with our text-critical methodology, we do not think that we can sufficiently justify doing this. As far as that ending is concerned, it can be noted that in *Grundriss* 8, sec. 163, Westendorf lists as *Besonderheiten* two cases of *.ti* endings with statives having 3rd person masculine singular reference, one in Smith (not our passage), but we do not want to lean too heavily on this. At the same time, we note that *dšr* needs to be taken as a stative and lacks a *.ti* ending, but other cases of the omission of this ending in Middle Egyptian as noted earlier make it too uncertain to use this as a criterion for identifying the antecedent/subject as *b3*(*3*)*.f*, as tempting as that would be. Still, perhaps the (erroneous?) *.ti* endings noted above in *Grundriss* 8 mean that the identification as *b3*(*3*) is not absolutely ruled out.

ṯ3w n ir(y?) n wt – For the problems in understanding the designation *ṯ3w n ir(y?) n*, see the discussion in Case #5.

dšr – To be taken as a stative, *dšr*(*w*). The absence of a *.ti* ending in such cases has been remarked on earlier and cannot be decisive for the identification of the word *b3*(*3*)*.f* vs. *irty.fy* in this passage; see above.

wnn irty.fy dšr(*w*) *ḏ3w mi irt ḥr pḫwy 3hd.s* – I understand this as a sentence headed by *wnn* as a manner nominalization. In this case the future sense that many grammars have ascribed to the geminating form *wnn* is clearly not applicable. Though this is not the place for an exploration of that entire issue, I think it is fair to say that examples such as the present one decrease the credibility of the future understanding of *wnn*.

Medical Commentary

Type of Injury

Case #19 represents a patient with a deeper penetrating stab wound to the temporal-zygomatic area with bone perforation (Visual Index IV, Temporal Area Fractures). Its clinical presentation includes evidence of orbital injury from damage to the external orbital wall, and of post-traumatic meningismus. Sub-conjunctiva eye hemorrhage is described by "his eye is bloodshot in his side that has that injury." Symptoms resulting from subarachnoid hemorrhage—"is painful so that how he has turned his neck is (only a) little"—would be expected in a penetrating cranial wound such as this. The patient has retained consciousness and is able to follow the examiner's commands.

Stab wounds are low-velocity injuries and have limited penetration. Symptoms of focal brain tissue damage occurring in the track of the offending weapon will vary depending upon the area affected. An intracranial vessel injury will result in extensive neurological damage, and possibly in death. In 1992 du Trevon and van Dellen[163] reported on modern cases of penetrating stab wounds of the brain in a total of 330 patients, 44 of these were in the temporal area. At the time of hospitalization the weapon had been removed in 76 percent of the 330 patients. As for level of consciousness, 25 percent were comatose and 30 percent were fully conscious at time of admission.

Evaluation today requires neurological exam, computer tomographic studies, and prompt surgical intervention, except for the dying.

Craniotomy with wound debridement of all affected tissues is mandatory. Hospitalization in neurosurgical intensive care, antibiotics, anticonvulsant medication would be standard treatment. Rehabilitation and speech therapy may be necessary.

Ancient Medical Methodology and Knowledge

In an orderly fashion, the Egyptian physician outlines the symptoms and signs of primary importance found upon examination of the patient. There is a wound in the temple. The patient is conscious and able to follow commands, showing signs of traumatic meningismus with a stiff neck, resulting from a penetrating cranial temporal wound that has produced subarachnoid hemorrhage, evidenced by the patient's pain when trying to turn his neck. It is possible that an associated neck injury could have occurred, but the likelihood of this alone accounting for neck rigidity is low. The eye on the same side as the penetrating injury is bloodshot, a finding

163. M. D. du Trevon and J. R. van Dellen, "Penetrating Stab Wounds to the Brain: The Timing of Angiography in Patients Presenting with the Weapon Already Removed," *Neurosurgery* 13/5 (1992): 905–12.

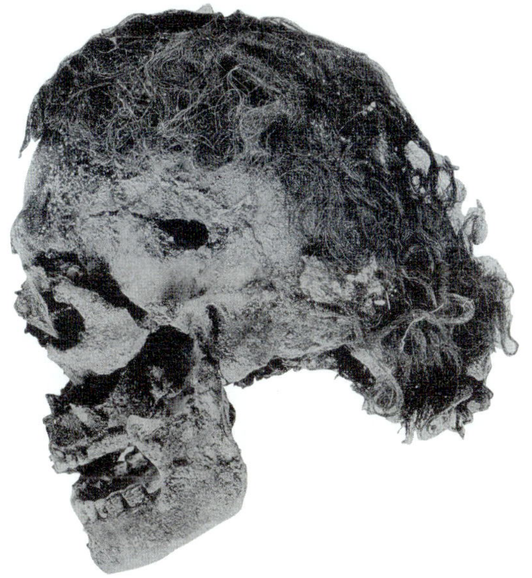

Fig. 20. Soldier #23, from Winlock, *Slain Soldiers of Neb-hep-et-Re Mentu-hotpe*, plate IX A, with perforating temporal stab wound.

attributed to the blow.[164] The traumatized eye color is compared to "the color of coriander berries." Furthermore, the explanation section expands upon the appearance of red and diseased eyes: "How both his eyes are (is) red (with blood?) and diseased like an eye at the end of its exhaustion." We can only speculate if this could refer to the appearance of the dead person's eyes(?), a condition the embalmer would have been familiar with. The condition of the eye is directly related to the blow inflicted in the temporo-zygomatic area, which most likely reached the orbit. There is no mention of limb paralysis or speech problems in this case, so we ascertain that the penetrating injury did not reach deep into the internal capsule and its "motor tracts," and also did not directly affect the areas of speech. It could also be a case in which the injury has occurred to the right side of the brain, or to the anterior and inferior left frontal region of the brain.

Despite the severe nature of this injury, the Egyptian physician issued the verdict, "a medical condition which I will handle/deal with."

From previous cases of head-injury treatment, we understand the patient was cared for with bed rest, under observation and with supportive care, until the critical period of the injury passed. During this time the wound was bandaged daily with ointment and honey dressings. Despite the optimistic verdict, this kind of patient could easily succumb to complications, mostly infectious. An example of this injury is shown in fig. 20. Soldier #23, from Winlock, *Slain Soldiers of Neb-hep-et-Re Mentu-hotpe*, plate IX A, with perforating temporal stab wound.

164. The reader is directed to appendix 2 for a compilation of the neurological symptoms and signs in the Edwin Smith Papyrus.

CASE #20:
Temporo-Zygomatic Stab Wound with Skull Perforation and Basilar Skull Fracture
(Plate VII:22–VIII:5)

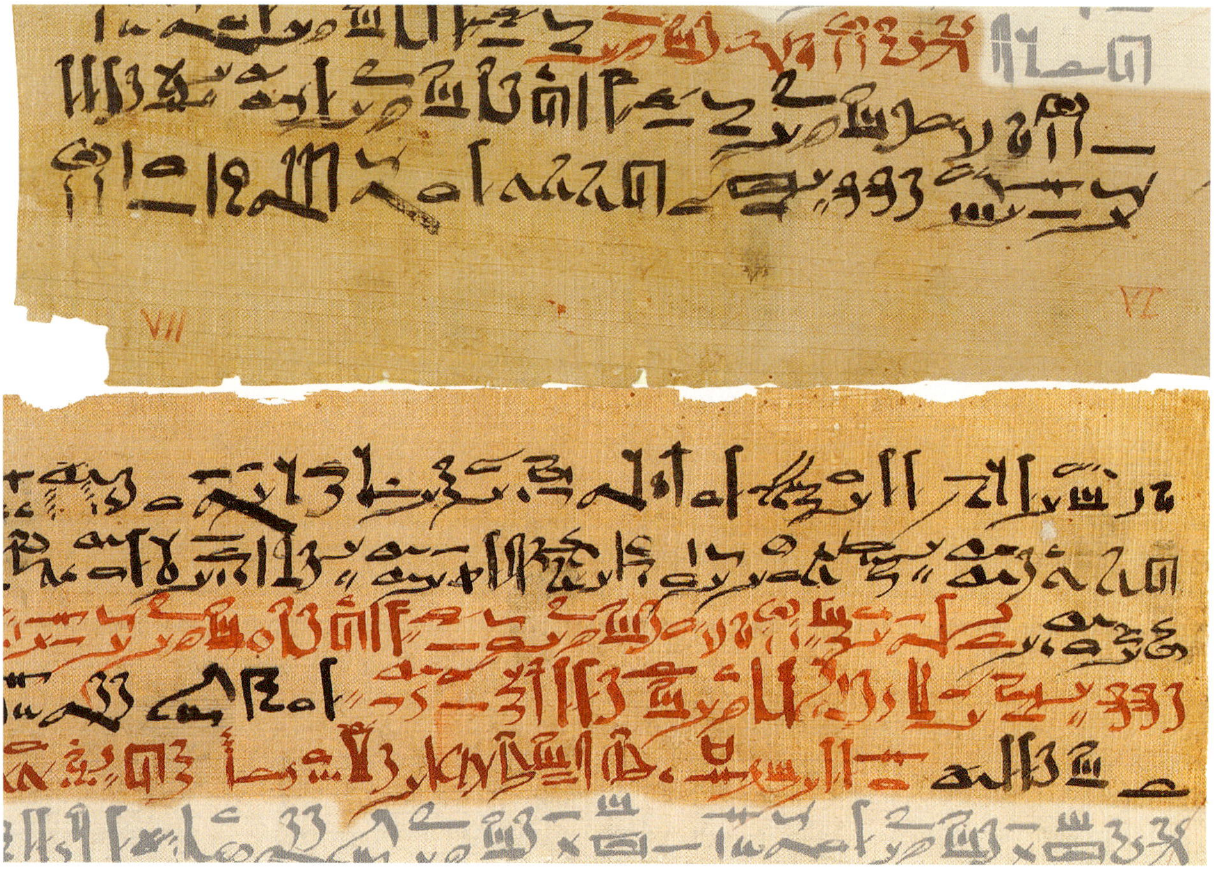

Courtesy New York Academy of Medicine.

22. 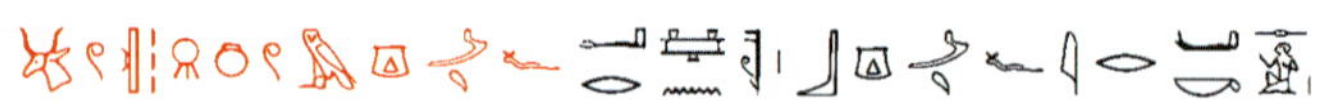

23. 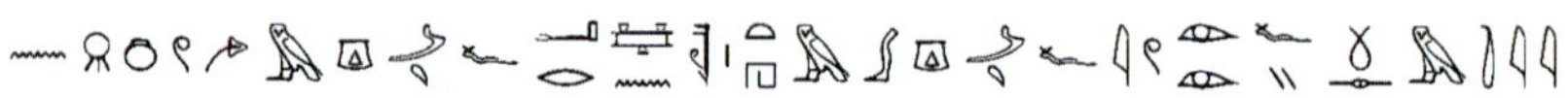

24. 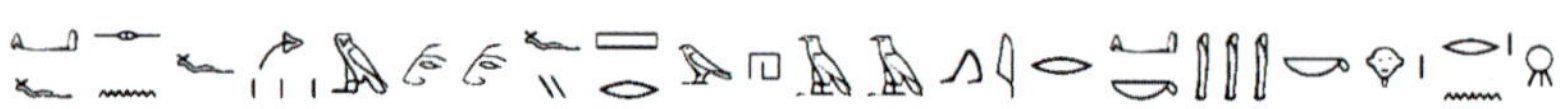

1. 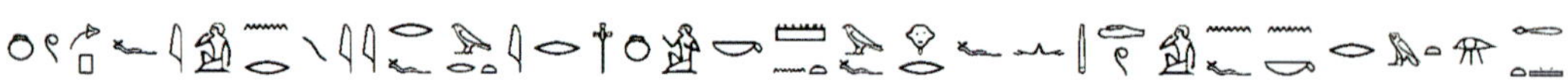

2. 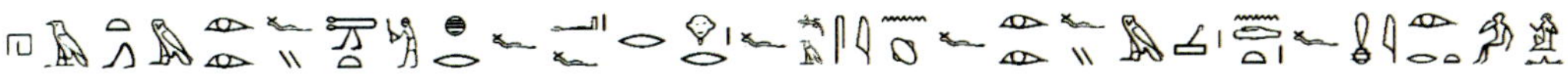

3. 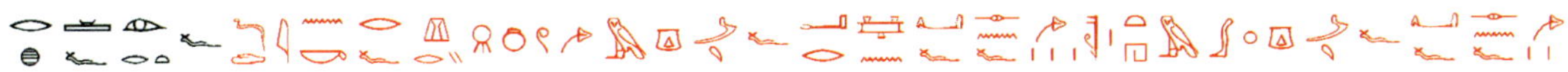

4. 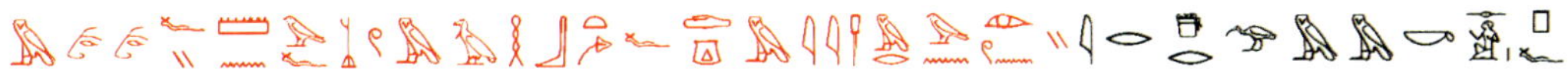

5. 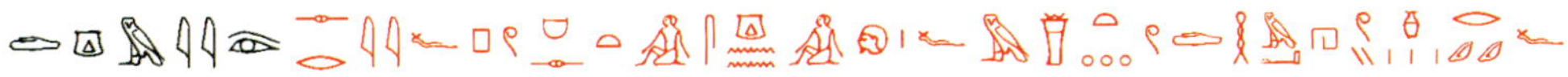

Transliteration

22§ *… šsȝw wbnw m gmȝ.f ʿr n ḳs thm gmȝ.f ir ḫȝ.k s*

23§ *n wbnw m gmȝ.f ʿr n ḳs hm gmȝ.f iw irty.fy šsm.ty*

24§ *di.f snf m msdty.fy šrr hȝȝ ir di.k ḏbʿw.k ḥr rȝ n*

1§ *wbnw pf inry r.f wrt ir nḏ.k mnt.f ḥr.f n mdw.n.f n.k rm<w>t ʿȝ<w>t*

2§ *hȝt m irty.fy iṯ.ḫr.f ʿ.f r ḥr.f ʿšȝ sin.f irty.fy m sȝ n ḏrt.f mi irrt ẖrd n*

3§ *rḫ.f irrt.f ḏd.in.k r.f ẖry wbnw m gmȝ.f ʿr n ḳs thm gmȝ.f di.f snf*

4§ *m msdty.fy mn.f ṯsw m nḫbt.f dgmy mḥr n irw.ny ir ḏr gmm.k s pf*

5§ *dgmy sry.f pw ḥmst s-gnn tp.f mrḥt wdḥ mhwy r msḏrwy.f*

Translation

Title:

Necessary knowledge and skills for a wound in his temple/zygomatic area, that penetrates to the bone and that perforates his temple:

Examination:

If you should examine a man for a wound in his temple/zygomatic area, that penetrates to the bone and perforates the bone of his temple/zygomatic area, both his eyes are bloodshot while he bleeds from both of his nostrils/nasal cavities, the drip/secretion being small.

If you put your fingers on the mouth of that wound so that it quakes/shifts at it very much, (and)

if you inquire about his injury, he cannot speak to you because of it,

while copious tears are dripping from both of his eyes.

Then he must take his hand to his face often that he might rub both his eyes with the back of his hand like what a child does, and he does not know what he does (or, who does not know what he does).

Diagnosis:

Then you are to say about him: "One who has a wound in his temple/zygomatic area, that extends to the bone and perforates his temple/zygomatic area, since he bleeds from both his nostrils/nasal cavities, while he suffers rigidity in the back of his neck

and is stuporous, a medical condition that cannot be handled/dealt with."

Treatment:

Now since how you find that man is: stuporous, it means: his treatment protocol(?) is "sitting upright."

Soothe his head with ointment and pour cream(?) into both his ears.

Notes

ʿr… ṯhm – Both active participles.

iw irty.fy šsm.ty – *iw* + noun + stative, an independent statement, not a circumstantial clause. Note the writing of the stative *šsm.ty* with double reedleaf, which greatly increases if not clinches the likelihood that in Case #19 above the same ending is to be read—even though the subject/antecedent in that passage is not written as a dual.

di.f – Circumstantial *sḏm.f*

šr h3ꜣ – I read *šr* not *šrr*, because no second *r* is written. I think that *šr* is probably the circumstantial *sḏm.f* of the adjective-verb, and *h33* a geminating (I tend to avoid the terms imperfective/perfective) active participle. I take the meaning to be "the drip/secretion/dripping or running substance being small." Loprieno and Gilula have claimed that the *sḏm.f* of the adjective-verb is prospective and have denied the existence of the circumstantial, but I think that there is clear evidence for it and it is accepted by Doret, *Narrative Verbal System*, 34, 117, 178; see also my review in *JARCE* 27 (1990): 223–24. I think that inter alia a passage such as *iw.f nḏm.f r-ʿwy* "he is well immediately" automatically contains the circumstantial *sḏm.f* in the compound statement of fact construction.

inry – Taking it in this passage as a stative with the sense of a stative of result; cf. above.

rmt ʿ3t – I prefer Breasted's rendition "copious," because I do not think this is a case of omitting the writing of the plural, I think that *rmt* is being treated as a "mass" rather than a "count" noun.

h3t – This is not an infinitive but a stative, *h3.t(i)*. The bare infinitive cannot provide a meaning such as "dripping"as a circumstantial, but would need to be preceded by a preposition, normally *ḥr*.

The noun Phrase + stative pattern here is dependent (circumstantial), not an independent statement.

sin.f – Taking this as a prospective *sḏm.f.*

irrt ḫrd ʿnd irrt.f – By far most likely taken as relative forms.

n rḫ.f irrt.f – This can be used as an "unmarked" or so-called "virtual" (I sometimes employ the term "indefinite") relative with the indefinite antecedent "a child," thus "a child who does not know that which he does."

iri is not an anomalous verb but normally classified as a normal 3ae inf. The writing of single and geminated *r* in the orthography of different periods has to be carefully borne in mind, but it is not irregular the way *ini*, *rdi* or *m33* is irregular.

di.f, mn.f – Circumstantial *sḏm.f*

sry – See discussion above.

mhwy – *Grundriss* 6:280 considers *mhwy/mhwt* "still undefinable" while noting that Breasted (*Edwin Smith* 1:287) thought that it "possibly means cream" and Lefèbvre (*GEC*) also translates it as "cream." This suggested meaning, which we use with a question mark, is compatible with the passages cited by Nunn and Manniche. The *Grundriss* entry (6:279–81) notes a wide range of employments throughout the medical papyri.

Medical Commentary

Type of Injury (Visual Index VIII)

Case #20 is the most severe of the penetrating wounds (*thm*) to the temporal area in the papyrus (Visual Index VIII). The offending object/weapon has produced an external opening of enough size for the physician to introduce his fingers into it, feeling the fractured bone fragments crepitate. The penetrating object has reached across the midline at the anterior floor of the skull base (fig. 4). This is responsible for active bleeding from the nose and injury to the orbits (Visual Index Va) causing both eyes to be blood shot. Blood spilling into the subarachnoid space[165] (fig. 1) is responsible for the symptoms of traumatic meningismus (rigidity in the back of his neck).[166]

The injury is most likely on the left side of the head and brain, as the patient demonstrates symptoms and signs of motor aphasia (the patient is unable to speak).[167] Speech is a cerebral cortical function predominantly located in the left hemisphere (Visual Indexes Vf and VIII). The patient also displays repetitive behavior rubbing his eyes: "Then he must take his hand to his face often that he might rub both his eyes with the back of his hand like what a child does, and he does not know what he does...." These symptoms are also consistent with his difficulty understanding and expressing himself (global aphasia) along with his frustration and confusion. The word *dgmy* , is used in the diagnosis to indicate an altered level of consciousness/response/sensibility, but no determinatives indicating exhaustion, weakness, or drowsiness are attached to it. However, the same word with the additional eye determinative is used in the treatment segment with the connotation that if you find that man stuporous he should be treated with the protocol used for severe craniocerebral injuries, including encampment/isolation, upright in the sitting position. (See the medical commentary to Case #22 for further discussion of the term *dgmy* and its variants.)

Case #20's penetrating injury is similar to van Dellen's Cases 6 and 8[168] in 1978, and Khalil's[169] Case 3 of 1988, in location and symptoms. In each of these three patients, the weapons penetrated deeply, to the midline of the brain along the skull base. In van Dellen's Case #6 there was penetration into the ethmoid air sinus and the patient had bleeding through his nose (epistaxis). The injury in van Dellen's Case #8 was produced by a knife blade penetrating the middle fossa, in a posterior direction and crossing the midline. That patient had stiff neck, hemiparesis, and aphasia. In Khalil's patient #3 there was a deep stab wound to the temporal region with a metal bar, the tip of which was above the sella turcica, reaching the midline. This patient was comatose, had pinpoint pupils and other signs of injury to the diencephalon and the upper brain stem.

With consideration to Case #20 in the Edwin Smith Papyrus as a representative "Case Type" and not necessarily a specific "Case History," we follow the likely trajectory of the weapon and the resultant structural intracranial injuries to arrive to the described symptoms. This is a temporo-zygomatic stab wound. The patient is aphasic but conscious and without obvious weakness. This suggests an injury to the primary speech areas of the dorsolateral frontal lobe and adjacent temporal lobe speech areas with damage to underlying white matter tracts. There appears to be no major damage to the anterior internal capsule as the patient has no evidence of limb paralysis. Preservation of consciousness suggests the direction of the weapon followed a slightly downward

165. Refer to Explanation C in Case #3 for an explanation of meningismus.

166. The reader is directed to appendix 2 for a compilation of the neurological symptoms and signs in the Edwin Smith Papyrus.

167. In most people, the left hemisphere of the brain is dominant, with the speech primary centers in the frontal and the temporal lobes. Damage to these areas produces aphasia, that is, the inability to express oneself, or to understand spoken speech. When both abilities are compromised "global aphasia" results.

168. J. R. van Dellen and R. Lipschitz, "Stab Wounds of the Skull," *Surgical Neurology* 10 (1978): 110–12.

169. N. Khalil, M. N. Elwany, and J. D. Miller, et al., "Transcranial Stab Wounds: Morbidity and Medicolegal Awareness," *Surgical Neurology* 35 (1988): 294–99.

and anterior or perpendicular path to the midline, sparing the Diencephalon and Brain stem. Bloodshot eyes in this case indicate orbital wall violation.

In contrast with high velocity missile injuries, the tissue damage in cranial stab wounds is a lower kinetic energy and tissue damage tends to be confined to the area of penetration and associated bleeding. Stab and other penetrating cranial wounds of this kind are less frequent in modern times than those produced by missiles and metallic fragments from explosive devices.

Evaluation and treatment of such cases today include plain radiographic and computer tomography studies. The trajectory of the weapon and its proximity to vascular structures, along with the presence of intracranial hemorrhage, if shown on CT scan, will determine the need for angiography. The surgical treatment of cranial stab wounds requires debridement of injured tissues along the weapon's tract, removal of associated hematomas and repair of the dura. Oftentimes, the weapon is still in place at the time of arrival to the medical facility and it is best to wait for its removal until the time of surgery. Special surgical needs may involve dural venous sinus repair and arterial lacerations management. The use of broad spectrum antibiotics is mandatory.

Even with the availability of rapid transportation to appropriate medical facilities, modern diagnostic technology, anesthesia, sterile techniques, neurosurgery, and antibiotics, the treatment of this type of injury still today carries significant mortality, 26 percent in recorded cases (1992) of du Trevon and van Dellen's cases.[170]

Ancient Medical Methodology and Knowledge

In the examination segment for Case #20 of the Edwin Smith Papyrus, the clinical information is detailed and precise, providing us the first known description of the symptoms and signs of what we consider aphasia.[171] This observation has been made by Elsberg, Courville, Horrax, Masdeu, and others, with its first extensive discussion by Minagar et al.[172]

In our patient of Case #20, prognosis for recovery is poor. Treatment by the sitting position is recommended on the basis of the patient's severe head injury, a remarkable measure still applicable to our current management of many severe head injuries (for discussion on the rationale for the use of sitting position in the treatment of head injuries, see Case #4 under ancient methodology and knowledge).

The purpose behind pouring cream (?) into both his ears is unclear. We are not aware of any practical usefulness of this measure, but it is known that milk in ancient Egypt was attributed with sustaining and regenerative attributes. It is also known from the Ebers Papyrus #854 and #856, and from #163 of the Berlin Papyrus that "the breath of life" entered through the right ear and the "breath of death" entered through the left. Whether there is any relationship with the practice prescribed in Case #20 is speculative.

170. du Trevon, M. D., and J. R. van Dellen, "Penetrating Stab Wounds to the Brain: The Timing of Angiography in Patients Presenting with the Weapon Already Removed," *Neurosurgery* 13/5 (1992): 905–12.

171. See Case #22 for discussion of aphasia.

172. C. A. Elsberg. "The Anatomy and Surgery of the Edwin Smith Surgical Papyrus," *Journal of Mount Sinai Hospital* 12 (1945): 141–51. C. B. Courville, "Injuries to the Skull and Brain in Ancient Egypt," *Bulletin of the Los Angeles Neurological Society* 14/2 (1949): 68. G. Horrax, *Neurosurgery: An Historical Sketch* (Springfield, IL: Thomas, 1952), 14. J. C. Masdeu, "Aphasia," *Archives of Neurology* 57 (2000): 892–95. A. Minagar, J. Ragheb, and R. E. Kelly, "The Edwin Smith Surgical Papyrus: Description and Analysis of the Earliest Case of Aphasia," *Journal of Medical Biology* 11 (2003): 114–17.

CASE #21:

Closed Head Injury with Temporo-Zygomatic Displaced Fracture and Basilar Skull Fractures into the Mastoid Area with Hyperacusis (Plate VIII:6–9)

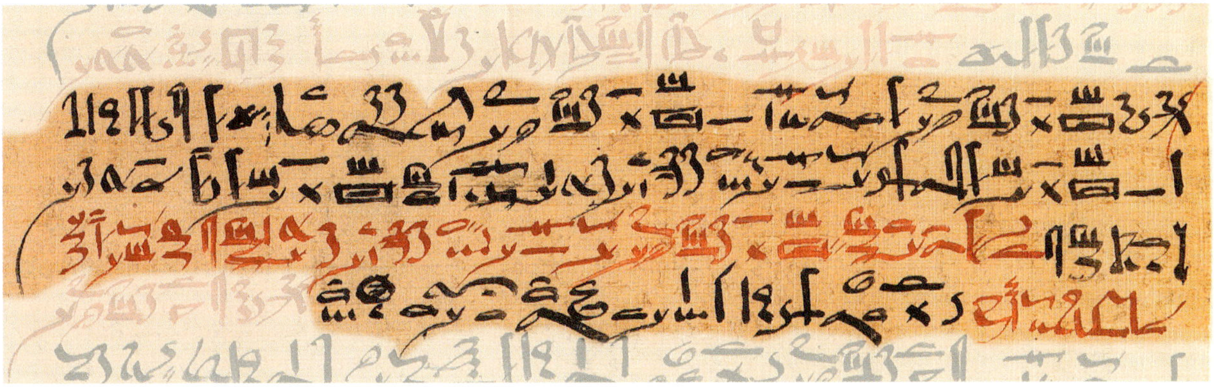

Courtesy New York Academy of Medicine.

6. 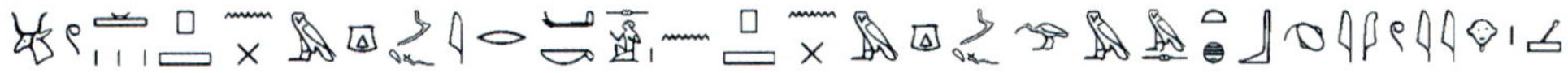

7. 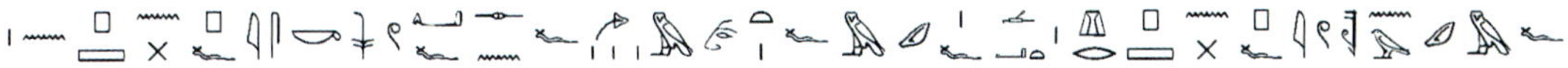

8. 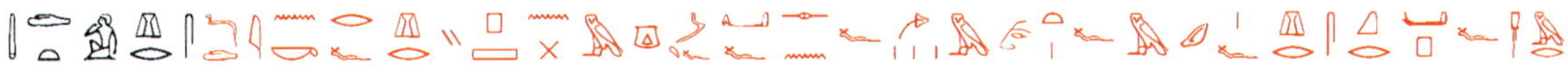

9. 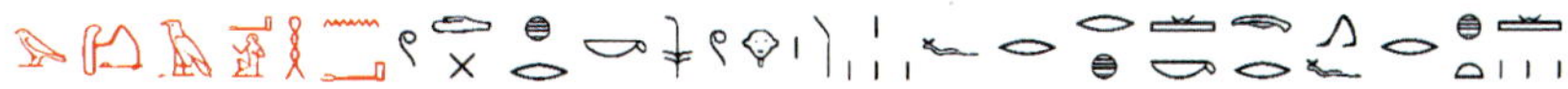

Transliteration

6§ *šsꜣw pšn m gmꜣ.f ir ḫꜣ.k s n pšn m gmꜣ.f gmm.k tḫb išwy ḥr-sꜣ*

7§ *n pšn pf isk sw di.f snf m šrt.f m msḏr.f wꜥt ḫr pšn pf jw ḳsn sḏm.f*

8§ *mdt ḫr.s ḏd.in.k r.f ḫry pšn m gmꜣ.f di.f snf m šrt.f m msḏr.f ḫr sḳr pf mḥr*

9§ *ꜥḥꜣ.i ḥnꜥ wḏ.ḫr.k sw ḥr mniw.f r rḫ.k spr.f r ḫt*

Translation

Title:

Necessary knowledge and skills for a split in his temple/zygomatic area:

Examination:

If you should examine a man for a split in his temple/zygomatic area, how you find the swelling (is): protruding/

swollen on the outside of that split fracture, while at the same time he bleeds from his nasal walls and from his one ear beneath that split, and it is painful when he hears speech because of it.

Diagnosis:

Then you are to say about him: "One who has a split in his temple/zygomatic area while he bleeds from his nasal walls and his ear because of that injury from a blow, a medical condition I will fight with."

Treatment:

Then you must place him on his bed under observation and support, until you know he arrives at a turning point.

Notes

pšn with crossed sticks determinative – Gardiner Sign-list Z 9–10 considers the crossed sticks sign to represent "two sticks crossed" and attributes to it a primary meaning of "break."

išwy – Stative

isk sw di.f – Cf. discussion above in Case #13.

iw ḳsn sḏm.f – I am not taking this as a *iw sḏm.f* construction. It could be taken that way if *sḏm.f* were identified as a nominal *sḏm.f*, which is a possibility ("How he hears is painful"). I prefer to take it (as also a similar sentence above) as *iw* + impersonal stative + circumstantial *sḏm.f*, if one wants to be very punctilious *iw ḳsn(w) sḏm.f*, "It is painful when he hears."

Medical Commentary

Type of Injury

This is a closed *pšn*, split/elevated fracture in the temporo-zygomatic area of the skull. In this type of injury there is bone plate separation where relatively larger sections of the outer skull plate have been broken and displaced. In addition to the swollen area protruding over the fractured site, this patient is bleeding profusely from his nose and from his ear, on the side of the injury. These signs indicate that fractures from the impact site have spread to the skull base in the middle and the anterior fossae (fig. 4, Case #4). As discussed above (Case #4), *pšn* injuries appear to result from tangential blows with heavy objects.

This patient is described as having the symptom of "Hyperacusis" a condition in which every sound is too loud: "it is painful when he hears speech, because of it." This peculiar symptom results from damage to the stapedius branch of the facial nerve as it courses through the temporal bone's mastoid segment (fig. 21).[173] This branch of the facial nerve powers the stapedius muscle, which attaches to the neck of the stapes ossicle in the middle ear. Contraction of this muscle pulls the stapes footplate away from the oval window at the middle ear, dampening loud sounds. When this nerve is injured, the paralyzed stapedius muscle is unable to attenuate vibrations of the oval membrane that are produced by loud sounds. Despite being a significant head injury, Case #21 does not mention alteration of level of consciousness, or other specific neurological symptoms.

The evaluation and treatment of this injury today would require the same general principles of treatment implemented in the evaluation and treatment of any severe closed head injury including cardio-respiratory

173. Nerve anatomy in the middle and inner ear.

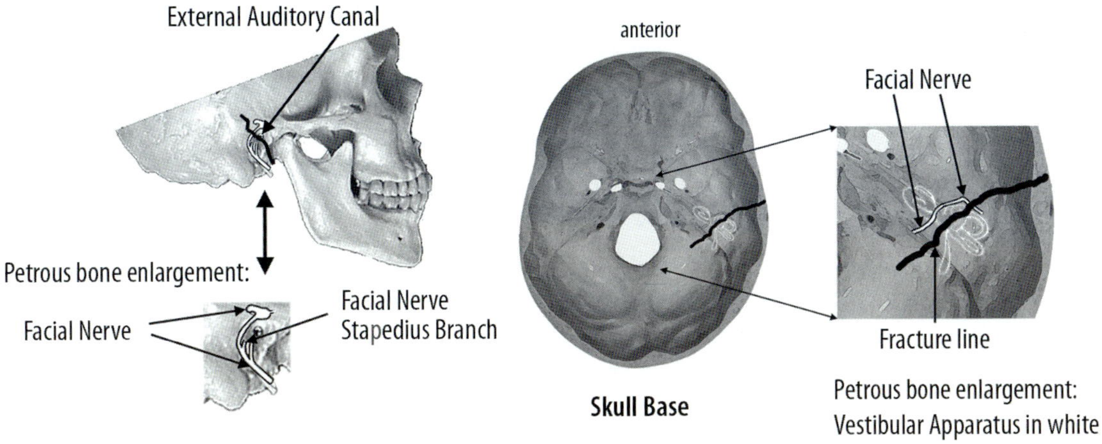

Fig. 21. Temporal fracture with hyperacusis.

support, immediate neurological assessment, and transportation to a neurosurgical facility. Whether surgery is needed or not, the patient would be closely managed in an intensive care neurological unit, probably kept on his bed. Intracranial pressure management may be necessary with antibiotic coverage until it is certain there is no spinal fluid leak from the ear or the nose. In addition to neurological and neurosurgical staff managing the patient's care, ophthalmology and ear, nose, and throat specialists would also be consulted.

Ancient Medical Methodology and Knowledge

The Egyptian physician's assessment of this closed head injury included documentation of important findings observed at the site of impact, and remotely, from the skull base fractures. Their documented awareness of the unique clinical symptom of painful hearing, known today as hyperacusis,[174] is an example of the ancient Egyptian physician's clinical acumen and knowledge base. Courville[175] in 1949, first annotated this extraordinary observation by the ancient Egyptian physician.

The verdict in Case #21, "a medical condition I will fight with," conveys the physician's intention to treat the injury, and, at the same time, uncertainty about the outcome. The Case #21 head injury was treated on his bed, until the patient's course defined itself, one way or another (see Case #4, Explanation C).

174. The reader is directed to appendix 2 for a compilation of the neurological symptoms and signs in the Edwin Smith Papyrus.

175. C. B. Courville, "Injuries to the Skull and Brain in Ancient Egypt," *Bulletin of the Los Angeles Neurological Society* 14/2 (1949): 53–82.

CASE #22:
Closed Head Injury to the Temporo-Zygomatic Area with Comminuted Fracture and Basilar Skull Fractures
(Plate VIII:9–17)

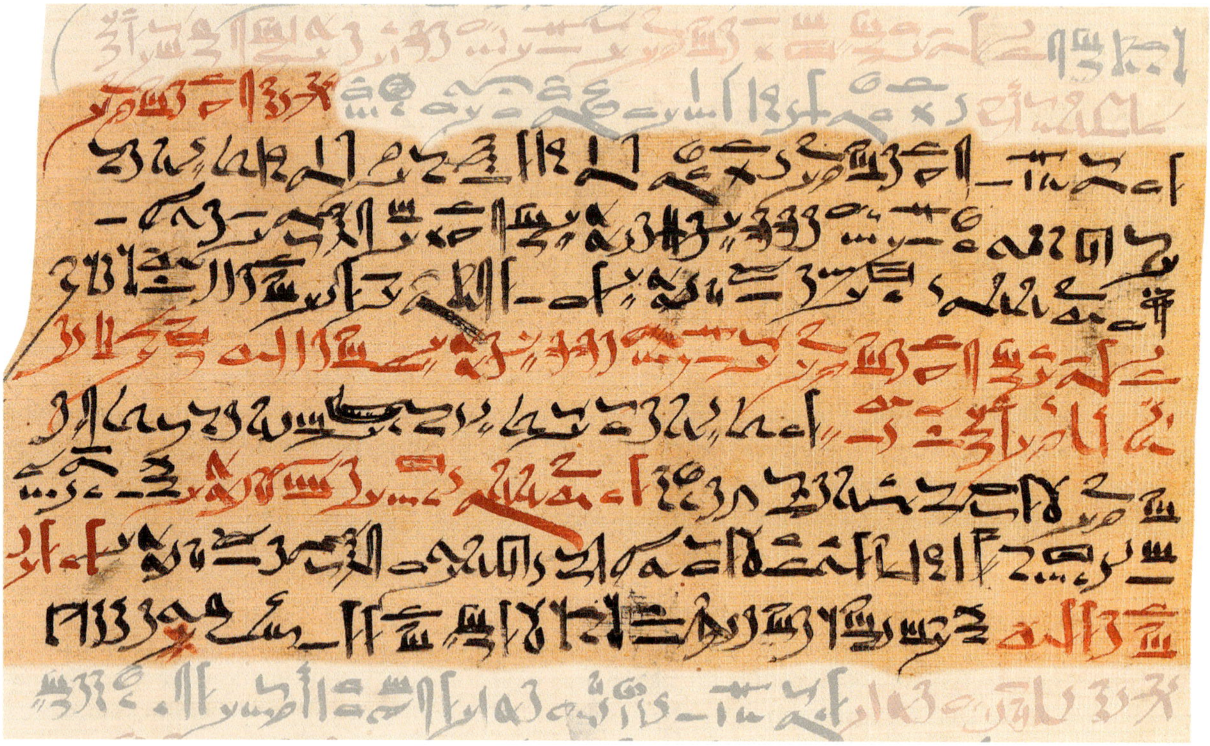

Courtesy New York Academy of Medicine.

9. 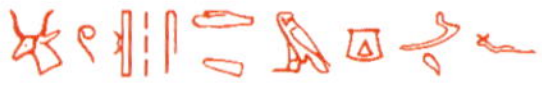

10. 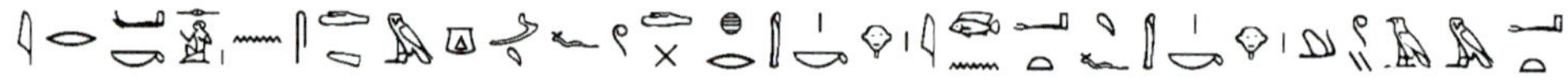

11. 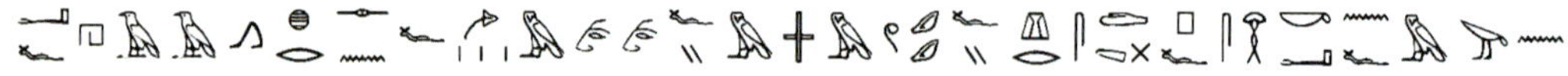

12. 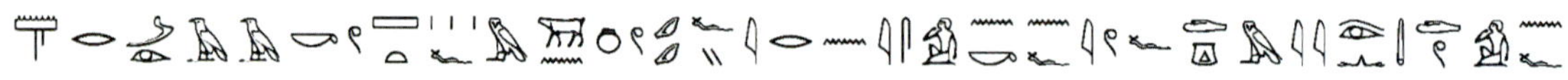

13. 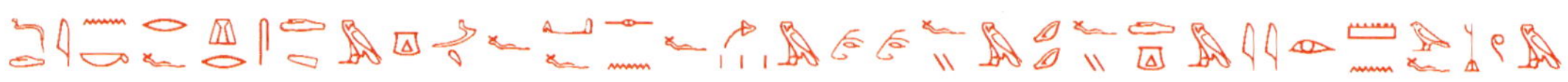

14. 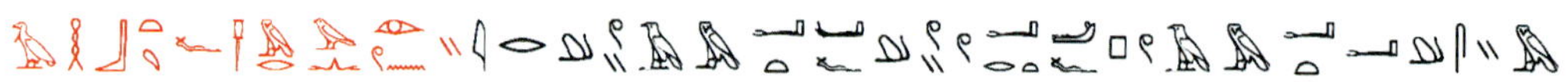

15. 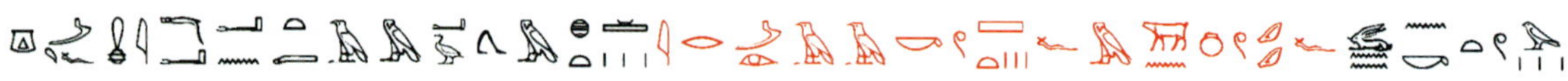

16. 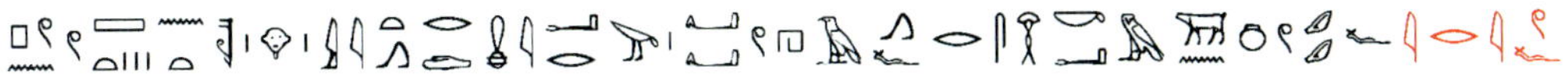

17. 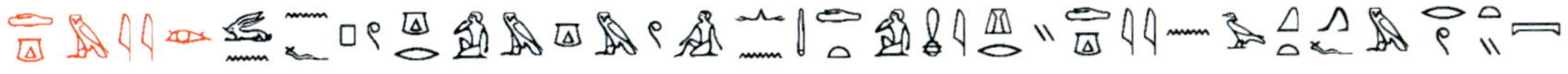

Transliteration

9§ … *šsȝw sd m gmȝ.f*

10§ *ir ḫȝ.k s n sḏ m gmȝ.f wd.ḫr.k ḏbꜥ.k ḥr inꜥt.f ḏbꜥ.k ḥr pḥwy ȝmꜥt.*

11§ *f hȝȝ.ḫr snf m msdty.fy m imyw msḏrwyfy ḫr sd pf sk n.f <sw> m sšm n*

12§ *ḥbs r mȝȝ.k wšt.f m-ẖnw msḏrwy.fy ir nis.n.k n.f iw.f dgmy n mdw.n.f*

13§ *ḏd.in.k r.f ḫr<y> sd m gmȝ.f di.f snf m msdty.fy m msḏrwy.fy dgmy mn.f ṯsw m*

14§ *nḥbt.f mḫr n irw.ny ir pḥwy ȝmꜥt.f pḥwy ꜥrt.f pw ȝmꜥt pḥ sy m*

15§ *gmȝ.f mi mḥ ꜥnt ȝmꜥ m ḫt ir mȝȝ.k wšt.f m-ẖnw msḏrwy.f wnn nktw*

16§ *pw n wšt nt ḳs ḥr iit r dmi r sšm dd.w hȝ.f r sk m-ẖnw msḏrwy.f ir iw.f*

17§ *dgmy wnn.f pw gr m gmw nn mdt mi ẖry dg<ȝ>y n ꜥḳt{f} m rwty*

Translation

Title:

Necessary knowledge and skills for a smashed in fracture in his temple /zygomatic area:

Examination:

If you should examine a man for a smashed in fracture in his temple/zygomatic area: then you must place your thumb on his chin and your finger on the end of his forked bone (ramus).

Then the blood comes down, out of his nostrils/nasal cavities and out of the inside of his ears from/under that crushed fracture.

Wipe <it> for him with a swab of cloth until you see its bone splinters inside of both his ears.

If you have called to him, he is stuporous, and he cannot speak.

Diagnosis:

Then you are to say about him: "One who has a smashed in fracture in his temple/zygomatic area, while he bleeds from both of his nostrils/nasal cavities and both of his ears, is stuporous and he suffers rigidity/stiffness in the back of his neck, a medical condition that cannot be handled/dealt with."

Explanation A:

As for "the end of his forked bone," it means the end of his lower jaw/mandible.

The forked bone ends in his temple/zygomatic area like the way the claw of a *ȝmꜥ* bird grasps onto something.

Explanation B:

As for "how you see {its} splinters of bone inside his ears," it means that there are small bits of bone splinters belonging to the bone of the face, coming away to adhere to the swab, that is made to descend, in order to clean out the inside of his ears.

Explanation C:

As for "he is stuporous," it means that he is being silent as in drowsiness, and not/without speaking, like one who has a fixed gaze because of that which has entered from outside.

Notes

sḏ – "smash fracture."

For the translation of the *sḏm.ḫr.f* form, see Depuydt, *Conjunction, Contiguity, Contingency*, 216–18.

iw.f dgmy – I would segment this passage as follows: "If you have called to him, he is stuporous ...." In other words, *iw.f* is more independent (*iw* + suffix-pronoun headed clauses are bivalent and can be either circumstantial or independent) and really acts as part of the apodosis. One could possibly say "(then) he is stuporous...."

n mdw.n.f – I would translate, as elsewhere, taking it as negation of ability, "he cannot speak."

di.f snf – Circumstantial *sḏm.f*, "while."

mn.f – Also circumstantial *sḏm.f*.

ꜣmꜥt pḥ sy – This is a noun in front extraposition (anticipatory emphasis) + participle + dependent pronoun subject, on the model of the sentence with adjectival predicate; see Gardiner, *EG*[3], sec. 374.

mi mḥ ꜥnt – Preposition *mi* + nominal *sḏm.f* or manner nominalization.

wnn nkwt ... – Nominal *sḏm.f*, in the classical Polotskyan sense of a "that-form": "that there are small fragments ..."

ḥr iit – *ḥr* + infinitive, the infinitive in an adverbial construction, this can be understood as "(in the act of) coming."

ddw hꜣ.f – Geminating passive participle + prospective *sḏm.f*, "which is caused to descend," literally, "which is caused that it (may) descend." There is no infinitive here and the *.f* is not an object but a subject. I think that a gloss such as Allen's (*AM*) "inserted" or Breasted's (*Edwin Smith*) "introduced" could be supplied in parentheses because it is a paraphrase of the Egyptian.

wnn.f – Nominal *sḏm.f* as "that-form" again, "that he is ..."+ stative. I am not inclined to accept Allen's "continually still" because I am very skeptical about the aspectual interpretation of the geminating *sḏm.f* form, both for *wnn* and in general, and I think it often proves to be either unlikely or unnecessary; but for an apparent counterexample see Case #43.

ꜥḳt{.f} m rwty – "because of that which has entered " (active participle) "from outside." If the *f* were to be included, it could be taken as a *sḏmty.fy* form, "one who shall enter," but the *f* is crossed out and the future form would not make as much sense. The Faulkner, *CDME*, 49 reference means that *ꜥḳ* + the preposition *n* means "to enter a state." So this is another case of "that which enters" the patient "from outside."

Medical Commentary

Type of Injury

As a *sd*, smash/comminuted fracture, Case #22 represents the most severe of the closed fractures of the temporal-zygomatic area (Visual Index IV, and fig. 22a and b). The findings provided by the patient's examination give us a clear idea of the extent of the damage to the temporal bone and facial skeletal structures of the skull base and also to the adjacent soft tissue of the region. The mandibular condyles have impacted into the anterior and inferior petrous portion of the temporal bone, shattering bone into the external auditory canals. Damage to bony and soft tissues of this region includes the eustachian tube, a soft tissue cartilaginous structure connecting the inner ear to the throat. Due to extensive damage to all of these structures, mobilization of the mandible by the examiner's hand produces active bleeding through the nostrils, ears, and mouth. Shattering of the petrous bone is confirmed by the examiner after clearing blood clots from the ear canal and finding bone splinters inside. Bleeding from the nose probably has originated, in this case, from the shattered areas of the temporal skull base, as it is precipitated with the jaw mobilization in the examination. In addition to traumatic meningismus (neck stiffness and bleeding from the nose and the ears) the patient has major neurological symptoms of brain injury, namely, stupor and aphasia. Although the injury has affected the entire head, aphasia suggests the primary damage has occurred to the left cerebral hemisphere. Our modern understanding of aphasia attributes speech integration primarily to functional circuitries between the dominant hemisphere's frontal lobe ("Broca's area") and those in the temporal lobe ("Wernicke's area"). Pure motor or pure receptive aphasias are rare, and a mix of both types is more common. The speech areas in the temporal lobe are primarily involved with speech reception, more than with pure formulation of speech. Global Aphasia is the most severe form, involving inability to communicate verbally and to understand the spoken word (Visual Indexes Vf and VIIIc). See summary discussion on the word *dgmy* below.

These types of injuries today are mostly due to motor-vehicle accidents. Condyle jaw fractures data from Fridrich, cited by Laub,[176] indicates that associated injuries occurred in 43 percent of patients. Of these, 39 percent had head injuries, 28 percent midface fractures, 12 percent nasal fractures, 16 percent ocular injuries, and 11 percent injuries to the cervical spine. The same source indicates that of all of the mandibular bone fractures, 26 percent were at the condyle. The most severe of condyle fractures result in its displacement into the middle cranial fossa of the skull base. Treatment of the injuries requires craniotomy, extensive facial bone reconstruction, and often a temporary tracheotomy (surgical procedure establishing direct airway communication to the trachea). The head injury management and prognosis will vary from case to case, but full neurological and neurosurgical facilities are required from the start. Ear, nose and throat, plastic surgery, ophthalmology, and rehabilitation specialties are necessary. While these forms of modern treatment have reduced the mortality rates, neurological recovery is limited.

Ancient Medical Methodology and Knowledge

Case #22 contains important anatomical and functional concepts. Explanation A: "As for 'the end of his forked bone,' it means the end of his lower jaw/mandible. The forked bone ends in his temple/zygomatic area like the way the claw of a plover bird grasps on something." Alluding to the anatomy of the mandibular ramus, the Egyptian physician compares the shape of the coronoid process and the condyle of the mandible to the shape of the claw of the *ꜣmꜥ* bird.[177] It is clear then that the Ama bird's foot has an opposing hind toe. Breasted notes (*Edwin Smith*, 294) that there is one depiction of this bird at a tomb of the Twelfth Dynasty (Baqt) at Beni Hasan, but neither he nor Nina Davies[178] were able to positively identify it. The *ama* bird painting has been

176. D. R. Laub, "Facial Trauma, Mandibular Fractures." Medscape Reference: http://emedicine.medscape.com/article/1283150-treatment; Burns and Blackwell, "Plastic Surgery," 2143.

177. The *ama* bird has been considered to be the Egyptian plover (*Pluvianus aegyptius*), but that bird is a resident of tropical sub-Sahara, and has three forward-oriented toes, not forming a true "claw."

178. Nina M. Davies, "Birds and Bats at Beni Hasan," *Journal of Egyptian Archaeology* 35 (1949): 18.

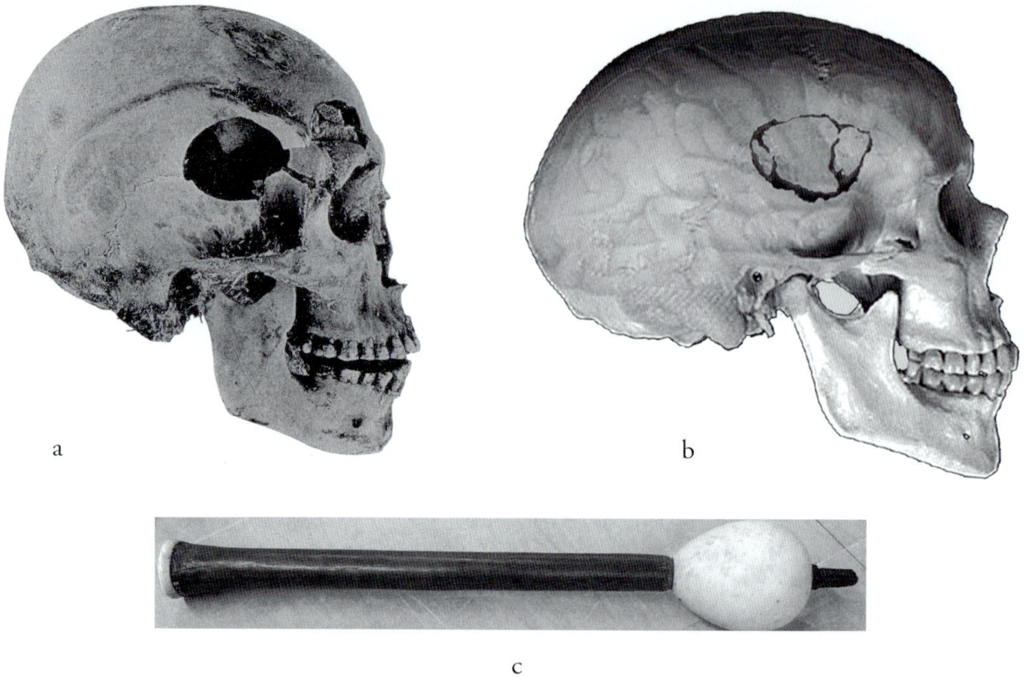

Fig. 22. a) Soldier #14, from Winlock, *Slain Soldiers of Neb-hep-et-Re Mentu-hotpe*, plate VIII C; b) Simulated injury with brain visualized. Drawing by the author (GSM); c) Mace, courtesy of the Royal Ontario Museum.

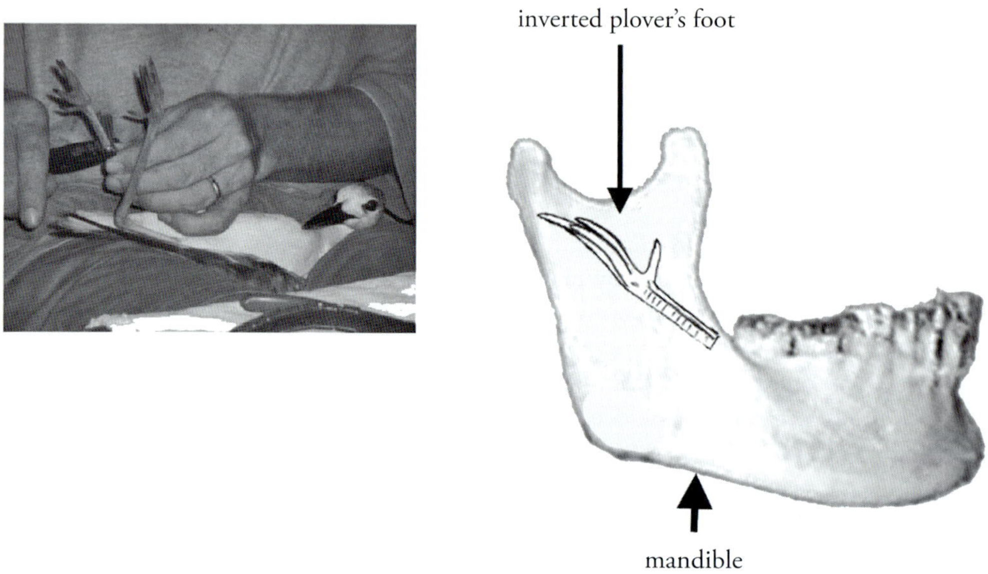

Fig. 23. Crab plover's foot inverted, projecting over mandibular ramus. Left: Banding crab plover (*Dromas ardeola*) feet detail (courtesy of "A Rocha Kenya"). Right: Mandible showing the inverted plover's foot.

copied by Wlkinson, Rosselini, Champollion, and Norman de G. Davies.[179] There are differences among these various renditions, but it is evident that the Ama bird is likely a shore or a wading bird, rather than a bird of prey. M. Gaillard is cited by Nina Davies, proposing the Ama bird to be the Little Bittern (*Ardetta minuta*). However, comparison of a known relief[180] of the Little Bittern with the Ama bird of Baqt's tomb painting reveals major discrepancies. Based on morphological and behavioral characteristics, other possibilities to be considered in the identification of the Ama bird are the Crab Plover (*Dromas ardeola*), the Gull-billed Tern (*Gelochelidon nilotica*), and the Sandpiper (*Tringa stagnatilis*). Of these, we favor the Crab Plover. This is a shore bird that breeds in the Red Sea, Somalia, and the Arabian Sea. This bird's feet have three partially webbed toes in the front, and a well-developed hind toe. In the inverted position, the shape of this bird's open "claw" indeed resembles the shape of the mandibular ramus with its condylar and coronoid processes (fig. 23). The inverted position of the plover's claw is indicated by the scribe's drawing the hieratic sign inverted.

To express an altered state of consciousness in this patient, the Egyptian physician utilizes again the term *dgmy*. This word has appeared in previous cases in which there is sufficient trauma to the head. This word appears in its various applications in the Edwin Smith Papyrus with and without determinatives, the latter being used pointedly in apparent connection to a variety of degrees of the alteration of consciousness.[181] From our analysis of the above, we propose the following conclusions:

- The word *dgmy* and related words appear singly or in various combinations in Cases #13, #17, # 20, #22, and #33. In all of these cases a significant brain trauma has occurred. These words refer to an altered state of responsiveness/consciousness in which listlessness or stupor predominate.
- As used in Case #20, the word , without determinatives, is used in the diagnosis to indicate an altered level of consciousness/response/sensibility. As used in Cases #13 and #17, *dgmy*, with determinative, is an altered level of consciousness/response/sensibility and motor activity. The later feature, reduced motor activity, is delineated by use of the determinative. In our opinion, this form of *dgmy* is most consistent with the modern term "torpid."

The determinative in signals an impaired consciousness and decreased responsiveness, as the predominant feature of *dgmy*, when used in describing the head injuries in Cases #20, #22 and #33. In these cases this term is most consistent with 'Stupor', detailed in this Case #22, Explanation C:" it means that he is being silent as in drowsiness , and not/without speaking like one who has a fixed gaze because of that which has entered from outside."

As used and discussed in Case #8, Explanation D, the implication of this statement is that of a person in which a spontaneous event with neurological consequences, as in the case of a stroke, has occurred. The neurological picture developing after a spontaneous brain injury (stroke) is equated with the neurological consequences caused from an external agent producing cranial trauma, as is in Case #22 (see Medical Commentary, discussion of Explanations C and D, Case #8). The Egyptian physician details his findings of injury to the skull base, detected by observing loose bone fragments in the external auditory canals. He readily acknowledges his observation of these splinters "belonging to the bone of his face" (Explanation B) to the skull base of the temporal bone. In this kind of injury it is no surprise that the damage to the adjacent brain, directly to the temporal lobes, has resulted in aphasia and loss of responsiveness.

179. Ibid., 13–20.
180. Patrick F. Houlihan, *The Birds of Ancient Egypt* (Warminster: Aris & Phillips, 1986), 20.
181. The reader is directed to appendix 2 for a compilation of the neurological symptoms and signs in the Edwin Smith Papyrus.

In Case #22, no treatment is recommended by the ancient Egyptian physician. Objectively, there was nothing that they could have done to effectively treat this case. A comminuted injury of this type is seen on the right side of the head of soldier #14 of Winlock's cache from Deir el-Bahari,[182] and in simulation in fig. 22b.

182. Winlock, *The Slain Soldiers of Neb-hep-et-Re Mentu-hotpe*, plate X A and B.

CASE #23:
Slashing Wound of the Ear
(Plate VIII:18–24)

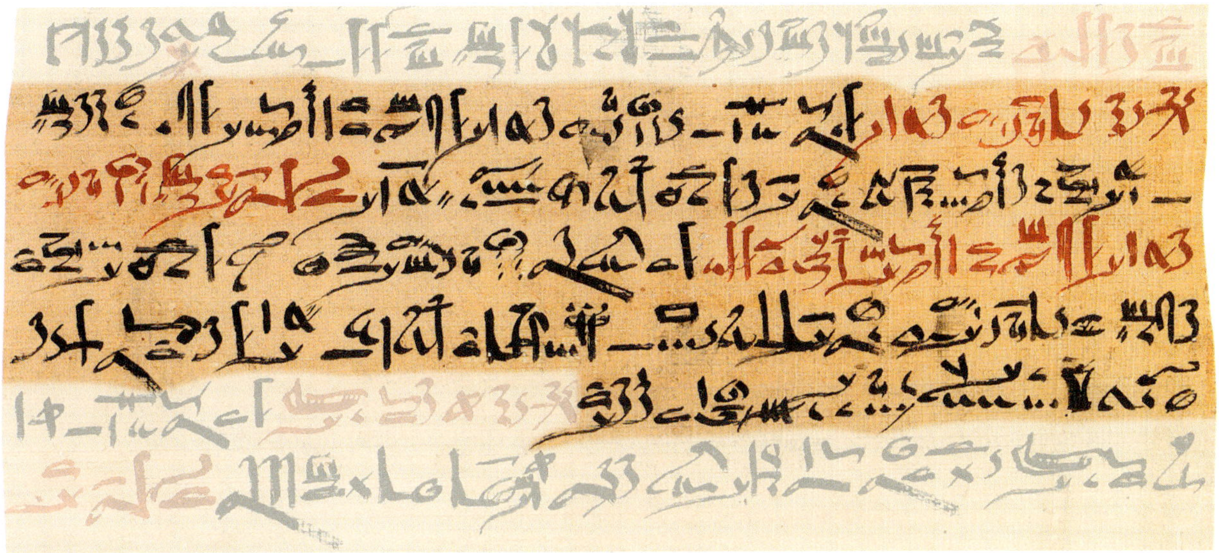

Courtesy New York Academy of Medicine.

18. 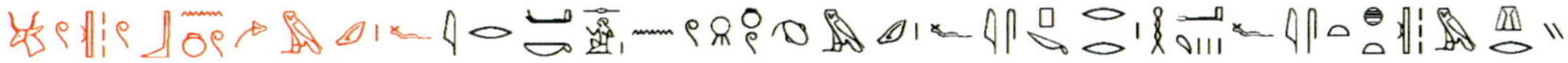

19. 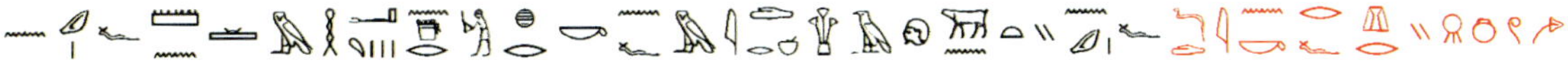

20. 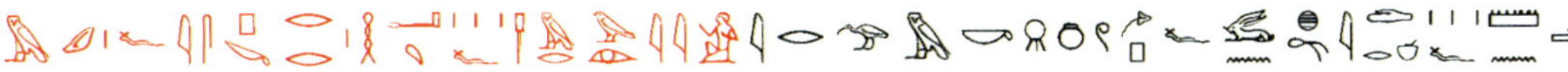

21. 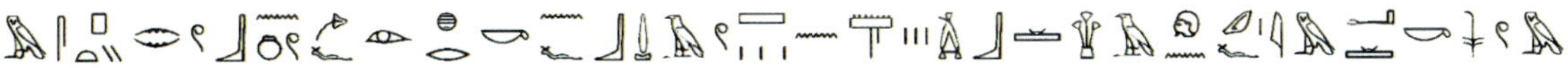

22. 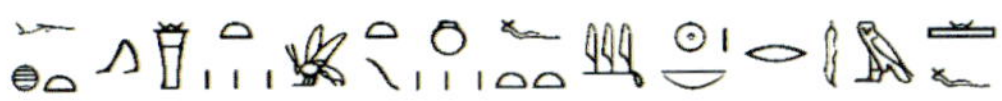

Transliteration

18§ *šs3w wbnw m msḏr.f y ir ḫ3.k s n wbnw m msḏr.f isp r r3 ḥꜥ.f isṯ ḫt m ẖry*

19§ *n msḏr.f mn m ḥꜥ nḏr.ḫr.k n.f m idr ḥ3 ḫnty n msḏr.f ḏd.in.k r.f ḫry wbnw*

20§ *m msḏr.f isp r r3 ḥꜥ.f mḥr iry.i ir gm.k wbnw pf wnḫ idrw.f mn*

21§ *m spty wbnw f ir.ḫr.k n.f bd3w n ḥbs ḏb3 ḥ3 n msḏr f im srwḫ.k sw*

22§ *m-ḫt mrḥt bit ftt rꜥ nb r nḏm.f*

Translation

Title:

Necessary knowledge and skills for a wound in his ear:

Examination:

If you should examine a man for a wound in his ear, (it being) cut through to the opening of its surface , although something of the lower part of his ear is (still) attached to the surface, then you must draw <it> together for him with stitching behind the hollow/inside of his ear.

Diagnosis:

Then you are to say about him: "One who has a wound in his ear, (it being) cut through to the opening of its surface, a medical condition which I will handle/deal with."

Treatment:

If you find that wound, its stitches loosened but (still) attached to the lips of his wound, then you must make for him stiff rolls of cloth and block up/pad the back of his ear therewith.

You should treat it thereafter with ointment and honey and a dressing every day, until it/he is well.

Notes

ỉsp(*w*) – The identification as a stative is possible because it is acting as a "virtual" (unmarked, indefinite) relative, that is, after an indefinite antecedent, "a wound." If it is stative then as a transitive verb it has to be passive in Middle Egyptian. Other translators render it as if they take it as an active participle.

ḥꜣ ẖnty n(*y*) *msḏr.f* – *ẖnty* is clearly the object of the preposition. Allen's (*AM*) and Breasted's (*Edwin Smith*) understanding is basically sound; perhaps we should translate "behind the hollow/inside of his ear."

wnẖ(*w*) *ỉdrw.f* – This is a passive *sḏm*(*w*)*.f* and is circumstantial.

bḏꜣw "stiff rolls" – see Faulkner, *CDME*, 86.

ḏbꜣ – Imperative.

Medical Commentary

Type of Injury

Case #23 describes a full thickness wound of the lower half of the auricle of the ear, involving the area of the concha cartilage that penetrates into the external auditory canal. The auricle is not completely detached. The position of the auricle of the ear on the side of the head makes it particularly vulnerable to injury.

Today the most common injury observed of this type is incomplete amputation of the ear. Auricular injuries if left untreated will invariably get infected producing additional tissue loss and external ear deformities.

Laceration repair of the auricle demands an intimate knowledge of its anatomy and histology. In the lower third of the auricle the ear's lobule is formed by skin layers with adipose tissue in between. The upper two-thirds of the auricle has a core layer of continuous cartilage, covered by a closely adherent layer of perichondrium. The cartilage itself is avascular, receiving nutrients through the covering perichondrium. The cartilage and perichondrium thickness varies from 1 to 3 mm. On the lateral surface of the ear, the skin covering is from .8 to 1.2 mm in thickness and adheres tightly to the cartilage. On the medial side, the soft tissues of the auricle measure from 1.2 to 3 mm in thickness, including a layer of subdermal adipose tissue that allows mobility of the skin over the perichondrium. The posteriomedial portion of the auricle has abundant blood supply.

Due to the auricle's peculiar histological arrangement, through-and-through laceration repair requires specific attention to the surgical technique[183] requiring suturing of the anterior and posterior portions of the laceration in multi-layer fashion. Closure begins from the depth of the wound outward. The posterior skin is first. As noted above, the skin of this area can be mobilized and often stretches sufficiently to allow coverage of most defects. The sutures should be placed through the skin and perichondrium, not through the cartilage itself, because the cartilage tears easily and does not hold sutures.[184] The cartilage needs only to be approximated. Suture material is in the 5-0 or 6-0 gauge (0.1 mm to 0.07 mm diameter, equivalent to American wire gauge 35-38, 38-40), using absorbable sutures to reduce tension from the wound edges. Anteriorly, the skin of the ear and the underlying cartilage adhere to each other and only skin closure is necessary using 5-0 or 6-0 nonabsorbable sutures.

Mastoid and bolster dressings are frequently applied over the laceration repair to support the cartilaginous skeleton and prevent perichondral hematomas.

An example of such a wound is found in Sir Charles Bell's painting of "Trooper 1st Royal Dragoons" (Visual Index III).[185]

Ancient Medical Methodology and Knowledge

Undoubtedly, the Egyptian physician was experienced in repairing auricle wounds. He specifically directs: "you must draw <it> together for him with stitching behind the hollow/inside of his ear." We interpret the ancient Egyptians' terms of hollow of the ear/inside the ear as synonymous. The area behind the hollow of the ear is the posterior or medial surface of the auricle. Pahor called attention to the Egyptian physician's knowledge in repairing an ear laceration "with stitching behind the hollow of his ear," the skin of that surface being "more amiable to such procedures."[186]

The histological layering of the posterior or medial ear auricle skin is thicker and can be mobilized over the adipose tissue, making the repair of these lacerations feasible, even with relatively crude needles and suture materials.

The use of oil and honey dressings would have prevented the wound from sticking to the dressings, kept the tissues supple, and reduced the chances of infection.

Given the frailty of the involved tissues and the surgical armamentarium available to the ancient Egyptians, it is not surprising that a consideration is given to the eventuality of the stitching becoming loose. It is at that stage that support of the auricle with padding behind the ear was considered necessary. It would have provided needed support to the repaired area, a measure we consider obligatory in treatment of these injuries today.

183. Steven P. Davison, Brooke N. Bosley, and Henry D. Sandel, "Ear Reconstruction and Salvage Procedures." Medscape Reference: http://emedicine.medscape.com/article/1288828-overview.

184. Trott, *Wounds and Lacerations*, 165–69.

185. In M. K. H. Crumplin and P. Starling, *A Surgical Artist at War: The Paintings and Sketches of Sir Charles Bell 1809–1815* (Edinburgh: The Royal College of Surgeons of Edinburgh, 2005), 42.

186. A. L. Pahor, "Ear Nose and Throat in Ancient Egypt," *The Journal of Otolaryngology and Otology* 106 (1992): 863–73.

CASE #24:
Mandibular Fracture(s)
(Plate VIII:24–IX:2)

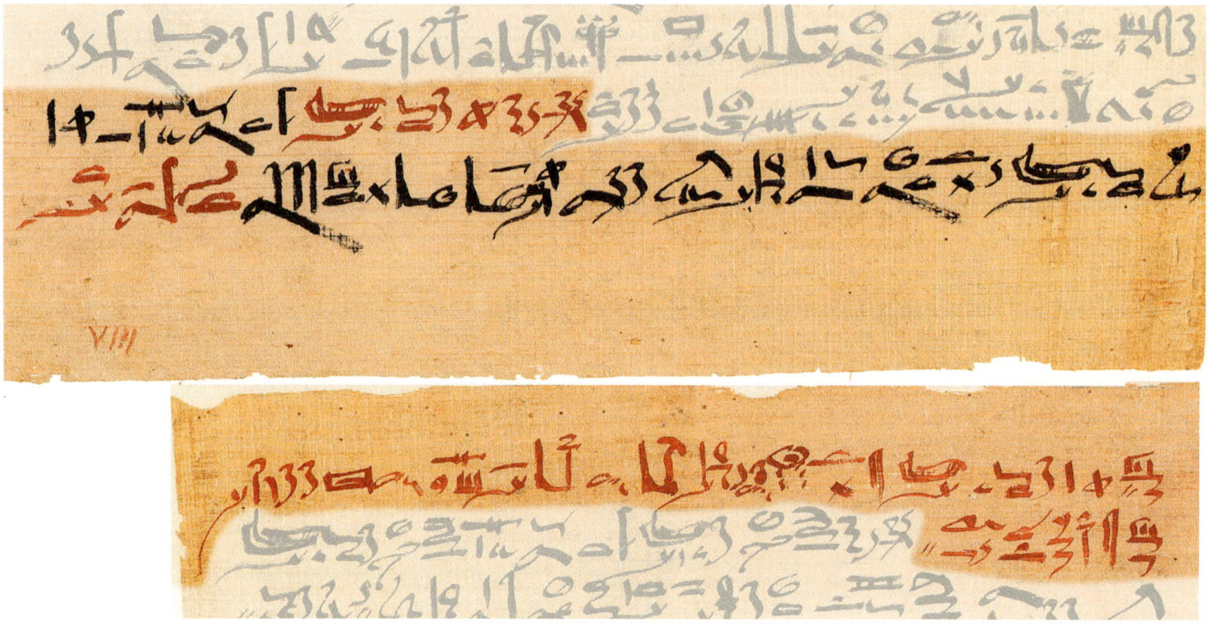

Courtesy New York Academy of Medicine.

22. 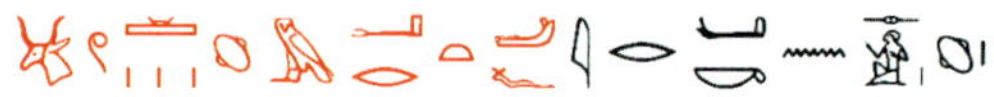

23. 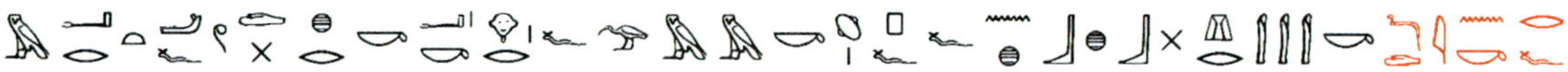

1. 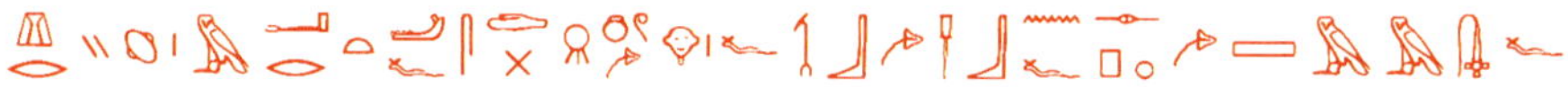

2. 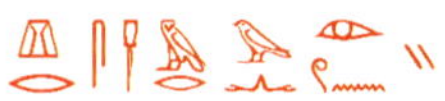

Transliteration

22§ … *šsꜣw ḥsb m ꜥrt.f ir ḫꜣ.k s n ḥsb*

23§ *m ꜥrt.f wd.ḫr.k ꜥ.k ḥr.f gmm.k ḥsb pf nḫbḫb ẖr ḏbꜥw.k ḏd.in.k r.f*

1§ *ẖry ḥsb m ꜥrt.f sḏ wbnw ḥr.f wꜣb(?) ꜣb.n.f sp(?) šmm.f*

2§ *ẖr.s mḫr n irw.ny*

Translation

Title:

Necessary knowledge and skills for a fracture in his lower jaw/mandible:

Examination:

If you should examine a man for a fracture in his mandible/lower jaw, then you must place your hand on it.

How you find that fracture (is): shifting/crepitating under your fingers.

Diagnosis:

Then you must say about him:

One who has a fracture in his mandible/lower jaw, a wound having been smashed over it;

the discharge(?), it has stopped(?)/"ceased moving" (or, it has remained??);

the coagulated diseased mass(?),

how it is hot (is) under it (i.e., under the lower jaw)—

Treatment:

a medical condition that cannot be handled/dealt with."

Notes

This is a very brief case but it contains a passage that presents both lexical and grammatical difficulties as well as uncertainties about the completeness and correctness of the text.

šd(*w*) *wbnw* – I take this as passive *sḏm*(*w*).*f*, which, as Hoch (*MEG*) reminds us, is a circumstantial.

wꜣb(*?*) *ꜣb.n.f sp* (*?*) – It is difficult if not impossible to pin down a clear and satisfactory meaning for the passage, and a long excursus is required to explore the uncertainties and options and to justify a possible, though at best only approximate, translation.

I think that *Grundriss* 7, 1:162 is on the right track taking the *wꜣs*-scepter + *b* + determinative as one word, and in reading it *wꜣb*, based on the apparently attested reading of the *wꜣs*-scepter as *wꜣb*(?) in Gardiner's sign list, S 40. Acknowledging Gardiner's uncertainty (though I think the reading is pretty evident), perhaps we should keep a question mark, *wꜣb*(?) *ꜣb.n.f sp*. As von Deines and Westendorf note, the apparent status of the words in question as hapaxes makes it very difficult to interpret the passage. They suggest either something like, "The discharge, it has ceased to flow" (also 7, 2:741–42), or alternatively, they suggest that *wꜣb*(?) could be a stative dependent on *wbnw*, something like "a wound having been smashed over it, it discharging/so that it is discharging." But it seems to me that this latter reading is more difficult to reconcile with the following "it has/having ceased to flow(?)" if that indeed is the meaning (which I suspect it is not; see below). I suggest that the present word *sp* is related to or even possibly a variant of *sp* "promoter/causer/stimulater of sickness" (*Wb*. 3:440), with a worm or wiggly snake determinative; note the similarly written word listed in *Grundriss* 7, 2:741. Von Deines and Westendorf realize that the *sp* with worm determinative "appears to be no real worm, but the designation for a worm-like clot/coagulated mass of diseased fluidity." It needs to be noted that the writing in *Grundriss* of the definitions of *sp* with worm determinative and *sp* in our passage in square brackets means that the meanings are uncertain (7, 1:III). It adds to the uncertainty that *ꜣb* in addition to "cease" can also mean "tarry, stay" (Faulkner,

CDME, 2); perhaps "cease moving" is the common denominator. Yet another possible "wild card" is the possibility of reading the face + stroke + *f* as "his face" rather than "upon/over it," but I am not pursuing this because it does not seem to lead to a clear solution for sorting out this passage.

When all of these possibilities and inferences are compared, I think that one reading worthy of serious consideration is to take the passage as two parallel clauses each featuring a noun in extraposition + a form of the Suffix Conjugation, first a *sḏm.n.f* and then a *sḏm.f*: *wꜣb ꜣb.n.f – sp šmm.f ẖr.s*: "The discharge(?), it has stopped(?)/remained(??); the coagulated diseased mass(?), how it is hot (is) under it." I think that the first clause could be analyzed as a statement of fact with noun + circumstantial *sḏm.n.f* (cf. Hoch, *MEG*, sec. 36 with *sḏm.f*), while the second clause features noun + manner nominalization + adverbial complement (*ẖr.s*). The only feminine antecedent available for the pronoun *.s* is *ꜥrt.f*, "his mandible/his lower jaw." However, I understand the preposition *ẖr* here spatially, "under." Thus the patient is hot under the (broken and injured/infected) chin, if this interpretation is correct.

Medical Commentary

Type of Injury

In our opinion, Case #24 represents two types of mandibular injuries, the description of which are interrupted by a scribal copying lapse.

The first injury is recorded in our examination section taken from the line 23 of plate VIII as a closed simple fracture (*ḥsb*) "shifting/crepitating ..." with no mention of a wound.

The second injury is recorded in our diagnosis section taken from the line 1 of plate IX as an open comminuted fracture with a wound smashed (*ḥsb* + *sd wbnw*) over the fracture.

The above discrepancy in which the closed simple fracture recorded in the examination suddenly changes in the diagnosis into an open comminuted fracture with a wound smashed over, and with infection, alerts us to the consideration of two different kinds of mandibular fractures (both *ḥsb* and *ḥsb sd wbnw*) being presented in this case, likely due to scribal error of omission, as we imagine he began copying the original document from line 23 of plate VIII accidentally to his first line of plate IX.

It looks to us as though our scribe in this situation has erred. The logical sequence observed in the Edwin Smith Papyrus of presenting simpler cases before complex cases for the same anatomical region would lead one to expect that the second injury recorded in this case would actually have followed in a separate case. There is in the papyrus, however, the absence of an appropriate record of "diagnosis" and "treatment" for the closed simple fracture and the absence of the "title" and "examination" findings for the open, comminuted, infected fracture. Thus, we see four segments missing between the end of the record (plate VIII) of the closed simple fracture and the beginning of the record (plate IX) of the open comminuted fracture. We can imagine here a distracted copyist.

The mandible's prominent location in the face makes it susceptible to fracture, and it is involved in 70 percent of patients with facial fractures.[187] The shape and rigidity of the mandible favors its breaking at multiple places upon impact. The trauma source and its direction can produce a variety of mandibular fractures.[188] A fist often produces single, nondisplaced fractures. Impacts from a pipe or similar rigid object produce localized

187. Jose E. Barrera, and Stephen G. Batuello, "Mandibular Body Fractures." Medscape Reference: http://emedicine.medscape.com/article/869123-overview.

188. D. B. Hoyt, R. Coimbra, and J. Acosta, "Management of Acute Trauma," in Townsend and Evers, *Sabiston Textbook of Surgery*, 494–95.

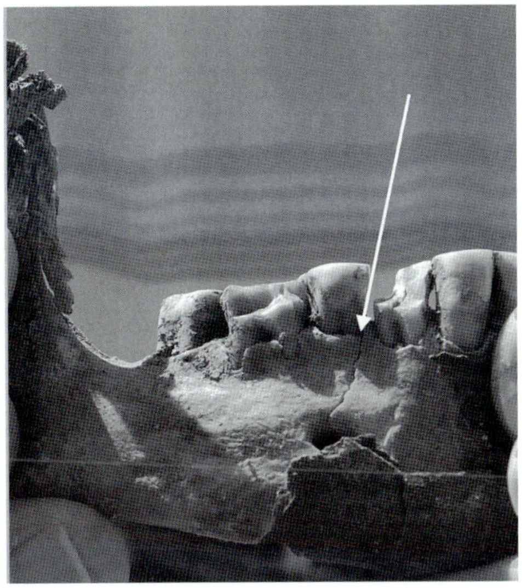

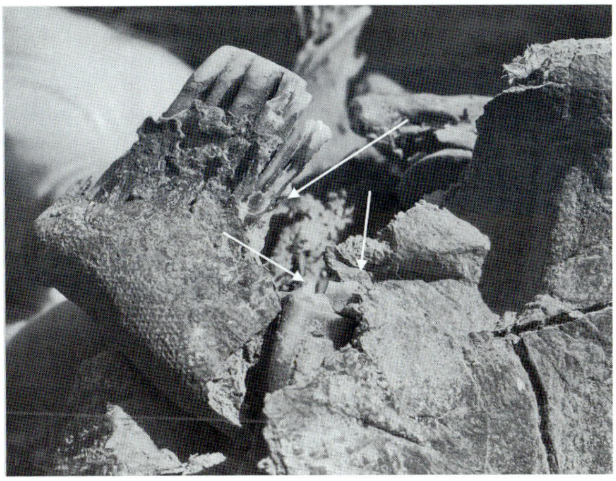

Fig. 24. Human remains, mandibular fractures. Left: *ḥsb* fracture. Right: *sd* fracture. (Specimens HRX-194-196-198.) Courtesy of the University of Arizona Egyptian Expedition, Tausret Temple Excavation, 2009–2010.

comminuted fractures and motor vehicle accidents are often responsible for multiple comminuted fractures. Direct impact to the chin often produces localized symphysis fracture and unilateral or bilateral condylar fractures.

Lacerations, hematoma, and ecchymosis are associated with mandibular fractures.[189] The examination usually reveals facial distortion and malocclusion of the teeth, and palpation of the fracture site may produce displacement and crepitation of the bone fragments. There may be associated injuries to neighboring structures like other facial fractures, basilar skull fractures, post-traumatic occlusion of the internal carotid artery, pneumothorax and subcutaneous cervical emphysema.

Proper evaluation in a medical facility today would include securing airway patency, general assessment of all injuries, radiographic and computer tomography scanning (CAT Scan). Consultation would be conducted with Ear, Nose, and Throat, or Oral Surgery specialties.

Until recently, the standard treatment of simple mandibular fractures was closed reduction or open reduction with wire osteosynthesis, requiring six weeks of immobilization with obvious complications, such as airway patency, obstacles to the provision of nutrition and hygiene, which would have made this treatment impractical, or impossible in antiquity. However, today closed reduction is still indicated in the management of grossly comminuted mandibular fractures, coronoid process and condylar fractures. Most complex facial fractures are currently treated by open reduction and fixation. The availability of plates, including absorbable materials with rigid and semi-rigid fixation have revolutionized and greatly enhanced surgical treatment possibilities, allowing for early mobilization, patient comfort, better nutrition and earlier return to daily life.[190]

The modern treatment of an open, infected fracture requires extensive debridement and infection control prior to any attempt to carry out complex surgical reconstruction.

The most common complication is infection or osteomyelitis, Staphylococcus aureus being the most common contaminant, but not excluding other bacteria, including anaerobic bacteria. Contributing factors to infec-

189. D. R. Laub, "Facial Trauma, Mandibular Fractures." Medscape Reference: http://emedicine.medscape.com/article/1283150-treatment.

190. Ibid.

tion are the presence of oral sepsis, teeth left in the fracture line, prolonged time to appropriate treatment, and comminuted fragments.[191]

In Case #24, the findings of mandibular fracture are confirmed. Considered as a closed simple fracture, there appears to be no problem that would warrant a poor prognosis, except for the difficulty to nourish the patient during his fracture healing and possible permanent malocclusion of his teeth. The features of an open, comminuted fractured jaw that has ceased draining and "the coagulated diseased mass" (suggesting necrosis) that has become infected, introduces the possibility of septic gangrene. Clostridial gas gangrene is a highly lethal necrotizing soft-tissue infection of skeletal muscle caused by toxin and gas producing clostridium species. The synonym clostridial myonecrosis better describes both the causative agent and the target tissue. Prior to the advent of antibiotics and mobile army surgical hospitals, as many as 5 percent of battlefield injuries were complicated by this condition.

For the development of *Clostridia* gangrene, inoculation and a low-oxygen environment are required. More than 50 percent of cases are related to trauma, with compound fractures being a favorable setting for infection. The infected site has a relatively low level of inflammation as such, and often there are no purulent secretions in the wound. However, muscle destruction progresses rapidly, spreading as fast as 2 cm per hour. Systemic toxic shock and renal failure lead to death, often within twelve hours. The disease untreated has 100 percent mortality, but if treated, mortality is reduced to 20 to 30 percent.[192]

Ancient Medical Methodology and Knowledge

As discussed above, it seems very probable that Case #24 was, inadvertently, composed of more than one clinical situation. The Egyptian physician's verdict in this case—"a medical condition that cannot be handled/dealt with"—is less consistent with that of a closed linear mandibular fracture than with an open, comminuted, and infected necrotic fracture. In ancient Egypt, physicians had neither the means to resolve deep infection, nor to restore successfully a fragmented comminuted jaw. Antibiotics, and maxillo/facial reconstructive surgery were unavailable until the twentieth century.

Two post-mortem examples of mandibular fractures are shown in fig. 24 from the mummified human remains material found by the University of Arizona Egyptian Expedition, at the excavation of Queen Tausret's memorial temple site in Luxor, Egypt (2009–2011 seasons).

Based on anatomical and functional information related to the Egyptian anatomical terms that appear in various cases in this papyrus—Amat, forked bone, Case #22, ramus; *gmꜣ*, zygomatic-temporal area, Cases #7, #18, #19, #20, #21, #22; *wꜣt*, cord, Case #7; *ʿrty*, mandible, lower jaw Cases #7, #22, #24, #25; and *wgyt*, jaw, Case #7—Peacock, Chapman, et al.[193] have replicated in human cadavers the facial bone defects evident in the mummified head of Djehutynakht,[194] circa 2000 B.C.E., in the collection of the Museum of Fine Arts, Boston. Using simple instruments to simulate what would have been available to the ancient physician (scalpel, mallet, 8-mm chisel, and two right angle retractors), and an intraoral approach, these authors were able to carry out

191. A. Lukosiunas, G. Sabalys, and R. Kubilus, "Prediction of Mandible Traumatic Osteomyelitis," *Stomatoloija, Baltic Dental and Maxillofacial Journal* 5 (2003): 65–69.

192. D. A. Anaya and E. P. Dellinger, "Necrotizing Soft-Tissue Infections: Diagnosis and Management," *Clinical Infectious Diseases* 44/5 (2007): 705–10.

193. Z. S. Peacock, P. H. Chapman, R. Gupta, and L. B. Kaban, "Replication of Ancient Egyptian Osteotomies of the Facial Skeleton: Insights into the Mummification Process," *International Journal of Oral Maxillofacial Surgery* 40/11 (2011): 1301–6.

194. P. H. Chapman and R. Gupta, "Reinvestigation of a Middle Kingdom Head Provides New Insights Concerning Mummification and Its Relationship to Contemporary Anatomic Knowledge and Funerary Ritual," *Journal of the American Research Center in Egypt* 43 (2007): 113–27.

sequential osteotomies of the maxillary sinus, the zygomatic-maxillary buttress, the inferior orbital rim to the zygomaticosphenoid suture and the zygomatic process of the temporal bone. These osteotomies made possible mobilization of the zygoma and zygomatic arch laterally. Then, by stripping of the masseter muscle at its origin, the mandibular coronoid process and the insertion of the temporalis muscle to it were exposed. Chiseling of the base of the coronoid process made the jaw completely mobile. Replication of the facial bones resection and detachments seen on Djehutynakht's mummified head, were confirmed by high resolution computer tomography scans with 3D reconstructions in the cadaver heads. It was clear that these osteotomies needed to be done sequentially, as resection of one area, made possible the exposure and resection of the next, following a strict order. Chapman and colleagues concluded "that the ancient Egyptians possessed a relatively sophisticated knowledge of the functional anatomy of the jaw and associated facial skeleton."

CASE #25:
Mandibular Dislocation
(Plate IX:2–6)

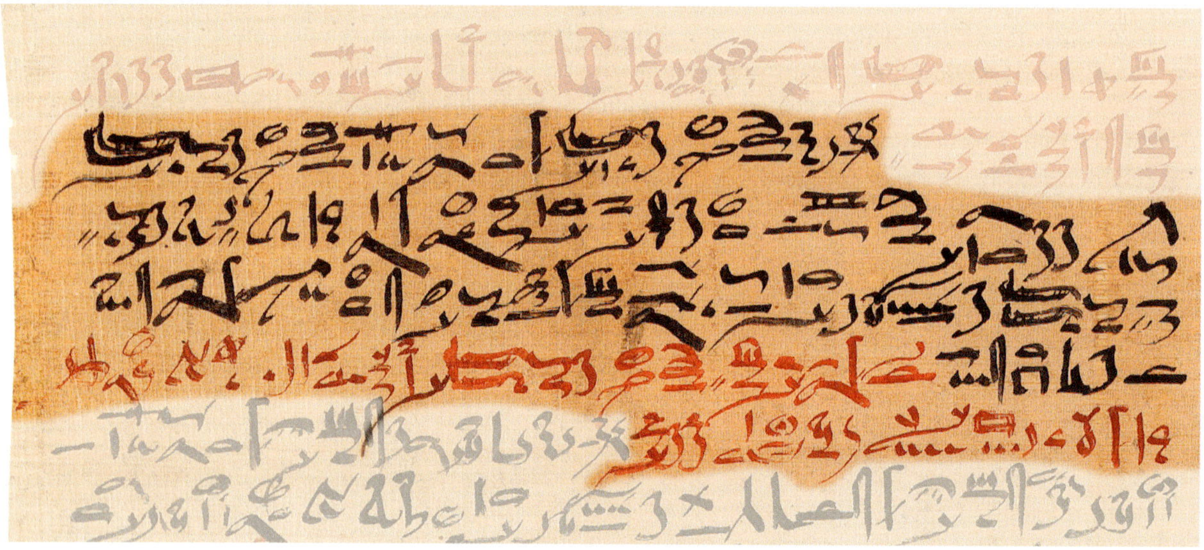

Courtesy New York Academy of Medicine.

2. 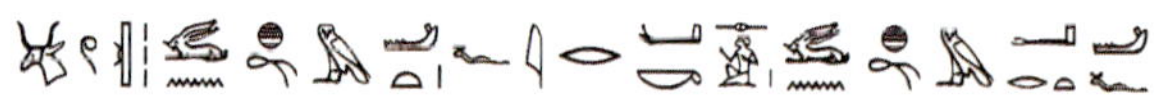

3. 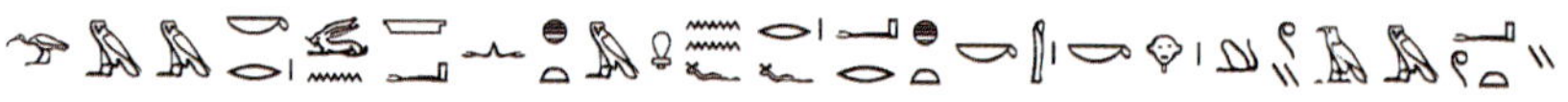

4. 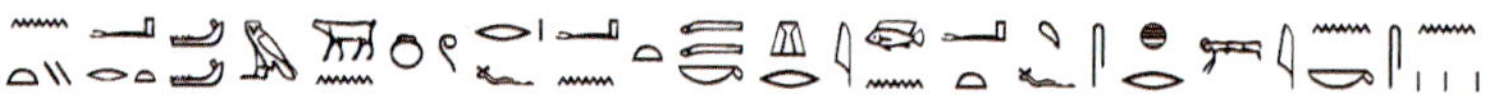

5. 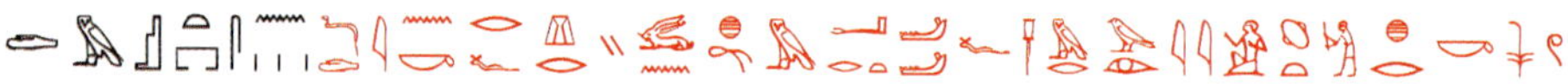

6. 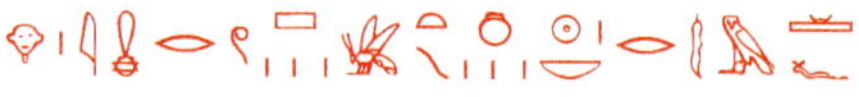

Transliteration

2§ *… šsꜣw wnẖ m ꜥrt.f i͗r ẖꜣ.k s <n> wnẖ m ꜥrt.f*

3§ *gmm.k rꜣ.f wn n ẖtm.n n.f rꜣ.f rdi͗.ḫr.k ḏbꜥ.k ḥr pḥwy ꜣmꜥwty*

4§ *nty <m> ꜥrt{y} m-ẖnw rꜣ.f ꜥnty.k ẖr i͗nꜥt.f sḫr.jn.k sn*

5§ *d(w)(?) m st.sn ḏd.i͗n.k r.f ẖry wnẖ m ꜥrt{y}.f mḥr i͗ry.i͗ wt.ḫr.k sw*

6§ *ḥr i͗mrw bji͗ rꜥ nb r nḏm.f*

Translation

Title:

Necessary knowledge and skills for a dislocation in his mandible/lower jaw:

Examination:

If you should examine a man (for) a dislocation in his mandible/lower jaw,

how you find his mouth (is) open, and his mouth cannot close for him.

Then you must put your thumb upon (each) of the two rear sections of the forked bones that are (in?) the mandible/lower jaw, in the inside of his mouth, and your two "claws" under his chin.

Then you are to cause them to fall back, so that they are put in their place(s).

Diagnosis:

Then you are to say about him: "One who has a dislocation in his mandible/lower jaw,

a medical condition which I will handle/deal with."

Treatment:

Then you must bind it (along) with alum(?) (or, a bandage with alum[?] shavings?) and honey every day until it/he is well.

Notes

wn(*w*) "open" – a stative.

nty <*m*> *ꜥrt*{*y*} – *m* is needed after *nty* because *nty* + a lone nominal predicate is not an attested relative clause in Middle Egyptian. This could be *m* of Predication, in which case the translation "that are the mandible/lower jaw" stands; or, if one wants to be pedantic, "that are (as) the mandible…"; or it could be "that are in the mandible …," hence my compromise translation with "(in?)," in parentheses.

ꜥrt{*y*} – For the explanation of the dual writing of "mandible/lower jaw," see Case #7.

d(*w*) (?) – *d* by itself is an attested writing of a verb also meaning "give, place, put," and can be read *d*(*w*); it need not be regarded as an abbreviation or truncated writing of *wdi* (see above). I take it as very clearly a stative and understand the sense here as a stative of result. As the stative of a transitive verb, the meaning comes out passive in Middle Egyptian. See also Case #12. In that passage, however, the *d* comes after a curl *w* of *sw*, where haplography of (*w*)*d* could be expected, and that is not the case here.

imrw – See Case #15: *Grundriss* 6:33–34 defines this as "an unknown mineral(?)," and regards *ibnw* (22–23) as alum, as do Aufrère, *L'univers minéral dans la pensée égyptienne*, 2:605–6, and Rainer Hannig, *Grosses Handwörterbuch Deutsch–Ägyptisch* (Mainz: von Zabern 2000), 27. Strangely, Aufrère seems to include no references to *imrw*.

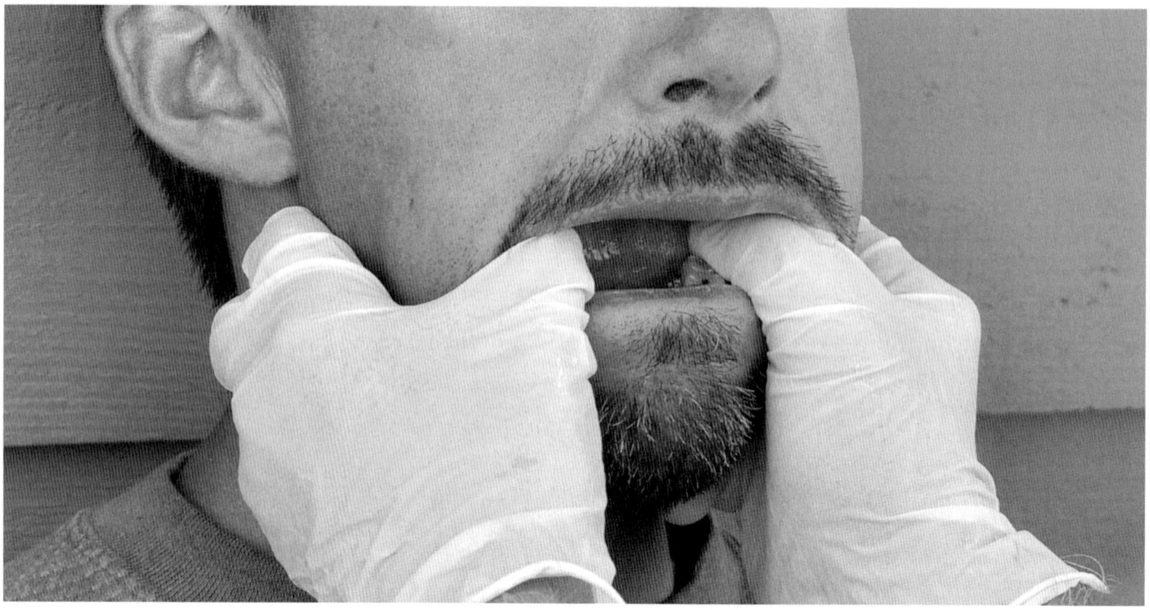

Fig. 25. Reduction technique for mandibular dislocation.

Medical Commentary

Type of Injury

This is a case of a dislocated jaw. Temporo-mandibular dislocations result from the mandibular condyle being displaced from its normal position in the temporal bone articular fossa. The dislocation can be unilateral or bilateral and often occurs after direct mandibular trauma or extreme opening of the mouth like laughing, yawning, intubation for general anesthesia, or during dental work. There is difficulty speaking and frequently there is pain in front of the ear. The dislocation mechanism is detailed by Chaudhry and Rosh:[195] "Most dislocations occur anteriorly and are secondary to an interruption in the normal sequence of muscle action when the mouth closes from extreme opening. The masseter and temporalis muscles elevate the mandible before the lateral pterygoid muscle relaxes resulting in the mandibular condyle being pulled anterior to the bony eminence and out of the temporal fossa. Spasm of the masseter, temporalis, and pterygoid muscles causes trismus and keeps the condyle from returning into the temporal fossa."

The current treatment of a mandibular dislocation is by manual reduction under sedation (fig. 25). The technique described by Newton[196] is as follows:

- Clinician faces the patient.
- Seat the patient on a chair against a wall and have him or her rest his or her head against the wall for support.

195. M. Chaudhry and A. J. Rosh, "Dislocation, Mandible: Treatment & Medication." Medscape Reference: http://emedicine.medscape.com/article/823775-treatment.

196. Philip M. Buttaravoli, and Thomas O. Stair, *Common Simple Emergencies*. Bowie, MD: Brady Communication Co., 1985. Online: http://www.ncemi.org/cse/cse0402.htm.

- Place gloved thumbs on the retro molar pad (i.e., behind the last molar) on either side of the mandible and grasp the inferior surface of the mandible with the fingers on each side.
- With elbows locked, exert downward pressure on the lower molars by bending your knees to free the condyle from its entrapped position anterior to the articular eminence.
- Ease the mandible posteriorly to return it to its anatomic position. Successful reduction is usually evident, as the teeth close rapidly due to masseter spasm, and a palpable (and sometimes audible) clunk occurs on reduction.

Note that the physician correctly placed his thumbs at the end of the rami, and not over the last molars. Current warning about this issue: "The physician must beware of having her or his thumbs trapped in an inadvertent human bite as the mandible relocates. Because of this risk, the common practice of wrapping both thumbs with gauze and pressing down on both molars is discouraged." The patient should avoid wide jaw opening for one to two weeks.

Ancient Medical Methodology and Knowledge

After the ancient Egyptian has found the patient with his mouth open and unable to close it, indicative of a dislocation in the mandible, he is instructed to proceed with reduction of the dislocation. The reduction technique for a dislocated jaw described step by step in Case #25 of the Edwin Smith Papyrus has remained unchanged to the present. The instructions are precise about placing of the physician's thumbs inside the mouth on the end of the rami, at the rear portion of the jaw beyond the molars, eliminating for the physician the potential hazard of being bitten. The rest of the fingers, forming a "claw," would grab the jaw under the chin and proceed with the maneuver to make the condyles fall back into the articular fossa of the temporal bone. Following successful reduction, the patient's mandible was to be supported with bandaging over medication, presumably an anti-inflammatory (alum?) and honey. It is uncertain why the use of honey in this instance.

Echoing Breasted's observation on the similarity of the technique of reduction of mandibular dislocations to that of Hippocrates, Stiefel et. al., propose that the Greeks derived their knowledge from the Egyptians.[197]

197. M. Stiefel, A. Shaner, and S. D. Schaefer, "The Edwin Smith Papyrus: The Birth of Analytical Thinking in Medicine and Otolaryngology," *The Laryngoscope* 116 (2006): 187.

CASE #26:
Upper Lip Full-Thickness Slash Wound
(Plate IX:6–13)

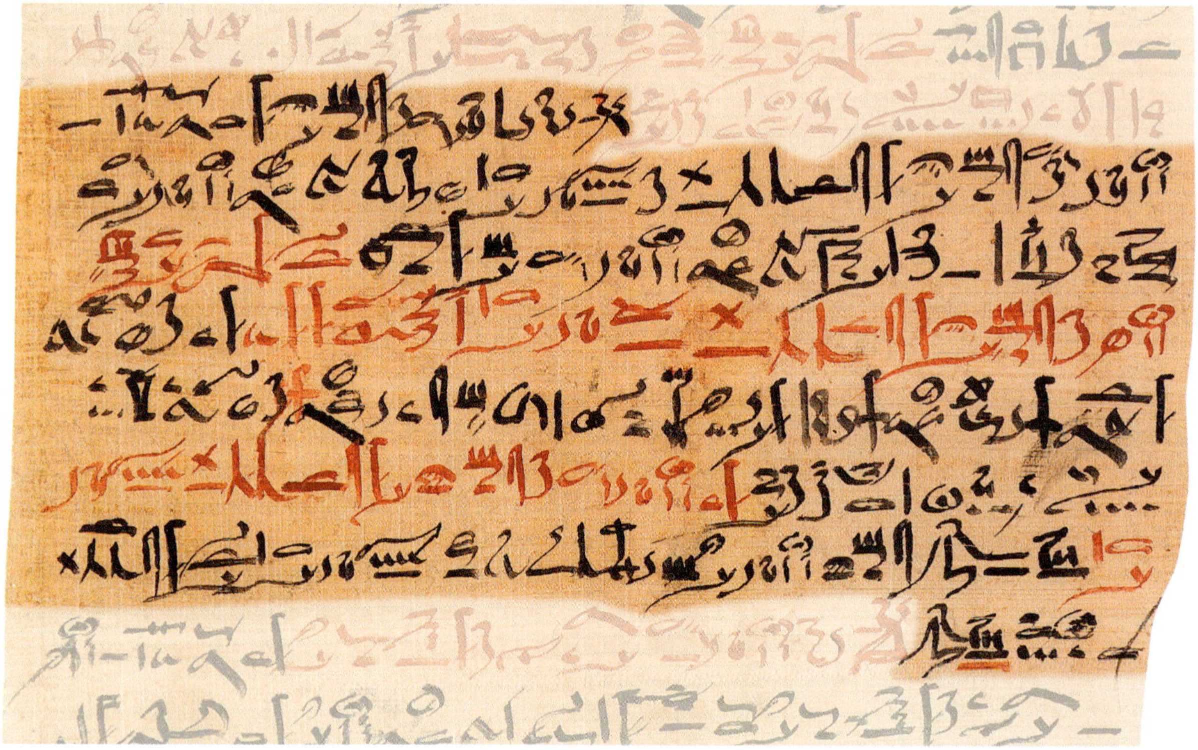

Courtesy New York Academy of Medicine.

6. 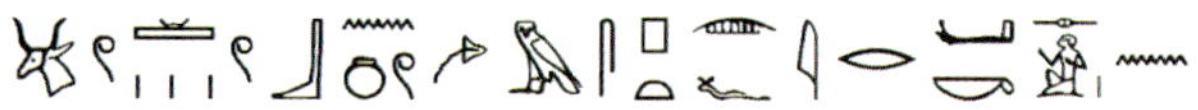

7. 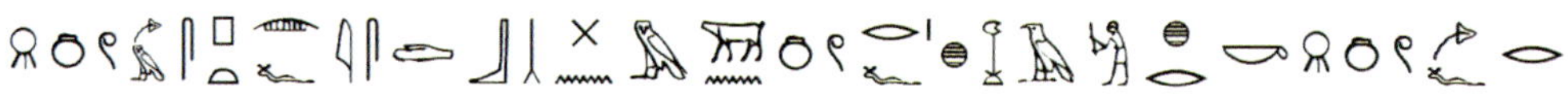

8. 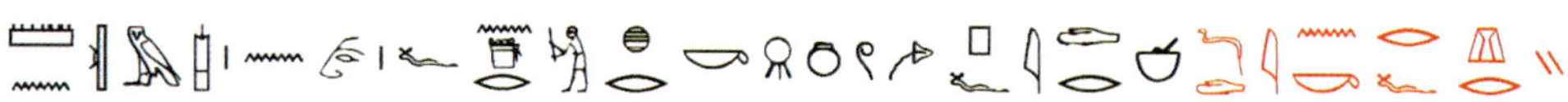

9. 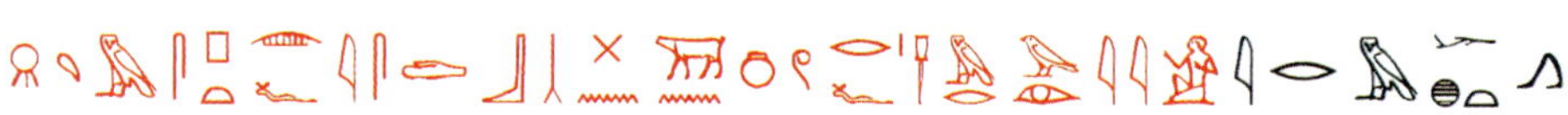

10. 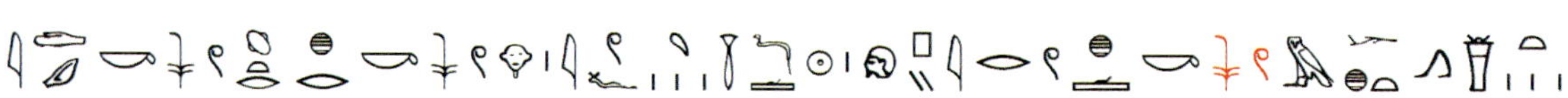

11. 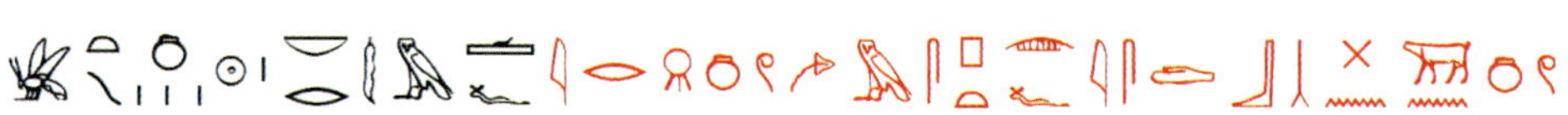

12. 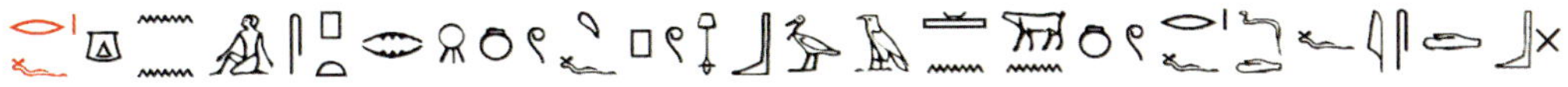

13. 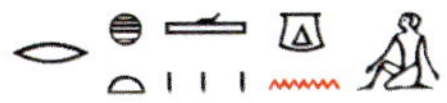

Transliteration

6§ *... šsꜣw wbnw m spt.f ir ḫꜣ.k s n*

7§ *wbnw m spt.f isdb n m-ḫnw rꜣ.f ḫꜣ.ḫr.k wbnw.f r-*

8§ *mn-m iwn n fnd.f nḏr.ḫr.k wbnw pf<m> idr ḏd.in.k r.f ḫry*

9§ *wbnw m spt.f isdb n ḫnw rꜣ.f mḥr iry.i ir m-ḫt*

10§ *[id].k sw wt.ḫr.k sw ḥr iwf wꜣḏ hrw tpy srwḫ.k sw m-ḫt mrḥt*

11§ *bit rꜥ nb r nḏm.f ir wbnw m spty.f isdb n ḫnw*

12§ *rꜣ.f gnn spty wbnw.f pw wbꜣ n ḫnw rꜣ.f ḏd.f isdb*

13§ *r ḫt gn*

Translation

Title:

Necessary knowledge and skills for a wound in his lip:

Examination:

If you should examine a man for a wound in his lip, it being pierced and collapsed through to the inside of his mouth, then you must examine his wound as far as the column of his nose.

Then you must draw together that wound <with> stitching/so that it is stitched(?).

Diagnosis:

Then you are to say to him: "One who has a wound in his lip, it being pierced and collapsed through to the inside of his mouth, a medical condition which I will handle/deal with."

Treatment:

After you suture it, you then must bind it (along) with fresh meat the first day.

You should treat it afterward with ointment and honey every day until it/he is well.

Explanation:

As for "a wound in his lip, it being pierced/which penetrates(?) through to the inside of his mouth," it means that the lips of his wound are pulpy/soft, they being open to the inside of his mouth"; he says: "being pierced through/which penetrates(?)," with respect to things that are pulpy/soft.

Notes

isdb – *Grundriss* 8, sec. 164 takes this as a stative. I took it as a stative in Case #14. This is my first rendition here, before the slash. After the slash I add a possible translation as an active participle, based on Faulkner's definition "penetrate" for *sḏb* (*CDME*, 259). Against this is the prevailing absence of the *i*-augment with active participles of triliteral verbs (for the attestation of augment in the participles see *Grundriss* 8, sec. 295 and Edel, *AG*, sec. 630). This objection would be reduced if the root *sdb* were analyzed as a causative. It is simpler and more straightforward to go with the stative. See the commentary to Case #14 for our understanding of this description as a "pierced (through) and collapsed" wound, which seems to be similar to what Allen (*AM*, 83, 89) intends with the terminology "obstructive wound."

n m (sic) *ẖnw* "to the inside" – There are two possibilities for analysis, with and without an emendation. Either the *m* is superfluous and is incorrectly included by the scribe because of influence of the preposition *m-ẖnw* "inside (of), within," or this is an instance of an unusual but attested use of a nominalized preposition or prepositional expression, with the compound preposition *m-ẖnw* being treated as a noun (Gardiner, *EG*^{3}, sec. 158.2), a construction that continues all the way into Coptic. It can be compared with the use of the phrase *zu Hause*, "at home," as a noun in current conversational German, where a place can be described as someone's "zu Hause." Maybe the superfluous *m* is more likely considering the number of cases in this text in which *m* is omitted; it seems to be subject to uncertainties or fluctuations at the hands of this scribe.

idr "<with> stitching" – Again there are two possible understandings, as *idr* can be either a noun or a verb (Faulkner, *CDME*, 36). Either *m* is omitted and we should read <*m*> *idr*, or *idr* is to be taken as *idr*(*w*), a stative of result, "so that it is stitched." I lean towards the former reading as simpler even though it involves an emendation.

gnn spty wbnw.f pw – "it means that the lips of his wound are soft" taking *gnn* as a nominal *sḏm.f* with the basic, "pristine" Polotskyan sense of a "that-form" that can function as a "that-clause."

Medical Commentary

Type of Injury

Case #26 is a through and through lip laceration pierced and collapsed through to the inside of the mouth, falling into the category of "*isdb*" wounds, injuries, which pierce through and through soft tissues that are not directly supported by bone. The lacerated wound edges would literally be folded into the oral cavity obstructing the wound. The location to the upper lip was inferred by Breasted (*Edwin Smith*, 306), who noted that exploration of the wound to "the pillar of the nose" could only be done in a wound of the upper lip. However, the treatment instructions in Case #26 could apply to the entire region formed by the lips.

Lip lacerations can cause severe cosmetic problems and they need meticulous repair. After wound debridement and removal of teeth fragments, skin closure proceeds with 5-0 nonabsorbable sutures by alignment of the lip's cutaneous "vermillion border" then the orbicularis oris muscle is closed with absorbable 5-0 sutures. It is also important to restore the mucosal border of the lip, dividing the intraoral portion of the lip from its extra-oral portion. The mucosa is sutured with 5-0 (0.1 mm diameter, equivalent to American wire gauge 35-38) absorbable material and the rest of the skin is sutured with 6-0 (0.07 mm diameter, equivalent to American wire gauge 38-40) nonabsorbable interrupted sutures. Local anesthesia is best administered remotely, as direct infiltration of the laceration will distort the lip, making it difficult to align its edges. Although the mouth is full of bacteria, infections are not frequent, but the use of oral antibiotics is customary for five to seven days. No dressings are applied to the lips today.

Ancient Medical Methodology and Knowledge

Points of interest in the ancient Egyptian physician directives in this injury are the mandate for thorough exploration of the "wound as far as the column of his nose" and to proceed with wound closure by stitching. We know from Case #11, that the lower portion of the "pillar of the nose" is the nasal septum cartilage inferior attachment to the nasal spine of the maxillary bone (fig. 11). Exploring to "the pillar of his nose" would cover its entirety. As for wound suturing, we have addressed in the above section the importance we attach today to proper lip wound reconstruction; it seems the ancient Egyptians thought the same way. Suturing of the wound would have controlled the bleeding. Local wound care was given by application of fresh meat on the first day and daily dressings with oil and honey dressings thereafter. The possible usefulness of applying fresh meat over a wound and of oil and honey dressings, have been discussed in detail in Case #1.

CASE #27:
Chin Full-Thickness Slash Wound
(Plate IX:13–18)

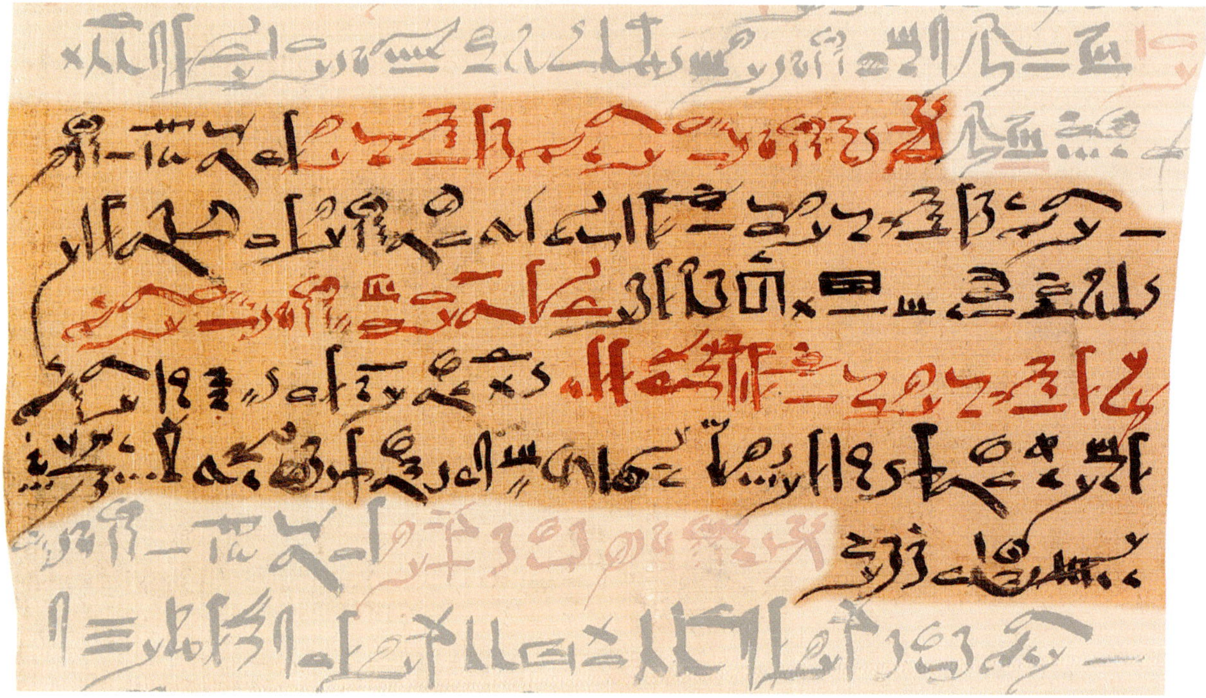

Courtesy New York Academy of Medicine.

13. 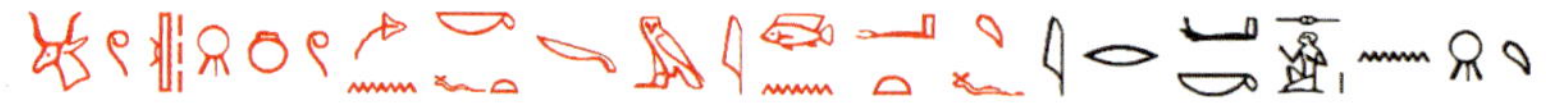

14. 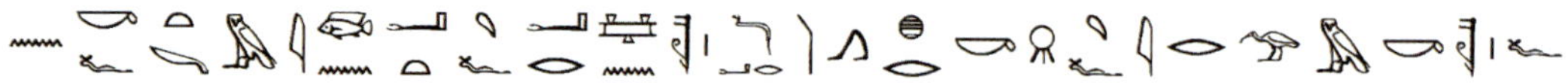

15. 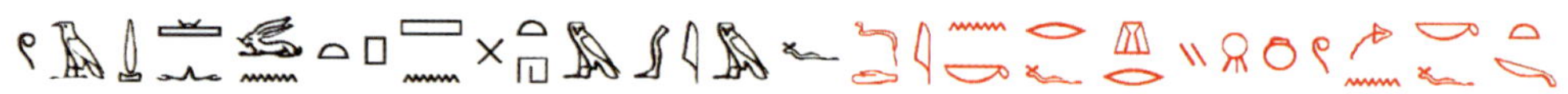

16. 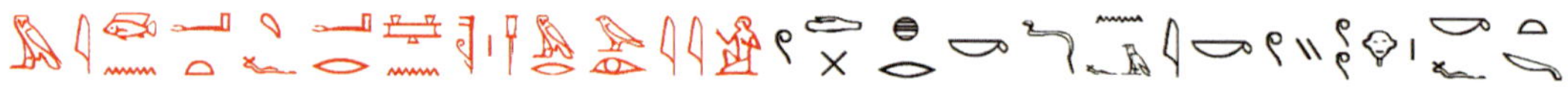

17. 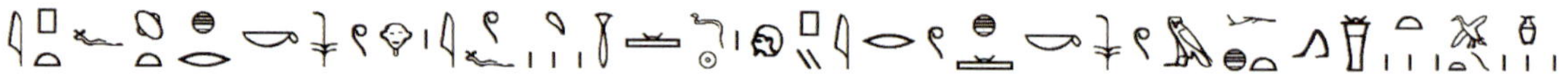

18. 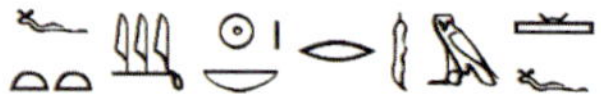

Transliteration

13§ *... šsꜣw wbnw n kft m inꜥt.f ir ẖꜣ.k s n wbnw*

14§ *n kft m inꜥt.f rꜥ n ḳs ḏꜥr.ẖr.k wbnw.f ir gm.k ḳs.f*

15§ *wḏꜣ n wnt pšn thm im.f ḏd.in.k r.f ẖry wbnw n kft*

16§ *m inꜥt.f ꜥr n ḳs mḥr iry.i wd.ẖr.k n.f ꜣirwy ḥr kft*

17§ *iptf wt.ẖr.k sw ḥr iwf wꜣḏ hrw tpy srwẖ.k sw m-ẖt mrḥt bit*

18§ *ftt rꜥ nb r nḏm.f*

Translation

Title:

Necessary knowledge and skills for a slash wound in his chin:

Examination:

If you should examine a man for a wound of a knife in his chin, that has penetrated to the bone, you have to palpate his wound.

If you find his bone intact, and there is no split or a perforation in it

Diagnosis:

then you are to say about him: "One who suffers from a slash wound in his chin, that has penetrated to the bone, a medical condition which I can handle/deal with."

Treatment:

You must apply to him a pair of bandages/linen strips over that slash wound.

Then you must bind it (along) with fresh meat the first day.

You should treat it afterward with ointment and honey and a dressing every day until it/he is well.

Notes

ꜥr – Not a relative form but an active participle. To be a relative form it would have to have its own subject or actor-expression conjugated like the *sḏm.f* or *sḏm.n.f*. The examples in Hoch, *MEG*, sec. 158 have this separate actor-expression. In the present passage, *wbnw* "wound" is the *antecedent* of the participle, not the subject/actor-expression of a relative form. It happens that with the participle, the antecedent and subject of the relative clause are the same, while with a relative form one is in the domain of relative clauses in which the antecedent is *not* the same as the subject of the relative clause. An example to illustrate this: antecedent + participle, "wound which penetrates," while a relative form would be, for instance, "wound which *he* inflicts."

ꜣirwy – See also D. Meeks, *Année Lexicographique* 1, 1. I agree, pace Hannig's suggestion, that nothing in the word itself indicates that the bandages are crossed or in fact what their physical arrangement is; that translation would be adding something that is not in the original. As far as I can see, the paired determinatives only indicate that one is dealing with a dual, that is, a pair of items.

Medical Commentary

Type of Injury

This is a cutting wound of the soft tissues of the chin that has reached the mandibular bone without producing a fracture. It is important to clarify that the bone is uninjured, in comparison with the open injury to the mandible incompletely described in the diagnosis section of Case #24. As with any other facial injury, there is a potential for chin lacerations to cause facial disfigurement, and, therefore, wound repair demands meticulous anatomical reconstitution. The chin has three distinct layers: skin, subcutaneous tissue, and muscle. Although the chin is separate from the lip, the two structures have an intimate muscular relationship in the sharing of the depressor and the orbicularis oris muscles of the mouth. The mentalis muscle is a small muscle with two attachment points, to the mandible below the incisors, and to the skin of the chin. Layer by layer repair is necessary using fine 4-0 size (0.15 mm diameter, or American wire gauge 32–34) absorbable suture material for muscle repair and subcutaneous suturing. Skin can be closed with 5-0 or 6-0 (0.1 mm to 0.07 mm diameter, equivalent to American wire gauge 35-38, 38-40) subcuticular closure, not uncommonly supplemented by liquid bandage adhesive or by steri-strips on the skin surface. The surgical site would be protected by light dressings.

Ancient Medical Methodology and Knowledge

The ancient Egyptian physician's recommendation for the treatment of this wound was to approximate the wound edges with two linen strips. As discussed above (Case #2), these cloth strips probably had adhesive properties. Dr. A. B. Luckhardt, advisor to James H. Breasted on medical issues in the Edwin Smith Papyrus, remarked in Case #27 (*Edwin Smith*, 312): "Wounds of the chin are likely to gape less than wounds of the lip, particularly if the wound of the chin is parallel with the course of the fibers of the *m. triangularis* and platysma. Hence we have stitching in the preceding case against taping in Case 27." The authors concur with this opinion. The approximation and apposition of the wound edges by taping would have resulted in good cosmetic effects. Wound treatment proceeded with their established routine of applying fresh meat the first day, followed by dressings with ointment and honey (see the medical commentary for Case #1). Sir. Charles Bell's Watercolor painting of a soldier wounded in the battle of Waterloo[198] depicts a wound to this area (Visual Index III).

198. M. K. H. Crumplin and P. Starling, *A Surgical Artist at War: The Paintings and Sketches of Sir Charles Bell 1809–1815* (Edinburgh: The Royal College of Surgeons of Edinburgh, 2005), 42.

CASE #28:

Anterior Neck Wound with Esophageal-Tracheal Fistula

(Plate IX:18–X:3)

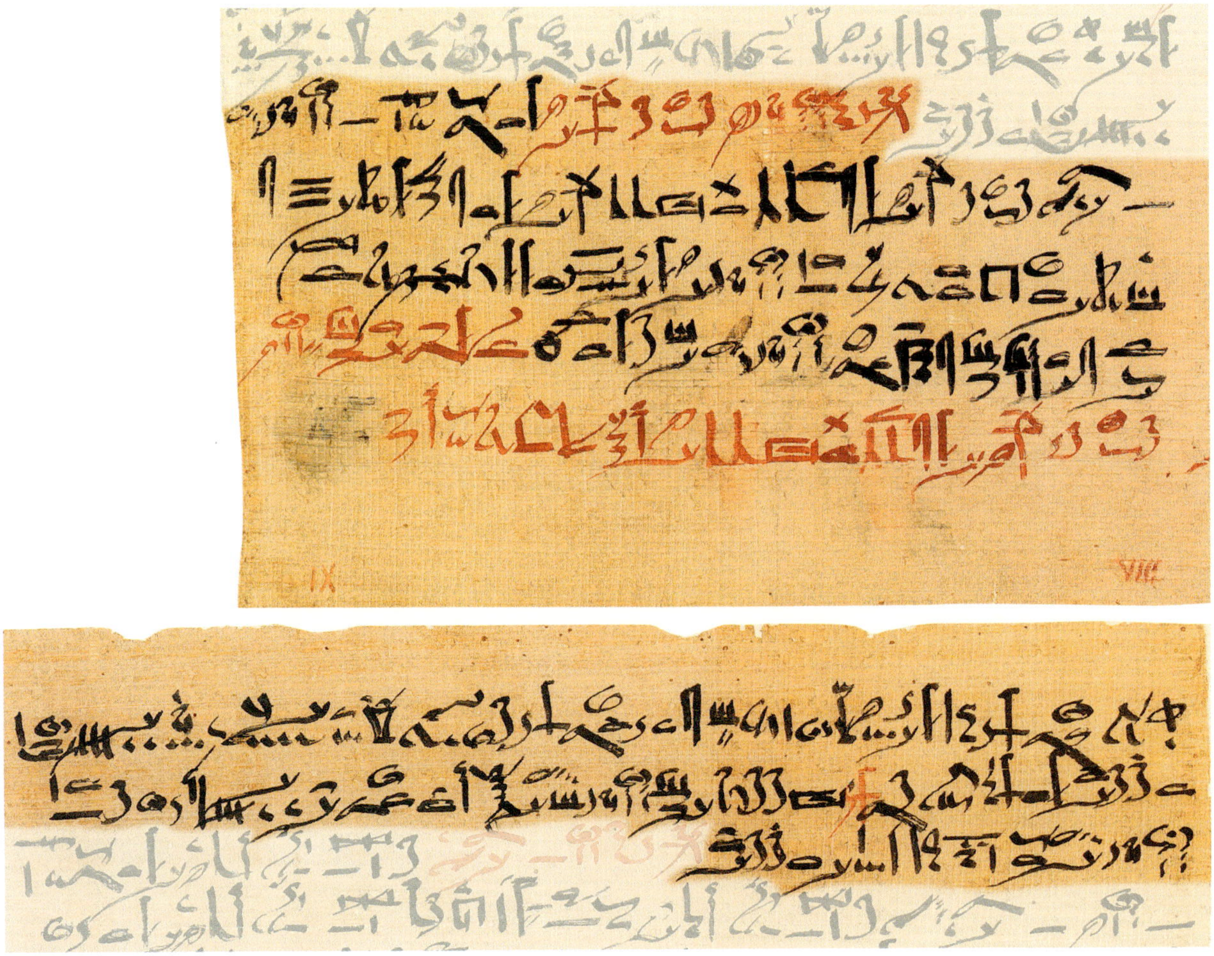

Courtesy New York Academy of Medicine.

18. 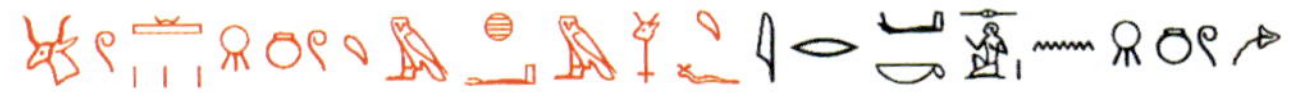

19. 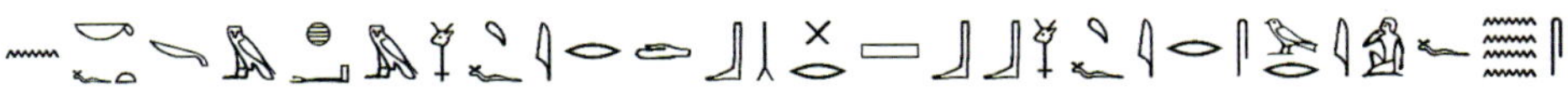

20. 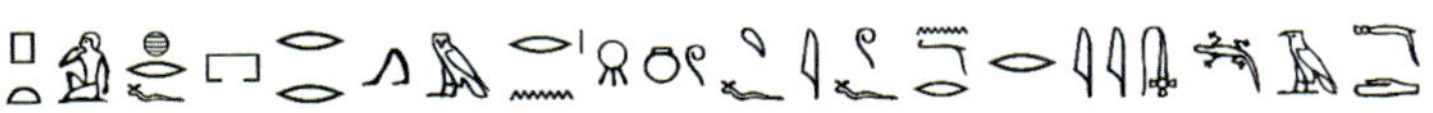

21. 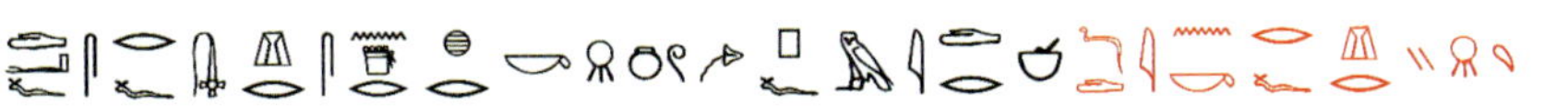

22. 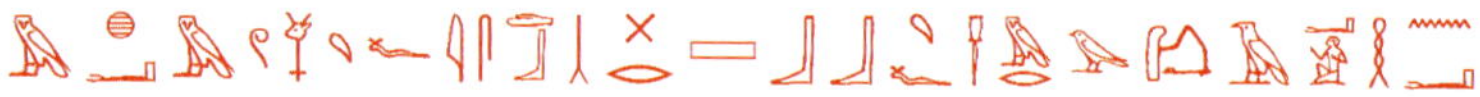

1. 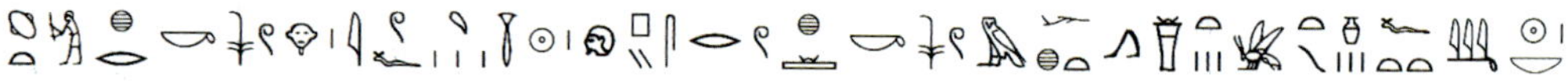

2. 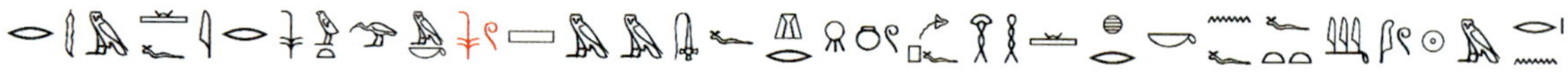

3. 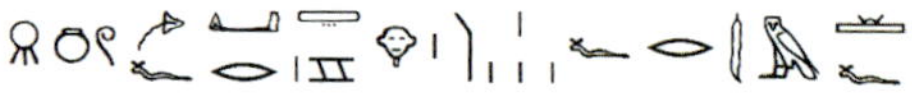

Transliteration

18§ … šs3w wbnw m ḫꜥm.f ir ḫ3.k s n wbnw

19§ n kft m ḫꜥm.f isdb r šbb.f ir swr.f mw

20§ s-tp.ḫr.f prr m r3 n wbnw.f iw.f nsry ꜥš3 šdd.f

21§ srf ḫr-s nḏr.ḫr.k wbnw pf m idr ḏd.in.k r.f ḫry wbnw

22§ m ḫꜥm.f isdb r šbb.f mḥr ꜥḥ3.i ḥnꜥ

1§ wt.ḫr.k sw ḥr iwf w3ḏ hrw tpy srwḫ.k sw m-ḫt <m> mrḥt bit ftt rꜥ nb

2§ r nḏm.f ir swt gm.k sw šmm.f ḫr wbnw pf w3ḥ.ḫr.k n.f ftt šw m r3 n

3§ wbnw.f di r t3 ḥr mniw.f r nḏm.f

Translation

Uncomplicated

Title:

Necessary knowledge and skills for a wound in the front of his neck:

Examination:

If you should examine a man for a slash wound in the front of his neck, pierced and collapsed through to his esophagus, if he drinks water, then he is caused to choke on what comes out of the mouth of his wound.

It is exceedingly inflamed, and why he takes on heat is because of it.

Then you must draw together that wound with thread/suture.

Diagnosis:

Then you are to say about him: "One who has a wound in the front of his neck, pierced and collapsed through to his esophagus, a medical condition I will fight with."

Treatment:

You have to bandage it (along) with fresh meat the first day.

You should treat it afterward <with> ointment and honey and a dressing every day until it/he is well.

Infected

Second Examination:

But if you should find him feverish because of that wound,

Second Treatment:

you must place in position for him a dry dressing in the mouth of his wound, and put him on the ground on his mooring post/resting place, until he is well.

Notes

isdb – For understanding as "pierced and collapsed," see notes above.

ir swr.f – The form after *ir* in the protasis is a prospective form and can be specifically identified as the active *sḏm(w).f*, as in Hoch, *MEG*, sec. 138; see the philological introduction. The same holds with *ir gm.k* below.

prr – Active participle. Many use the terms imperfect and imperfective but I prefer to avoid them as per my discussion in "Participles, Relative Forms and Gemination in Middle Egyptian," and I would simply say geminating active participle.

šmm.f – Since *šmm* is a 2ae gem. verb, *šmm.f* can be a circumstantial *sḏm.f* and that is how I take it, "(He being) feverish."

ftt šw – Here the word "dry" is specified, hence a "dry dressing" is specifically required.

Medical Commentary

Uncomplicated

Type of Injury

Case #28 represents a stab wound to the front of the neck (fig. 26a and b) that produced a tracheo-esophageal cutaneous fistula, which at the first stage of being examined, showed signs of inflammation and possible infection. We have no indication of a time interval between injury and the physician's consultation. This injury is categorized as an *isdb* wound involving soft tissues not supported by bone, being "pierced and collapsed through," in this case, to the esophagus.

The initial evaluation of penetrating injuries to the neck is simplified by their location in an anterior-posterior plane and in the cranio-caudal direction[199] (fig. 26a). The neck is anatomically divided in anterior and posterior triangles outlined by the sternocleidomastoid muscle, with the major aero-digestive structures in the anterior triangle. In the cranio-caudal direction the neck is divided in three zones. Zone I extends from the sternal notch to the cricoid cartilage. Zone II extends from the cricoid cartilage to the angle of the jaw. Zone III extends from the angle of the jaw to the base of the skull. The injury in Case #28 appears to correspond to the

199. D. B. Hoyt, R. Coimbra, and J. Acosta, "Management of Acute Trauma," *Sabiston Textbook of Surgery* (18th ed.; ed. Beauchamp Townsend and Mattox Evers; Philadelphia: Elsevier, 2008), 489–93.

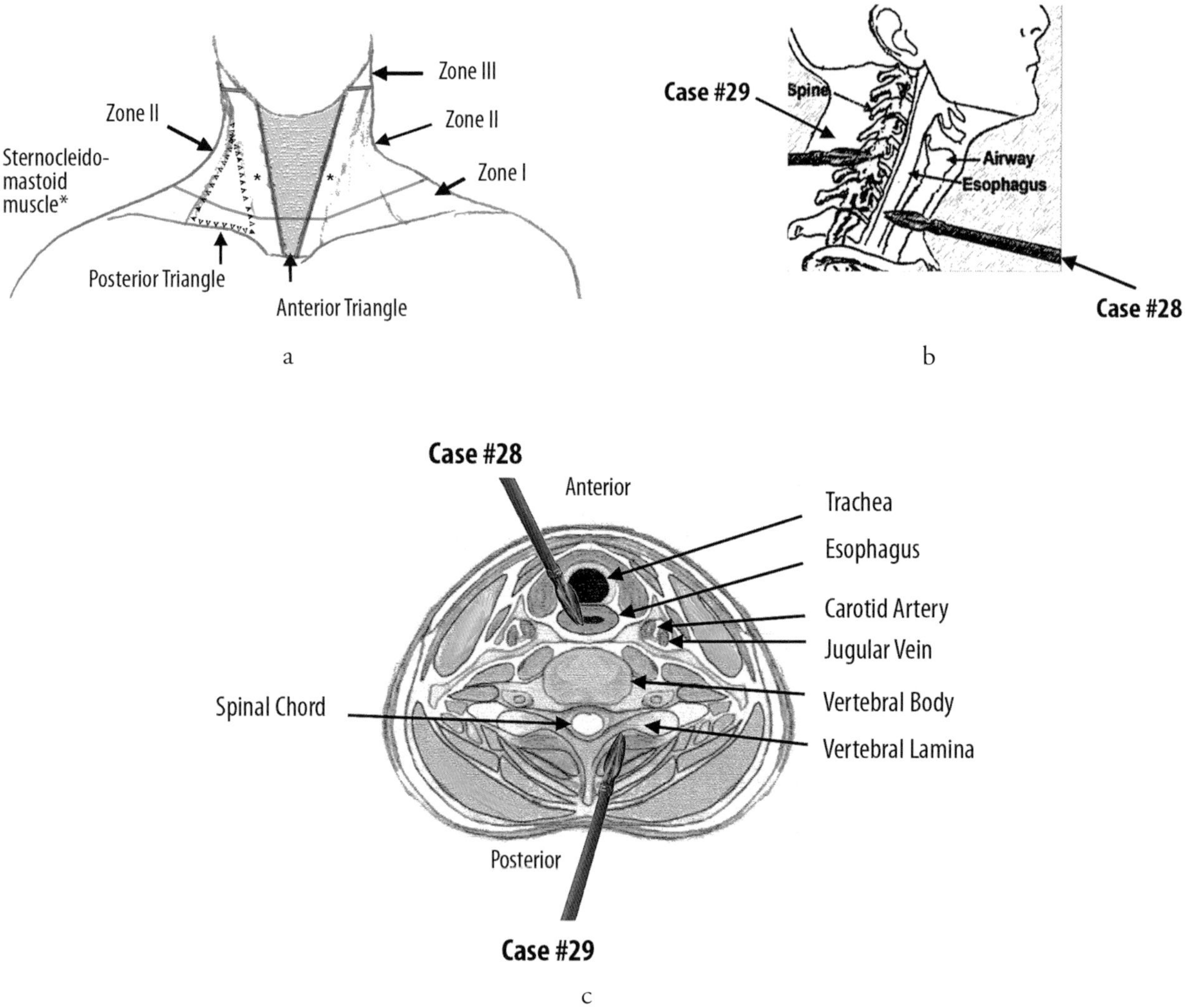

Fig. 26. Penetrating cervical injuries: a) Anatomic triangles and zones of the neck; b) Direction of injury, Cases #28 and #29; c) Neck cross-section lower cervical spine, direction of injury cases #28 and #29.

anterior triangle, central Zone II (figs. 26a, b, and c). This is the area demarcated by the sternocleidomastoid muscle posteriorly, the mandible superiorly, and the midline anteriorly. The vertebral body constitutes the back of this space, and is traversed by the pharynx, esophagus, larynx, trachea, carotid and vertebral arteries, jugular veins, and brachiocephalic veins. Due to these compacted multiple anatomical structures traversing this area as they connect the head with the chest, a penetrating wound can cause major and complex injuries, many of them lethal. There also are other structures of importance in this area, the injury of which is not life threatening, such as the thyroid and parathyroid glands, the thoracic duct, vagus, phrenic and recurrent laryngeal nerves. Injuries to Zone I have the highest mortality and morbidity.

Today over 95 percent of penetrating neck wounds are caused by gunshot wounds and knives. Current data indicates that 20 to 30 percent of the penetrating neck wounds result in laryngeal, tracheal, or esophageal injuries. However, vascular injuries occur in penetrating neck wounds in 25 to 56 percent of cases, arterial lacerations account for the highest number of deaths.

In our Case #28, the fact that no major hemorrhaging or death occurred indicates that the major vascular cervical bundle formed by the carotid and vertebral arteries and the jugular veins had been spared. The entry wound, whether by an arrow or a knife, would have been anywhere from the surface anterior midline and no more than two inches laterally, with its point impacting the anterior surface of the vertebral body from the midline to one inch laterally. An injury such as described in the Edwin Smith Papyrus Case #28 carries a mortality of 11 to 19 percent.[200]

The emergency treatment of such injury today requires maintenance of the airway patency by endotracheal intubation. Due to the tracheal injury, endotracheal intubation may have to be done with the assistance of a flexible bronchoscope, or it may require a tracheostomy distal to the tracheal tear. A nasogastric tube is inserted once the airway is secured. Once in a stable condition, the patient should be transferred to a trauma center for complete evaluation of the injury and for surgical decisions. High resolution CT (computer tomography) scanning and CT angiography would be most informative in determination of vascular, tracheal and esophageal injury in the trajectory of the weapon. Further evaluation may require endoscopic procedures. Antibiotic coverage and tetanus booster would be mandatory. Patients with penetrating injuries to Zone II are often taken directly to surgery.[201] Workup of the aero-digestive tract is completed during surgery. The esophageal injuries are repaired primarily with muscular tissue interposed between the trachea and esophagus.

Ancient Medical Methodology and Knowledge

In Case #28, the offending weapon was likely a knife or an arrow. The presence of inflammation and local heat indicates that this wound was at least several hours old. We do not have a description of what wound layers were sutured, but, it is probable that four thousand years ago, only the skin, platysma muscle, and, at most, the superficial aponeurosis had been included in one layer. It is unlikely that deep structures such as the trachea or esophagus would have been amenable at that time to repair. Closing the surface wound in this case eliminated communication of the esophageal wound to the outside, but would not have prevented choking when swallowing. Additionally, it would have favored development of deep infection.

Infected

Type of Injury

This is the original tracheo-esophageal penetrating wound described above, but it has now become infected: "But if you should find him feverish because of that wound."

Today, infections of this kind of wound occur rarely and would be due to missed foreign material during debridement, or in the occasional case when conservative treatment was elected on the basis of negative CT scanning for the presence of a foreign body, such as in Barrett, et.al.'s case of retained bamboo.[202] Mandatory surgical

200. J. A. Asencio, S. Chahwan, W. Forno, "Penetrating Esophageal Injuries: Multicenter Study of the American Association for the Surgery of Trauma," *Journal of Trauma* 50/2 (2001): 289–96; David B. Levy and Brian S. Gruber, "Neck Trauma." Medscape Reference: http://emedicine.medscape.com/article/827223-overview.

201. W. R. Smythe, S. I. Reznik, J. B. Putnam, Jr., "Lung (Including Pulmonary Embolism and Thoracic Outlet Syndrome)," in Townsend and Evers, *Sabiston Textbook of Surgery*, 1729.

202. George Barrett, Catherine Williams, and David Thomas, "Delayed Presentation of a Penetrating Neck Injury: Diagnostic and Management Difficulties with Retained Organic Material," *Journal of the Royal Society of Medicine Short Reports* 1/2 (2010): 19. Online: http://www.ncbi.nlm.nih.gov/pmc/articles/PMC2984346/.

exploration or re-exploration would be required with removal of all infected material and wound irrigation with delayed repair.

Ancient Medical Methodology and Knowledge

In this evolving clinical scenario, our patient has developed fever that the ancient Egyptian physician attributes to the wound. His recommended treatment at this stage is to insert dry linen dressing (wicks?) in the wound, presumably to keep it draining to the outside and, furthermore, to place the patient at rest, with supportive care, until he is well.

The combination of a tracheo-esophageal cutaneous fistula and serious infection explains the uncertain verdict, "a medical condition I will fight with." Even without initial infection, the fistulous communication between the alimentary tract and the airway would have persisted, despite the surface suturing, resulting in complications and in poor prognosis for life.

Figure 27a is an example of this kind of injury depicted in the battle reliefs of Ramesses II at the First Pylon, Luxor Temple. Figures 27b and 27c are illustrations of two such injuries from the battle reliefs of Sety I, at the northwest exterior wall in the Hypostyle Hall of the Temple of Karnak.

CASE #29:

Cervical Stab Wound, Perforating a Vertebra

(Plate X:3–8)

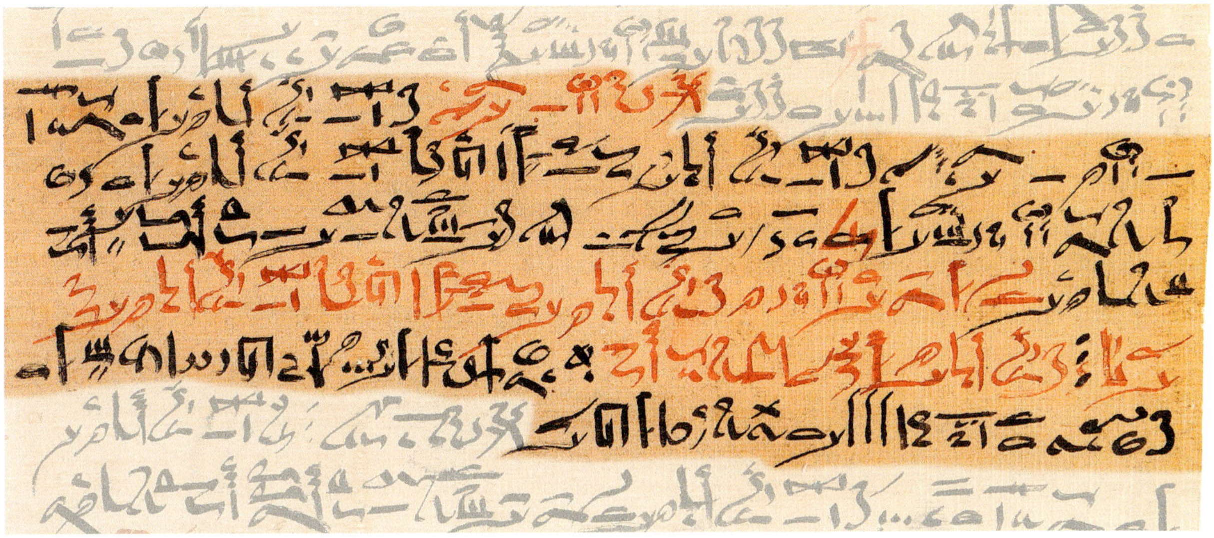

Courtesy New York Academy of Medicine.

3. 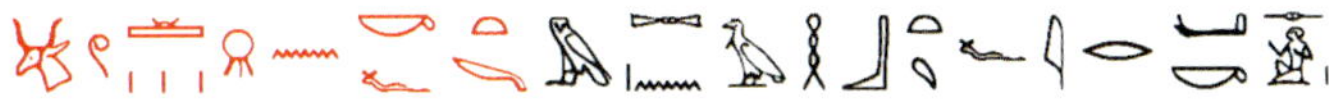

4. 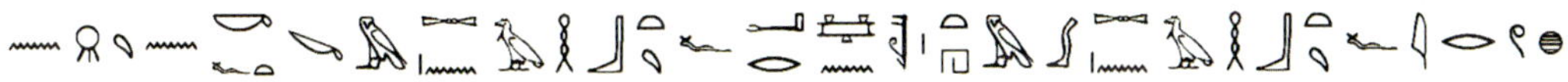

5. 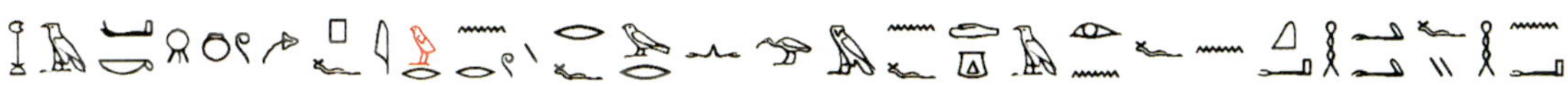

6. 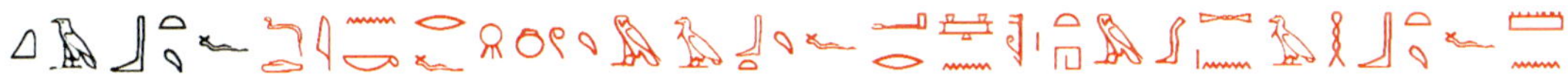

7. 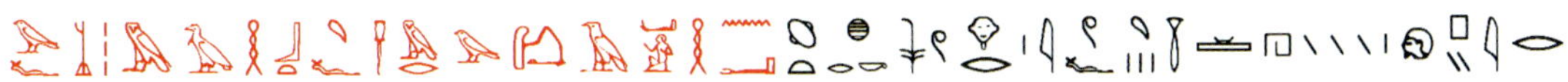

8. 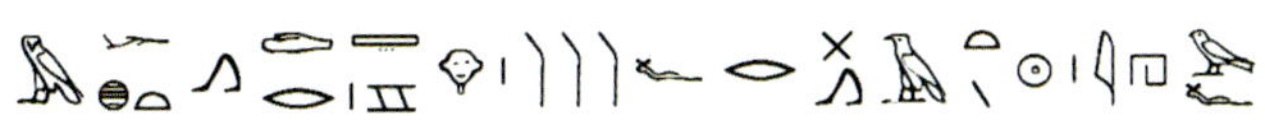

Transliteration

3§ *… šsꜣw wbnw n kft m ṯs n nḥbt.f ir ḫꜣ.k s*

4§ *n wbnw n kft m ṯs n nḥbt.f ꜥr n ḳs thm ṯs n nḥbt.f ir*

5§ *wḫꜣ.k wbnw pf iw {r}nrw r.f wr n gm.n.f dgꜣ.{n}.f n ḳꜥḥwy.fy ḥnꜥ*

6§ *ḳꜣbt.f ḏd.ỉn.k r.f wbnw m nḥbt.f ꜥr n ḳs thm ṯs n nḥbt.f mn.f*

7§ *ṯsw m nḥbt.f mḥr ꜥḥꜣ.ỉ ḥnꜥ wt.ḫr.k sw ḥr ỉwf wꜣḏ hrw tpy ỉr*

8§ *m-ḫt d(w) <sw> r tꜣ ḥr mnỉw.f r swꜣ ꜣt ỉh.f*

Translation

Title:

Necessary knowledge and skills concerning a slash wound in a vertebra of the back of his neck:

Examination:

If you should examine a man for a slash wound in a vertebra of the back of his neck, that has penetrated to the bone, that has perforated a vertebra of the back of his neck,

if you empty out that wound and (it/there) is crepitating/quaking extremely concerning it, and he cannot look to both his shoulders and his chest,

Diagnosis:

then you are to say about it/him: "A wound in the back of his neck, that has penetrated to the bone, that has perforated a vertebra in the back of his neck, while he suffers rigidity in the back of his neck: a medical condition I will fight with."

Treatment:

Then you must bind it (along) with fresh meat the first day.

Afterward, lay (him) down on his bed (under observation and support) until the (critical) period of his injury passes.

Notes

n kft and the mineral *kf* – See earlier notes.

wbnw n kft "slash wound," as attributive genitive – See earlier notes.

thm – I agree with the understanding "penetrate, perforate the bone." This is to be carefully differentiated from *sdb/ỉsdb* meaning "pierced and collapsed through," with reference to soft tissue.

ꜥr and *thm* – Best taken as active participles.

ỉr wḫꜣ.k – *ỉr* + Active *sḏm(w).f* forming the protasis of a conditional sentence.

ỉw nrw – A number of comments are called for in the identification and parsing of this construction. (1) I think that the scribe's correction from *ỉr nrw to *ỉw nrw* shows that he expected another conditional *ỉr* or was influenced by the conditional *ỉr* that he had just written and then corrected himself. Many literate people writing in their native languages have made this kind of error; it belongs to the domain of linguistics known as "pragmatics," which includes the occasional disparities between "competence" and "performance." (2) I do not think that *ỉw nrw* is a variant of the form with prothetic reedleaf *ỉnrw*, because I do not think that *ỉw* is being used as a variant of prothetic *ỉ-* this early, nor do I think the *w* is erroneous and should be emended out; therefore I think it should be taken as the word *ỉw* (this point came up in the notes to a previous case). (3) I think that *nrw* is the stative, which as noted earlier can occur both with and without the *ỉ-* augment; therefore this construction is *ỉw* + impersonal stative.

n gm.n.f dg3.n[sic]*.f* – The expected construction is *n gm.n.f dg3.f* as in Cases 3 and 4. With some misgivings I am proposing to emend *n gm.n.f dg3{.n}.f.* Westendorf lists this passage as *Fehlerhaft* (*Grundriss* 8, sec. 243, p. 176) in a discussion of *sḏm.n.f* interchanging with *sḏm.f.* If one tries to take it literally as a *sḏm.n.f,* one ends up with something like "He cannot have looked at," which in any case is difficult to parallel and seems labored in its sense though perhaps it cannot altogether be ruled out.

mn.f – Circumstantial *sḏm.f*

d – Possibly if not likely the attested verb *d*(*w*), not necessarily an abbreviated writing of *wd*; see notes above.

r sw3 3t ih.f – *r* + *sḏm.f* as elsewhere in this text.

Medical Commentary

Type of Injury

Case #29 is a stab injury to the back of the neck that has reached the spinal column and has perforated (*thm*) bone. The patient is in pain as his wound is being examined and "emptied out." The patient's neck is rigid due to "muscle guarding" and he avoids moving it around. Even though the bone has been perforated, there is no evidence that neurological damage has occurred to the spinal cord or nerve roots. In ancient Egypt, such a penetrating type of wound could have been caused by a dagger, a spear, an arrow, or a spike (fig. 26). In Case #29 there is no evidence that the offending weapon was left in the wound.

Medical literature search from 1959 to 2006 by Shashlaie, et al.[203] on nonmissile penetrating injuries to the spine reveals the following:

- The most common offending weapon is the knife in 72–84 percent.
- The spinal injury was inflicted from behind to the victim's cervical spine in 27 to 30 percent of cases, and to the thoracic spine in 54–63 percent.
- Most often the weapon has been removed by the attacker, rarely breaking or staying lodged in the vertebrae.[204]
- One-third of patients with these injuries to the spine do not have neurological injury.

Today the spinal stab injured patient would be transferred with appropriate precautions avoiding motion of the injured area to a trauma center, where the first task would be assessment of neurological condition and possible associated injuries to lungs and blood vessels. Imaging studies by radiographs and CT scanning would be done regularly. MRI scanning would only be used once the presence of retained metal has been ruled out, in order to avoid the danger of possible magnetization, and movement, of fragments.

These types of spinal injuries are generally stable and internal fixation is rarely necessary. Debridement of the tissue path for removal of foreign material is mandatory, particularly when the offending weapon has a blunt tip, such as a screwdriver, which can easily deposit hair and cloth fibers at the wound's depth. Broad spectrum antibiotics and post-operative imaging studies are indicated to check for retained fragments.

203. K. Shashlaie, D. J. Chang, J. T. Anderson, "Nonmissile Penetrating Spinal Injury," *Journal of Neurosurgery: Spine* 4 (2006): 400–409. Online: http://thejns.org/doi/pdf/10.3171/spi.2006.4.5.400.

204. Ibid.

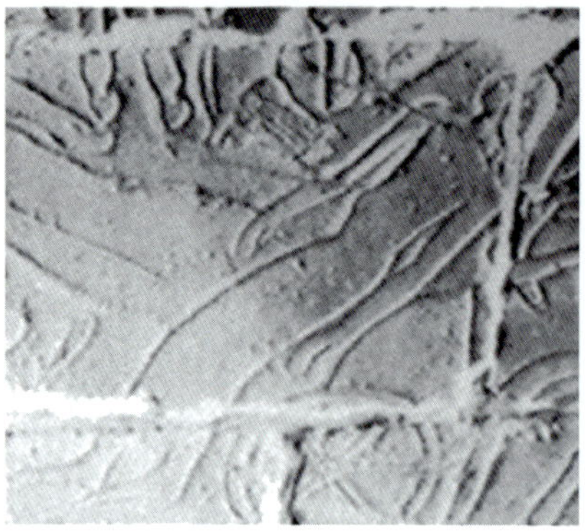

a) Battle relief of Ramesses II, First Pylon, Luxor Temple. Battle of Kadesh.

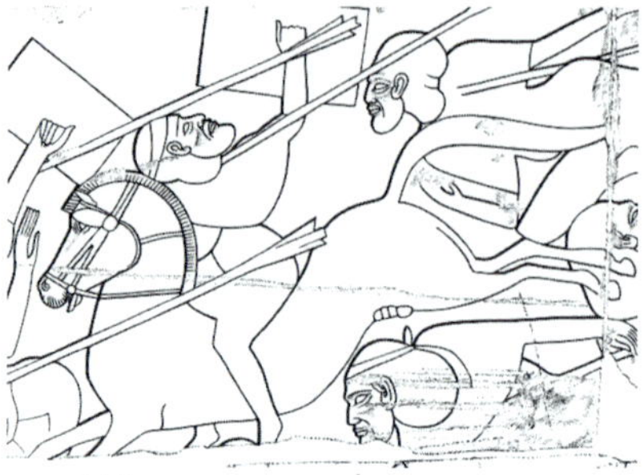

b) Battle relief of Sety I, Temple of Karnak, Hypostyle Hall, Luxor. Courtesy of The Oriental Institute of the University of Chicago.

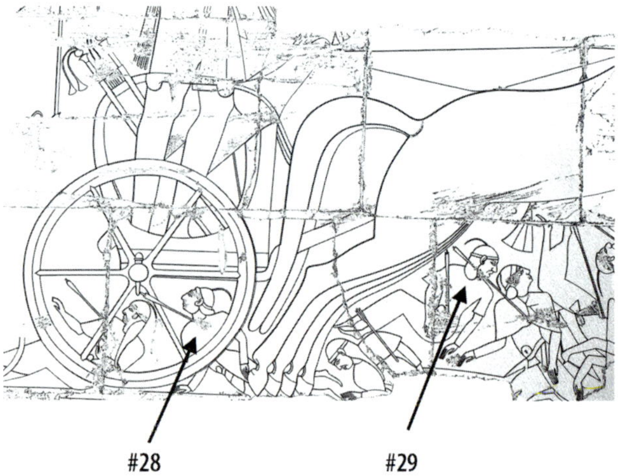

c) Battle reliefs of Sety I, Hypostyle Hall, Temple of Karnak, Luxor. Battle of Kadesh. Courtesy of The Oriental Institute of the University of Chicago.

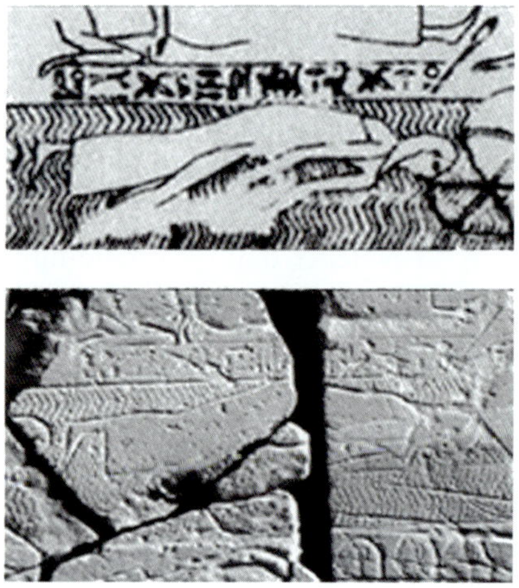

d) Drawing and stone relief of the battle of Kadesh, Ramesseum, Second Pylon, Luxor. From W. Wreszinski, *Atlas zur Altägyptischen Kulturgeschichte*, 92.

Fig. 27. Battle relief examples of injuries in Cases #28 and #29: a) courtesy of the author; b) and c) courtesy of The Oriental Institute of the University of Chicago; d) from W. Wreszinski, *Altas zur altägyptischen Kulturgeschischte* (Leipzig: Hinrichs, 1923).

Ancient Medical Methodology and Knowledge

The Egyptian physician's clinical evaluation of this stab wound begins with exploring and emptying the wound ("if you empty out that wound and (it/there) is crepitating/quaking extremely concerning it …," by which he ascertains that the wound has penetrated to the bone, and has produced a perforation in the bone as well as palpable fragments that crepitate during examination.

This penetrating injury to the posterior cervical spine has caused neck rigidity, preventing the patient from moving his neck freely: "and he cannot look to both his shoulders and his chest." The verdict is that this is an injury to contend with, a decisive but guarded opinion. Treatment is then established by local application of fresh meat over the wound (for the purposes discussed in the medical commentary to Case #1) and by placing the patient lying down, under observation, to be cared for until the critical period of his injury passes.

We have illustrations of these type of injuries in the battle reliefs of Sety I, at the northwest exterior wall in the Hypostyle Hall, Temple of Karnak [205] (fig. 27c) and in Ramesses II's relief of the battle of Kadesh on the Second Pylon of the Ramesseum Temple (fig. 27d).[206]

205. Gonzalo M. Sanchez, "A Neurosurgeon's View of the Battle Reliefs of King Sety I: Aspects of Neurological Importance," *Journal of the American Research Center in Egypt* 27 (2000): 143–65.

206. Gonzalo M. Sanchez, "Injuries in the Battle of Kadesh," *KMT* 14/1 (2003): 58–65.

CASE #30:

Cervical Wrenching/Sprain with Disc Injury

(Plate X:8–12)

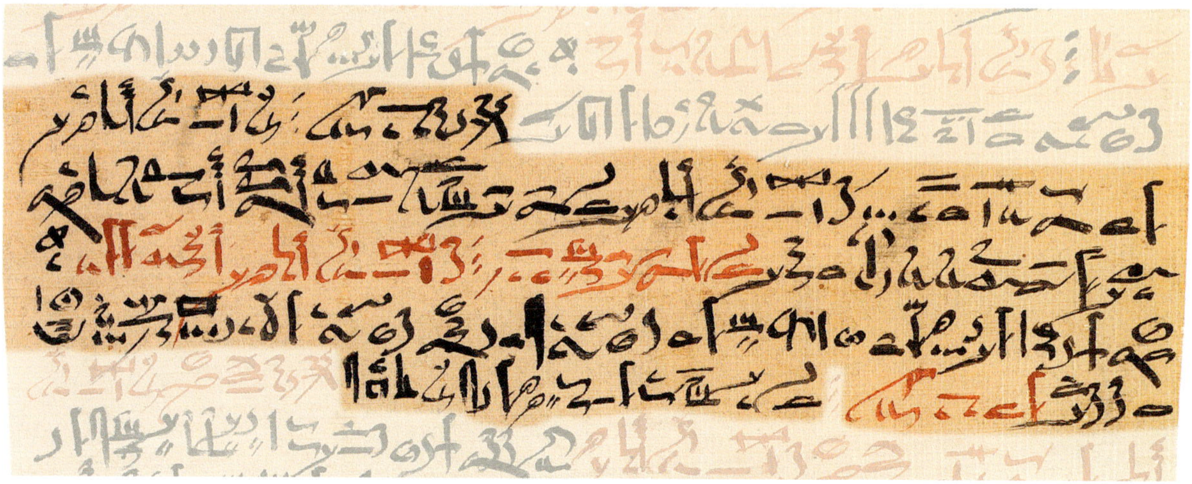

Courtesy New York Academy of Medicine.

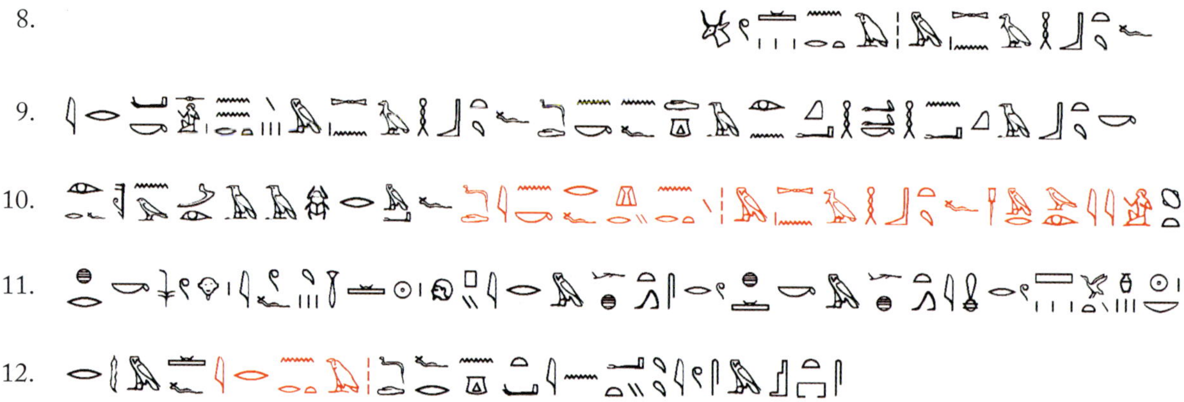

Transliteration

8§ *… šsꜣw nrwt m ṯs n nḥbt.f*

9§ *i͗r ḫꜣ.k s n nrwt m ṯs n nḥbt.f ḏd.<j>n.k n.f dgꜣ n ḳꜥḥwy.k<y> ḥnꜥ ḳꜣbt.k*

10§ *i͗rr.f ḳsn mꜣꜣ ḫpr mꜥ.f ḏd.i͗n.k r.f ẖry nrwt m ṯs n nḥbt.f mḥr i͗ry.i*

11§ *wt.ḫr.k sw ḥr i͗wf wꜣḏ hrw tpy i͗r m-ḫt srwḫ.k {m-ḫt} i͗mrw bi͗t rꜥ nb*

12§ *r nḏm.f i͗r nrwt ḏd.f r ngt i͗n ꜥty i͗w.s m st.s*

Translation

Title:

Necessary knowledge and skills for a wrenching/sprain in the vertebral column of the back of his neck:

Examination:

If you should examine a man for a wrenching/sprain in the vertebral column of the back of his neck, then you are to say to him: “Look towards both your shoulders and your chest.”

How he does so (is) how the looking which transpires with him/happens to or through him is painful.

Diagnosis:

Then you are to say concerning him: “One who has a wrenching/sprain in the vertebral column of the back of his neck, a medical condition which I will handle/deal with.”

Treatment:

You must bind it (along) with fresh meat the first day.

Afterward, you should treat <with> alum(?) (or, a bandage with alum[?] shavings?) and honey every day until he/it is well.

Explanation:

As for “the wrenching/sprain,” he says about the wrenching apart by an intervertebral joint, while it is (still) in its place.

Notes

ḏd .<ỉ>n.k – Accepting emendation to *sḏm.in.f* form as elsewhere in this text.

ỉrr.f ḳsn m33 … – I understand this as a true *Wechselsatz*, or sentence comprising a balanced pair of nominal forms/manner nominalizations, conveying that the one is commensurate with the other: How the patient does this (looks at his shoulders and chest) is how (the way that, the extent to which) the looking is painful. *ḳsn* is the nominal *sḏm.f* of the adjective-verb.

ḫpr – Active participle. *ḫpr m-ꜥ* usually means “transpire or come about with, happen to,” or in the most active possible sense in which it could be taken, “happen through.” Thus Breasted (*Edwin Smith*, 1:320) is not really incorrect but “done” is not what I would consider the word choice that best expresses the essential meaning of *ḫpr*. In the Shipwrecked Sailor passage that Breasted cites, the meaning should be understood as “which also happened to me,” as explained to me in class by Prof. R. J. Williams; see also my article “A Rare Use of *ḏs* + Suffix Pronoun in Middle Egyptian,” 33–35.

<*m*> *ỉmrw* – An *m* is needed before the noun, and this omission is well paralleled in this text. For the word *imrw* see also Case #15.

ỉw.s … – I take this as a circumstantial clause and not as a quotation that the authority is saying; thus syntactically I stay closer to Breasted’s translation. The circumstantial clause explains when it is appropriate to use the word *nrwt*.

Medical Commentary

Type of Injury

Of utmost importance in understanding this case is to ascertain that the injury refers to a cervical intervertebral disc. The key Egyptian word appearing in Case #30 and Case #48 is *ʿty*. James H. Walker, Physician and Egyptologist,[207] provides his opinions and conclusions regarding joints:

> The fact that *ʿty* is only found in connection with joints such as the intervertebral joints in the neck, and not with the major joints in the limbs, may not be pure coincidence ... the use of *ʿty* may have been restricted to such non-synovial joints, joints in which the bones are directly held together by ligaments and/or cartilage and which do not possess a sizable synovial cavity. It is quite possible, on the other hand, that the use of *r3-ʿty* was restricted to synovial joints, those joints in which the bones are only indirectly joined, they being separated from one another by an intervening cavity (*r3*).

Dr. Walker goes further, comparing ancient Egyptian concepts with our own:

> Reflected in the terms *ʿty* and *r3-ʿty* is an important difference between Egyptian perceptions of the body and its joints and our modern perceptions. To the Egyptians, the ligaments, cartilages and cavities or potential spaces between the bones were more important than the bones themselves. Joints were viewed as the sites at which the body naturally divides into its many separate entities and at which, of course, it can be readily be divided up artificially. We, on the other hand, perceive the ends of the bones on either side of the joint cavity to be the most important in the definition of a joint and, indeed, it is they which are being "joined." To us, a joint is an anatomical complex which unites the disparate parts of the body; joints are the sites at which the body is held together so as to maintain its integrity as a whole, as a single unit. This conceptual difference has important implications for the study of Egyptian anatomical terms, particularly those which denote portions of, or structures belonging to, the limbs.[208]

In considering injuries to the spinal column and in particular the specific mechanisms of various injuries, we need briefly to analyze its basic functional anatomical features. The spine is functionally composed of various supporting columns. The anterior column is formed by the vertebral bodies and the intervertebral discs. The interspinous ligaments, the facet joint capsules, and the spinous processes comprise the posterior column. Some consider the existence of a middle column that includes the backs of the discs and the backs of the vertebral bodies, the posterior longitudinal ligament, and the pedicles. Anatomical and physiological concepts of the cervical spine are shown in fig. 28.

Our understanding of pathogenesis and pathophysiology of injuries most often occurring to the cervical intervertebral disc can easily be identified in the text of Case #30: "the wrenching apart by an intervertebral joint, while it is (still) in its place." According to Argenson et al.'s schema for the classification of lower cervical spine injuries,[209] the mechanism of production of a sprain is forced flexion and extension of the vertebral column, acting upon the sagittal spinal axis, located posteriorly on the vertebral body. Forced flexion compresses the vertebral bodies and the intervertebral discs, while distracting the interspinous ligaments and the facet joint capsules (fig. 29). This forced flexion to the neck is what damages the intervertebral disc.

Interestingly, the Egyptian physician in Case #30 shares Argenson's terminology for this type of injury as a "sprain," as a form of "whiplash injury."

207. Walker, *Studies in Ancient Egyptian Anatomical Terminology*, 30–31.

208. Ibid. Long quotation from Dr. James H. Walker with permission from the Australian Centre for Egyptology (9/8/2011).

209. C. Argenson, F. de Pereti, A. Ghabris, P. Eude, J. Lovet, and I. Hovorka, "Classification des Lesions Traumatiques du Rachis Cervical Inferieur," *Maîtrise Orthopédique* 61 (1997). Online: http://www.maitrise-orthop.com/viewPage.do?id=86.

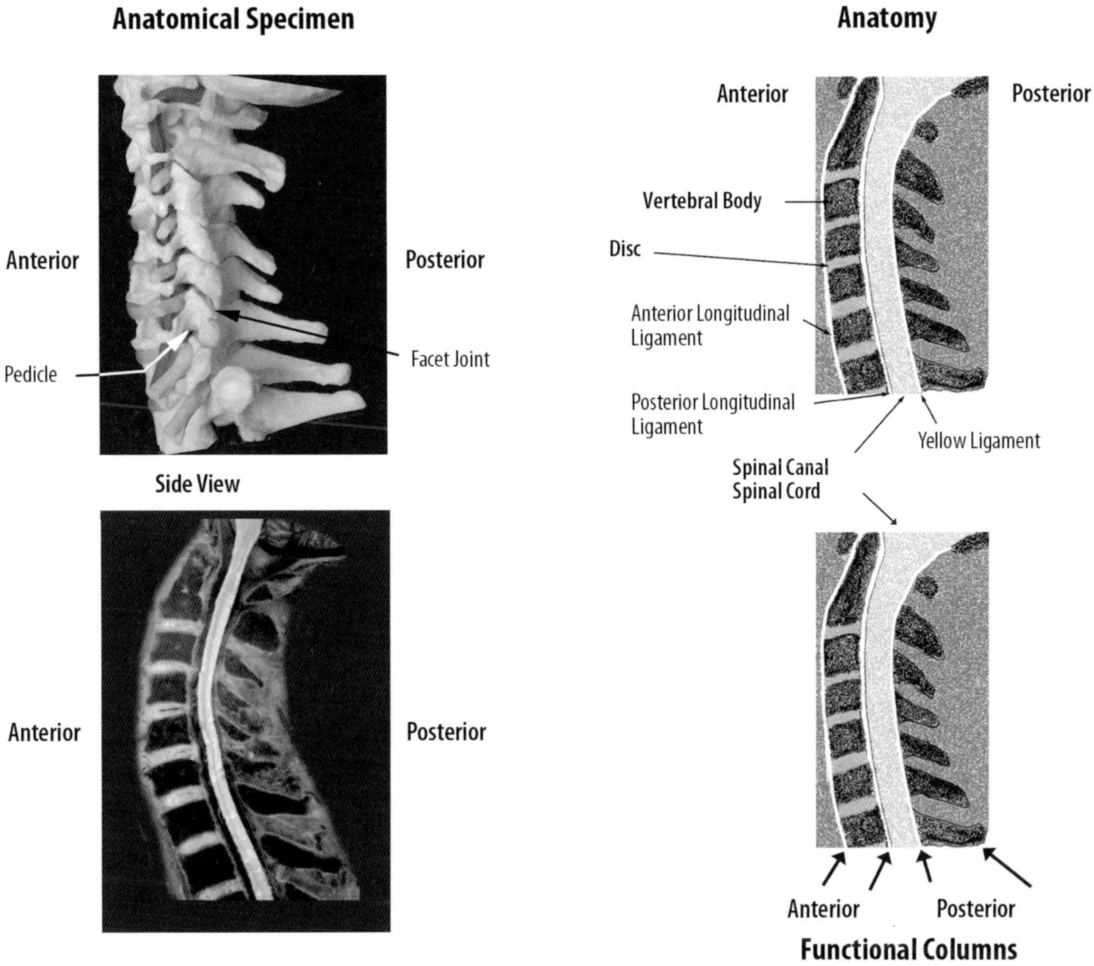

Fig. 28. Cervical spine anatomy and current functional concepts.

Cervical sprains and herniated discs would have been relatively common injuries in construction workers and in the military. In our day, the most common sources of neck injuries are from motor-vehicle accidents, followed by sporting events.

Often in this kind of injury, pain is the only symptom. In more severe cases, damage can occur to the nerve roots and/or the spinal cord. Nerve root symptoms are mainly manifested by arm pain, and numbness and weakness, affecting the skin and muscle distribution for that particular nerve root. Spinal-cord symptoms of lower limb spasticity from cervical disc injury are rare and would be seen in conjunction with nerve root symptoms. Today, treatment of lesser cervical sprains and herniated discs begins with neck immobilization and is followed by a thorough neurological examination. Evaluation also requires cervical spine x-rays. CAT scanning is optional, but often required.

Once this type of injury is determined to be mechanically stable, treatment consists of analgesics, muscle relaxants, and temporary neck bracing, followed by physical therapy. Fifty percent of these patients recover fully within six weeks. Others may require surgical intervention.

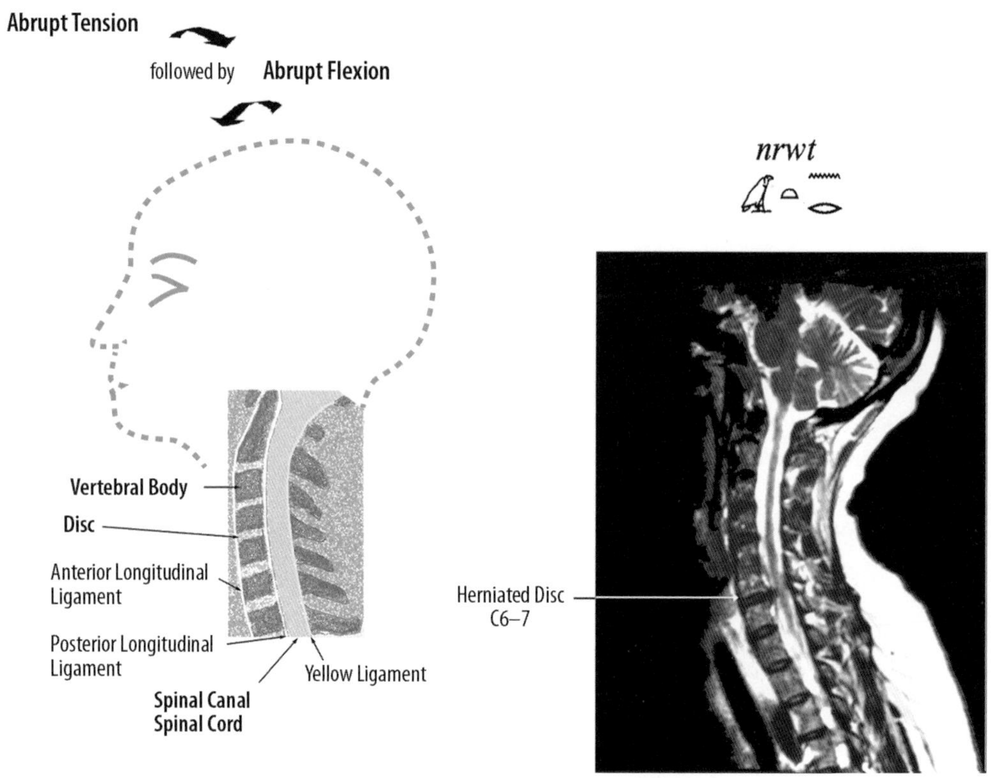

Fig. 29: Cervical sprain/injured disc, mechanism of injury.

Ancient Medical Methodology and Knowledge

The Egyptian physician precisely identifies, by use of the term *ʿty* in designating the joint, the site of this injury. This is a term that applies only to "nonsynovial" joints.[210] In the spine, the intervertebral discs are such nonsynovial joints. The Egyptian physician clarifies that there is no associated vertebral dislocation: "he says about the wrenching apart by an intervertebral joint, while it is (still) in its place."

The only symptom noted in Case #30 is neck pain when the patient follows the physician's command: "Look towards both your shoulders and your chest." According to Meltzer, the manner in which this finding is written, ("I understand this as a true *Wechselsatz*, or sentence comprising a balanced pair of nominal forms/ manner nominalizations, conveying that the one is commensurate with the other: How the patient does this [looks at his shoulders and chest] is how [the way that, the extent to which] the looking is painful.") is clinically important as it indicates that the patient's degree of neck pain while following the physician's command to turn his head to look at his shoulders or his chest, is proportional to the extent that he turned his neck. In Case #30, there are no symptoms or signs of nerve root, or spinal-cord damage.

The injury, in Case #30 is deemed treatable. On the first day the neck is bandaged with fresh meat. Afterwards the neck is treated by topical applications of honey and alum. Without an open wound, the reasoning

210. Non-synovial joints are also called synarthrosis. In contrast with synovial joints they have no joint space. Nonsynovial joints provide structural integrity, with minimal movement.

for using fresh meat and honey, usually employed in ancient Egypt (see Case #1) to support healing and for antibacterial purposes, respectively, is uncertain. We may presume that the aluminum sulfate and potassium sulfate constituents of alum were probably used for their anti-inflammatory properties. Whether these topical medications had much effect is unknown, but the bandaging to keep them in place would have had a similar effect to a soft cervical collar.

CASE #31:

Cervical Vertebral Dislocation with Spinal Cord and Head Injuries

(Plate X:12–22)

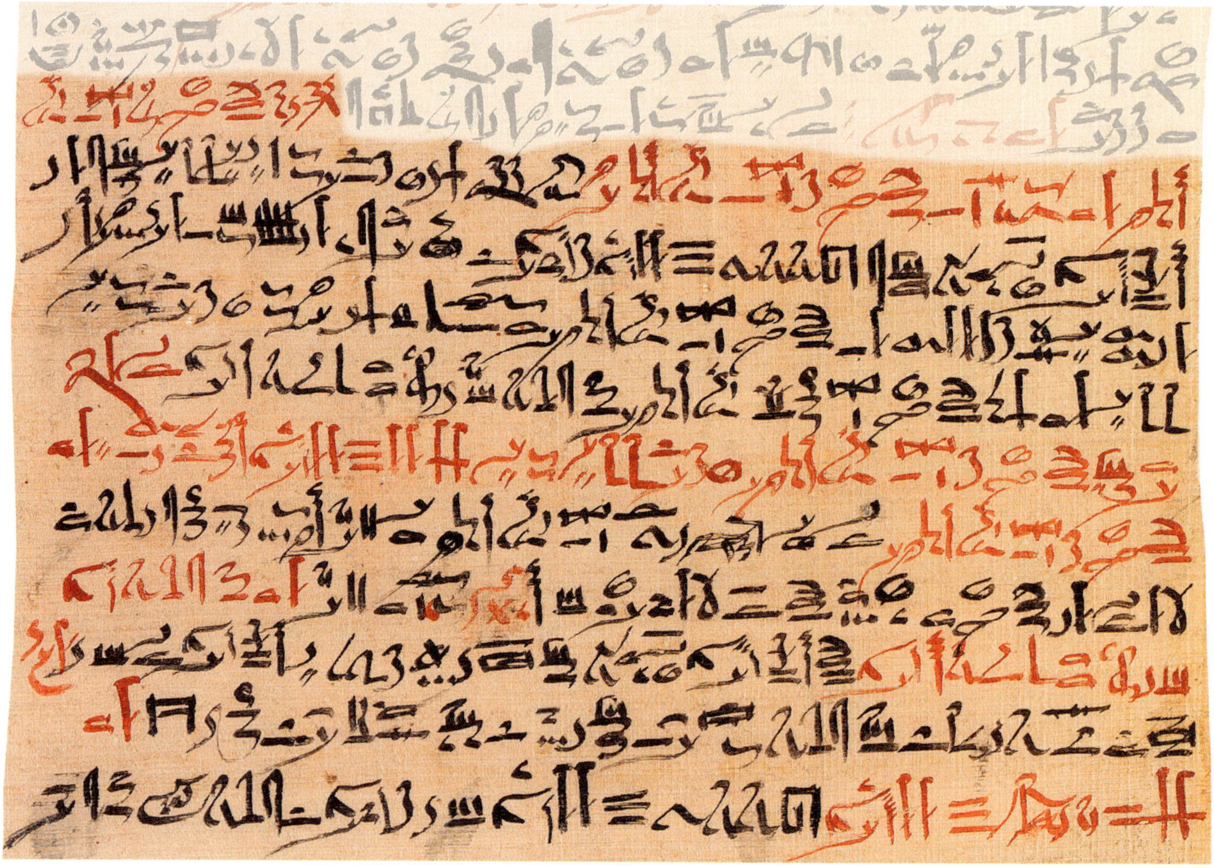

Courtesy New York Academy of Medicine.

12.
13.
14.
15.
16.
17.

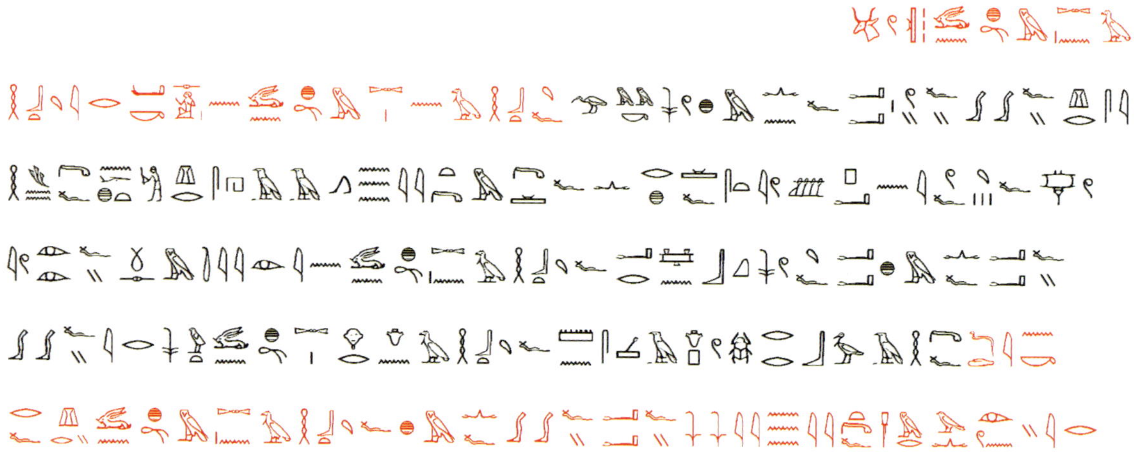

18. 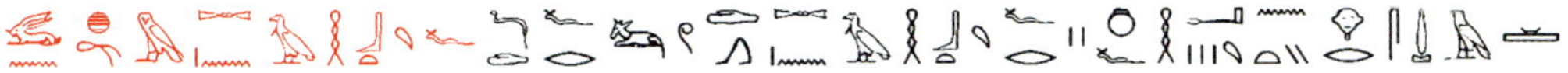

19. 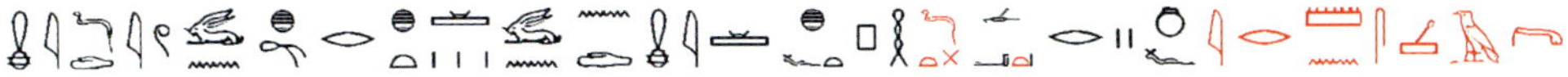

20. 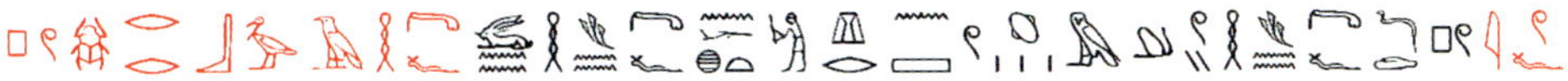

21. 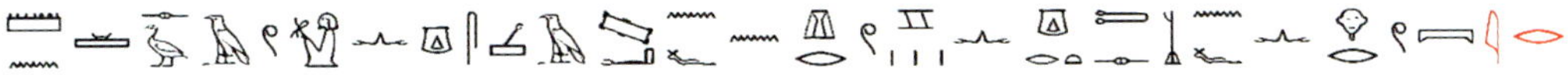

22. 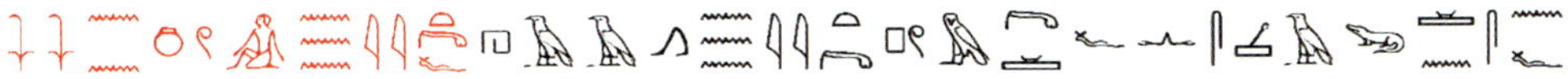

Transliteration

12§ *… šsꜣw wnḫ m ṯs n*

13§ *nḥbt ir ḫꜣ.k s n wnḫ m ṯs n nḥbt.f gmm.k sw ḫm.n.f ꜥwy.fy wꜥrt <wy>.fy ḫr.s iw*

14§ *ḥnn.f nḫt ḫr.s hꜣꜣ mwyt m bꜣḥ.f n rḫ.f st iw šsp.n iwf.f ṯꜣw*

15§ *iw irty.fy šsm.ty in wnḫ ṯs n nḥbt.f ꜥr n bksw.f dd ḫm.f ꜥwy.fy*

16§ *wꜥrty.fy ir swt wnḫ ṯs ḥr ib n nḥbt.f mnsꜣ pw ḫpr r bꜣḥ.f ḏd.in.k*

17§ *r.f ḫry wnḫ m ṯs n nḥbt.f ḫm.f wꜥrty.fy ꜥwy.fy nny mwyt.f mḥr n irw.ny ir*

18§ *wnḫ m ṯs n nḥbt.f ḏd.f r iwd ṯs n nḥbt.f r snw.f ḫꜥ nty ḥr.s wꜣḏ*

19§ *mi ḏd iw wnḫ r ḫt wnn dmi ḫft pḥḏt wꜥt r snw.f ir mnsꜣ*

20§ *pw ḫpr r bꜣḥ.f wnn ḥnn.f nḫt ḫr nšw m pḥwy ḥnn.f ḏd pw iw.f*

21§ *mn sꜣw n gsꜣ.n.f n ḫrw n grt ṯs.n.f n ḥrw ir*

22§ *nnw mwyt.f hꜣꜣ mwyt pw m bꜣḥ.f n sꜣ<ḳ>.n.s n.f*

Translation

Title:

Necessary knowledge and skills for a dislocation in the vertebral column of the back of the neck:

Examination:

If you should examine a man for a dislocation in the vertebral column of the back of his neck, how you find him (is): unaware of both his arms and his legs, as a result of it. His penis is stiff because of it. How urine drips from the end of his penis (is) without his knowing it(?), his internal organs have become gaseous and both his eyes are bloodshot. It is a dislocation of the vertebral column of the back of his neck which extends to his thoracic spine, that causes him to be unaware of both his arms and his legs.

If however, a vertebra in the middle of the back of the neck is dislocated, it means that/it comes to pass that an involuntary discharge/ejaculation occurs at the end of his penis.

Diagnosis:

Then you are to say about him: "One who has a dislocation in the vertebral column of the back of his neck, he being unaware of his legs and his arms, while his urine dribbles/his urine is incontinent, a medical condition that cannot be handled/dealt with."

Explanation A:

As for "a dislocation in the vertebral column of the back of his neck," he is speaking about one vertebra of the back of his neck separating from its counterpart, the flesh/surface that is on it being sound, like saying: "it is dislocated" about things which had been joined when one is detached/severed from its counterpart.

Explanation B:

As for "it means/it comes to pass that an involuntary discharge/ejaculation occurs at the end of his penis," how his penis is (is) stiff and subject to issue/emission from the end of his phallus.

That is to say, it (the penis) remains stationary, it cannot tilt down to the genital region, neither, moreover, can it lift upward.

Explanation C:

As for "his urine dribbles/is incontinent," it means that urine drips from his penis and it cannot hold back for him.

Notes

wnḫ m ṯs n nḥbt – Brawanski maintains that *m* is to be understood as "of" rather than "in," but that is because he takes *ṯs* as referring to a single vertebra; "in" makes perfectly good sense when *ṯs* applies to the "vertebral column."

ḫm.n.f – "unaware/unconscious of." Brawanski notes the use of the *sḏm.n.f* form, which he calls "past," and says that Breasted proceeds from a scribal error. This might seem reasonable in light of the use of *ḫm.f* in the *sḏm.f* below, but it is not at all what Breasted does. Breasted cites a quotation from the Shipwrecked Sailor in which the *sḏm.n.f* of this verb is translated as a past, but that is a matter of context. Breasted proceeds to explain correctly, and showing admirable grammatical acuity for his time, that "It is interesting, and grammatically important to notice that the *n*-form of the verb, *ḫmy-n-f*, is employed with a permansive meaning parallel with that of the following pseudo-participle (*dgm-y*)" (*Edwin Smith*, 1:339). "Permansive" means "stative," and is what Akkadian grammarians used to call the Akkadian stative, which Erman first identified with the Egyptian form we now normally call the stative, but which Breasted and many others have called the pseudo-participle or pseudoparticiple. (The history of this nomenclature is somewhat convoluted and probably not necessary to expound fully here.) This is echoed in more modern terminology by Gilula (review of H. Satzinger, *Die negativen Konstruktionen im Alt- und Mittelägyptischen. Journal of Egyptian Archaeology* 56 [1970]: 206): "the negative *n sḏm.f* as a negative correlative of Old Perfective [= stative, ESM] is confined primarily to the verb *rḫ* "to know," ... and to its partner *ḫm* 'not to know.'" The use of the *sḏm.n.f* of *ḫm* "not know" to express a present tense or present state as felicitously described by Breasted, can be explained if it is parallel to *rḫ* "know," which is considered the result of a previous action or process and universally acknowledged by grammarians to use *sḏm.n.f* to express the present (Gardiner, *EG*[3], sec. 414.4; Edel, *AG*, sec. 538). Grammars do not specify the verb *ḫm* as having the same characteristic, but it seems highly likely to me that this could be the case, not only because of the parallel meanings of "know" and "not know," but because it is very sensible that from the Egyptian point of view "not knowing" could be the result of "having lost knowledge or awareness of," especially when used in cases such as "not knowing" one's body, faculties, etc. This need not be invalidated by the fact that there are many examples attested of *ḫm.f*, such as one cited below in this same case, just as there are many examples of *rḫ.f*. One final point is that *ḫm.n.f* can function here as the adverbial complement of the manner nominalization *gmm.k sw* because it is the circumstantial *sḏm.n.f* of *ḫm*.

iw ḥnn.f nḫt(w) – This is an independent clause, not a clause of circumstance. A sense of strong contrast, which could enable it to be translated subordinately, is not present here.

ḥnn – This word does not only refer to the circumcised penis. When the Egyptians were fighting the Sea Peoples and Libyans and other campaigns of the Ramesside period, the texts sometimes state that the "body count" trophies that were cut from the corpses of the enemy were the hands of circumcised enemies and the phalli of uncircumcised enemies. One such text is the Great Historical Inscription of Merneptah at Karnak, where for example in line 46 *ḥnyw ḳrnwt* "penises (with) foreskins" or "uncircumcised penises" are listed, with a writing that is a variant spelling of Classical Egyptian *ḥnn* or *ḥnnw*.[211] For the possible etymological connection between *ḥnn* or *ḥnnw* "penis" and *ḥnn* "hoe," see E. Meltzer, "An Observation on the Hieroglyph 𓌸," *Journal of Egyptian Archaeology* 56 (1970): 193–94.

nnw – Faulkner, *CDME*, 134.

hꜣꜣ … n rḫ.f st – *hꜣꜣ* is a manner nominalization, and with some hesitation (shown by the question mark) I am translating the negative clause *n rḫ.f st* as the adverbial complement, although such clauses are not included by Doret among constructions attested as adverbial complements. This is because there seems little point in emphasizing the phrase "from the end of his penis," and because Satzinger has proposed that there are circumstantial *n sḏm.f* negations, though Gilula is skeptical (review of Satzinger, *Die negativen Konstruktionen,* 206).

bꜣḥ.f – I am translating "the end of his penis" to recognize the difference between *bꜣḥ* and *ḥnn*.

ꜥr and *dd* are both active participles. The entire passage *in … wꜥrty.fy* is a participial statement.

ḫpr is a stative; it can be transliterated *ḫpr(w)*. The contruction is noun + *pw* + stative.

mnsꜣ – For this word, see also Edmund Meltzer, "Wenamun 2, 46," *Journal of the Society for the Study of Egyptian Antiquities* 17 (1987): 86–88.

ḫm.f … nny … – These are both circumstantial *sḏm.f*. The *sḏm.f* of *ḫm* has been remarked on above.

iw wnḫ(w) – *iw* + impersonal stative.

ḫft pḥdt – I do not take this as a *sḏmt.f* form, since there is no construction *ḫft* + *sḏmt.f* in Middle Egyptian, and it cannot be preposition + Infinitive since the infinitive of *pḥd* has no *–t* ending. It is a passive, *ḫft pḥd.t(w)*, as taken by Breasted (*Edwin Smith,* 1:329), and is normally transitive. Breasted remarks that it can be found intransitively, referring to the bursting of a cyst, and this is cited by Faulkner, *CDME*, 93.

ir mnsꜣ pw ḫpr(w) … – I think that this entire passage is quoted from above to be explicated, not only the word *mnsꜣ*. Moreover, I think that the reason there is no *pw* "this means that" in the following clause is that the similar construction in this clause was felt as the same by the scribe or interfered with the composition of the second one.

wnn – manner nominalization. I am still a bit uncertain about the segmentation, where the "nexus" belongs in this sentence.

nḫt(w) – stative.

iw.f mn(w) sꜣ(w) – I wonder whether a pun on the word *mnsꜣ* is intended, since word play was a proclivity of Egyptian writings.

gsꜣ … n ḫrw – According to Faulkner, *CDME*, 292, this expression means "sink down."

211. See Colleen Manassa, *The Great Karnak Inscription of Merneptah: Grand Strategy in the 13th Century BC* (Yale Egyptological Studies 5; New Haven: Yale Egyptological Seminar, 2003), 52, 176, 178, plate 11.

hꜣꜣ ... – Nominal *sḏm.f*, which I am taking in the "pristine" Polotskyan sense of a "that" clause.

Medical Commentary

Type of Injury

Case #31 represents a greater degree of cervical trauma than Case #30. This is a fracture dislocation of the lower cervical spine producing spinal cord injury in which several plausible mechanisms of injury can be involved (fig. 30). Without explicitly documenting the spinal cord itself, the ancient Egyptian physician relates spinal column injury to the neurological symptoms of spinal-cord injury.[212] The severity of the spinal-cord injury in this case is manifested by quadriplegia, anesthesia of the body below the level of the spinal-cord injury, urinary incontinence, intestinal ileus, and priapism, all of which are indicative of spinal-cord physiological transection.

To create this injury, shearing would have occurred across the anterior and posterior elements of the cervical spine, disrupting bone, discs, and ligaments, including the facet joints. The injury to the facet joints (see fig. 28 for normal anatomical details), in our current case, was probably not a typical bilateral facet dislocation expected in flexion injuries. The one clinical clue suggestive of the true mechanism of injury to the cervical spine in Case #31 is the injury to the front of the head as evidenced by, "and both his eyes are bloodshot." This is a finding frequently seen in cranio-facial trauma when there are fractures to the anterior skull base. Evidence of a frontal injury in conjunction with a cervical dislocation as seen in Case #31, suggests a cervical-extension trauma mechanism.

From Allen and Ferguson's cervical spine injury phylogeny,[213] two possible extension injury mechanisms need to be considered: "distractive extension" and "compressive extension." The clinical features in Case #31 suggest that it was the result of a "distractive-extension" injury. In its lowest degree, a DES1 injury (Distractive Extension Grade 1), there is failure of the anterior spinal ligamentous complex. In a DES2 injury (Distractive Extension Grade 2), there is, in addition, failure of the posterior ligamentous complex. The combined ligamentous injuries result in a posterior dislocation of the upper vertebral body into the spinal canal, damaging the spinal cord (fig. 30).[214] In the cervical "Compressive Extension" Grade 2 (CES2) injuries the initial damage is to the posterior vertebral elements, fracturing the articular pillar, the ipsilateral pedicle, and the lamina. At this stage there is no failure of the anterior anatomical constrains. CES2 injuries are often associated with spinal-cord injury, although there is no evidence of a major vertebral body dislocation.

Case #31, as demonstrated above, indicates that the Egyptian physicians had substantial concepts about physiology and that they were already aware of the functions of the spinal cord.[215] The Egyptian physician made an attempt, albeit inaccurate, to differentiate clinically a cervico-thoracic injury from a mid-cervical injury.[216] The

212. The reader is directed to appendix 2 for a compilation of the neurological symptoms and signs in the Edwin Smith Papyrus.

213. B. L. Allen, R. L. Ferguson, T. R. Leheman, and R. P. O'Brien, "A Mechanistic Classification of Closed Indirect Fractures and Dislocations of the Lower Cervical Spine," *Spine* 7 (1982): 1–27. Lower cervical spine injuries were divided into "phylogenies" based on the mechanism of injury, and each category is arranged by progression in severity.

214. Argenson, C., F. de Pereti, A. Ghabris, P. Eude, J. Lovet, and I. Hovorka, "Classification des Lesions Traumatiques du Rachis Cervical Inferieur," *Maîtrise Orthopédique* 61 (1997): http://www.maitrise-orthop.com/viewPage.do?id=86.

215. C. M. Helgason, "Commentaries on the Significance for Modern Neurology of the 17th Century B.C. Surgical Papyrus," *Canadian Journal of Neurological Sciences* 14 (1987): 560–63. J. T. Goodrich, "Cervical Spine Surgery in the Ancient and Medieval Worlds," *Neurosurgical Focus* 23/1 (2007): 2–4. Joost J. van Middendorp, Gonzalo M. Sanchez, and Alwyn L. Burridge, "The Edwin Smith Papyrus: A Clinical Reappraisal of the Oldest Known Document on Spinal Injuries," *European Spine Journal* 19/11 (2010): 1815–23. Online: http://www.springerlink.com/content/vk460l07q7028186/fulltext.pdf.

216. In discussing the "the middle vertebra of his neck," Brawanski suggests it might instead refer to the vertical axis of the vertebral column, in which case it could allude to a forward shift of the dislocating spine. A. Brawanski, "Die Wirbelsäulenverletzungen des Papyrus

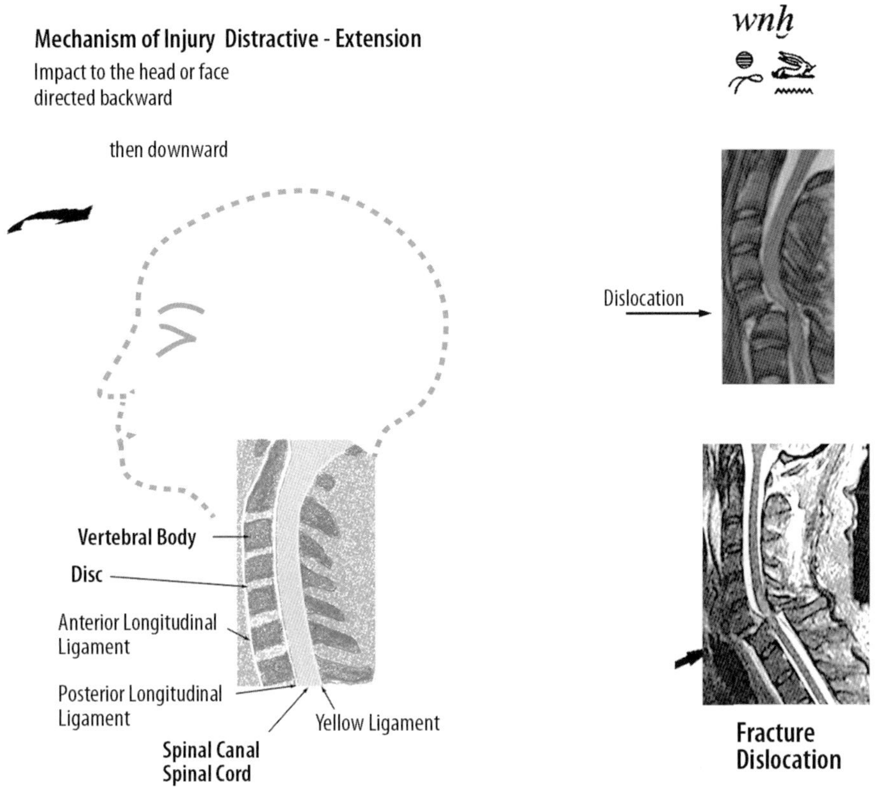

Fig. 30: Cervical vertebral dislocation, mechanism of injury.

initial portion of the examination paragraph refers to an injury at the cervico-thoracic junction, specifically using the term *bḳsw* = thoracic spine. Injury to this area is manifested by quadriplegia, anesthesia of the body below the level of the spinal cord injury, priapism, urinary incontinence, and intestinal ileus. Next, the Egyptian physician refers to a higher cervical injury: "If however, a vertebra in the middle of the back of the neck is dislocated, it means that/it comes to pass that an involuntary discharge/ejaculation occurs at the end of his penis." The ancient Egyptian has described symptom grouping variants related to the cervical spine dislocations, attempting to differentiate the anatomical level of cervical spine injury. Today we can differentiate various levels of spinal injury on the basis of the neurological exam. An injury to the lower cervical spine may spare some of motor and sensory tracts to the proximal upper limbs, with certain "awareness" of the upper extremities preserved.[217] Although inaccurate, it is a remarkable clinical effort of the ancient Egyptian physicians to seek differential anatomical-pathological diagnosis of the cervical spine based on differences in neurological sequelae.

The mechanisms of cervical injury in antiquity and modern times have been considered in Case #30.

Today, a patient such as this would immediately be immobilized and transported to a trauma center where proper neurological assessment and management of the dislocation would be carried out both by nonoperative and operative means, with the primary goal of spinal stabilization, and decompression of the spinal cord by

Edwin Smith (Fälle 29–33)," *Studien zur altägyptischen Kultur* 32 (2004): 66–71. We believe the Egyptian concept of the cervical spine was that of a structure composed of seven vertebrae. Therefore, the injury in "a vertebra in the middle of the back of the neck is dislocated," probably means exactly what it says: a dislocation of a vertebra in the middle of the cervical spine, in contrast with the previous injury that occurred below, at the cervico-thoracic junction. See Walker, *Studies in Ancient Egyptian Anatomical Terminology*, 155.

217. Van Middendorp, et al., "The Edwin Smith Papyrus: A Clinical Reappraisal."

chemical and surgical means as appropriate. Extensive rehabilitation will be necessary in most cases. The present evaluation and treatment of spinal-cord injuries is evolving. There are great hopes in the research of spinal-cord regeneration stimulated at molecular levels, and of genetically manipulated stem cells, and other projects. But, so far, a cure for spinal-cord injury does not exist.

Ancient Medical Methodology and Knowledge

This particular case reveals a great deal of understanding by the Egyptian physician of the anatomical and functional subtract, and ability to explain the mechanism of this spinal injury and the fundamental anatomical pathology of this kind of vertebral dislocation (Explanation A): "As for 'a dislocation in the vertebral column of the back of his neck,' he is speaking about one vertebra of the back of his neck separating from its counterpart, the flesh/surface that is on it being sound, like saying: 'it is dislocated,' about things which had been joined when one is detached/severed from its counterpart." Additionally, he observed and documented the neurological functional consequences of a severe cervical spinal injury:

- limb paralysis: "how you find him (is): unaware of both his arms and his legs, as a result of it … It is a dislocation of the vertebral column of the back of his neck which extends to his thoracic spine, that causes him to be unaware of both his arms and his legs." In our opinion, being "unaware" refers to a sense of nonexistence of that part of the body, from the ancient Egyptian perspective of considering the human body as an association of different parts (Walker, "Egyptian Medicine and the Gods," 83) working together. Non-awareness would then encompass absence of both motion and sensation, in other words, nonexistence of that bodily entity.
- urinary incontinence: "How urine drips from the end of his penis (is) without his knowing it…." And in Explanation C: "As for 'his urine dribbles/is incontinent,' it means that urine drips from his penis and it cannot hold back for him."
- bowel distension (ileus): "his internal organs have become gaseous."
- priapism: "His penis is (is) stiff …" In Explanation B: "That is to say, it (the penis) remains stationary, it cannot tilt down to the genital region, neither, moreover, can it lift upward."
- spontaneous ejaculation: "it means/it comes to pass that an involuntary discharge/ejaculation occurs at the end of his penis …"

As discussed in the preceding section, the Egyptian physician attempted a clinical differentiation of a lower cervical spine injury, from one occurring at the mid-cervical level, attributing the presence of spontaneous ejaculation to the latter. The ancient Egyptian physician's effort to link various symptoms with a specific anatomical level of cervical spinal injury, was not, in the end correct, but was testimony to his sense of diligence, and to his astute observations.

The treatment outlook for a complete spinal-cord injury as presented in this case, was understandably poor: "(this is) a medical condition that cannot be handled/dealt with."

CASE #32:

Cervical Vertebral Compression Fracture

(Plate XI:1–9)

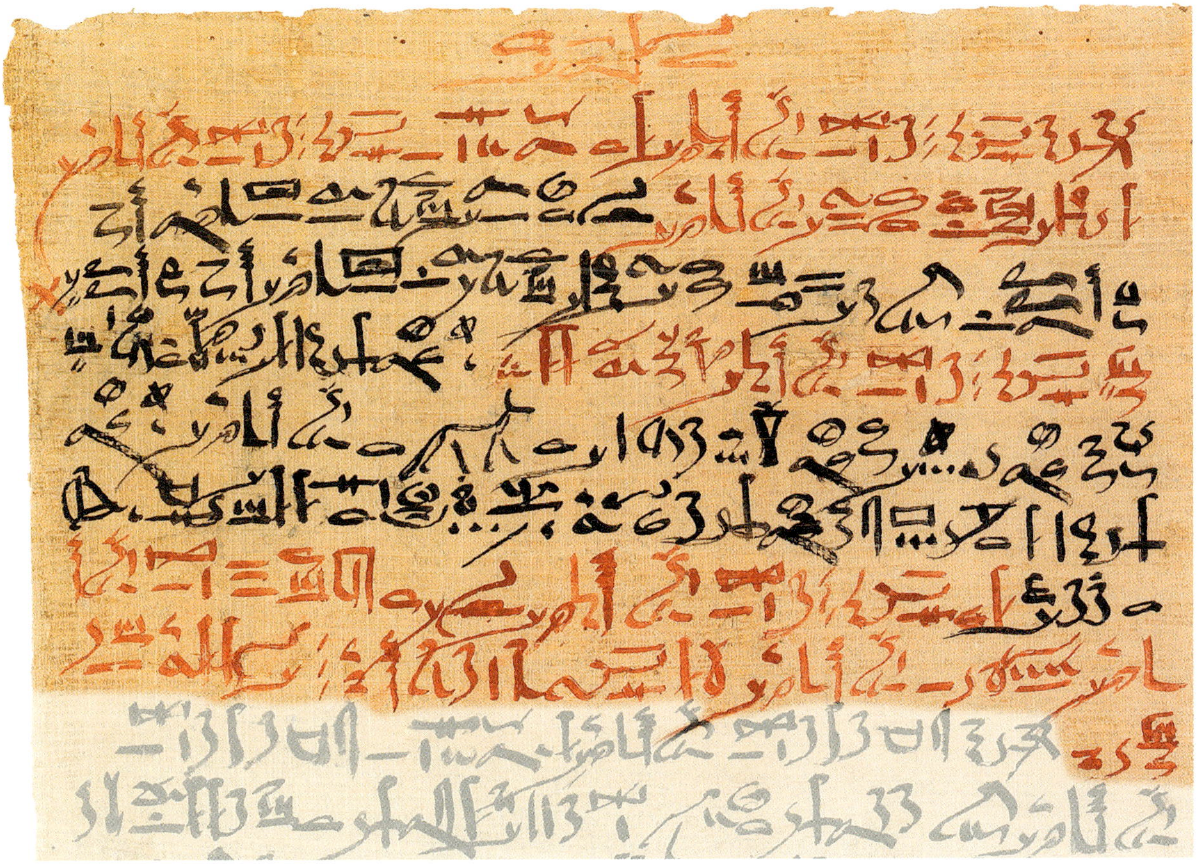

Courtesy New York Academy of Medicine.

1. 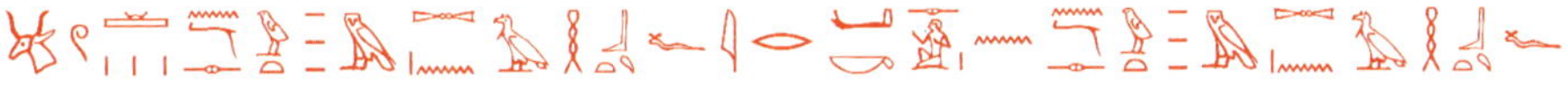

2. 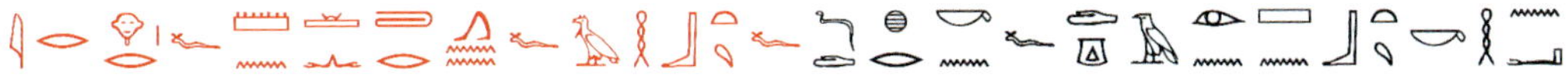

3. 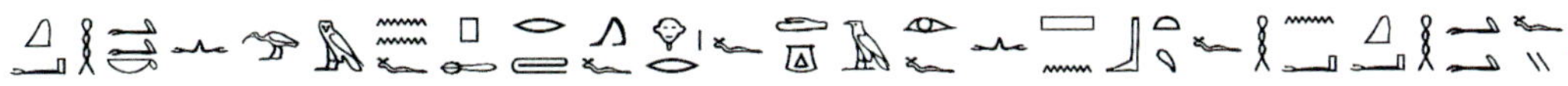

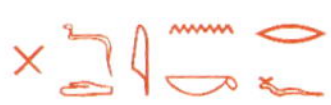

4. 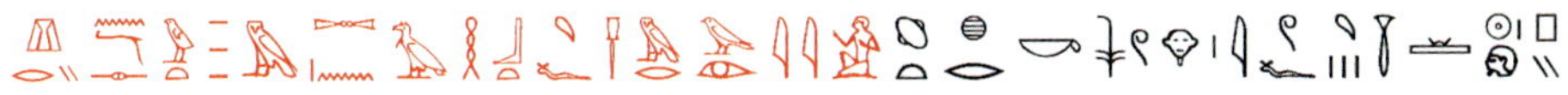

5. 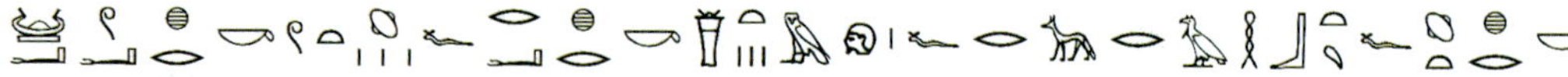

6. 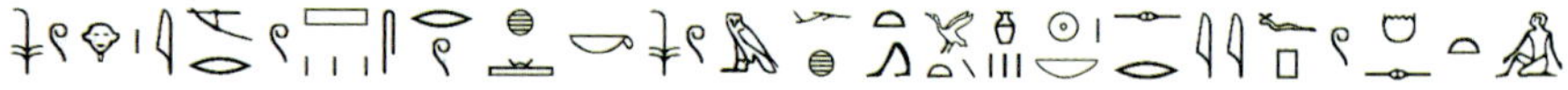

7. 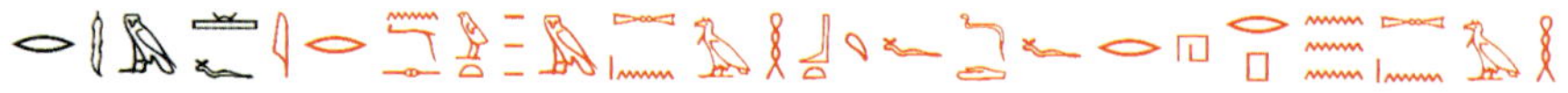

8. 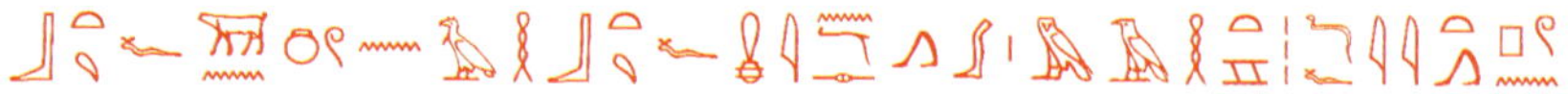

9. 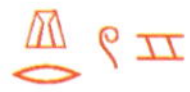

Transliteration

1§ *šs3w nswt m ṯs n nḥbt.f ir ḫ3.k s n nswt m ṯs n nḥbt.f*

2§ *iw ḥr.f mn n pḫr.n n.f nḥbt.f ḏd.ḫr.k n.f dg3 n šnbt.k ḥnʿ*

3§ *ḳʿḥwy.k n gm.n{ n}.f pḫr.f ḥr.f dg3.f n šnbt.f ḥnʿ ḳʿḥwy.fy <ḏd.jn.k r.f>*

4§ *ḫry nswt m ṯs n nḥbt.f mḥr iry.i wt.ḫr.k sw ḥr jwf w3ḏ hrw tpy*

5§ *wḥʿ.ḫr.k wt.f rdi.ḫr.k mrḥt m tp.f r s3b r nḥbt.f wt.ḫr.k*

6§ *sw ḥr imrw srwḫ.k sw m-ḫt bit rʿ nb sry.f pw ḥmst*

7§ *r nḏm.f ir nswt m ṯs n nḥbt.f ḏd.f r hrp ṯs n nḥbt.f*

8§ *ḫnw n nḥbt.f mi ns rd m 3ḫt ḏfyt pw n*

9§ *ḫrw*

Translation

Title:

Necessary knowledge and skills for a sinking in a vertebra of the back of his neck:

Examination:

If you should examine a man for a sinking in a vertebra in the back of his neck, and his face is fixed, and his neck cannot turn for him, then you must say to him: "Look to the front of your chest and to your two shoulder joints," and he cannot turn his face that he may look to the front of his chest and his two shoulder joints.

Diagnosis:

Then you are to say about him: "One who has a sinking in a vertebra in the back of his neck, a medical condition which I will handle/deal with."

Treatment:

Then you must bind it (along) with fresh meat the first day.

Then you must loosen his bandages, and then you must apply ointment to his head in order to run/flow down onto the back of his neck.

Then you must bandage it (along) with alum(?) (or, a bandage with alum[?] shavings?) and you should treat him afterward with honey every day.

His treatment protocol is sitting upright until he is well.

Explanation:

As for "a sinking in a vertebra of the back of his neck," he says concerning/with respect to the depressing of a vertebra of the back of his neck <in(?)> the inside of the back of his neck being like the way a foot sinks into cultivated soil; it is a compressing/penetration downwards.

Notes

nswt – I am following the *Grundriss* (7, 1:480) definition as simply as possible; thus also Brawanski, "Die Wirbelsäulenverletzungen des Papyrus Edwin Smith (Fälle 29–33)," 71–72. Allen's (*AM*, 93) translation "settling" is similar.

kꜥḫwy.k – Gardiner notes that the *y* in the euphonic suffix-pronoun *.ky* after a dual noun is written "sometimes" (*EG*³, sec. 75.2). Thus, it can be considered optional and its omission cannot be considered an error or incomplete writing.

n gm.n{n}.f – I think that Breasted was most probably correct in considering the second *n* in *gm.n{n}.f* redundant or superfluous, though I resist emendations as much as possible. I do not think that the two passages *n pẖr.n n.f nḥbt.f* and *n gm.n{n}.f pẖr.f ḥr.f* are precisely parallel. In the second passage, both the verb *gmi* and the verb *pẖr* have *.f* as subject, which are obviously coreferential and both refer to the patient. I do not think that one can parallel a construction **gm.n pẖr.f* without a subject on the *gm.n* form. (No such examples are cited by Gardiner, *EG*³, sec. 486–488; the example in Gardiner, sec. 184.1 is from Edwin Smith and typical of the examples we have seen until now.) Therefore I doubt strongly that the passage could be understood as **n gm.n n.f pẖr.f.* Westendorf in *Grundriss* 8, sec. 241 takes *n pẖr.n n.f nḥbt.f* as we do, "nicht kann sich ihm sein Nacken drehen." Brawanski's translation is similar but does not explicitly include the phraseology "kann nicht" (p. 71). Allen on the other hand seems to take both passages as having a superfluous *n*, "he cannot turn his neck" and "it is impossible for him to turn his face" (*AM*, 93). That, I think, is unlikely and stretches the bounds of scribal error.

r sꜣb r nḥbt.f – Breasted encloses "as far as" in half brackets marking it as uncertain despite his ingenious argumentation and his overly categorical statement that the jackal is "doubtless" a writing of one particular verb. Breasted refers it to the verb *sꜣb*, the same verb listed in *Wb.* 3:420–21, "(wie ein Schakal) durchziehen …" and with a very similar description. It should perhaps be noted that Breasted was one of the foreign scholars who worked on the *Wörterbuch* project. Despite Brawanski's following of Breasted's translation (*Edwin Smith*, 1:72), I cannot find anywhere a listing for or identification of a compound preposition *r-sꜣb-r*, and indeed *Wb.* does not propose one. I think that Allen is correct in taking *sꜣb* here as a verb meaning "run, flow," as *Wb.* 4:420 (with the same writing, as a jackal, in the Eighteenth Dynasty), also Faulkner, *CDME*, 209 "drip," also *Grundriss* 7, 2:709. Brawanski notes Westendorf's and Grapow's translation in accordance with this latter understanding, "sodaß … herabrinnt" (72), although he does not adopt it.

For the sense of the second *r*, see Gardiner, *EG*³, sec. 163.1.

imrw – See above. Note the writing with the *mr* hoe rather than the *mi* sign remarked on earlier.

sry.f pw – For *sry*, see above. The *pw* construction need not be translated "it means that" here—this is not an explanation or a gloss—but simply as an ordinary nominal sentence.

r ḥrp – *r* is "concerning, with respect to" after the verb *ḏd*.

<*m*?> *ẖnw* – With some hesitation I am following a suggestion of Brawanski (p. 32) implying (though he does not discuss this explicitly) that the preposition *m* is omitted before *ẖnw*.

... *mi* ... – This is a circumstantial not an independent clause.

ns – This is a manner nominalization. The verb is biliteral (*Grundriss* 7, 1:479), not 3ae inf., so there is no gemination.

ḏfyt – Faulkner, *CDME*, 322 also gives "penetration."

n ẖrw – Note that here this term cannot refer to the pubic region.

Medical Commentary

Type of Injury

This is a cervical vertebral body compression fracture, without dislocation (fig. 31). This type of injury results from compression/flexion forces acting upon the head and neck. The direction of the force is downward and back. Today the majority of cervical injuries of this type are the result of motor vehicle accidents, falls, and high-impact sports.

In the Allen and Ferguson phylogeny, compression-flexion injuries are labeled as "CF," and graded in five stages of progressive severity. The clinical symptoms in Case #32 are consistent with a compression-flexion cervical spine injury Stage 1 or 2.[218] At this stage of a CF injury, the anterior vertebral body loses height from compression failure giving a "beaked" appearance on x-ray. In the CF Stage 3, an oblique fracture develops in the vertebral body from its anterior surface, progressing downward to the inferior plate. The fractured bone has a "tear-drop" appearance in radiographs and there is no vertebral subluxation, that is, no misalignment of one or more vertebrae.

The primary symptom in CFS1 and CFS2 is neck pain spontaneously and when attempting movement. At these stages neurological symptoms or findings are infrequent. They are considered stable and treatment is conservative. At higher CF injury stages spinal-cord injury is common, at CFS3 in 25 percent of the cases, and at CFS5 in 91 percent. A CFS3 Stage is potentially unstable, if the intervertebral disc and the posterior ligaments are damaged. Stage 3 requires surgical stabilization.

The highest danger to the spinal cord is at the time of injury, but, because an unstable spine can cause additional spinal-cord damage, any cervical spine injury is considered unstable and the neck must be immobilized and the patient transported to an emergency facility. No examination of neck motion should be attempted until screening x-rays or CT scanning proves there is no cervical vertebrae instability. A complete neurological examination must be completed and repeated at intervals. The primary goal after stabilization is pain control, which can be achieved with medication and physical therapy modalities to relieve muscle pain, like the use of cold and heat.

The prognosis for a mechanically stable cervical compression fracture in which there is no evidence of spinal cord damage is excellent. The same applies to those injuries in which there is no spinal cord injury but that require stabilization. These fractures may take three to six months to heal.

We believe the site of injury in the vertebra is at the vertebral body. Brawanski, however, has proposed that the injury as described, is a fracture of the spinous processes instead, and regards a moderate extension injury fracturing the spinous processes at the back of the vertebra to be the mechanism of injury in this case. He does

218. Allen, et al. "A Mechanistic Classification of Closed Indirect Fractures." Lower cervical spine injuries were divided into "phylogenies," based on the mechanism of injury, and each category is arranged by progression in severity.

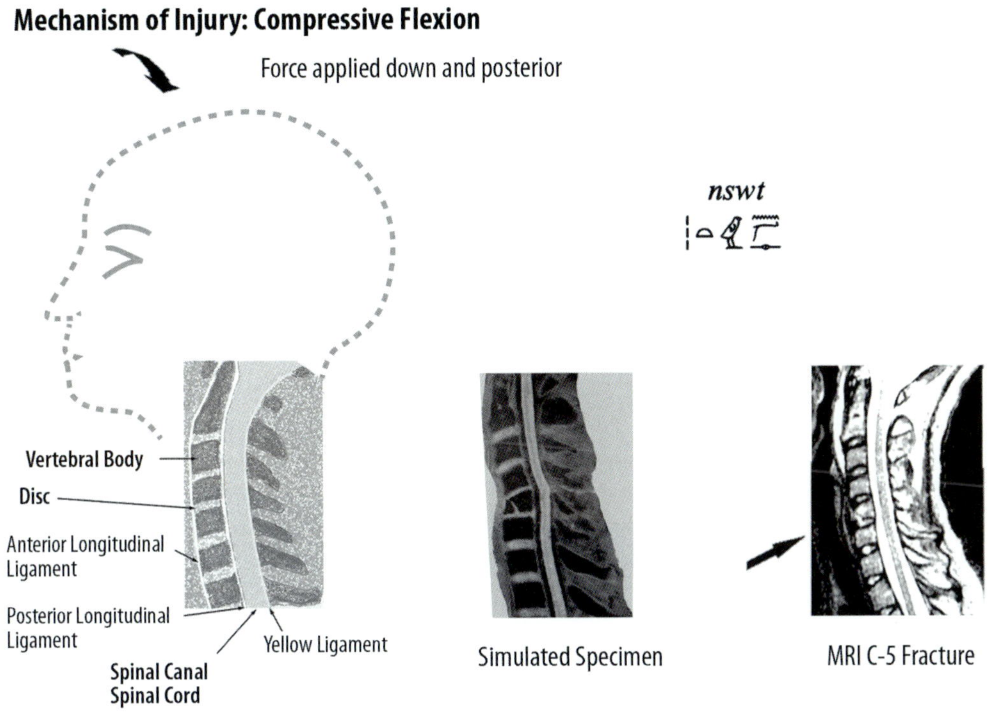

Fig. 31. Cervical compression fracture, mechanism of injury.

call attention to the fact that these types of injuries are not usually accompanied by vertebral body displacement or by neurological deficit.[219] My disagreement with Brawanski's assertion is based on the Egyptian physician's scrupulous description of pathological anatomy: "'a sinking in a vertebra of the back of his neck,' he says concerning/with respect to the depressing of a vertebra of the back of his neck <in(?)> the inside of the back of his neck being like the way a foot sinks into cultivated soil; it is a compressing/penetration downwards." This statement seems specifically, and, more appropriately, to apply to the solid vertebral body, sinking down into the next vertebral body: "a penetration downwards." The thin and narrow cervical spinous processes would crumble on impact. Additionally, the Egyptian's specific term for the spinous process[220] of the vertebra, *ʿḥʿt,* does not appear in the text of Case #32.

Ancient Medical Methodology and Knowledge

As in previously considered cervical spine injuries, Case #32 gives us another example of the ancient Egyptian physician's excellent understanding of cervical fractures. Using the analogy of a foot sinking on cultivated ground, the Egyptian physician accurately describes the mechanism of this injury and the pathological appearance of the anteriorly compressed vertebrae.

219. Brawanski, "Die Wirbelsäulenverletzungen des Papyrus Edwin Smith (Fälle 29–33)," 71–72.
220. Walker, *Studies in Ancient Egyptian Anatomical Terminology*, 267.

It is evident in this case that the patient is not suffering from paralysis because there is no mention of "unawareness" of arms and legs. As in Case #30, the patient is asked in Case #32, to look at his chest and shoulders, but here, the patient could not (or would not) move his neck, due to rigidity from neck pain. In Cases #31 and #33, where there is limb paralysis indicated by "unawareness"of limbs, the ancient Egyptian physician does not ask those paralyzed patients to move their neck. Today, we would by no means ask a patient with a cervical spine injury to move his neck and risk spinal-cord injury.

Treatment of this injury required the neck to be initially wrapped with fresh meat. This initial measure provided warm moisture (fresh muscle is 70% water) and mild pressure over the soft tissues, and, when bandaged over, some physical support not unlike that a modern soft cervical collar. The use of meat as specified here and elsewhere in this papyrus was to be limited to the first day. It is known today that after eighteen to twenty-four hours, the pH of fresh meat reaches its lowest value (5.4 to 5.7),[221] then, it begins to rise, and, after the pH reaches 6.5, decomposition begins. The meat was removed after the first day by loosening the bandages and ointment was applied "to run/flow down onto the back of his neck." Clearly, even in the application of oil, neck manipulation was avoided. Afterwards neck bandaging was done with daily use of alum and honey, until the patient healed. The patient was treated sitting upright. We do not have in this case specific instructions about using brick supports (to keep the head in a neutral position) as in some head injury cases in this papyrus. It is possible that such measure was part of a treatment protocol while having a patient in the sitting position.

221. Measuring the pH value of Meat: http://www.eutechinst.com/techtips/tech-tips35.htm.

CASE #33:
Cervical Burst Fracture with Spinal Cord Injury and Brain Contusion
(Plate XI:9–17)

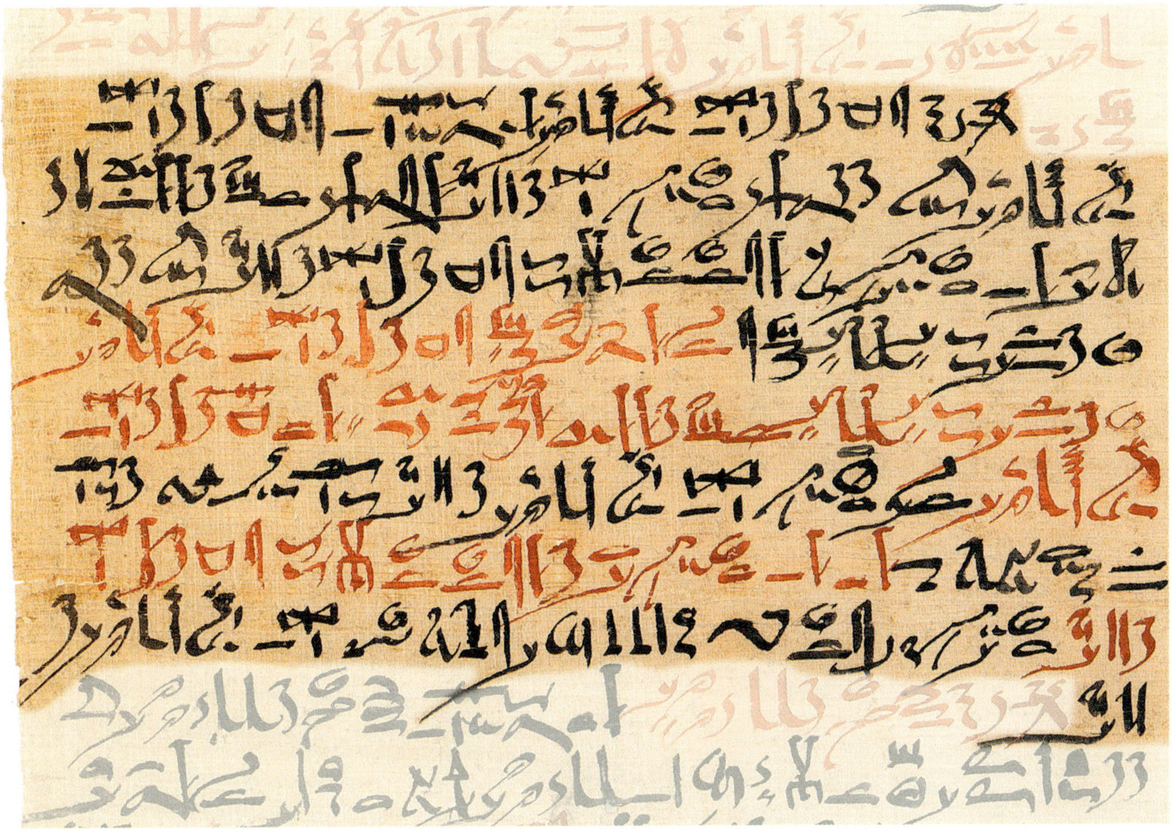

Courtesy New York Academy of Medicine.

9. 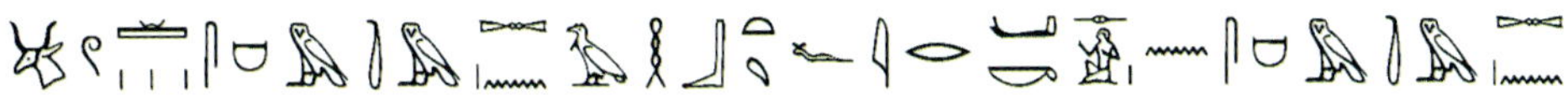

10. 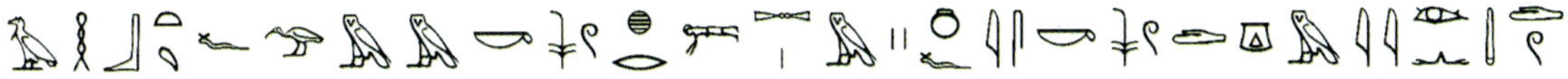

11. 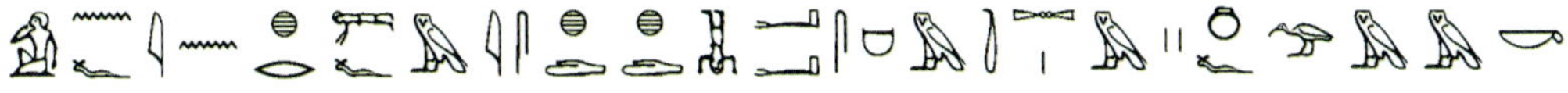

12. 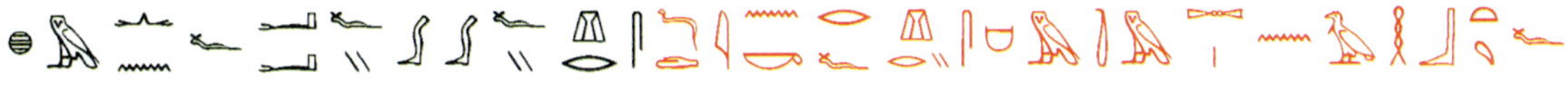

13. 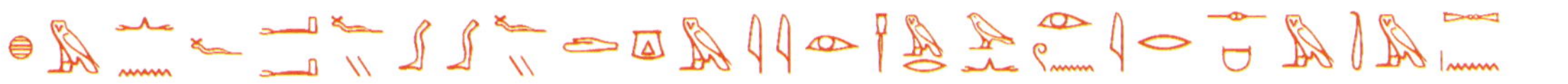

14. 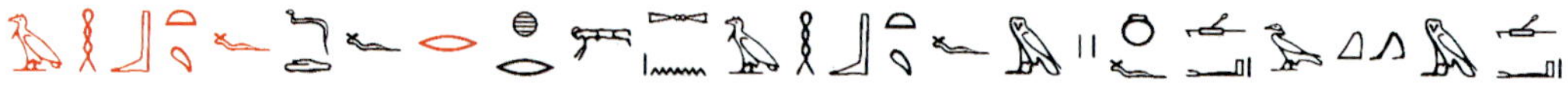

15. 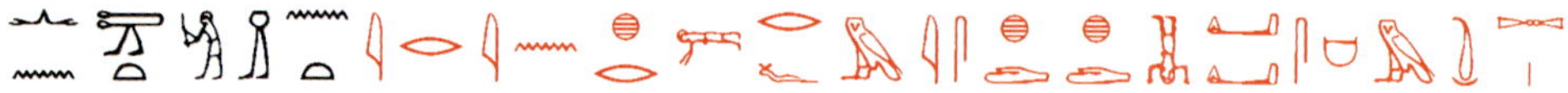

16. 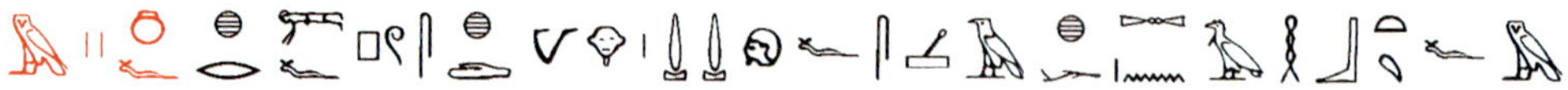

17. 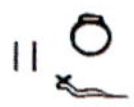

Transliteration

9§ *... šsꜣw sḥm m ṯs n nḥbt.f ir ḫꜣ.k s n sḥm m ṯs n*

10§ *nḥbt.f gmm.k sw ḫr ṯs m snw.f isk sw dgmy n mdw*

11§ *.n.f in ḫr.f m isḫdḫd dd sḥm ṯs m snnw.f gmm.k*

12§ *ḫm.n.f ꜥwy.fy wꜥrty.fy ḫr.s ḏd.in.k r.f ḫry sḥm m ṯs n nḥbt.f*

13§ *ḫm.n.f ꜥwy.fy wꜥrty.fy dgmy mḫr n irw.ny ir sḥm m ṯs n*

14§ *nḥbt.f ḏd.f r ḫr ṯs n nḥbt.f m snnw.f wꜥ ꜥḳ m wꜥ*

15§ *nn iṯt int ir in ḫr{r}.f m isḫdḫd dd sḥm ṯs*

16§ *m sn.nw.f ḫr.f pw sḫd ḥr ḏꜣḏꜣ.f sꜣḫ ṯs n nḥbt.f m*

17§ *snw.f*

Translation

Title:

Necessary knowledge and skills concerning a crush in a vertebra of the back of his neck:

Examination:

If you should examine a man for a crush in a vertebra of the back of his neck, how you find it/him (is): one vertebra falling into its counterpart, while he is stuporous and he cannot speak.

It is his falling/the way he falls head downward/on his head (literally "as one who has fallen head downward/on his head." that causes a vertebra to crush into its counterpart. How you find (him) (is) unaware of both his arms and his legs because of it.

Diagnosis:

Then you are to say about him: "One who has a crush in a vertebra in the back of his neck, (he being) unaware of both his arms and legs, and stuporous: a medical condition that cannot be handled/dealt with."

Explanation A:

As for "a crush in a vertebra in the back of his neck,"

sḥm

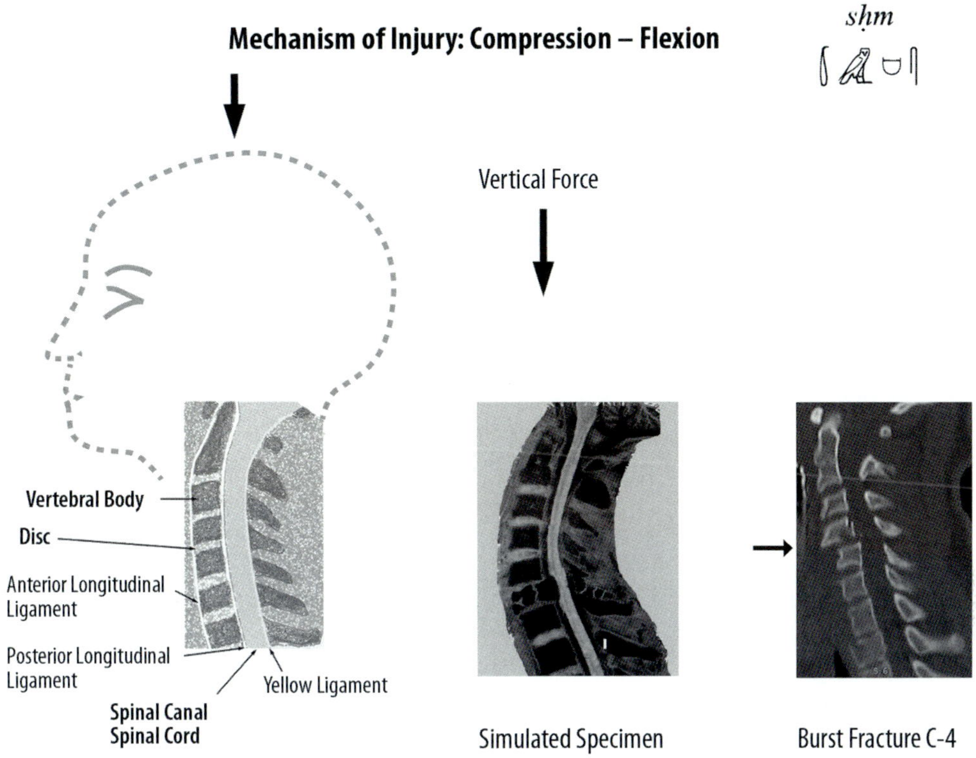

Fig. 32. Cervical burst fracture, mechanism of injury.

he says: "concerning the falling of one vertebra of the back of his neck into its counterpart, (it is) one entering into the other one without moving back and forth."

Explanation B:

As for "it is his falling/the way he falls head downward/on his head that causes one vertebra to crush into its counterpart," it means, his falling/the way he falls head downward, upon the vault of his head, which forcibly drives one vertebra of the back of his neck into its counterpart.

Notes

sḥm m ṯs "a crush in a vertebra" – Brawanski translates similarly, "*Quetschung eines Wirbel*" ("Die Wirbelsäulenverletzungen des Papyrus Edwin Smith [Fälle 29–33]," 73). Allen (*AM*, 93) also takes *sḥm* as a noun, "contusion," but I think this translation is weaker than the pathology indicates. Also, he uses the title "A Shifted Neck Vertebra," the same as Case #32, which, if not an error, seems to miss the point of the case.

gmm.k sw – For the ambiguity of *sw*, which could refer to the patient or the vertebra, see Brawanski, ibid. The verb of course is a manner nominalization.

ẖr ṯs – While translators have agreed in understanding this as an anterior event or relative past, the form seems to be a circumstantial *sḏm.f* which is a concomitant circumstance, and to translate "having fallen."etc. I think one would have to emend to a circumstantial *sḏm.n.f, ḫr<.n>.f*. The passive *sḏm(w).f* would also provide an anterior circumstance, but there is no need or warrant for using a passive verb in this passage. Therefore I am translating a simultaneous circumstance although this might seem a bit awkward. The clause is clearly circumstantial, the first of two circumstantial clauses which are complements to the manner nominalization.

isk sw – This also introduces a circumstantial clause as just alluded to.

in … – This sentence is a participial statement. I take *ḫr.f* "his falling" as probably another manner nominalization, "how/the way he falls." The verb *ḫr* is biliteral and does not geminate. I take *m isḫdḫd* as literally "as one who has fallen on his head," similarly to Brawanski, "Die Wirbelsäulenverletzungen des Papyrus Edwin Smith (Fälle 29–33)," 74 and *Grundriss* 7, 2:792; these authors correctly identify it as a participle. This meaning is also explained in the explanation section of the text itself.

gmm.k – Another manner nominalization.

ḫm.n.f – Circumstantial *sḏm.n.f* as complement to the manner nominalization. For the understanding of this form, see the notes to Case #31 above.

ḫm.n.f (second time) – Also a circumstantial *sḏm.n.f*.

in … – In Explanation B, a participial statement as above.

ḫr.f written as *ḫ* + *r* + det. + *r* + *f* in the repetition – Rather than simply seeing this writing as an erroneous addition of an extra *r*, I wonder if it could be an example of an orthography indicating that the *r* of *ḫr* was pronounced before the suffix-pronoun *.f*, while it might have been lost in free final position. For similar instances see Gardiner, appendix A, p. 432 with notes 3–4. This type of orthography can be identified as early as the Old Kingdom and becomes extremely common in Late Egyptian.

s3ḫ – Active participle. I am not taking *ḫr.f* … as an independent sentence. In Old Egyptian there are participial statements without *in*, which can be found in later times (such as the name *rꜥ-ms-sw* "Ramesses," and probably also an example in the first hymn to Senwosret III from Kahun, cited but explained differently by Gardiner, *EG*^{3}, sec. 486; and in Case #1, p. 35 above).

Medical Commentary

Type of Injury

Case #33 represents a combined injury from a direct blow to the top of the head and the cervical spine. The injury has resulted in signs of encephalopathy and spinal-cord injury. The patient is quadriplegic and has anesthesia of the body below the level of the spinal-cord injury, having "unawareness" of his arms and his legs.[222]

The cervical spine fracture is a burst fracture of the vertebral body, causing its fragmentation and expansion when vertically compressed by the impact, the spine being neutral or in a slightly flexed position (fig. 32). In these injuries, the fracture line begins at the upper end-plate of the vertebral body and spreads radially through the vertebral body, resulting in its mechanical failure and fragmentation, often with retropulsion.[223] In the most severe cases, the posterior component of the fragmented vertebral body is pushed backwards into the spinal canal, thereby damaging the spinal cord. In the Allen-Ferguson classification, vertical compression cervical frac-

222. The reader is directed to appendix for a compilation of the neurological symptoms and signs in the Edwin Smith Papyrus.

223. A. O. Mekhail, P. M. Steinmetz, and E. C. Benzel, "Subaxial Cervical Spine Burst Fractures," *The Cervical Spine* (ed. Charles R. Clark; 4th ed.; Philadelphia: Lippincott Williams & Wilkins, 2005), 683–95.

tures are staged in grades of progressive severity from VCS1 to VCS3.[224] These injuries accounted for 14 percent of the cervical fractures.

We need to point out that the theoretical mechanisms of fracture of the cervical spine rarely occur in a pure form, often having rotational and/or tilting components, all of which result in variables in the anatomical injuries produced for the individual case. Dr. Brawanski's excellent review presents Case #33 as being a compression fracture and/or a burst fracture.[225] Compression fractures of the anterior vertebral body are more likely to occur in a compression flexion injury to the cervical spine, producing an anterior wedge-shaped fragment. Vertical compression fractures of the vertebral body could show "cupping" of either bony end-plate in Grade I injuries (VCS1), cupping of both plates in VCS2 injuries, and a burst fracture with radial fragment displacement in VCS3 fractures, impacting into the spinal canal and the spinal cord. In our opinion, Case #33 is a burst fracture case, based on the specific use of the Egyptian word "*sḥm*," which means "crushing," and on the Egyptian physician's Explanation B: "As for 'it is his falling/the way he falls head downward/on his head that causes one vertebra to crush into its counterpart ..." (the classic mechanism of injury for a "burst fracture" in a patient who has suffered a spinal cord injury).

Explanation A details the anatomical pathology of the injured vertebra: "concerning the falling of one vertebra of the back of his neck into its counterpart, (it is) one entering into the other one without moving back and forth," suggesting this may be a mechanically stable fracture. Determination of mechanical stability in the management of cervical fractures is necessary to prevent potential injury or further injury to the spinal cord. Stability of cervical fractures is dependent upon the structural damage that has occurred to the vertebral elements, as understood in the functional concept of three existing columns in the spine (fig. 28). The anterior column is formed by the anterior longitudinal ligament, the anterior two-thirds of the vertebral bodies, and the discs. The middle column is formed by the posterior third of the vertebral bodies, discs, and the posterior longitudinal ligament. The posterior column is formed by the pedicles, laminas, ligamentum flavum, and the spinous processes. When any two columns are disrupted, the spine is considered unstable. There are, however, a number of variants in assessment of stability. The mechanical stability of the fracture in Case #33 will depend on the integrity of the posterior longitudinal ligament and the posterior vertebral column.

The patient in Case #33 has also suffered a head injury by landing on his head and is described as being stuporous. No other information is provided in regard to the head injury.

Today's management of these injuries consists of applying the general principles for head and cervical spine trauma. After securing of the airway and adequate circulation, neck and head immobilization, the patient is transported to an emergency facility for Neurosurgical evaluation and imaging investigation of the traumatized areas. A cervical burst fracture may need to be decompressed and surgically immobilized. Often the surgical approach needs to be from directions, front and back. The patient would probably be referred to a spinal cord rehabilitation facility for extensive rehabilitation. Extensive and promising international research in the treatment of spinal cord injury is ongoing.

---

224. B. L. Allen, R. L. Ferguson, T. R. Leheman, and R. P. O'Brien, "A Mechanistic Classification of Closed Indirect Fractures and Dislocations of the Lower Cervical Spine," *Spine* 7 (1982): 1–27. Lower cervical spine injuries were divided into "phylogenies" based on the mechanism of injury, and each category is arranged by progression in severity. D. G. Anderson, and A. R. Vaccaro, "Classification of Lower Cervical Spine Injuries," *The Cervical Spine* (ed. Charles R. Clark; 4th Edition; Philadelphia: Lippincott Williams & Wilkins, 2005), 651–59.

225. Brawanski, "Die Wirbelsäulenverletzungen des Papyrus Edwin Smith (Fälle 29–33)," 75.

Ancient Medical Methodology and Knowledge

Once more, the master clinician from ancient Egypt shows his comprehensive knowledge on the subject, providing the pupil with a complete clinical picture of the severity of this burst fracture and resulting neurological dysfunction. The anatomical-pathological details of this injury and production mechanisms, by the patient falling head downward are identified. The resulting effects from the head and cervical spine injury are succinctly given as stupor and quadriplegia.

In ancient Egypt, this type of vertebral compression injury could have occurred in head-downward falls. situations that would favor this type of injury would include construction accidents with falls from a height or battle injuries with direct blows to the top of the head.

Not unexpectedly, the verdict in Case #33 is not one in which successful treatment would have been possible and no treatment segment is included. Nonetheless it is quite certain that supportive treatment was provided, as we have repeatedly seen in other severe injury cases in the Edwin Smith papyrus.

CASE #34:
Sterno-Clavicular Dislocation (Bilateral?)
(Plate XI:17–XII:2)

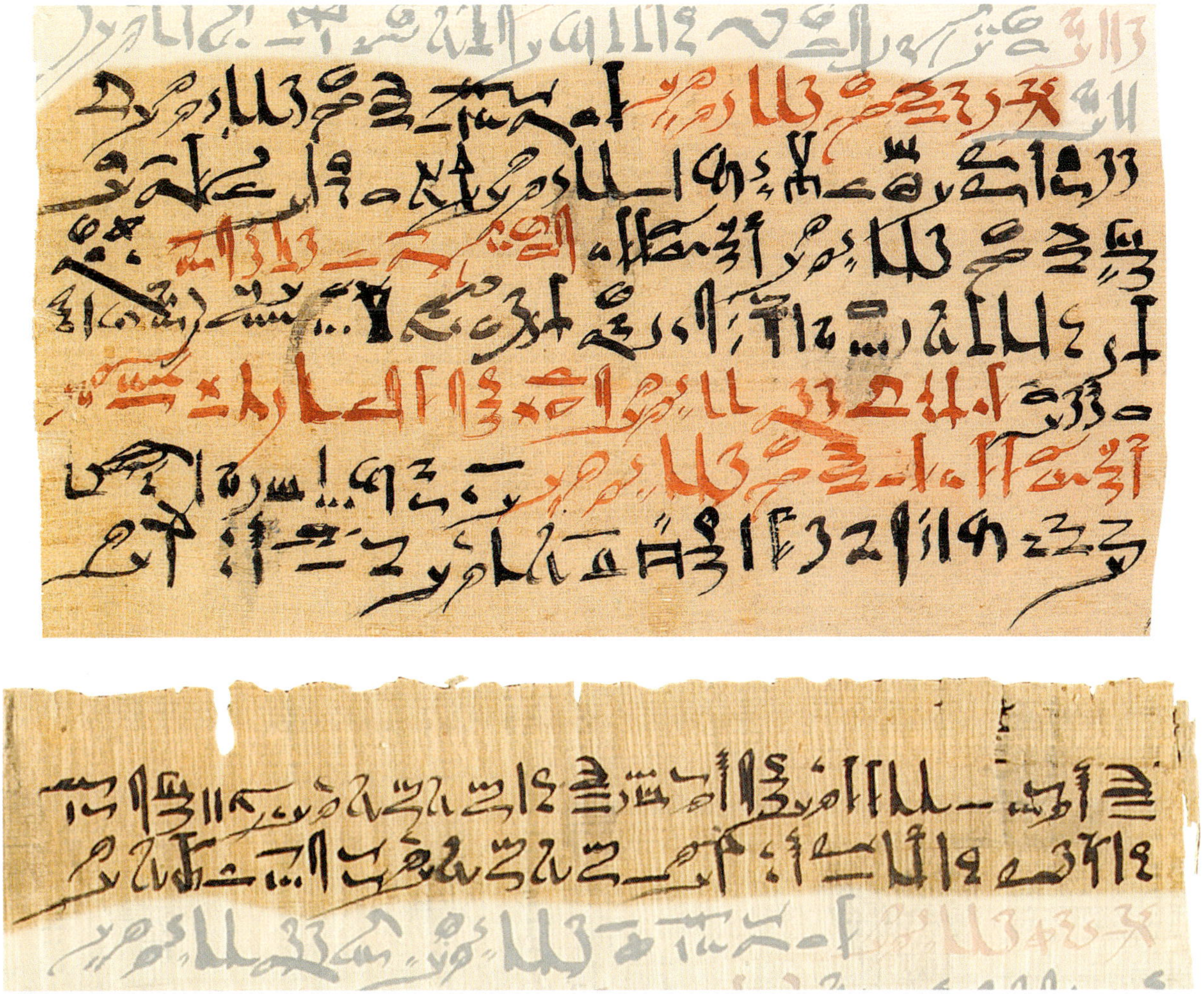

Courtesy New York Academy of Medicine.

17. 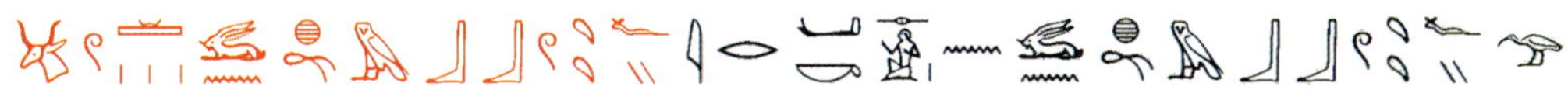

18. 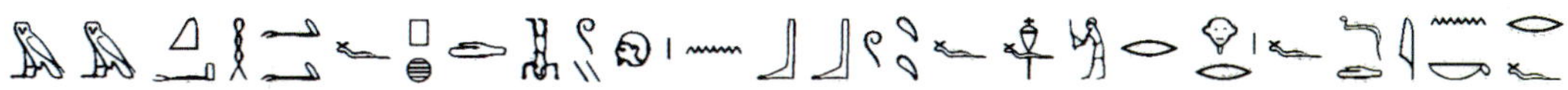

19. 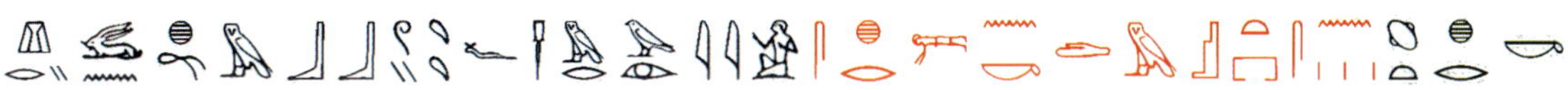

20. 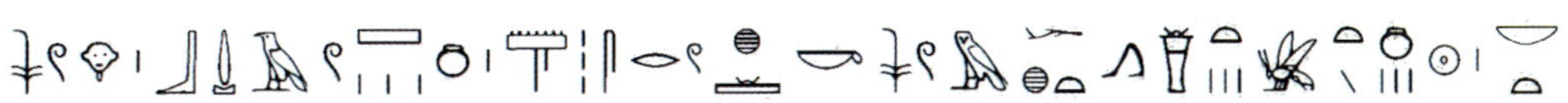

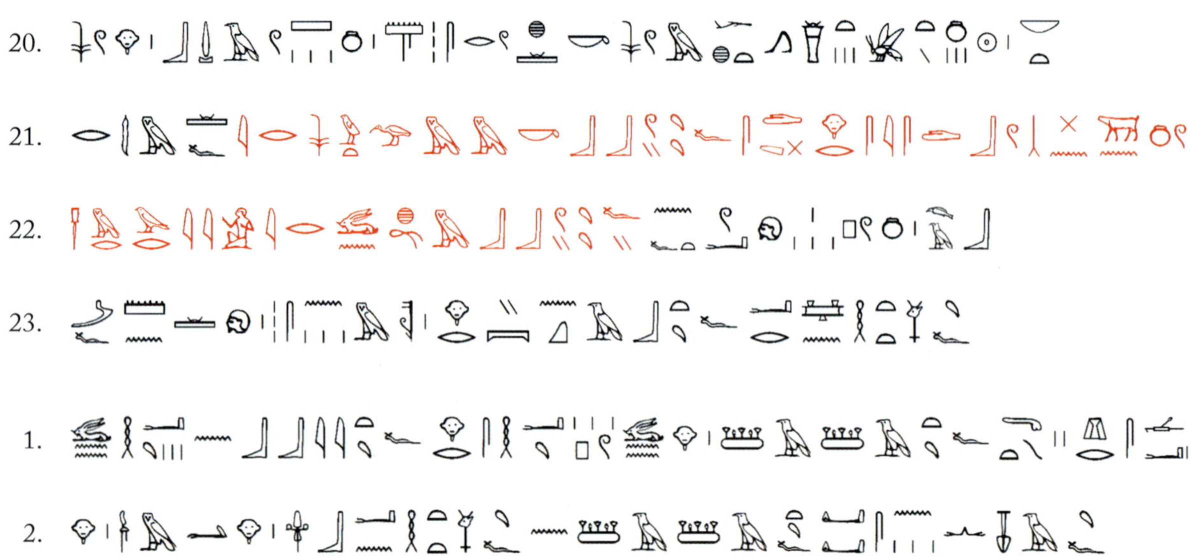

Transliteration

17§ … *šs3w wnḫ m bbwy.fy ir ḫ3.k s n wnḫ m bbwy.f*

18§ *gmm ḳᶜḥwy.f p<3> ḫd.wy tp n bbwyf ḫsf r ḥr.f ḏd.in.k r.f*

19§ *ḫry wnḫ m bbwy.f mḥr iry.i sḫr.<i> n.k <sn> d(w) m st.sn wt.ḫr.k*

20§ *sw ḥr bḏ3w nw ḥbsw srwḫ.k sw m-ḫt mrḥt bit rᶜ nb{t}*

21§ *r nḏm.f ir swt gmm.k bbwy.f sḏ. ḥr.s isdbw n ḫnw*

22§ *mḥr iry.i ir wnḫ m bbwy.fy nft tpw pw nw ḫ3b<wy>*

23§ *.f mn tpw.sn m ḳs ḥrj n ḳ3bt.f ᶜr n ḥtyt.f*

1§ *wnn ḥᶜ n bbyt.f ḥr-s ḥᶜ pw wnn ḥr š3š3t.f mt snw ḫr-s wᶜ*

2§ *ḥr wnmy <wᶜ> ḥr i3by n ḥtyt.f n š3š3t.f dd.sn n sm3.f*

Translation

Case #34A

Title:

Necessary knowledge and skills for a dislocation in both of his collarbones:

Examination:

If you should examine a man for a dislocation in both of his collarbones, whose shoulder joints and arms are found drooping downward (or, how <you> find both of his shoulder joints and arms (is): drooping downward??), the head(s) of his two collar-bones twisted towards his face,

Diagnosis:

then you are to say about him: "One who has a dislocation in both of his collarbones, an injury/medical condition which I will handle/deal with."

Treatment:

Then you are to cause (the collarbones) to fall back, so that they are lying in their place(s).

Then you must bind it over stiff rolls of cloth, and you should treat him afterward with ointment and honey every day until he is well.

Case #34b: Posterior Clavicular Dislocation

Second Examination and Diagnosis:

But, if how you find his two collarbones (is): smash fractured over it (and) pierced through and collapsed to the inside—a medical condition which I will handle/deal with."

Explanation:

As for a dislocation in his collarbones: it means that the heads of his clavicles have been detached, while their heads are attached to the upper bone of his sternum, penetrating to his trachea, over which is the skin of the hollows above his collarbones; that is, the skin which is on his upper chest, two blood vessels (being) under it: one upon the right side and (one) upon the left side of his trachea of his upper chest; how they give (blood) (is) to his respiratory tract.

Notes

gmm – Breasted considers this form "an error for *gmm-k*" (*Edwin Smith* 1:343). This is a distinct possibility in my view. Allen takes another option which I think yields a viable translation without emendation, "whose shoulders are found drooping" (93). This is the construction of the passive participle, here a geminating passive participle, with what Gardiner calls a "retained object" (sec. 277). See also examples in Adriaan de Buck, *Egyptian Readingbook: Exercises and Middle Egyptian Texts* (3rd ed.; Leiden: Nederlands Instituut voor het Nabije Oosten, 1970), 20–23. Though this is a possible reading of the passage without emendation, the manner nominalization *gmm.k* is far more standard for this type of clause. Therefore I have adopted the retained object as my preferred rendition but with the emended manner nominalization version in parentheses. Please note that there is no feasible grammatical mechanism known for having some participles or "concrete" relative forms act as manner nominalizations or Emphatic Forms, despite an attempt by Westendorf to suggest this possibility; see Meltzer, "Participles, Relative Forms and Gemination in Middle Egyptian," 231–32 and Junge's comment in "How to Study Egyptian Grammar," 391–92.

tp… – This is a circumstantial not an independent clause.

kꜥḥwy.f, bbwy.f – As remarked previously, the two-tick *y* on the suffix-pronoun after a dual is optional.

sḫr.<i>n.k – Accepting the emendation to the *sḏm.in.f* form.

d(w) – As in previous cases, without a preceding *w* to serve as a haplography, I do not consider this an "abbreviated" writing of *wd* but a writing of the different, similarly employed verb *d(w)*. Again I take the sense of the stative here as a stative of result.

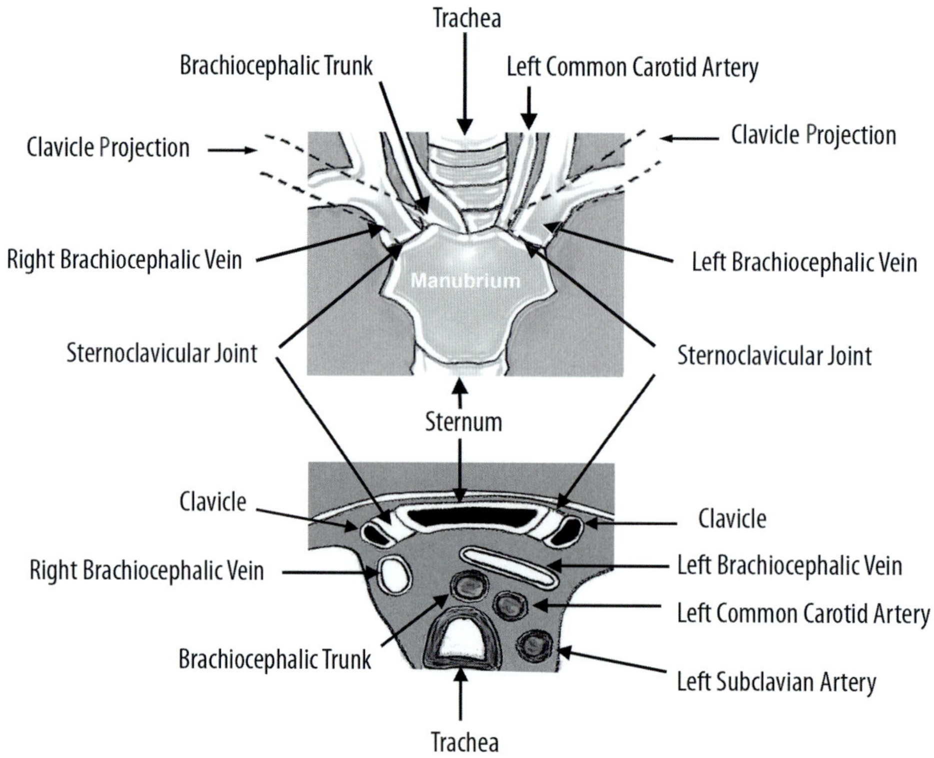

Fig. 33. Sternoclavicular joints, trachea, and adjacent vessels.

rʿ nb{t} – This error is facilitated by the obsolescence of feminine *–t* in free final position (Gardiner, *EG*³, 34 n. 1a, 432 note 4).

isdbw – See previous discussion (p. 126).

nft tpw – *nft* before the subject *tpw* cannot be a stative. The only obvious possibility is passive *sḏm(w).f*. Note that the passive *sḏm(w).f* is an ambivalent form which is frequently circumstantial or adverbial (and was so identified by Polotsky in *Egyptian Tenses*) but can also be attested as a nominal form (Doret, *Narrative Verbal System*, 177, table 11). Here I am taking it as a "that" clause and am adjusting the time reference to the past or anterior field, that is, what in the active verb would be expressed with the *sḏm.n.f*.

mn tpw.sn – This is a circumstantial clause and the form is a circumstantial *sḏm.f*.

ʿr n – Faulkner, *CDME*, 45 does list a noun *ʿr* "proximity," but I see no justification for its autonomous use to mean "in proximity." I would want to emend an <*m*> before *ʿr* for this meaning, and I am reluctant to do this. I think that *ʿr* can be a stative *ʿr(w)* because the verb is intransitive (see the Faulkner listing). As a participle its syntax would be very awkward. Thus I prefer the Breasted/Allen type of translation, "penetrating/extending to," probably "penetrating."

wnn followed by *ḥʿ* is a geminating relative form with *ḥʿ* as the separately expressed subject or actor, and the entire construction is that of Gardiner, *EG*³, sec. 383.

wnn (second occurrence) – Geminating active participle.

mt snw … – This is a circumstantial not an independent clause.

one … (one) – It makes sense that the right and left refer to the two blood vessels.

dd.sn – This is a manner nominalization or nominal *sḏm.f* of *rdi*, "how they give (blood) (is) to his respiratory tract."

n written with negative arms – A well-attested scribal variant; see also p. 244 below.

Medical Commentary

Type of Injury

It should be stated that bilateral clavicular dislocations, anterior or posterior, are rare. As discussed in Case #25, referring to the mandible, it appears that the "dual" was employed by the Egyptians when discussing paired anatomical structures. It would then be that Case #34 refers to a single clavicular injury, anterior or posterior.

The sternoclavicular joint is a saddle-type joint that provides free movement of the clavicle in nearly all planes. The strength and stability of the sternoclavicular joint resides in its enclosing capsule and supporting ligaments. Because only approximately 50 percent of the medial end of the clavicle articulates with the manubrium of the sternum, the sternoclavicular joint has little inherent stability. The capsule surrounding the joint is weakest inferiorly.

There is discrepancy in the explanation between: a) "as for a dislocation in his collarbones: it means that the heads of his clavicles have been detached," and b) "while their heads are attached to the upper bone of his sternum, penetrating to his trachea...." The first portion of the papyrus' explanation with the heads of the clavicles dislocated corresponds with the context of Case #34a. The second portion, in which the heads of the clavicles are said to be attached to the sternum, but the fragmented portion of the clavicle is pushed backwards into the area of the trachea and large vessels in the superior mediastinum, is consistent with the injury described in Case #34b.

Bilateral Sternoclavicular Anterior Dislocation

Anterior sternoclavicular dislocations are much more frequent than posterior dislocations with a ratio of 9 to 1.[226] Anterior dislocations often are the result of an impact to the shoulder from the front causing it to rotate backwards and to the medial end of the clavicle to snap forward.

The physical examination of a case of bilateral anterior sterno-clavicular dislocation will show the patient with his/her arms and shoulders slumping downward, with marked protrusion of the heads of the clavicles, which is particularly evident when observed from below.

Today, the treatment of most cases of anterior dislocation is nonoperative. The currently advocated technique for closed reduction[227] is as follows:

- Place the patient in a supine position on the stretcher.
- Place a 3 to 4 inch thick bolster (rolled sheet or sandbag) between the scapula and spine (to help separate the clavicle from the manubrium).
- Have an assistant abduct (to 90°) and extend (10–15°) the shoulder on the affected side and apply traction.
- If reduction does not occur, apply pressure to the medial clavicle in a posterior and inferior direction.

226. John P. Rudzinski, "Sternoclavicular Joint Injury." Medscape Reference: http://www.emedicine.com/emerg/topic783.htm.
227. Ibid.

Bilateral Sternoclavicular Posterior Dislocation

Case #34b is a posterior sternoclavicular comminuted fracture-dislocation of the proximal portion of the clavicle produced by a direct smash blow without an open wound. The *isdb* injury that we believe has the meaning of piercing through and collapsing to the inside, refers to the posterior penetration of the fractured clavicle into the upper mediastinum, towards the trachea. These injuries are accompanied by a 25 percent complication rate due to injuries to the anatomical structures of the anterior mediastinum, which are immediately posterior to the sterno-clavicular joints and on each side of the trachea (fig. 33). These are:

- the subclavian veins
- the right and left brachiocephalic veins
- the left carotid artery
- the right brachiocephalic arterial trunk

This penetrating injury into the upper mediastinum was not accompanied by an open wound. If this had been the case, the patient would have been gravely ill with life threatening complications, such as pneumothorax, major arterial or venous hemorrhaging, or mediastinal thrombosis, entities which the ancient Egyptians would not have been able to treat. Nonetheless, his verdict in Case #34b is "a medical condition that can be handled/dealt with."

Symptoms in this kind of injury are pain at the base of the neck, and pain when taking a deep breath. Swelling is minimal and the usual prominence of the proximal end of the clavicle is absent.[228] Pain on examination of the area shows exquisite tenderness medially.[229] Respiratory distress and sudden death may occur.

Today, the treatment of posterior clavicular dislocation may be postponed if respiratory and/or vascular complications need to be treated first. Closed reduction of posterior sternoclavicular dislocation may fail or produce injury to the upper mediastinum structures, which can be disastrous. Reduction is carried out in the operating room under general anesthesia by a surgical team consisting of traumatologist and cardiovascular and orthopedic surgeons. With the arm abducted > 90 degrees, traction is applied, while reducing the clavicular dislocation by manipulation. Immobilization with plaster figure of eight bandage follows.

Open reduction and internal fixation may be required.

Ancient Medical Methodology and Knowledge

Anterior Sternoclavicular Joint Dislocation

Case #34a is an anterior sternoclavicular joint dislocation. Its pathological subtract and clinical presentation are precisely given by the Egyptian physician: "how <you> find both of his shoulder joints and arms (is): drooping downward??), the head(s) of his two collar-bones twisted towards his face." The Egyptian physician does not elaborate here on details of his reduction technique, although this is explained in subsequent cases. Our text in Case #34a merely instructs: "Then you are to cause (the collarbones) to fall back, so that they are lying in their place(s)," binding the area afterwards with stiff rolls of cloth and daily topical applications of honey. Technical details of binding to this area are given more explicitly in the treatment of clavicular fractures in Case #35.

228. Fred L. Allman, "Fractures and Ligamentous Injuries of the Clavicle and Its Articulation," *Journal of Bone and Joint Surgery, American Volume* 49/4 (1967): 782.

229. Rudzinski, "Sternoclavicular Joint Injury."

Posterior Sternoclavicular Joint Dislocation

Case #34b is a closed fractured clavicle with posterior displacement, pierced through, and collapsed to the inside towards the trachea. There is no open wound. The ancient physician decides this injury is treatable: "a medical condition which I will handle/deal with," but does not elaborate further.

The master physician alerts the student to the existence of important adjacent anatomical structures behind the fractured clavicular heads: "two blood vessels (being) under it: one upon the right side and (one) upon the left side of his trachea of his upper chest" and the potential consequences of vascular injury at this site from bleeding into the airway and lungs: "how they give (blood) (is) to his respiratory tract."

Our interpretation of this text and our medical conclusions vary from other authors in the issue of identity of the *mtw*. Breasted initially thought these were large blood vessels, but his medical consultant Dr. Arno Luckhardt forcefully stated these structures were the bronchi, based on Breasted's own translation about these *mtw*: "they lead to the lungs." This assertion by Luckhardt was made, despite his own observation that the bronchi branch off the trachea at the level of the third or the fourth ribs, which eliminates these as being the bronchi The *mtw* in the text of Case #34 are at the same level of the trachea, and on each side of it, indicating the brachiocephalic veins and trunks. We believe Breasted's initial impression was correct, these *mtw* are blood vessels.

The final conclusion of the explanation segment must be revisited in order both to reveal the description of the pathogenetic mechanism of serious injury in this case, and for further speculation concerning the anatomical and physiological concepts held by the ancient Egyptians.

Ebers #854a, previously cited in the medical commentary to Case #1, reads: "As for the air that enters at the nose, it enters to the heart and lungs, and they convey to the whole body" establishing that air reaches the heart and lungs and then it is distributed to the rest of the body. On this reference, John Nunn remarks: "if for 'air' we substitute 'oxygen' (in solution and chemical combination in blood), the whole concept is remarkably close to the truth."[230] We do not have further description on what happens to the air at the heart and lungs, and there is some evidence that the ancient Egyptians thought that some vessels contained air.[231] But it is also clear that air belonged to the airway and blood was present in the blood vessels. Ebers Papyrus #876 deals with vessel bleeding requiring cauterization.[232]

The Paragraph #855k of the Ebers Papyrus describes a situation consistent with congestive heart failure. In this clinical entity acute ventricular heart failure due to pulmonary venous hypertension occurs with flooding of the lung's alveoli by serous fluid and blood. The symptoms are acute respiratory distress, profuse sweating with blood tinged frothy sputum and can become rapidly fatal. In Ebers #855k the heart is described as flooding with blood of the lung making a direct reference to the abnormal situation of the presence of blood in the respiratory tract. From a traumatic source, Case #34b speaks of a potential serious vascular injury in a clavicular posterior dislocation hemorrhaging into the trachea and lungs.

230. Nunn, *Ancient Egyptian Medicine*, 55.

231. Ebers Papyrus #855e. Grapow, *Grundriss* 5:7.

232. Gonzalo M. Sanchez and T. Siuda, "Ebers Papyrus Case #873 - A Probable Case of Neurofibromatosis," *The South Dakota Journal of Medicine* 55/12 (2000): 529–35.

CASE #35:
Clavicular Fractures
(Plate XII:2–8)

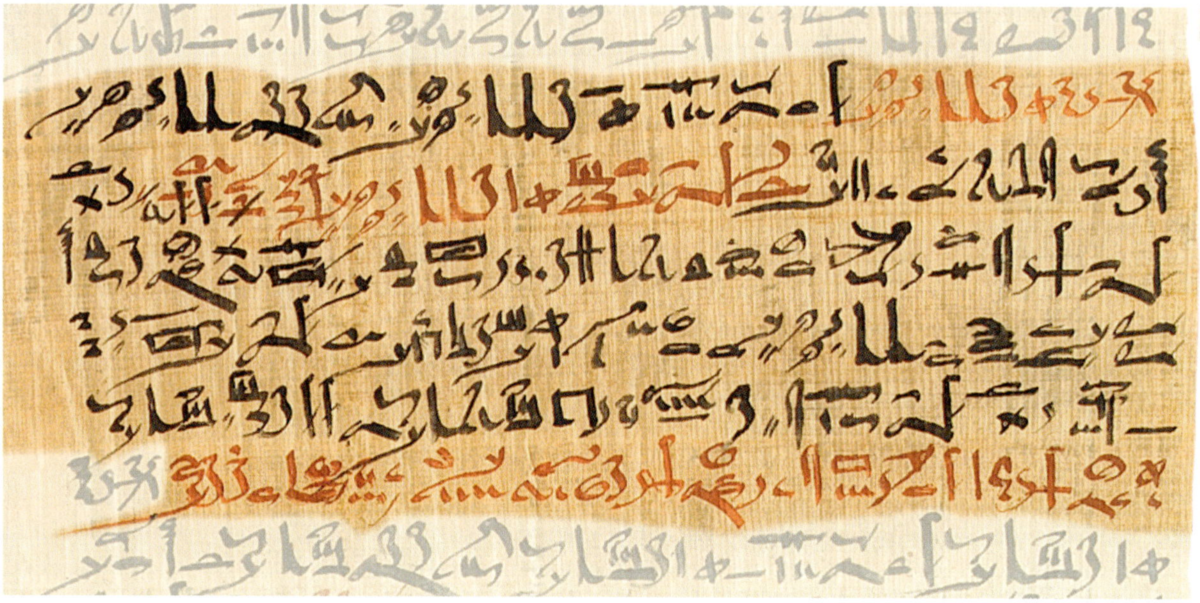

Courtesy New York Academy of Medicine.

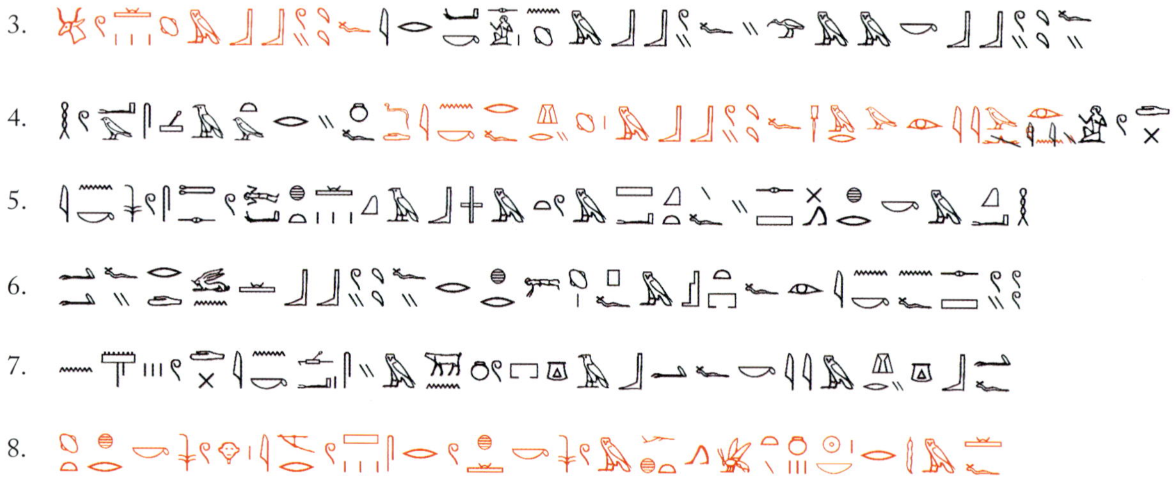

Transliteration

3§ … *šs3w ḥsb m bbwy.f ỉr ḫ3.k s n ḥsb m bbwy.fy gmm.k bbwy.fy*

4§ *ḥwꜥ s3t r snw.f ḏd.in.k r.f ẖry ḥsb m bbwy.fy mḥr {n ỉrw.ny} ỉry.i wd.*

5§ *i͗n.k sw sṯꜣs.w ḫt ḳꜣb i͗mytw mšꜥḳty.fy sš.ḫr.k <sw> m ḳꜥḥwy.*

6§ *fy r dwn bbwy.fy r ḫr ḥsb pf m st.f i͗r.i͗n.k n.f sšwy*

7§ *n ḥbsw wd.i͗n.k wꜥ s<n>y m-ẖnw gbꜣ.f ky m-ẖry gbꜣ.f*

8§ *wt.ḫr.k sw ḥr i͗mrw srwḫ.k sw m-ḫt <m> bi͗t rꜥ nb r nḏm.f*

Translation

Title:

Necessary knowledge and skills for a fracture in his collarbones:

Examination:

If you should examine a man for a fracture in his collarbones, how your find both of his collarbones (is): shortened,

(each) being pushed out of alignment with respect to its counterpart.

Diagnosis:

Then you are to say about him: "One who has a fracture in his collarbones: an injury/medical condition which {cannot be handled/dealt with} I will handle/deal with."

Treatment:

Then you lay him so that he is stretched out (with) something folded between his shoulder blades.

Then you must spread out by means of his two shoulders, in order to stretch apart his collar-bones so that/until that break falls into its place.

Then you make for him a double strip(?) of cloth.

Then you place one of the two of them on the inside of his upper arm and the other on the underside of his upper arm.

Then you must bind it (along) with alum(?) (or, a bandage with alum[?] shavings?), and you should treat it afterward <with> honey every day until it/he is well.

Notes

ḥwꜥ(w) sꜣt(w) – statives. The translation of *sꜣt(w)* as a subordinate form is more appropriate.

Prognosis – As previous translators note, *i͗ry.i͗* is corrected from an originally written unfavorable prognosis.

sṯꜣsw – Taking this as a stative of result.

sš. ḫr.k – This verb is ambiguous in its reading and can be transliterated either *sš* or *sn* (Faulkner, *CDME*, 246; cf. *Wb.* 3:483) and could be given as: *sš*(?)/*sn*(?), though this is not noted in the *Grundriss* (7, 2:797) listing.

r ḫr ḥsb – Both "so/in order that" and "until" (the choice of both Breasted and Allen) are possible, so I have indicated them as alternatives in the translation.

sšwy – Both *Wb.* 4:76 and *Grundriss* 7, 2:733 list this word (the form listed in the lemma is singular not dual) under *swš* (in *Wb.* under the vertical *s*). The plain meaning seems to be two strips or double strip of cloth; the meaning "sling" is unlikely as explained in the medical commentary.

s<n>y – Accepting this emendation.

m ẖnw … m ẖry – I am translating this so as to distinguish it from the simple meaning "inside, in the interior" for *m-ẖnw*, which would clearly be impossible, and the simple writing of "under," which would be done with the preposition *ẖr*. For *m* with the meaning "on" or as a parallel/variant of *ḥr*, cf. *Grundriss* 7, 1:340.

imrw – See the discussions above. I am reflecting Brawanski's discussion in the alternative translation, with a question mark.

<m> bit – The preposition *m* has to be supplied.

Medical Commentary

Type of Injury

This is a (*ḥsb*) fracture produced by direct blows to the collar bone (Visual Index II), from falling on an outstretched arm, or falling sideways against the shoulder. Seventy-two to eighty percent of all fractures occur in the middle third of the clavicle (fig. 34).[233]

The symptoms are pain and tenderness over the fracture site, and when moving the shoulder or the arm. On physical examination, the clavicle is shortened and its proximal segment is pulled upwards by the sternocleidomastoid muscle. Due to the subcutaneous position of the clavicles the fragment pulled superiorly appears prominent, creating a very obvious deformity.

Current treatment of most clavicular fractures is immobilization. Operational Medicine. The FMST Student Manual - 2008 Web Edition of the United States Marine Corps, Field Medical Training Battalion. Under its "Manage Musculoskeletal Injuries" section, details the field management of these fractures, with general and specific rules for splinting.[234]

Ancient Medical Methodology and Knowledge

Case #35 sets forth fractures of the two collar bones, which would be an unusual occurrence. Breasted (*Edwin Smith*, 350) makes the point of a possible scribal error writing the dual *bbwy,* or perhaps that it was a figure of speech, meaning "either one of the two." We have also addressed this issue in regard to anatomical concepts of the ancient Egyptians in Cases #25 and #34, in that it appears that they used "dual" when discussing paired anatomical structures.

The clinical description is accurate as provided by the Egyptian physicians for the collar bones appearing "shortened, (each) being pushed out of alignment with respect to its counterpart."

Their recommended technique for reduction and realignment of these fractures, followed by immobilization, is still valid today. The specific arrangement of the two strips of cloth suggests these were intended to be used as modern swathes (long broad strips or linen belts) or as splints, in Breasted's opinion. One of these strips was applied to the inside of the arm (the medial surface of the arm, close to the chest wall), the other under the arm (behind the arm of the patient lying on his back). The arrangement of the two linen splints would form a cradle for the arm. Further support would be provided by bandaging this over to the chest, effectively stabilizing the fractured clavicle. Although there are no instructions indicating that the bandage bound the arm to the chest,

---

233. L. J. Rubino, M. W. Lawless, and B. P. Kleinhenz, "Clavicle Fractures." Medscape Reference: http://emedicine.medscape.com/article/1260953-overview.

234. Online: http://www.operationalmedicine.org/TextbookFiles/FMST_20008/FMST_1407.htm.

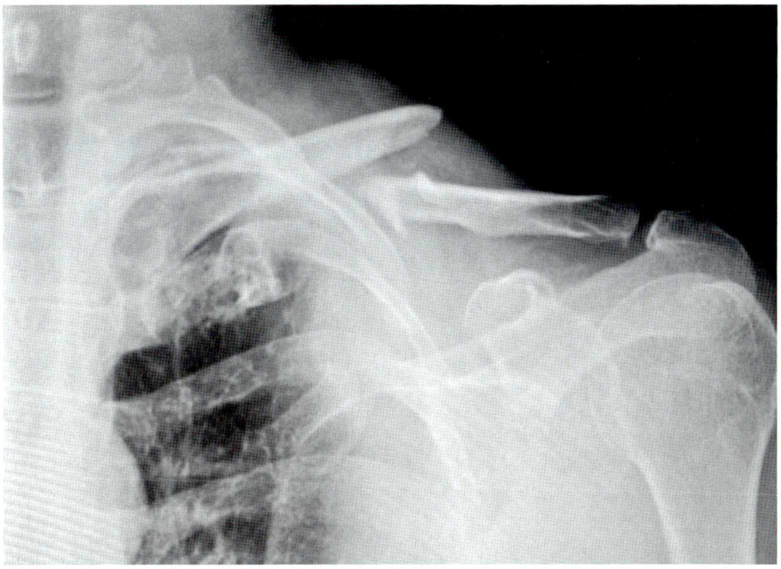

Fig 34. Fractured clavicle.

it is the only way that a fractured clavicle could be effectively treated. Wrapping a bandage over the upper arm itself would do nothing to help the muscular traction effects of gravity on the outer segment of the fractured clavicle.

A possible alternative use of the linen strips would have been as a sling. However, nothing is mentioned in Case #35 about placing the strips of linen in such a way as to provide support under the elbow and under the flexed forearm, and of knotting the two strips around the opposite side of the neck. These are the necessary technical instructions to be followed for the sling to serve its intended support of the upper extremity in the affected side.

Bandaging included their established treatment routine for injuries of using daily applications of alum and honey.

CASE #36:
Linear Fracture of the Humerus
(Plate XII:8–14)

Courtesy New York Academy of Medicine.

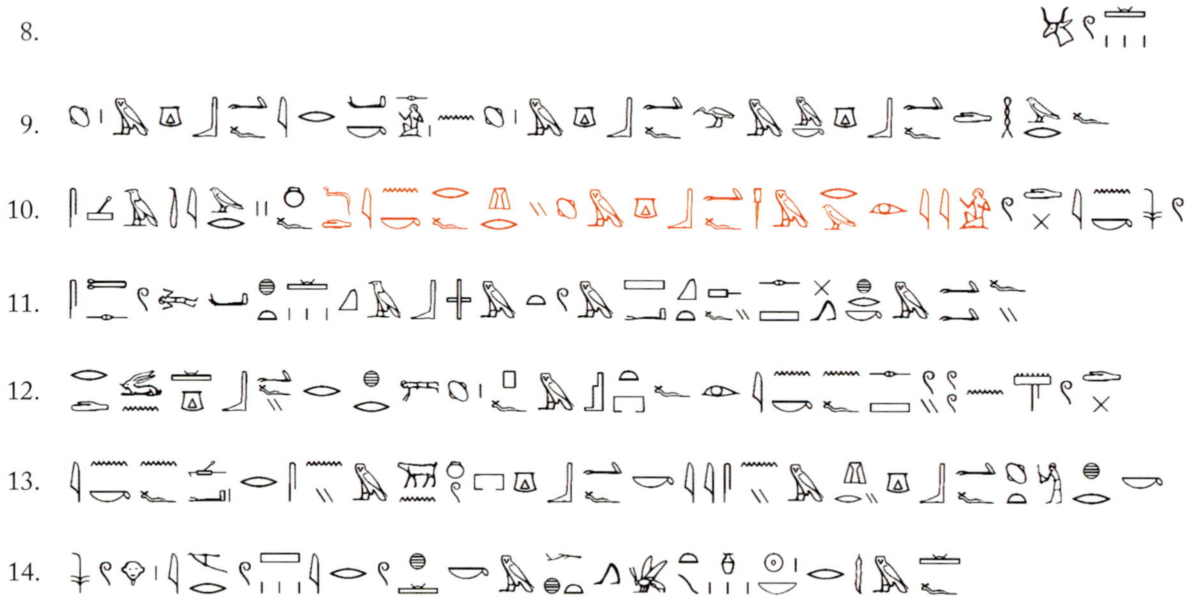

Transliteration

8§ … *šs3w*

9§ *ḥsb m gꜣb.f ỉr ḫꜣ.k s n ḥsb m gꜣb.f gmm.k gꜣb.f dḥ r.f*

10§ *sꜣt.ỉ r snw.f ḏd.ỉn.k r.f ẖry ḥsb m gꜣb.f mḥr ỉry.ỉ wd.ỉn.k sw*

11§ *sṯꜣs.w ḫt ḳꜣb ỉmytw mšꜥḳt<y>.fy sš.ḫr.k m ḳꜥḥwy.fy*

12§ *r dwn gꜣb<wy>.fy r ḫr ḥsb pf m st.f ỉr.ỉn.k n.f sšwy n ḥbs wd.*

13§ *ỉn.k n.f wꜥ r sny m-ẖnw gꜣb.f ky sny m-ẖry gꜣb.f. wt.ḫr.k*

14§ *sw ḥr ỉmrw srwḫ.k m-ḫt <m> bỉt rꜥ nb r nḏm.f*

Translation

Title:

Necessary knowledge and skills for a fracture in his humerus/his upper arm:

Examination:

If you should examine a man for a fracture in his humerus/his upper arm, how you find his upper arm/his humerus (is): dangling down with respect to him and pushed out of alignment with respect to its counterpart.

Diagnosis:

Then you are to say about him: "One who has a fracture in his humerus/his upper arm: a medical condition which I will handle/deal with."

Treatment:

Then you are to lay him so that he is stretched out (with) something folded between his shoulder blades.

Then you must spread out by means of his shoulders, in order to stretch apart the two segments of his humerus/his upper arm, so that/until that break falls into its place.

Then you make for him a double strip(?) of cloth.

Then you shall lay for him one pertaining to(?) the two of them on the inside of his humerus/upper arm, and the other of the two of them on the underside of his humerus/upper arm.

Then you must bind it (along) with alum(?) (or a bandage with alum[?] shavings?) and treat afterward <with> honey every day until it/he is well.

Notes

Many of the forms and expressions in this Case were already discussed in Case 35 which often has similar or identical wording. Notes that would be the same are not repeated here.

sꜣt.ỉ – The *ti* sign is not written in error but comprises the last consonant of the verbal root, *t*, + the ending which here appears as *.ỉ*. See *Grundriss* 7, 2:713. For the ending *.y* with this form, see Gardiner, *EG*[3], sec. 309.

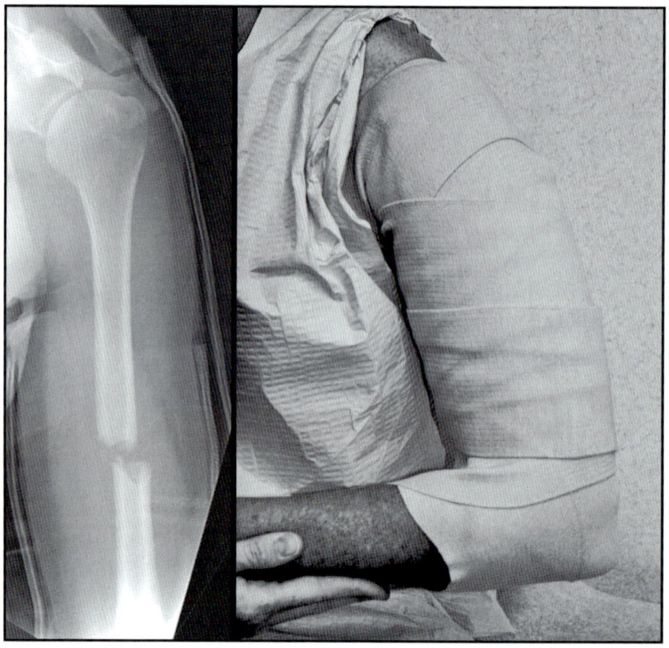

Fig. 35. Fractured humerus with coaptation splint.

r sny – I am translating the preposition *r* as "pertaining to." I think it is relevant that the preposition *r* acquires the significance of possession in the derived expression *iry* or *irw* as a periphrasis of the 3rd-person suffix-pronouns (Faulkner, *CDME*, 25, Gardiner, *EG*[3], sec. 113.2; cf. Meltzer, "Problems of Adjectival Constructions in Old and Middle Egyptian," 30–31). The preposition does not appear in the corresponding expression in Case 35. It also is not repeated in *ky.sny* in the present sentence. The pronoun is fully written both times in the present passage.

Medical Commentary

Type of Injury

This is a closed linear fracture (*ḥsb*) of the humeral shaft (fig. 35) produced by blunt trauma to the arm, or shoulder, or by falling on an outstretched, abducted arm.

These patients present with local pain, swelling, and shortening of the arm. Crepitus and pain might be produced by manipulation, but the large muscles surrounding the humerus prevent direct palpation of the fracture.

Successful treatment of closed fractures can be achieved in more than 90 percent[235] of cases by placing the limb in a hanging arm cast, or a coaptation splint[236] for one to three weeks. These devices are most effective with the patient upright, either, standing or sitting, allowing gravity to assist in fracture reduction. The fractured arm is then supported in a functional brace (fig. 35).

235. M. W. Lawless, "Midshaft Humerus Fractures." Medscape Reference: http://emedicine.medscape.com/article/1239985-treatment.
236. A coaptation splint is a small splint fitted to a fractured limb to prevent overriding of the fragments of bone.

Ancient Medical Methodology and Knowledge

This is a closed fracture of the humeral shaft which was treated by reduction through stretching the upper arm: "Then you must spread out by means of his shoulders, in order to stretch apart the two segments of his humerus/his upper arm, so that/until that break falls into its place." The reader will notice that the same reduction technique was used here as for the preceding case of a clavicular fracture. Nunn[237] assesses this to be a scribal error. However, in a recumbent patient with a folded roll between his shoulder blades, as prescribed in this case, the shoulders would be elevated off the bed allowing the rest of the upper extremity to hang alongside. Thus, gravity would facilitate reduction and realignment of the fractured humeral shaft. Therefore the authors do not concur that scribal error is evident here.

Support to the fractured humerus also used the same technique of immobilization as that described in Case #35 for a fractured clavicle. The placement of a strip of cloth/splint to the inside of the arm (the medial surface of the arm, close to the chest wall) would have been particularly important here to support the fractured shaft as it leaned on the chest wall. The posterior strip or cloth/splint applied behind the upper arm (in the recumbent patient) would complete forming a stiff supporting cradle, over which a bandage with alum and honey was applied, binding it to the chest. Effective humeral fracture stabilization would have been obtained by this immobilizing technique, just as it was for the fractured clavicle.

The ancient Egyptian physicians successfully used here the same technique in our Case #36 as in the prior Case #35, but with different objectives. In the clavicular fracture, immobilization of the upper extremity by binding it to the chest would effectively take away the traction effects on the outer fragment of the fractured bone, allowing it to heal in the proper alignment. In the humeral fracture, direct external support of the fractured humeral shaft would be provided by the strips of cloth/splints placed on the inner, and the posterior aspects of the upper arm. Lateral and anterior support to the fractured area would be obtained by bandaging over it, immobilizing it against the chest, but still allowing the now reduced effect of gravity to help keep the fracture properly aligned.

Still another method of immobilizing the fractured humerus in Case #36 would have been direct bandaging over the two strips of cloth/splints, wrapping the upper arm itself. In that case, additional support to the arm would have been necessary with a sling. No prescription for such treatment is noted in this case.

In ancient Egypt, injuries of this nature would have occurred during close combat with clubs or maces, or in civilian life in construction accidents. Multiple examples of healed humeral shaft fractures were found in specimens from the Nubian excavations, undertaken before the raising of the First Aswan Dam, and documented by Jones in 1908.[238] Of the long-bone fractures found in human remains from the tombs of the pyramid builders at Giza, the most frequently affected bones were the ulna, radius, humerus, and fibula. Most of these fractures had evidence of complete healing and good bone realignment.[239]

237. Nunn, *Ancient Egyptian Medicine*, 176.

238. F. W. Jones, "Some Lessons From Ancient Fractures," *British Medical Journal* (1908): 455–58, cited by Nunn in *Ancient Egyptian Medicine*, fig. 8.8. This photograph shows healed fractures of six long bones with excellent alignment, including a humeral shaft.

239. Zahi Hawass, "The Discovery of the Tombs of the Pyramid Builders at Giza." Online: http://guardians.net/hawass/buildtomb.htm.

CASE 37:
Compound Fracture(s) of the Humerus
(Plate XII:14–21)

Courtesy New York Academy of Medicine.

14.
15.
16.
17.
18.
19.
20.
21.

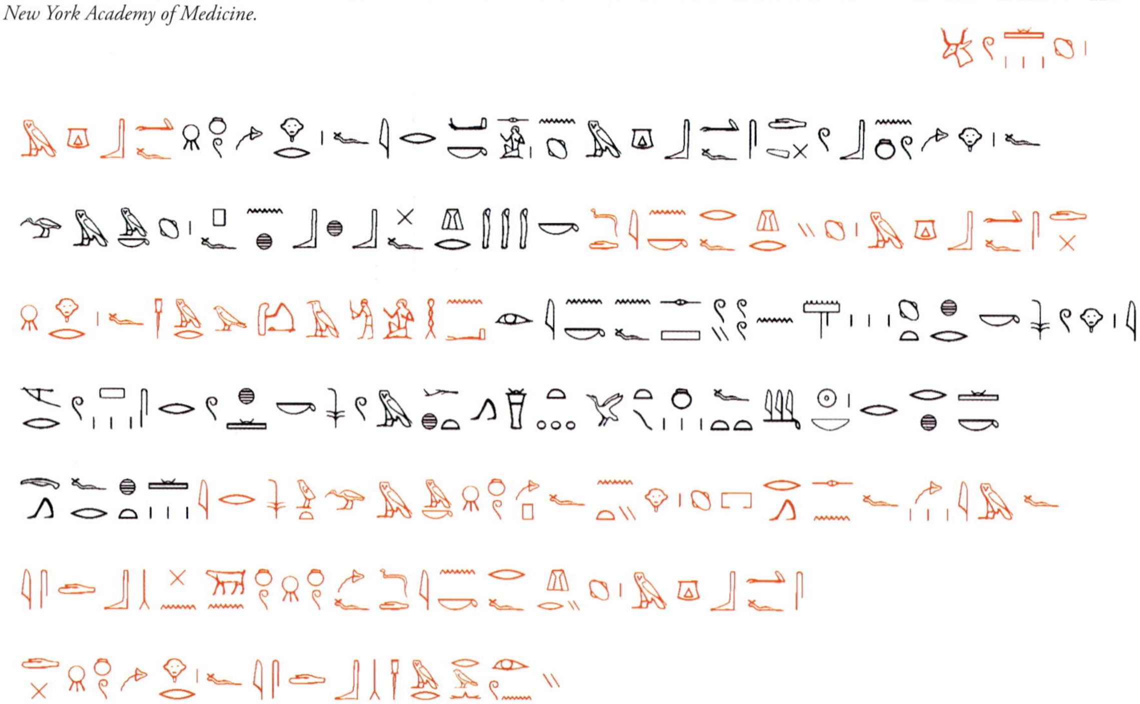

Transliteration

14§ … *šsꜣw ḥsb*

15§ *m gbꜣ.f wbnw ḥr.f ir ḫꜣ.k s n ḥsb m gbꜣ.f sḏ wbnw ḥr.f*

16§ *gmm.k ḥsb pf nḫbḫb.f ẖr ḏbꜥw.k ḏd.in.k r.f ẖry ḥsb m gbꜣ.f sḏ*

17§ *wbnw ḥr.f mḥr ꜥḥꜣ.i ḥnꜥ ir.in.k n.f sšwy n ḥbsw wt.ḫr.k sw ḥr*

18§ *imrw srwḫ.k sw m-ḫt mrḥt bit ftt rꜥ nb r rḫ.k*

19§ *spr.f r ẖt ir swt gmm.k wbnw pf nty ḥr ḥsb pr snf im.f*

20§ *isdb n ẖnw wbnw.f ḏd.in.k r.f ẖry ḥsb m gbꜣ.f*

21§ *sḏ wbnw ḥr.f isdb mḥr n irw.ny*

Translation

Comminuted Fracture of the Humerus (Plate XII:14–19)

Title:

Necessary knowledge and skills for a fracture in his humerus/upper arm with a wound on it:

Examination:

If you should examine a man for a fracture in his upper arm, a wound having been smashed over it. How you find that fracture (is): shifting/crepitating under your fingers.

Diagnosis:

Then you are to say about him: "One who has a fracture in his upper arm, a wound having been smashed over it—a medical condition I will fight with."

Treatment:

Then you make for him a double strip of cloth.

Then you must bandage it (along) with alum(?) (or a bandage with alum[?] shavings?) and you should treat him afterward with ointment and honey, and a dressing every day until you know he arrives at the turning point.

Compound Comminuted Fracture of the Humerus Piercing through from Inside (plate XII:19–21)

Examination:

But if how you find that wound which is over the fracture (is): blood issuing from within it, pierced through and collapsed to the inside of his wound,

Diagnosis:

then you are to say about him: "One who has a fracture in his upper arm, a wound having been smashed over it, pierced through and collapsed, a medical condition that cannot be handled/dealt with."

Notes

sd(*w*) *wbnw ḥr.f* – Passive *sḏm*(*w*)*.f*, hence I am translating as an anterior circumstance. This is the case for all repetitions of this form. Since "a fracture" is indefinite, the following circumstantials can also be taken as the indefinite or unmarked or so-called virtual relative, yielding "a fracture over which a wound has been smashed/ smash fractured)." In the title, *ḥsb … wbnw ḥr.f* has the same structure, "A fracture …" (indefinite antecedent) + "(with) a wound on it" (circumstantial, noun + Prepositional Phrase, as relative).

nḫbḫb.f – Circumstantial *sḏm.f* as complement to the manner nominalization.

wbnw pf nty ḥr ḥsb "that wound which is over the fracture" – Note the marked or definite relative clause with *nty*, following the definite antecedent *wbnw pf* "that wound," in contrast to the indefinite or unmarked relative clauses after an indefinite antecedent.

pr snf – Circumstantial *sḏm.f* as (first) complement to a manner nominalization.

sšwy, ỉmrw – see above.

ỉsdb – stative. For the meaning of this word, see previous notes. I think the proposed meaning fits very well here.

Medical Commentary

Comminuted Fracture of the Humerus

Type of Injury

The injury in Case #37a is a closed humeral linear fracture (*ḥsb*) produced by a severe direct blow. There are traumatized soft tissues (*sd*) over the fracture site. There is shifting of the broken fragments felt upon examination of the arm.

Today, after splinting of the fractured arm, the patient would be transported to an emergency care facility for treatment. The treatment of most closed humeral fractures is nonsurgical. After surface wound care, reduction and immobilization of the fracture are primary. In cases in which vascular or neurological injuries are present, open exploration and repair are mandatory.

Ancient Medical Methodology and Knowledge

The treatment for the fracture in Case #37a is simply stated as: "Then you make for him a double strip of cloth." This form of treatment for fracture immobilization has already been described in Cases #35 and #36, the same is implied here, using their established protocol of alum and honey. The high success of the ancient Egyptian physician in treating long-bone fractures is evident upon inspection of the many healed fracture specimens obtained from the Nubian graves[240] and the Giza cemeteries of the pyramid builders.[241]

240. J. F. Nunn, *Ancient Egyptian Medicine*, 177. Nunn refers to Wood Jones's 1908 publication "Some Lessons from Ancient Fractures." In this work, Woods gives an extensive account of fractures found in six thousand bodies during the excavation of the areas south of the first cataract.

241. Hawass, "The Discovery of the Tombs of the Pyramid Builders at Giza." Online: http://guardians.net/hawass/buildtomb.htm.

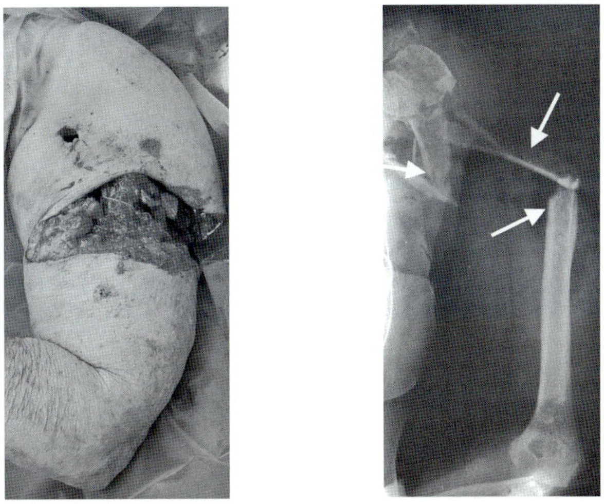

Fig. 36. Compound, comminuted humeral fracture. White arrows indicate fragmented humerus.

Compound Comminuted Fracture of the Humerus Piercing through from Inside

Type of Injury

Case #37b, an open fracture of the humerus in which there is soft tissue damage with active bleeding, is a considerably more severe injury than Case #37a, and constitutes a true orthopedic emergency. At the fracture site, the covering soft tissues have been damaged from the inside, by broken and jagged bone (fig. 36). The fracture in this case is equivalent to a Grade III Type A, or Type C injury, in Gustillo/Anderson's Open fracture Classification.[242] In Grade III A, the soft tissue covering the fractured bone is adequate. In Grade III C there is arterial injury.

Today, after immediate splinting of the fractured arm, the patient would be given antibiotics and transferred to a medical facility where orthopedic surgery is readily available. In the operating room, aggressive debridement and lavage are followed by a stable fixation of the fracture. It has been shown that in clean cases, internal fixation with plates or intramedullary nails are possible and safe. Early soft tissue covering is highly desirable. If the wound is contaminated, external fracture immobilization can be carried out with wound debridement every 48 hours, until the wound is clean. Vascular injuries need immediate repair. Nerve repair can be delayed until there is certainty that the wound is not infected.[243] Open fractures Grade III A carry an infection rate of 7 percent and an amputation rate 2.5 percent. Open fractures Grade IIIC have an infection rate of 25 to 50 percent and an amputation rate 25 percent.

Ancient Medical Methodology and Knowledge

In Case #37b, the severity and extent of damage to the humerus and secondary soft tissue injury produced by jagged edges of the fractured bone would likely injure muscles, nerves, and blood vessels. The soft tissues in Case #37b have suffered an *isdb* type[244] of injury, pierced through and collapsed at the fracture site and there

242. "Open Fractures." Online: http://www.rcsed.ac.uk/fellows/lvanrensburg/classification/commonfiles/open.htm.

243. M. W. Lawless, "Midshaft Humerus Fractures." Medscape Reference: http://emedicine.medscape.com/article/1239985-treatment.

244. See the medical commentary to Case #14 for an explanation of *isdb*: "… can be understood as a piercing injury of tissue not supported by bone, whose soft lacerated, and now, disorganized tissue layers, infold (Case #14, Case #26), or outfold (Case #37b), obstructing the wound itself."

is active bleeding. In these injuries wound contamination would be almost certain. The combination of these factors would make this injury a condition beyond the treatment capabilities of the ancient Egyptian physician, and, indeed, their treatment verdict is "a medical condition that cannot be handled/dealt with."

CASE #38:
Closed Displaced Fracture of the Humerus
(Plate XII:21–XIII:2)

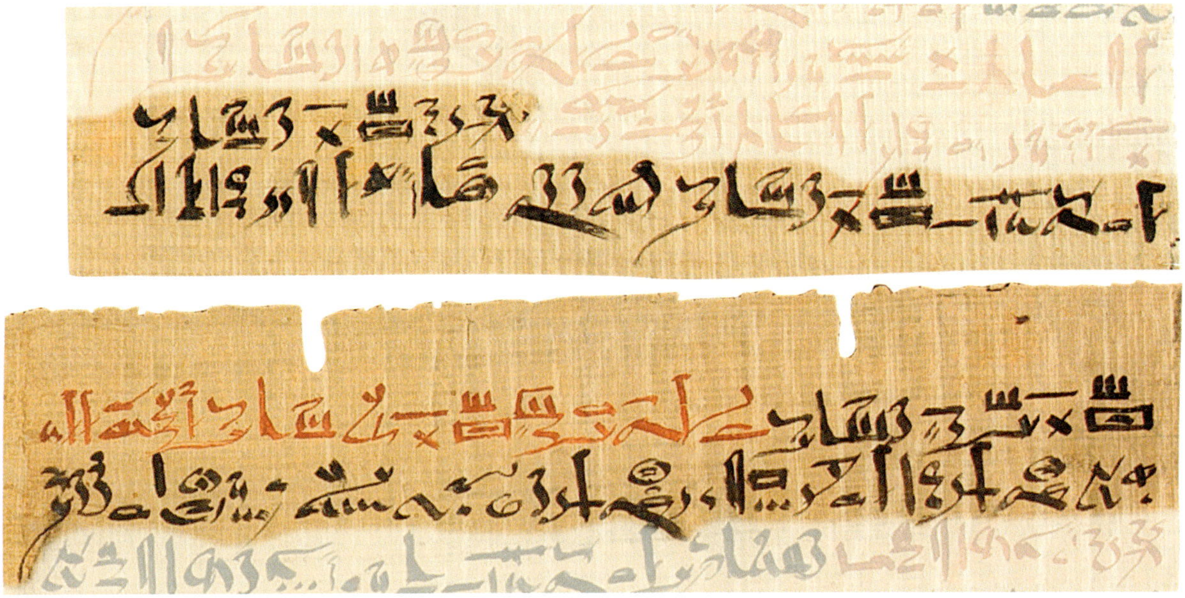

Courtesy New York Academy of Medicine.

21. 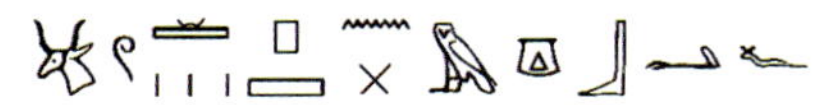

22. 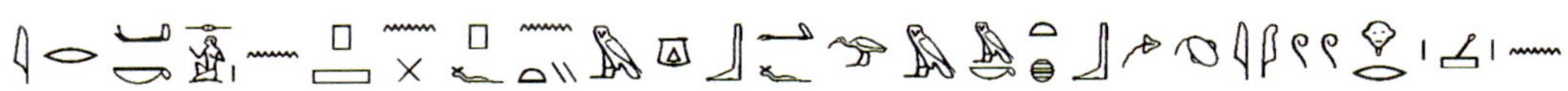

1. 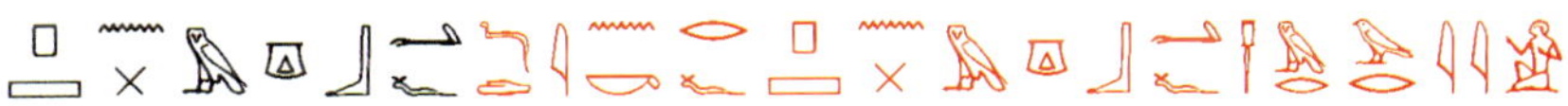

2. 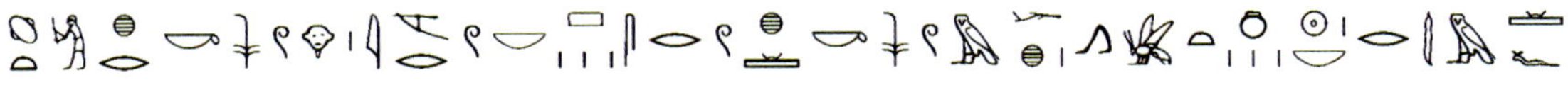

Transliteration

21§ *… šsꜣ.w pšn m gꜣb.f*

22§ *ir ḫꜣ.k s n pšn m gꜣb.f gmm.k ṯḫb išww ḥr-sꜣ n*

1§ *pšn pf nty m gꜣb.f dd.in.k r.f ẖry pšn m gꜣb.f mḥr iry.i*

2§ *wt.ḥr.k sw ḥr imrw srwḫ.k sw m-ḫt <m> bit rʿ nb r nḏm.f*

Translation

Title:

Necessary knowledge and skills for a split fracture in his humerus/upper arm:

Examination:

If you examine a man for a split fracture in his humerus/upper arm, how you find a swelling (is): protruding on the outside of that split which is in his upper arm.

Diagnosis:

Then you are to say concerning him: "One who has a split fracture in his humerus/upper arm, a medical condition which I will handle/deal with."

Treatment:

Then you must bind it (along) with alum (?) (or, a bandage with alum[?] shavings?) and you should treat it afterwards <with> honey every day until it/he is well.

Notes

pšn pf nty m gbꜣ.f – Note the definite antecedent *pšn pf* followed by a marked or definite relative clause with *nty*.

imrw – See above.

<*m*> "<with>" – Must be supplied as above.

Medical Commentary

Type of Injury

Case #38 is a *pšn* fracture such as that described in Case #4 (head trauma), where Explanation A delineates it as a split or segmental fracture.[245] Our Case #38 represents such an injury to the humerus, which is split and partially displaced (fig. 37). The local swelling over the fracture, is, at least in part, formed by hemorrhaging from the bone and periosteum. The general symptoms and findings in patients with humeral shaft fractures are arm pain, deformity, and swelling, with shortened arm. There is motion and crepitus upon fracture site manipulation. As a closed wound, there is better prognosis than had it been an open fracture, where infection is always a threat.

Today, splinting of the fractured arm and transportation of the patient to an emergency facility for complete evaluation of the fracture would be followed by an Orthopedic Surgeon's evaluation.[246] Most closed fractures of the humeral shaft are successfully treated with closed methods, resulting in union rates of more than 90 percent. The fractured arm would be placed in a coaptation splint (fig. 35) or in a hanging arm cast for one to

245. A segmental fracture is "a bone break in which several large bone fragments separate from the main body of a fractured bone. The ends of the fragments may pierce the skin, as in an open fracture, or may be contained within the skin, as in a closed fracture." See http://medical-dictionary.thefreedictionary.com/segmental+fracture.

246. M. W. Lawless, "Midshaft Humerus Fractures." Medscape Reference: http://emedicine.medscape.com/article/1239985-treatment.

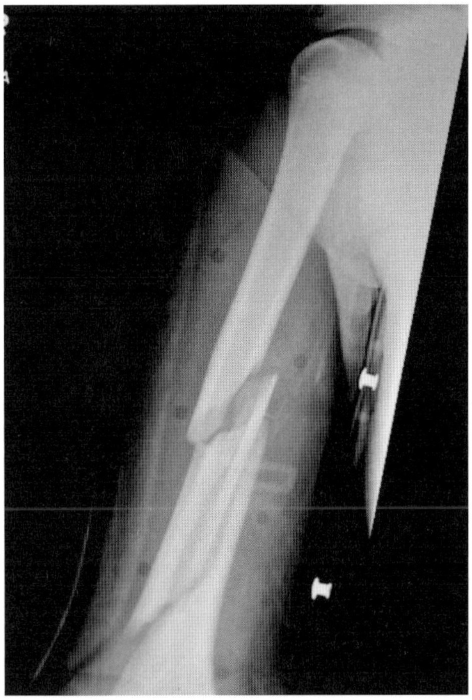

Fig. 37. Humeral *pšn* type of fracture.

three weeks, and then in a functional brace. The fracture in Case #38, however, appears to fall into the category of segmented fracture with extensive bone fragmentation and displacement. Today's treatment for these injuries is surgical with instrumented devices that allow better reconstitution of segmented bone fragments.

Whether these fractures are treated by closed or open methods, the humeral shaft heals well, allowing adequate arm function, even if foreshortened or not in the ideal fragment alignment. The following healing deformity parameters of a healed humerus are still compatible with good use of the limb:

- Angulation of 30° of varus/valgus
- Foreshortening of up to 3 cm.
- 20° of anterior/posterior curvature malrotation[247]

Ancient Medical Methodology and Knowledge

Although the *pšn* type of fracture can occur in either an open or a closed situation, Case #38 is a closed, comminuted fracture with large fragments, likely a common injury in ancient Egypt. These kinds of fractures would occur in war from mace blows, chariot-related accidents, and in construction work from falls. Having diagnosed a splintered, displaced humeral fracture, and understanding the anatomical pathology of this injury, the Egyptian physician treated it by realignment and immobilization, bandaging it over with alum.

247. M. W. Lawless, "Midshaft Humerus Fractures." Online: http://emedicine.medscape.com/article/1239985-overview.

CASE #39:
Infected Chest Wound with Abscesses
(Plate XIII:3–12)

Courtesy New York Academy of Medicine.

3. 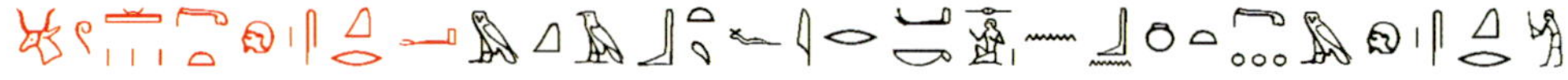

4. 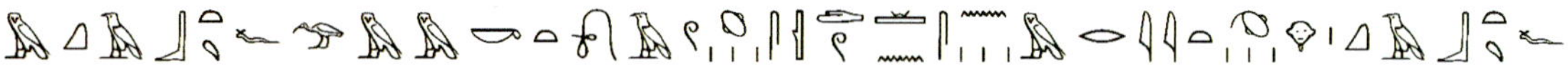

5. 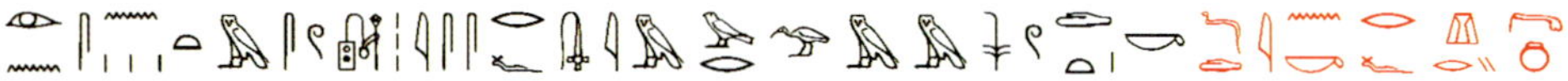

6. 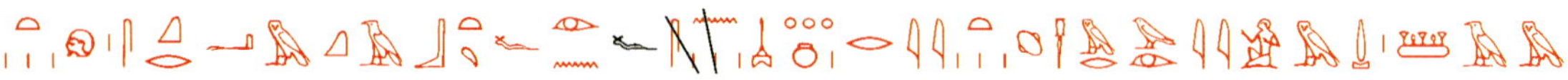

7. 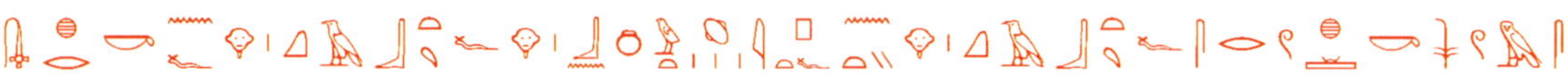

8. 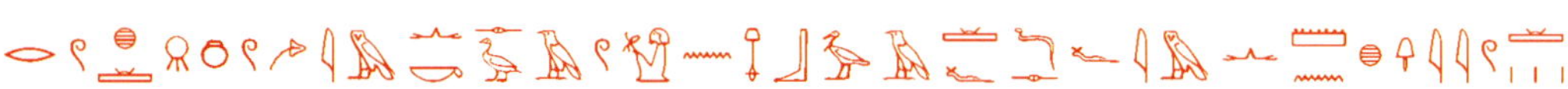

9. 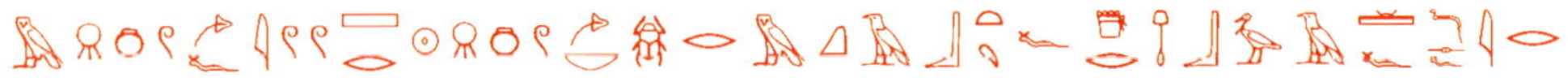

10. 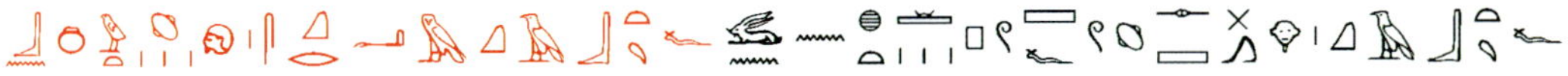

11. 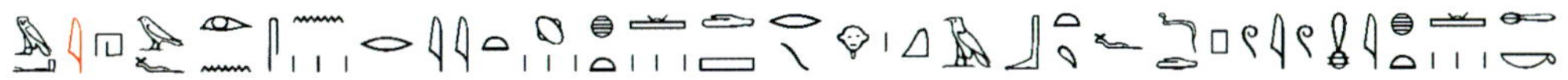

12. 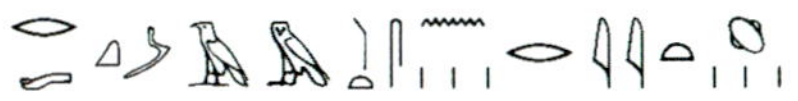

Transliteration

3§ *šsꜣw bnwt tp sḳr m ḳꜣbt.f ir ḫꜣ.k s n bnwt m-tp sḳr*

4§ *m ḳꜣbt.f gmm.k twꜣw sḳd.n.sn m ryt ḥr ḳꜣbt.f*

5§ *ir.n.sn ṯmsw isk srf jm wr gmm sw ḏrt.k ḏd.in.k r.f ẖry bnwt*

6§ *tp sḳr m ḳꜣbt.f ir.n.f wḏʿw nw ryt mḫr iry.i m ḏꜣ šꜣm.*

7§ *ḫr.k n.f ḥr ḳꜣbt.f ḥr bnwt iptf nty ḥr ḳꜣbt.f srwḫ.k sw m*

8§ *srwḫ wbnw im.k sꜣw n wbꜣ.f ḏs.f im n mnḫyw*

9§ *m wbnw.f iw wšr wbnw nb ḫpr m ḳꜣbt.f ḏr wbꜣ.f ḏs.f ir*

10§ *bnwt tp sḳr m ḳꜣbt.f wnn ẖt pw šf.w sš ḥr ḳꜣbt.f*

11§ *m-ʿ ỉh.f ir.n.sn ryt ẖt dšr ḥr ḳꜣbt.f ḏd pw iw mi ẖt <ꜣ>ẖ<ʿ>.k*

12§ *r ʿnt ḳmꜣt.sn ryt*

Translation

Title:

Necessary knowledge and skills for a discharging abscess atop the wound from a strike in his chest:

Examination:

If you should examine a man for a discharging abscess on top of a wound from a strike in his chest, how you find the rising collections (is): having spread with pus over his chest and having created redness, while the heat within is great the way your hand finds it.

Diagnosis:

Then you are to say about him: "One who has discharging abscesses atop a wound from a strike in his chest, it having made/which has made secretions of pus, a medical condition which I will handle with the firedrill."

Treatment:

Then you must cauterize because of it: on his chest, on those abscesses which are on his chest.

You should treat him by treating the wound.

You should not prevent its opening by itself therein, because of the efficaciousness/beneficial effects for his wound.

Every wound that occurs in his chest dries up as soon as it opens itself.

Explanation:

As for abscesses atop an injury from a strike in his chest, it means the things are swollen and spread over on his chest because of his affliction, they having made pus and red things on his chest.

It means: "It is like the things you scratch from a fingernail, which will create pus."

Notes

sḳd.n.sn … *ir.n.sn* – Circumstantial *sḏm.n.f.*

gmm sw ḏrt.k – Nominal *sḏm.f.*

ir.n.f – Circumstantial *sḏm.n.f.* Once again this can serve as an indefinite or unmarked relative after an indefinite antecedent.

bnwt iptf nty – Also as earlier, note the definite antecedent *bnwt iptf* followed by *nty* introducing a definite or marked relative clause.

im.k … *im, n mnḫyw* … – I think that the second *ỉm* should be taken as the adverbial word *im*, and the negative arms as a word reading *n*. I do not think it can be identified as the negative *n* however, and I follow *Grundriss* 8, sec. 370 in taking it as a writing of the preposition or conjunction *n*. (For the use of negative *n* for ordinary *n*, see p. 223 above.) There are several reasons for this in addition to what seems to be the reasonableness of the translation: (1) *ỉm* cannot be in a prepositional relationship with *mnḫyw* interrupted by negative *n*—there are no parallels for such syntax that I am aware of; (2) I do not think that negative *n* + a noun, be it an ordinary substantive or a nisbe adjective used nominally, is attested as a construction that means "that is not." The *Grundriss* translation offers a clear syntactic construction, preposition *n* + a noun; *Grundriss* and I end up with the same basic meaning, "Do not prevent its opening, because of the beneficial effects of the opening."

ḫpr – Active participle.

m-ꜥ ih.f – This goes with the preceding, not the following clause. Despite the arguments of some scholars and the admitted attestation of exceptions, free adverbial elements in sentence-initial position should be avoided. Although the discussion is not concluded, I have presented a response to John Gee's article "Fronted Adverbials" in *Bulletin of the Egyptological Seminar* 18 (2008): 83–90, at the Annual Meeting of ARCE in Chicago, April 2011: "Once Again Initial Adverbials and the Standard Theory." The bottom line is that fronted adverbials are not a random assortment or cross-section of adverbials but predominantly at least are expressions of time or expressions containing a full or "heavy" form of a preposition (e.g., *in-gꜣw-n* instead of *n-gꜣw-n*). When we segment *m-ꜥ ih.f* with the preceding, the syntax of these clauses sorts itself out very clearly, as seen in the identification of the following form.

ir.n.sn – Circumstantial *sḏm.n.f.*

ỉw mi ḫt … – *ỉw* before the prepositional phrase marks it as a strongly independent statement, not a mere phrase. This is a sentence like the famous example *ỉw mi sḫr nṯr* in Sinuhe, which we have discussed above (along with the analogous construction of *ỉw* + impersonal stative).

ḫt <*ꜣ*> *ḫ*<*ꜥ*>*.k* – Allen uses the translation as the verb "to scratch" (*AM*, 97). The verb form is a relative form; masculine forms following the word *ḫt* have been noted earlier.

ḳmꜣt.sn – This is not a *sḏmt.f* form, because there is no independent *sḏmt.f* in Middle Egyptian, only the negative *n sḏmt.f* and *sḏmt.f* after certain prepositions. This has been generally agreed since the 1970s, see, e.g., W. Schenkel, "Das Ende des narrativen *sdm.t=f*," *Göttinger Miszellen* 4 (1973): 23–28. For the meaning "and (which) create," which seems to be Allen's understanding, a participle would do and a form *ḳmꜣt.sn* is meaningless. As a relative form, *ḳmꜣt.sn* would mean "that which they create," with *sn* as the additional actor-expression required by the relative form. I take *ḳmꜣt.sn* in this passage as a writing of *ḳmꜣty.sn*, the *sḏmty.fy* form or future (with rare exceptions active) participial form, sometimes called "verbal adjective," hence "which will create." I think that by using this form, the ancient Egyptian physician is indicating knowledge (rather impressive knowledge it seems to me) of a causal sequence: things that one scratches from a fingernail will create pus.

Medical Commentary

Type of Injury

This is a soft tissue infection with multiple abscesses having developed over a chest wound. A traumatic abscess is a collection of pus caused by bacterial skin flora implanted by contaminated objects such as needles, knives, bullets, or even, as the text indicates, a fingernail. The most common bacteria causing abscesses are Staphylococcus aureus, streptococcus, and *Escherichia coli*. Dead cells release cytokines triggering an inflammatory response that draws large numbers of white blood cells to the area and increases the regional blood flow. Pus is formed by dead white blood cells and bacteria that accumulate in an encapsulated cavity formed by healthy surrounding tissue to contain the infection. However, this also prevents immune cells from reaching the bacteria.

The symptoms and findings of a skin and subcutaneous abscess are local redness, pain, and swelling. Often there is a "punctum," a round spot of different color from the surrounding tissue allowing for spontaneous opening of the abscess or for surgical draining.

Once the abscess has evolved from serous inflammation to a softer purulent stage the treatment is surgical drainage removing all necrotic tissue and foreign bodies. Any dead space needs to be eliminated, keeping the abscess open until it is completely empty. The treatment today is supplemented by antibiotics.

Ancient Medical Methodology and Knowledge

Case #39 is an extraordinarily simple presentation of the ancient Egyptian physicians's concepts related to infection, 1700 years before Celsus[248] identified them in the first century AD as "tumor, rubor, calor, dolor." Case #39 not only preconditions the development of abscesses to tissue injury produced by a strike, but observes, recognizes, and identifies three of Celsus's cardinal signs and symptoms of inflammation as rising collections, redness, and heat. The papyrus compares the appearance of the spreading of multiple soft tissue abscesses with the pattern seen in infection dissemination occurring from nail scratching, a conclusion undoubtedly derived from clinical experience.

The ancient Egyptian physician in Case #39 established the indispensable principle in the treatment of any abscess, its drainage. Furthermore, the papyrus specifically recommends the use of cauterization (with a firedrill), a technique that would be effective both as a sterile procedure and one that favors the skin margins to remain open until the infection resolves. The Egyptians were aware that an abscess needs to be drained in order to be cured, a medical concept much later expressed by the Roman aphorism *ubi pus, ibi evacua* "where there is pus, there evacuate it." The rest of the treatment appears to fall into an established protocol: "You should treat him by treating the wound."

---

248. Aulus Cornelius Celsus, *De Medicina*. Online: http://en.wikipedia.org/wiki/De_Medicina. In the First Century AD the Roman Physician Celsus defined inflammation by the signs: tumor, calor, rubor, dolor, meaning respectively: swelling, heat, redness, pain. This is a basic nonspecific immune response in which the body reacts to infection or other injury.

CASE #40:

Chest Wound Perforating the Manubrium of the Sternum

(Plate XIII:12–17)

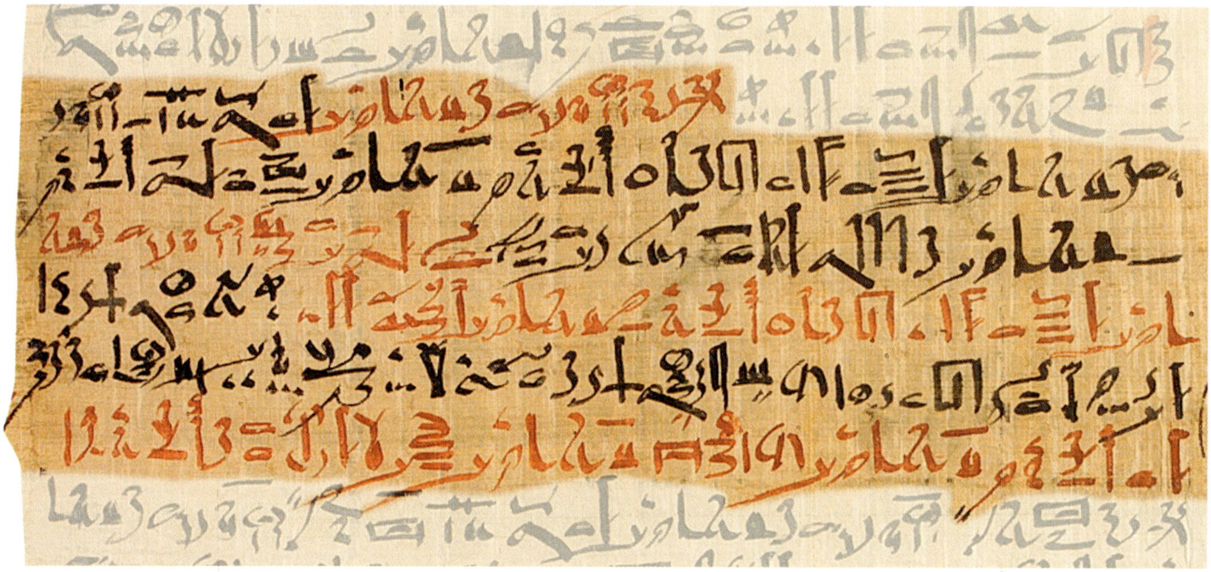

Courtesy New York Academy of Medicine.

12.
13.
14.
15.
16.
17.

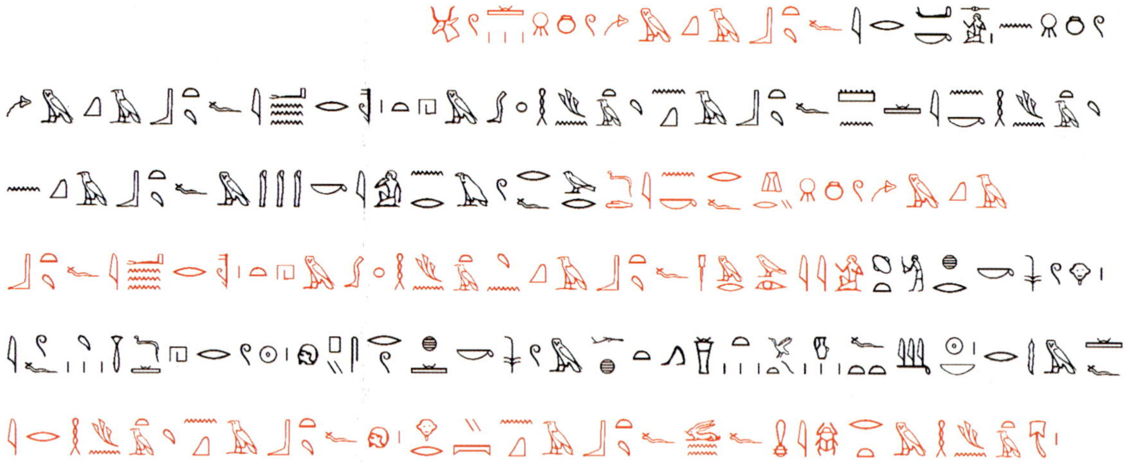

Transliteration

12§ … *šs3w wbnw m ḳ3bt.f ir ẖ3.k s wbnw*

13§ *m ḳ3bt.f iʿ r ḳs thm ḥnt3 n ḳ3bt.f mn.in.k ḥnt3*

14§ *n ḳ3bt.f m ḏbʿw.k inrw r.f wr ḏd.in.k r.f ẖry wbnw m ḳ3bt.f*

15§ *ỉꜥ r ḳs thm ḥntꜣ n ḳꜣbt.f mḥr ỉry.i wt.ḫr.k sw ḥr*

16§ *ỉwf wꜣḏ hrw tpy. srwḫ.k sw m-ḫt mrḥt bỉt ftt rꜥ nb r nḏm.f*

17§ *ir ḥntꜣ ḳꜣbt.f tp ḥry n ḳꜣbt.f wnn.f mỉ ḫprt m ḥntꜣ*

Translation

Title:

Necessary knowledge and skills for a wound in his breastbone:

Examination:

If you should examine a man for a wound in his sternum, penetrating to the bone and perforating the manubrium of his sternum, then you are to press the manubrium of his sternum with your fingers, so that it/he quakes/shifts greatly concerning it.

Diagnosis:

Then you are to say about him: "One who has a wound in his breastbone, penetrating to the bone and perforating the manubrium of his sternum: a medical condition which I will handle/deal with."

Treatment:

You must bandage it (along) with fresh meat the first day.

Then you should treat it afterward <with> ointment and honey and a dressing every day until it/he is well.

Explanation:

As for the manubrium of his breastbone, (it is) the upper end of his sternum; how it is (is) like that which occurs in a hedgehog(?).

Notes

ỉꜥ (apparently for *ꜥr*, see below), *thm* – These cannot be infinitives, which are syntactically incapable of functioning as this passage would demand, nor can they be statives, because *thm* is a transitive verb and its stative should not have active meaning in Middle Egyptian. They are active participles.

ỉꜥ is given in *Grundriss* 7, 1:25 in Case 40 only (twice) as a variant or alternant of *ꜥr*. The writing is identical to *ỉꜥỉ* "wash," but the latter would make no sense in the present context. I do not think the initial *ỉ* is an augment; I think the writing stems from a verb *ỉꜥ* "ascend, arise" (Faulkner, *CDME*, 10) which parallels *ꜥr* and seems to be a doublet of it. (Cf. also *ḏꜣi* and *ḏꜣr*, both meaning "subdue"; Faulkner, *CDME*, 309 with a cross-reference at *ḏꜣi*.) The choice of this verb is perhaps facilitated by the use of the preposition *r* that follows, with the possibility that the *r* + *r* combination could lead to the elision of one *r* (though admittedly this does not happen in the instances written *ꜥr r* that we have seen previously). For derivatives from these two rather synonymous verbs, cf. the words *ỉꜥ* "tomb" (Faulkner, *CDME*, 10) and *ꜥr* "staircase" (*Wb.* 1:208); also A. Badawy, "The Ideology of the Mastaba Tomb in Egypt," *Journal of Near Eastern Studies* 15 (1956): 180–83. Though this must be extremely tentative, one wonders whether the consistent use of *ỉꜥ* rather than *ꜥr* in this passage reflects the use of a different source for this case, in which *ỉꜥ* was preferred, or even just possibly the dictation of a different speaker? The latter is suggestive because the writing *ỉꜥ* + three water lines looks as if the scribe might have misunderstood *ỉꜥ* "extend,

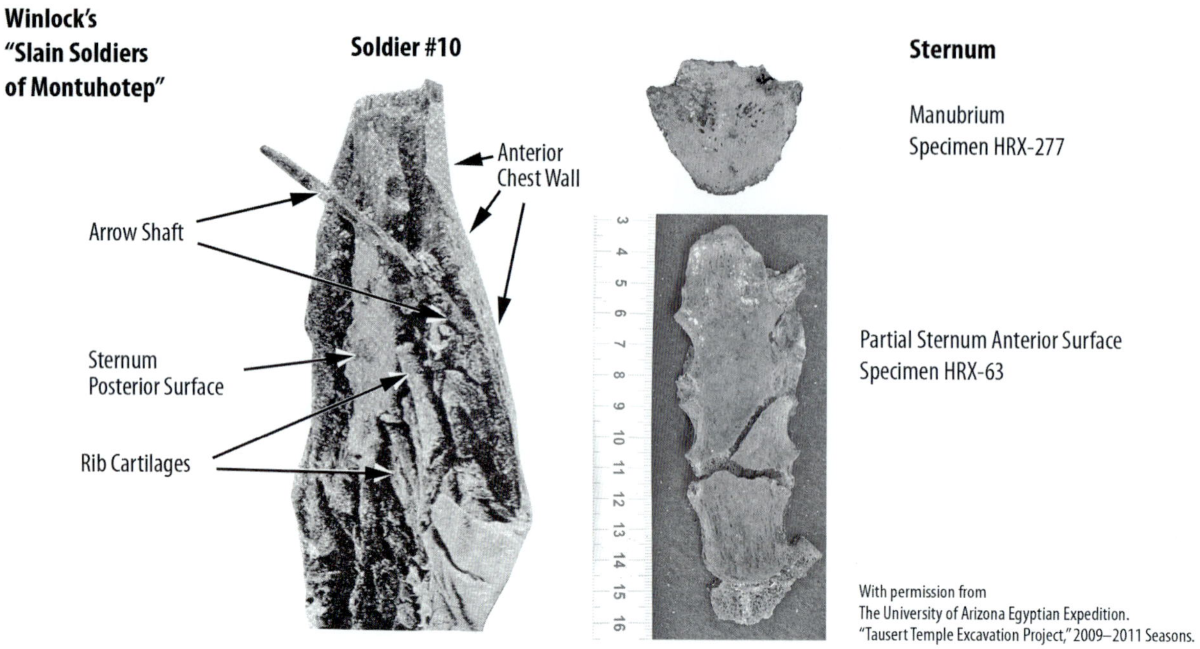

Fig. 38. Left: Arrow injury chest wall and sternum, soldier #10, from Winlock, *Slain Soldiers of Neb-hep-et-Re Mentu-hotpe*, plate VII B. Right: Human remains, University of Arizona Tausret Temple Excavation, Luxor 2010.

penetrate" as *ỉʿ* "wash," which would be an example of a *Hörfehler*; it is not a misunderstanding that could occur in copying a text.

mn.in.k is a *sḏm.in.f.* form.

inrw – Not a noun but a stative, which I am taking as a stative of result.

"<with> ointment ..." – *m* is omitted as in other cases previously.

wnn.f – Manner nominalization; *mi* ... is the complement.

ḥprt – Active participle.

ḥntꜣ – I am adding a question mark, because *Grundriss* 7, 2:611 translates it with a question mark and Faulkner, *CDME*, 173 gives the meaning as "porcupine(?)." I think that the word *ḥntꜣsw* "lizard" (Coptic ϩⲁⲛⲧⲟⲩⲥ, reportedly surviving in Egyptian Arabic as *handus* or *handuz* according to Černý and Vycichl),[249] is related; see Meltzer, "Problems of Adjectival Constructions in Old and Middle Egyptian," 246.

Medical Commentary

Type of Injury

This is a low-velocity penetrating (*thm*) injury of the anterior chest wall, which has injured and penetrated the manubrium of the sternum (Visual Index II), which is covered by soft tissue layers of skin, subcutaneous tissue, a thin fascia layer, and periosteum. Severe pain over the fracture site is common in these injuries, arising

249. J. Černý, "Language and Writing," *The Legacy of Egypt* (2nd ed.; ed. J. R. Harris; Oxford: Oxford University Press 1971), 209. W. Vycichl, "Coptic Dialect Geography Based on Inscriptions," *Enchoria* 8 (1978) 65*/111.

mostly from the direct injury and from hemorrhaging at the level of the periostial layer, which is richly innervated. Pain is readily reproducible by palpation, but bone crepitation would only be present if there is significant bone fragmentation and instability.

In Case #40, the injury and penetration seem limited to, but not through, the sternum. Although in Case #40 we have no indication of heart or great vessel injury, the heart and major vessels of the anterior mediastinum would have been injured if the sternum had been penetrated,[250] as is the case in penetrating stab wounds that slip over the top or lateral margins of the sternum.

The best-known case of a penetrating chest wound in antiquity is a near-lethal wound to Alexander the Great that occurred in 326 BC while campaigning in India.[251] Despite his high-quality body armor, an arrow pierced his breastplate. In the process of treating his king, the surgeon Critobulus first had to saw off the arrow shaft before the breastplate could be removed. Strong bleeding and fainting followed extraction of the arrow. These types of injuries have not been survivable until the 1930s. Unfortunately, these injuries are not mere ancient history. Today, assaults and drug-related stabbings are commonly seen in our large US metropolitan area emergency rooms.

Today, upon initial cardiovascular and airway stabilization, the patient is transferred to an emergency medical facility where clinical assessment includes radiological studies and often a chest CT (computer tomography) scan. The treatment of a chest-wall injury without cavity penetration is simple debridement and closure. Observation for a period of six hours is mandatory with another chest x-ray study prior to discharging the patient, to eliminate the possibility of a delayed pneumothorax,[252] which today occurs in 7 percent of chest-wall injuries.

Ancient Medical Methodology and Knowledge

In ancient Egypt the low-velocity penetrating sternal injury would have been produced in warfare by missiles (arrows, javelins, sling shots) and in close combat by knives and daggers.

Once the injury was evaluated as a perforation to the sternum, the ancient Egyptian physician considered it as treatable. It is logical to consider that in ancient Egypt, the most serious injuries to these areas, those that would have penetrated the chest cavity/lung/heart/great vessels, would have been lethal in a very short time.

The treatment measures implemented in Case #40 consisted of initial wound covering with fresh meat on the first day, followed by daily dressings with honey and oil, the form of wound treatment that conformed to a standard wound-care protocol for superficial open wounds seen in prior cases in this papyrus.

As often done, the use of comparison or illustration with everyday subjects is used in Case #40 in the Explanation section where the ancient Egyptian physician provides an anatomical comparison between the sternal manubrium and the shape of an animal that is unclear to us in translation, but, perhaps, that of a lizard or of a hedgehog.

Soldier #10 of Winlock's cache of human remains shows an injury by the sternal margin, from the reverse direction (see fig. 38a). An arrow penetrates the left shoulder, passes through the chest and exits along the right lateral margin of the sternum, between two rib cartilages. The sternum specimens shown in fig. 38b are from the mummified human remains material found by the University of Arizona Egyptian Expedition, at the excavation of Queen Tausret's memorial temple site in Luxor, Egypt (2009–2011 seasons).

250. T. M. Fallum, S. M. Siram, and M. Righini, "Stab Wounds to the Chest: A Retrospective Review of 100 Consecutive Cases," *Journal of the National Medical Association* 82/2 (1990): 111. Online: http://www.ncbi.nlm.nih.gov/pmc/articles/PMC2625943/.

251. Salazar, *The Treatment of War Wounds in Graeco-Roman Antiquity*, 204–8.

252. Pneumothorax is the penetration of air into the pleural space, which normally has negative pressure. Intrapleural air disrupts respiratory and cardiac functions by reducing lung filling capacity.

CASE #41:
Infection of a Wound of the Chest
(Plate XIII:18–XIV:16)

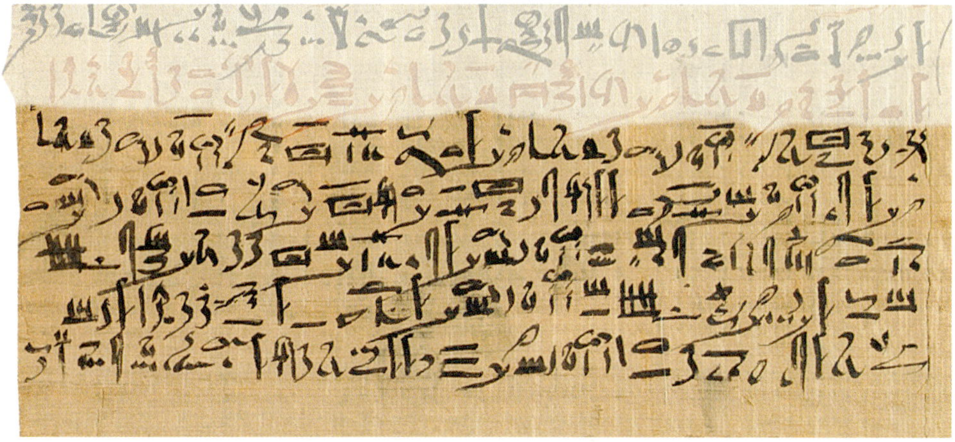

Courtesy New York Academy of Medicine.

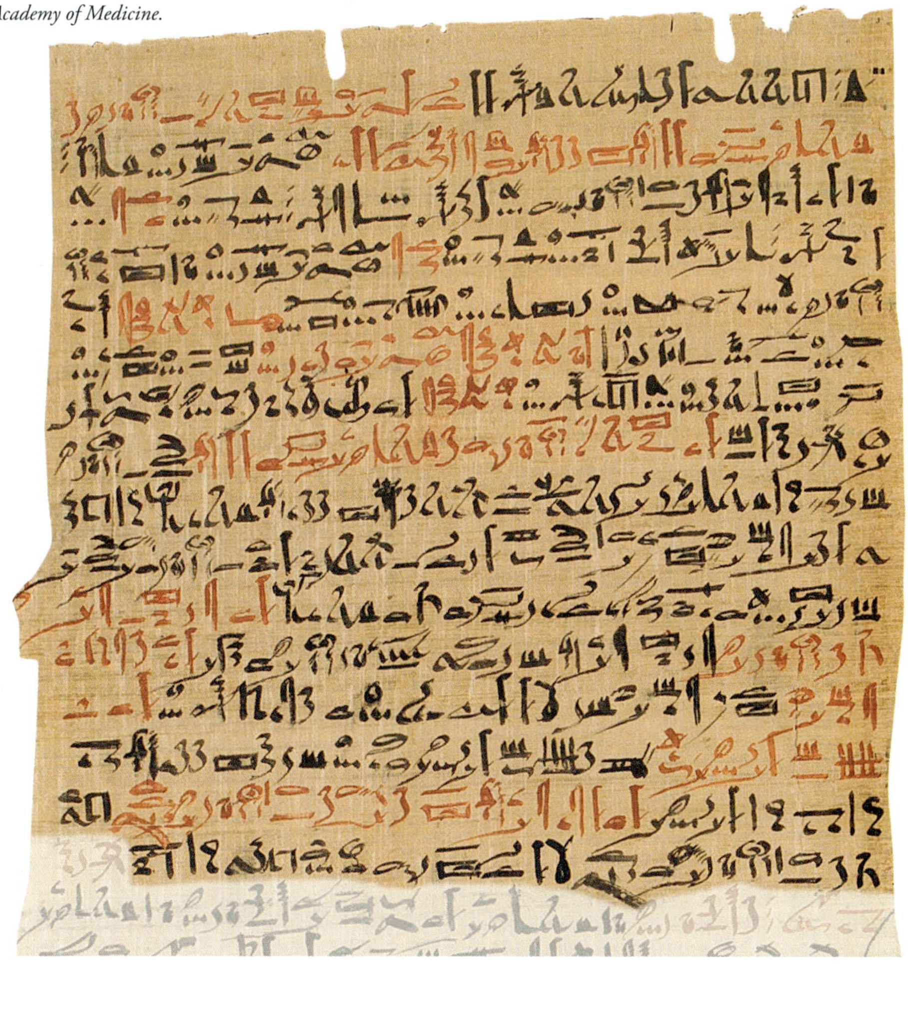

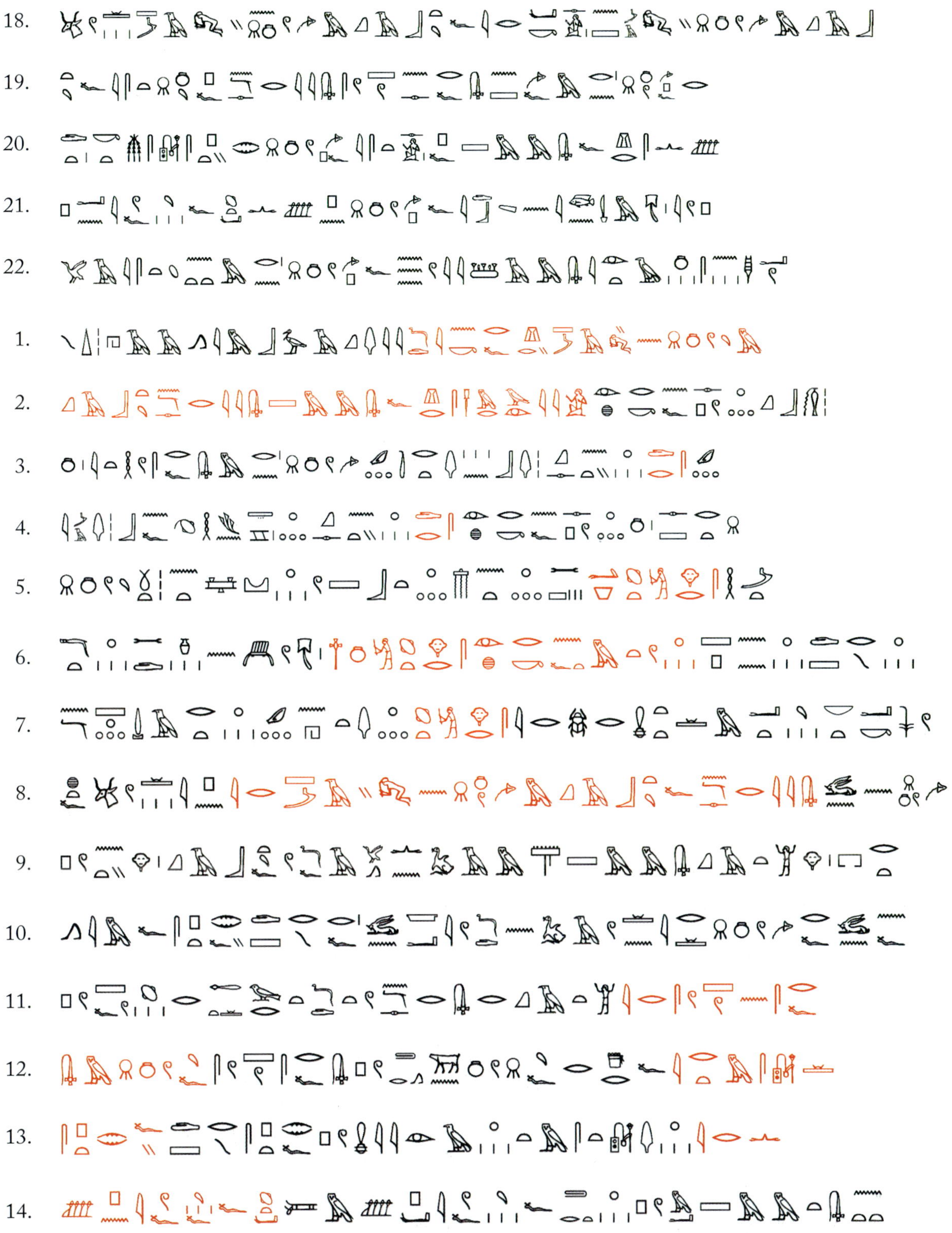

15. 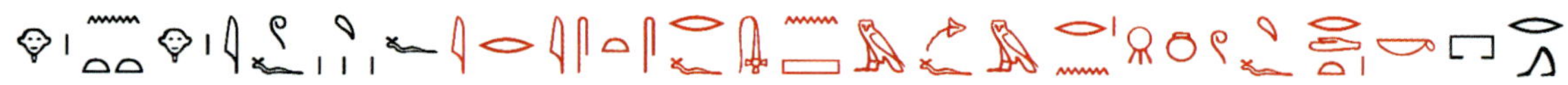

16. 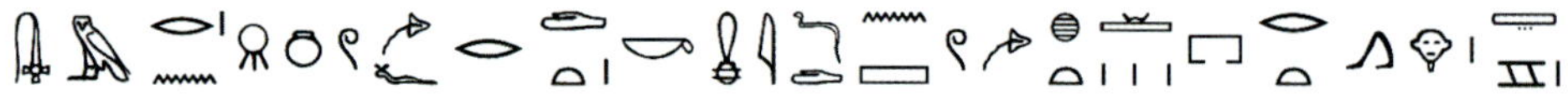

Transliteration

18§ *šs3w šm3y wbnw m ḳ3bt.f ir ḫ3.k s n šm3y n wbnw m ḳ3bt.*

19§ *f isṯ wbnw pf nsry swš n srf nš.f m r3 n wbnw pf r*

20§ *ḏrt.k tms spty wbnw pf isṯ s pf šmm.f ḫr.s n*

21§ *šsp.n iwf.f wt n šsp.n wbnw pf idb n inm iw*

22§ *p3 ist ntt m r3 n wbnw pf mwy š3m irtyw.sn ʿḥʿ.w*

1§ *h33 im b3ḳy ḏd.in.k r.f ḫry šm3y n wbnw m*

2§ *ḳ3bt nsry šmm.f ḫr.s mḥr iry.i ir.ḫr.k n.f spw ḳbw*

3§ *nw itḥ srf m r3 n wbnw ḏrdw ṯrt nbs ḳsnty dr.s ḏrdw*

4§ *im3w bnf ḥni- t3 ḳsnty dr.s ir.ḫr.k n.f spw nw sšrt*

5§ *wbnw šst nt w3ḏw wšbt ṯḥnt ʿḏ. nḏ wt ḥr.s ḥm3t*

6§ *mḥt ʿḏ n ni3w nḏ wt ḥr.s ir.ḫr.k n.f tmtw špnn dšrt*

7§ *nsš ḏ3rt ḏrdw nht wt ḥr.s ir ḫpr mitt m ʿwt nbt swrḫ.k sw*

8§ *ḫft šs3w ipn ir šm3y n wbnw m ḳ3bt.f nsry wnn wbnw*

9§ *pw nty ḥr ḳ3bt.f wḏf nn ṯʿm šmmt ḳ3t ḥr prt*

10§ *im.f spty.fy dšr r3.f wn iw ḏd.n ṯ3w.n ir mḏ3t n wbnw r.f wnn.f*

11§ *pw šfw r ʿ3t wrt ḏd.tw nsr r ḳ3t ir swš n srf*

12§ *m wbnw.f swš srf pw pḫr ḫnw wbnw.f r-ḏr.f ir ṯms*

13§ *spty.fy dšr spty.f pw mi irtyw ṯmst prt ir n*

14§ *šsp.n iwf.f wt tm šsp iwf.f pḫrt pw m-ʿ šmmt ntt*

15§ *ḥr {ntt ḥr} iwf.f ir isṯ srf nš.f m r3 n wbnw.f r ḏrt.k pr*

16§ *srf m r3 n wbnw.f r ḏrt.k mi ḏd nšw ḫt prt ḥr t3.*

Translation

Title:

Necessary knowledge and skills for infection of a wound in his chest.

Examination:

If you should examine a man for infection in a wound in his chest

while that wound is infected

and while a convergence of heat flows out from the mouth of that wound to your hand, the two lips of that wound being ruddy,

while that man is febrile because of it,

and his flesh cannot accept a bandage, and that wound cannot acquire a margin of (new) skin,

and the manifestation/type of emergence that is in the mouth of that wound is liquid,

their state/condition being burning,

while the secretions that drip there from are oily.

Diagnosis:

then you are to say about him: "One who has infection in a wound in his chest, which is inflamed-hot/infected and because of which he is febrile:

a medical condition which I will handle/deal with."

Treatment:

You must prepare for him the cooling remedies for drawing out the heat from the mouth of the wound:

leaves of willow, zizyphus (leaves), and *ḳsnty* mineral. Apply to it.

leaves of *im3* trees, ox bile, ground rushes, and *ḳsnty* mineral. Apply to it.

You must prepare for him a remedy for drying the wound:

powder of malachite, *wšbt* and crushed frit.

Grind. Bandage (along) with it.

Northern natron salt, and fat of ibex.

Grind. Bandage (along) with it.

You must prepare for him a powder of

red poppy (extract), *nšš* <seeds>, carob beans, and pulverized sycamore leaves.

Bind (along) with it.

If the same occurs in any body part, you should treat it according to these instructions.

Explanation A:

As for a nonhealing wound in his chest which is inflamed-hot/infected

it means that the wound which is on his chest is lingering/has stopped healing,

without closing over,

while high fever is coming from it,

its lips being red and

its mouth open.

The "Compilation of What Pertains to Wounds" has said regarding it, it means that it is very greatly swollen and inflamed, one says/(there) is said "rising."

Explanation B:

As for "the convergence of heat in his wound," it means that "the convergence of heat from inflammation/infection pervades the inside of his wound in its entirety."

Explanation C:

As for "ruddyness, its lips being red," it means that "its lips are like the color of red tree fruit."

Explanation D:

As for "his flesh cannot accept a bandage," it means that "his flesh fails to accept the remedy because of the fever that is in his flesh."

Explanation E:

Now, as for "heat, while it flows out from the mouth of his wound to your hand" while the heat comes out from the mouth of his wound to your hand, like saying something spews which comes forth onto the ground."

Notes

šmꜣy – cf. previous notes. (From Edwin Smith, case #15 "disease-demons, disease-bringing entities," "infection," concept Case #41 Explanation A.)

nsry – stative

swš n srf nš.f, s pf šmm.f – noun or noun phrase + *sḏm.f.* Following Doret, *Narrative Verbal System*, 26, 34, 115 (table 1), I take this as a circumstantial *sḏm.f* (as noted previously, *šmm* is a 2ae gem., verb, not 3ae inf.), and one in which the meaning of the clause is circumstantial, not a construction in which initial element + noun = indicative. This is reinforced by the alternation of this construction with simple circumstantial *sḏm.f* and with noun + stative, and the addition of the nonenclitic particle *isṯ/ist.*

tms spty – Circumstantial *sḏm.f.*

n šsp.n … n šsp.n … – I take these two clauses as parallel; I see no convincing justification for translating the second one as a past circumstantial or imparting the notion of causality. The Egyptian physician's view of the causality is given in Explanation D.

iw pꜣist … mwy – *iw* + noun + stative is an independent, not a circumstantial, clause, unless a meaning of strong contrast is present (in which case one can have a "whereas," or concessive, clause), which is not the case here. The definition of *pꜣist* in *Grundriss* 7, 1:257 as "appearance at a *wbnw*-wound" is enclosed in brackets indicating that it is uncertain, and moreover it does not denote "appearance" per se, but AN appearance that the authors cannot identify. (Just as, *mutatis mutandis*, when *Wb.* defines a word as "noun" or "verb," it does not mean that it was the ancient Egyptian word for "noun" or "verb," but that it is a noun or verb that cannot be identified.)

šꜣm irtyw.sn – Circumstantial *sḏm.f*

ꜥḥꜥw … bꜣḳy – Though the adjective-verb back-formed from a nisbe-adjective is rare (see Meltzer, "Problems of Adjectival Constructions in Old and Middle Egyptian," II.4), *bꜣḳy* must be one, because syntactically a stative is required and a simple adjective, be it nisbe or qualitative, will not work. As in other cases, the clause noun or noun phrase + stative is circumstantial, not independent.

šmm.f ẖr.s – Circumstantial *sḏm.f* as indefinite or unmarked relative with indefinite antecedent.

ḳsnty and *wšbt* do not appear in Aufrère, *L'univers minéral dans la pensée égyptienne.*

d(*w*) *r.s* –"Put on it/Apply to it" of Breasted (*Edwin Smith*, 1:256) and Allen (*AM*, 99). I would opt for the verb *d*(*w*) rather than *wdi*, as explained in previous notes, though these are to all intents and purposes synonymous and even interchangeable in some of the expressions in which we found them.

nḏ "grind."

ḥsmn – Aufrère (*L'univers minéral dans la pensée égyptienne*, s.v.) defines as "natron salt."

tmtw – Without more explicit data, I am going with the *Grundriss* 7, 2:955 definition, "powder."

šmmt kꜣt ḥr prt im.f – A circumstantial clause, not independent.

ṯꜣw... – On the title of this work and related expressions, see previous notes.

pr srf... – I am taking this as a circumstantial *sḏm.f*, paraphrasing the circumstantial clause which is being defined in the explanation. It does not geminate and I do not feel justified in emending a manner nominalization though the sense would be very felicitous.

I think that, when correctly identified, the series of circumstantial clauses makes a very elegant and clear syntactic pattern.

Medical Commentary

Type of Injury

The patient in Case #41 has a chest wound, not affecting the bony structure of the chest, which has become infected. The wound infection is at the stage of Cellulitis, which is a diffuse and severe inflammation of the connective tissue of skin and subcutaneous layers produced, in this case, by traumatic introduction of bacteria normally present in the skin, most commonly Staphylococcus aureus and group A β-hemolytic streptococci. Traumatic tissue destruction and the presence of foreign bodies provide the ideal environment for infection to develop, triggering an inflammatory response that results in local swelling, increased local temperature, redness, and pain. Spreading infection through the lymphatic system may produce lymphadenopathy. Although Cellulitis has been considered as an entity not forming purulent drainage, the division between Cellulitis and abscess is indistinct. Cellulitis may evolve into abscess formation and may also spread through the blood stream causing bacteremia, which is manifested by the development of generalized fever.

Today, Cellulitis is treated with appropriate antibiotics. The recovery varies from hours to months.

Ancient Medical Methodology and Knowledge

This is a case of a chest wound that is not healing (described by the Egyptian term *šmꜣy*) and that has become infected. In Case #41, the nonhealing chest wound has developed all of the characteristics of Cellulitis, and the patient has become febrile as a result. Describing the clinical signs of the developing infection in the wound, Explanation A details three of the four classic signs of localized inflammation, which were much later described by Celsus.[253] The wound is not healing, is remaining open, and it is greatly inflamed and swollen, or rising. The wound is hot, red, and has an oily discharge (not a purulent discharge). Explanation B attributes the whirl of heat coming from the mouth of the wound to the process of inflammation that "pervades the inside of his wound in its entirety." The heat flowing out of the mouth of the wound to the examiner's hand is described in explanation E: "like saying something spews which comes forth onto the ground."

253. See note 247 in Case #39.

Explanation D clarifies that the flesh does not accept a bandage because of the high fever in the flesh. That is, because it is infected, the flesh rejects the bandage.

As indicated above, in Case #41, fever is a systemic symptom directly attributed to the presence of Cellulitis. The Egyptian physician has deduced, in the papyrus record, that fever is an outcome/result of the localized wound infection, what we now call infectious Cellulitis. The ancient Egyptian concept of infection needs to be understood as derived from observing that the wound became inflamed and hot. It is not equivalent to our additional understanding of these processes being the consequence of bacterial proliferation.

The historical importance of the medical legacy of the ancient Egyptian physician towards understanding the pathogenetic concept of infection, prior to the identification of bacteria as the causative agent, should be underscored. Using the word *šmꜣy* with the A-14 determinative 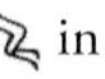 in Case #41, referring to an infectious Cellulitis developing in a wound that fails to heal normally, implies a direct association to disease bringing entities. The word *šmꜣy* is apparently related to *šmꜣw* "disease-demons, disease-bringing entities" (Faulkner, *CDME*, 266; *Wb*. 4:471). This is in turn considered to be related to *šmꜣw* "foreigners, wanderers" (Faulkner, *CDME*, 266; *Wb*. 4:470). (See the notes section in Case #15.)

In Case #41 the infected chest wound is treated in two sequential steps, each with specific goals of first drawing the heat away from the wound by using topical applications without bandaging, and secondly drying out the wound using ingredients which are ground and bandaged over the wound.

The materials and sequence used in these prescriptions outlined in the treatment segment, were, in all probability, arrived at by experience. Our retrospective analysis of their effects derives from modern chemistry and pharmacology and from the current experience with these substances by many African countries in which such prescriptions are still in use.

The topical prescriptions for cooling the wound/drawing the heat from it appear to be prescribed for sequential use. First, is a combination of leaves of willow and zizyphus with the unknown element "*ḳsnty*." The willow leaves would provide analgesic, anti-inflammatory and antiseptic effects,[254] while zizyphus would be astringent and soothing.[255] The *ḳsnty* component has mineral determinatives, but, at present, remains an unidentified substance. It could have been a vehicle for the other materials, but the similarity of its name with "*ḳsnt*" (pain) raises the possibility of this being a commonly used substance receiving its vernacular name for practical applications. The second prescription includes more antimicrobial components in *ỉmꜣ* tree leaves (Maerua crossofolia)[256] and in ox

254. J. M. Campbell and A. R. David. "The Application of Archaeobotany, Phytogeography and Pharmacognosy to Confirm the Pharmacopoeia of Ancient Egypt 1850–1200 BC," *Pharmacy and Medicine in Ancient Egypt* (ed. Jenefer Cockitt and Rosalie David; BAR International Series 2141; Oxford: Archaeopress, 2010), 20–29. Hidayat Hussain, et al., "Chemical Constituents and Antimicrobial Activity of *Salix subserrata*," *Records of Natural Products* 5/2 (2011), 133–37. Online: http://www.acgpubs.org/RNP/2011/Volume%205/Issue%201/18_RNP-1007-266.pdf.

255. Zizyphus spina-christi. Online: http://www.worldagroforestrycentre.org/sea/Products/AFDbases/af/asp/SpeciesInfo.asp?SpID=18002.

256. Sydney H. Aufrère, "Plants, Gardens and Horticulture in Their Relationship to Egyptian Culture and Cosmology." Online: http://www.clusiusstichting.nl/aufrere.html. Essam Abdel-Sattar, Fathalla M. Harraz, and Sabah H. El-Gayed, "Antimicrobial Activity of Extracts of Some Plants Collected from the Kingdom of Saudi Arabia," *Journal King Abdulaziz University: Med. Sci.* 15/1 (2008): 25–33. Online: http://malsuraihi.kau.edu.sa/Files/320/Researches/52140_22272.pdf. See also "Maerua crassofolia Forssk," Prelude Medicinal Plants Database. Online: http://www.africamuseum.be/collections/external/prelude/view_mu?id=225592. Cf. also R. Germer, *Handbuch der altägyptischen Heilpflanzen*, 25–27. This highly useful compendium should be consulted for all of the plant names in the papyrus.

bile.[257] The *im3* tree leaves would also provide analgesia.[258] The *ḳsnty* mineral and ground rushes complete the formula.

The next phase in the topical treatment of the infected wound is to dry it. The open wound is now at a different phase of cellulitis. Again, the prescriptions were to be used sequentially. The combination of malachite powder,[259] *wšbt* (possible aluminum and potassium sulfate[260]) and frit[261] (silica,[262] copper oxide[263]) provides powerful antiseptic/antibacterial effects. Frit and *wšbt* provide also astringent action. Next northern salt is mixed with ibex fat and applied to the wound as a greasy ointment. This provides a more powerful astringent substance on the wound than frit and *wšbt* previously used. Lastly is a preparation consisting primarily of a potent analgesic in the red poppy[264] and a local anesthetic in the sycamore leaves extract,[265] equivalent to that of Xylocaine. In this prescription, there also are anti-inflammatories (red poppy, flax[266]) demulcents (flax and carob beans[267]) and a mild astringent (carob beans).

Overall, these prescriptions would have served their intended purpose, in accord with the wound condition and the specific pharmacological needs at the various stages of its evolution. The physician's verdict in Case #41 expresses confidence in his management of this chest soft tissue infection. The treatment section of this case specifies that these general instructions are to be applied in this type of infection occurring at any part of the body.

---

257. Hoffman, Alan F., and Lars Eckmann, "How Bile Acids Confer Gut Mucosal Protection against Bacteria," *Proceedings of the National Academy of Sciences of the United States of America* 103/12 (2006): 4333–34. Online: http://www.ncbi.nlm.nih.gov/pmc/articles/PMC1450168/. A. I. Prieto, F. Ramos-Morales, and J. Casadesus, "Bile-Induced DNA Damage in *Salmonella enterica*," *Genetics* 168 (2004): 1787–94. M. Begley, C. G. Gahan, and C. Hill, "The Interaction between Bacteria and Bile," *FEMS Microbiology Reviews* 29/4 (2005): 625–51. Online: http://www.ncbi.nlm.nih.gov/pubmed/16102595.

258. J. Bellakhdar, "Médecine traditionelle et toxicology ouest-serharienne, contribution à l'ètude de la pharmacopèe marocaine." Prelude Medicinal Plants Database: http://www.metafro.be/prelude/view_mu?id=225592.

259. Majno, *The Healing Hand*, 111–15.

260. Potassium alum. Online: http://en.wikipedia.org/wiki/Potassium_alum.

261. A. Lucas, *Ancient Egyptian Materials and Industries* (3rd ed.; London: Edward Arnold, 1948), 550.

262. M. Vallet-Regi and F. Balas,"Silica Materials for Medical Applications," *The Open Biomedical Engineering Journal* 2 (2008): 1–9.

263. Jeffrey Gabay, Gadi Borkow, Joseph Mishal, Eli Magen, Richard Zatcoff, and Yonat Shemer-Avni, "Copper Oxide Impregnated Textiles with Potent Biocidal Activities," *Journal of Industrial Textiles* 35/4 (2006): 323–35. Online: http://jit.sagepub.com/content/35/4/323.short.

264. M. Krajnik, Z. Zylicz, F. Finlay, J. Luckza, A. A. van Sorge, "Potential Use of Topical Opioids in Palliative Care Report of 6 Cases," *Pain* 80 (1999): 121–25.

265. S. G. Zaku, F. A. Abdulrahaman, P. A. Onyeyili, O. C. Aguzue, and S. A. Thomas, "Photochemical Constituents and Effects of Aqueous Root-Bark Extract of *Ficus sycomorus* L. (Moracaea) on Muscular Relaxation, Anaesthetic and Sleeping Time on Laboratory Animals," *African Journal of Biotechnology* 8/21 (2009): 6004–6. Online: http://www.academicjournals.org/AJB/abstracts/abs2009/2Nov/Zaku%20et%20al.htm.

266. Online: http://sites.google.com/site/forgetmenotps/list-of-oils-used-in-soap. "Flaxseed," Medline Plus. Online: http://www.nlm.nih.gov/medlineplus/druginfo/natural/991.html.

267. Ceratonia siliqua. Online: http://en.wikipedia.org/wiki/Ceratonia_siliqua.

CASE #42:

Traumatic Costochondritis

(Plate XIV:16–22)

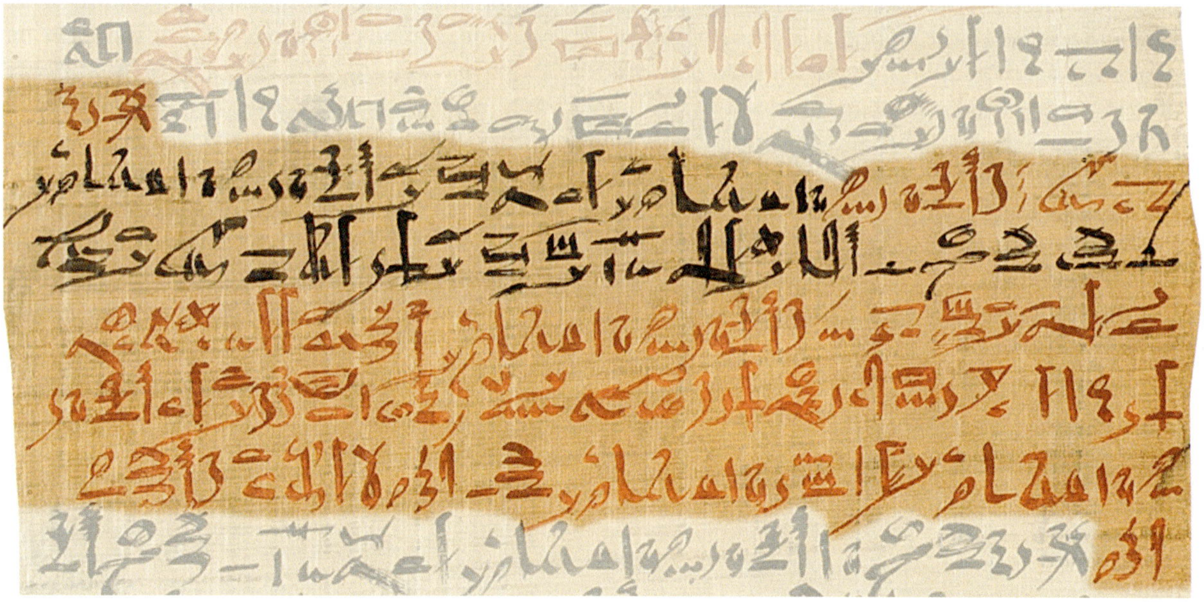

Courtesy New York Academy of Medicine.

16.
17.
18.
19.
20.
21.
22.

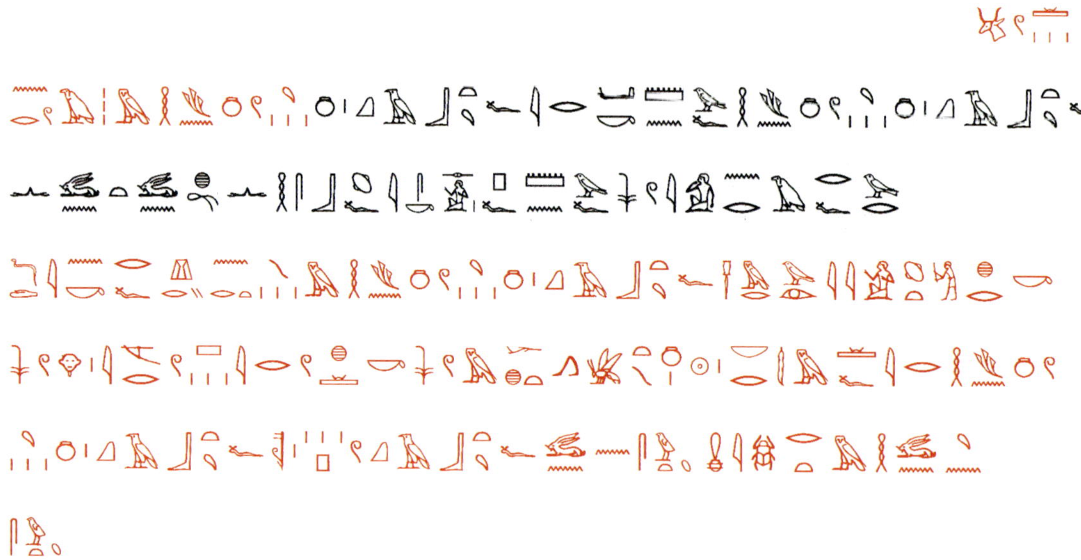

Transliteration

16§ … *šsꜣw*

17§ *nrwt m ḥnw nw ḳꜣbt.f ir ḫꜣ.k mn<t>.f<m> ḥnw nw ḳꜣbt.f*

18§ *n wnt wnḫ n ḥsb.f isk s pf mn.f sw inr r.f wr*

19§ *ḏd.in.k r.f ẖry nrwt m ḥnw nw ḳꜣbt.f mḫr iry.i wt.ḫr.k*

20§ *sw ḫr imrw srwḫ.k sw m-ḫt <m> bit rꜥ nb r nḏm.f ir ḥnw*

21§ *nw ḳꜣbt.f ḳsw pw nw ḳꜣbt.f wnn swt mi ḫprt m ḥwn n*

22§ *swt*

Translation

Title:

Necessary knowledge and skills for sprains in the ribs of his chest:

Examination:

If you examine <a man> who is suffering in the ribs of his chest, and there is no dislocation, it not having been broken, while at the same time that man is suffering from it and shivering/shuddering greatly concerning it.

Diagnosis:

Then you are to say about him: "One having sprain in the ribs of his chest, a medical condition which I will handle/deal with."

Treatment:

Then you must bind it (along) with alum(?) (or, a bandage with alum[?] shavings?), and you should treat him afterward <with> honey every day until he/it is well.

Explanation:

As for "the ribs of his chest," it means the bones belonging to his chest; how the costal region is (is) like what occurs in a piece of meat of the costal region/rib roast.

Notes

<s> mn.f … – Rather than to emend *mn<t>.f<m>*, I think it more likely that the word *s* "man" was omitted, and if it is added no other emendation is needed. *mn.f* is a circumstantial *sḏm.f*, which according to this emendation is acting as an indefinite or unmarked relative modifying the indefinite antecedent "a man." The verb *mn* "suffer from/in" requires no preposition (Faulkner, *CDME*, 107), so *<m>* need not be emended. Admittedly the most common pattern is "If you examine a man" followed by *n* "for …," but this is not absolutely invariable, and the emendation proposed here seems to me the most economical and elegant option and in effect emends as little as possible though some emendation is necessary.

n ḥsb(w).f – Passive *sḏmw.f* as an adverbial form.

s pf mn.f – Noun + circumstantial *sḏm.f* in a pleonastic circumstantial clause with *isk*; see above.

inr – Stative.

imrw – See above.

swt etc. – I follow *Grundriss* 7, 2:723 in the understanding of this word.

wnn – a nominal *sḏm.f* used as a manner nominalization. *swt* is the subject of *wnn*; I cannot understand *ḳsw* ... *wnn swt mi* ... to mean "the bones ... being the costal region, are like ...," which requires *wnn* to be a stative and an <*m*> of predication to be emended before *swt*, because neither *iw* nor *wnn* occurs followed directly by a noun in a statement of equivalence.

ḫprt – active participle.

Medical Commentary

Type of Injury

Case #42 is one of costochondritis, an inflammatory process of the costal cartilages that attach to the ribs, and/or, to the sternum (Visual Index II). The costochondral joints are the articulations between the ribs and costal cartilage. There is a cup-like depression at the anterior end of the rib that receives the lateral end of each costal cartilage that is held together by periosteum. There is normally no movement at these joints. The joints between costal cartilages of ribs six to nine are synovial joints and the articulation between the costal cartilage of ribs nine and ten is fibrous. In 90 percent of such cases more than one cartilage is involved. The source of costochondritis is not well defined and may involve more than a single factor. Repetitive minor trauma occurring during physical activities to which an individual is not accustomed, as in painting walls, or participating in sporting events anew are considered the most likely causes.

The symptoms of costochondritis are pain and tenderness over the inflamed cartilage. The pain can be severe and is exacerbated by trunk motion, deep breathing, and physical exertion. The inflammatory process in this case is not accompanied by fever as it is due not to infection but is simply secondary to the trauma.

The treatment today consists of decreasing motion by taping, splinting, and orthotic devices that hold the ribs still. These devices help reduce pain by diminishing motion of the chest wall, thereby favoring shallow breathing and allowing the surrounding tissues to heal. Customarily, analgesics and anti-inflammatories are also administered.

Ancient Medical Methodology and Knowledge

As a society that depended heavily upon intensive manual labor, injuries such as these would have been common in ancient Egypt. Using the method of illustration by use of everyday objects that we see in this papyrus with some frequency, the text describes the costal region by likening it to a rib roast from an animal.

The Egyptian physician through physical examination eliminates dislocation or rib fractures and diagnoses this injury as a sprain causing significant suffering and severe pain.

Considering this condition as treatable, chest binding is recommended, first with alum, then with topical application of honey.

CASE #43:
Sternocostal-Costochondral Dislocation
(Plate XIV:22–XV:6)

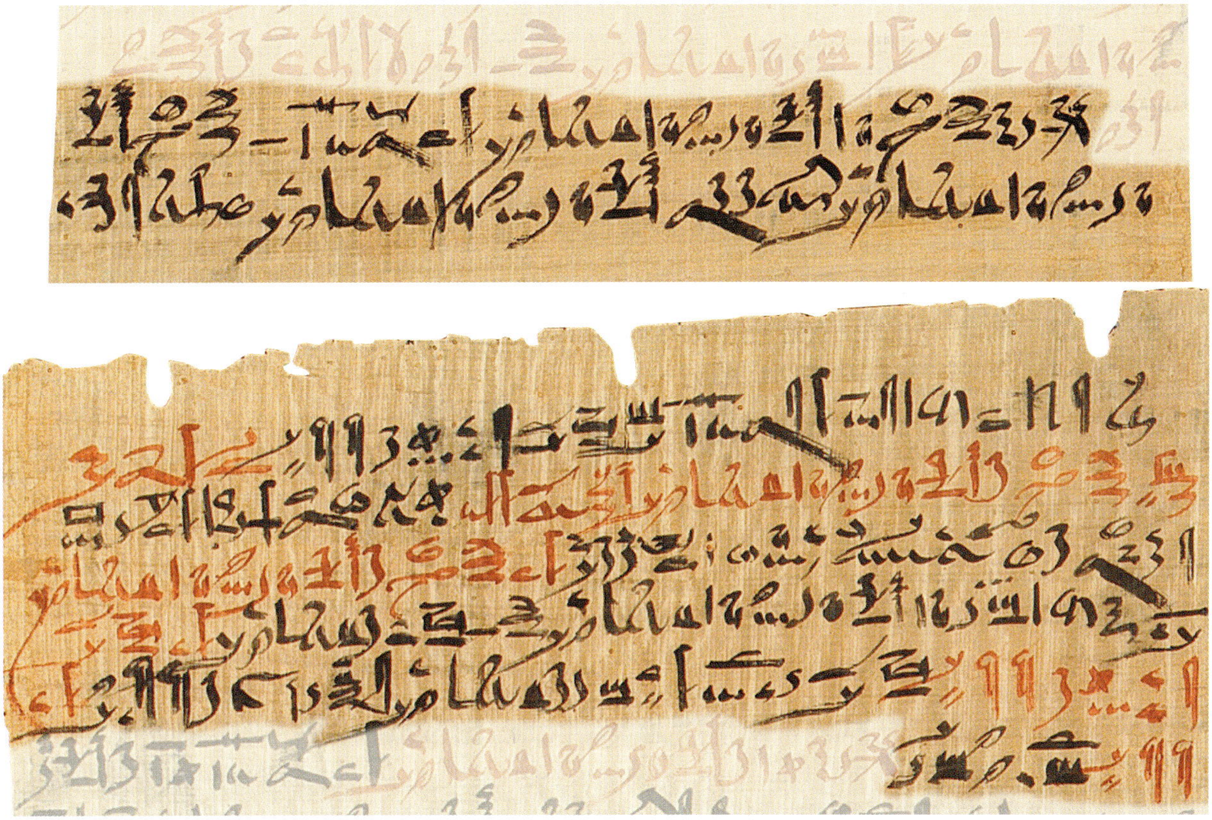

Courtesy New York Academy of Medicine.

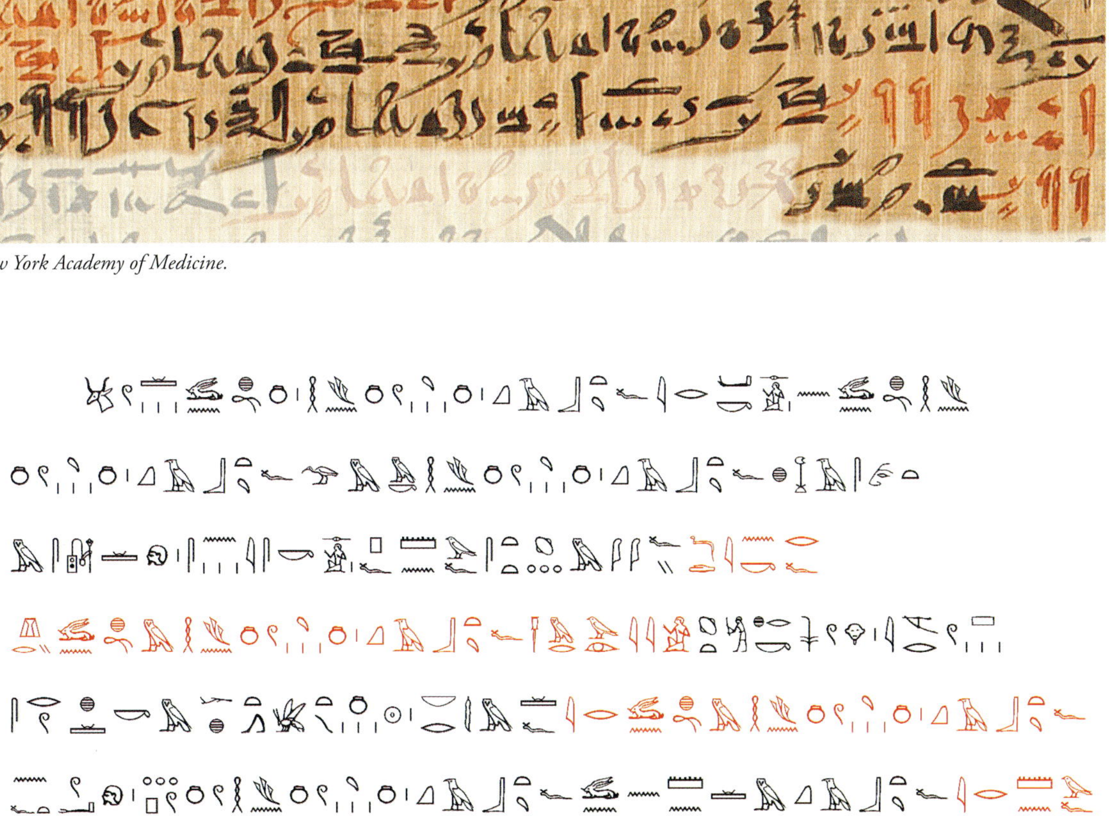

22.
23.
1.
2.
3.
4.

5. 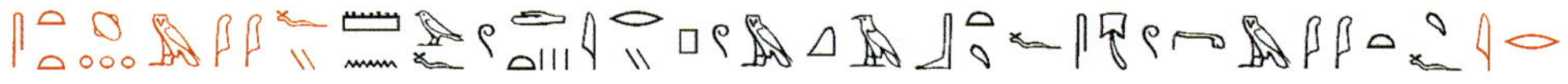

6. 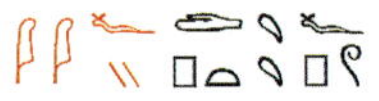

Transliteration

22§ … *šs3w wnḫ n{w} ḥnw nw ḳ3bt.f ir ḫ3.k s n wnḫ <n> ḥnw*

23§ *nw ḳ3bt.f gmm.k ḥnw nw ḳ3bt.f ḫ3s*

1§ *tms tp<w>.sn isk s pf mn.f stwt m šw<ty>.fy ḏd.in.k r.f*

2§ *ḫry wnḫ m ḥnw nw ḳ3bt.f mḫr iry.i wt.ḫr.k sw ḥr imrw*

3§ *srwḫ.k m-ḫt <m> bit rʿ nb r nḏm.f ir wnḫ m ḥnw nw ḳ3bt.f*

4§ *nft tpw pw nw ḥnw nw ḳ3bt.f wnn mn m ḳ3bt.f ir mn.f*

5§ *stwt m šw<ty>.fy mn.f wdwt iry pw m ḳ3bt.f st.w m šwt<y>.f ir*

6§ *šw<ty>.fy dp.ty.f pw*

Translation

Title:

Necessary knowledge and skills for a dislocation of the ribs of his chest:

Examination:

If you should examine a man for a dislocation the ribs of his chest, how you find the ribs of his chest (is): bent/arched forward, their heads being reddened,

while that man suffers from shooting pains in both sides of his chest.

Diagnosis:

Then you are to say about him: "One who has a dislocation in the rib sections of his chest:

a medical condition which I will handle/deal with."

Treatment:

Then you have to bind it (along) with alum(?) (or, a bandage with alum[?] shavings?), and you should treat afterwards <with> honey every day until he/it is well.

Explanation A:

As for "a dislocation in the ribs of his chest," it means the heads of the ribs of his chest having been detached, that are normally fixed in his chest.

Explanation B:

As for "while he suffers from shooting pains in both sides of his chest," it means, he suffers from their displacements in his chest, so that they are surging in both sides of his chest.

Explanation C:

As for "both sides of his chest," it means "his two flanks" (Breasted, *Edwin Smith* 1:546; Walker, *Studies in Ancient Egyptian Anatomical Terminology,* 276)

Notes

wnḫ nw (sic) *ḥnw* – Breasted was correct to consider the use of *nw* an error, though he does not seem entirely clear about the nature of the error. It is plural, whereas the antecedent is singular, and thus if the scribe wanted to use the Indirect Genitive, the correct choice would be <*n*(*y*)>. The precise motivation for the use of direct or indirect genitive is often obscure despite some apparently clear-cut syntactic rules and the proposals of some scholars such as Bakir; see Meltzer "Problems of Adjectival Constructions in Old and Middle Egyptian," ch. 4.

"*ḫꜣs*"– I have thought for decades that *ḫꜣm* and *ḫꜣb*(*b*) are related, and I think it is at least as likely that *m* and *b* are third consonants or "determinants" (not the same as a determinative[!!] but a consonant that expands and perhaps specializes a biliteral root) added to a biliteral kernel or simplex *ḫꜣ* having to do with crookedness, as it is that they are phonetic (dialectal?) variants though that too is possible. If one provisionally accepts a biliteral root *ḫꜣ*, this probably militates in favor of the reading of a verb *ḫꜣs*, because it would likely be related to the word *ḫꜣs* "curl on front of Red Crown(?)" (Faulkner, *CDME,* 185) as well as *ḫꜣs* "creek(?), runnel(?)," and perhaps *ḫꜣs* "scramble(?)," listed there. On "determinants," see, for Semitic, Sabatino Moscati, et al., *An Introduction to the Comparative Grammar of the Semitic Languages: Phonology and Morphology* (Wiesbaden: Harrassowitz, 1969), 72–75; for Egyptian we have cited literature on biliteralism above, of which we shall only mention again Edel, *AG,* sec. 423–45. It is not true that the Smith passage is the only occurrence of this sequence or that it is a unique occurrence or a hapax; a nearly identical writing occurs in Papyrus Ebers, differing only in the lack of the initial phonetic complement *ḫ*, and with suffix-pronoun, reading *ḫꜣs.f.* Von Deines and Westendorf (*Grundriss* 7, 2:649) note that it is unclear whether the Ebers occurrence is an ordinary noun or an infinitive. They also note that the context and determinative enable a sense "nose-like, arched/curved forward." They try to move beyond an uncertain general definition, but without sufficient certainty to list it as the lemma of the word in their dictionary. The verb form is a stative.

tms – This is not a predicate adjective, but the circumstantial *sḏm.f* of the adjective-verb, and another clear example refuting the claims that this form does not exist; see my comment in my review of Doret, *Narrative Verbal System,* 223–24.

mn.f – Circumstantial *sḏm.f.*

ỉsk s pf mn.f – With the particle *ỉsk* and the noun (or noun Phrase) + circumstantial *sḏm.f* construction, this is what I have called a pleonastic circumstantial clause (see above).

ỉmrw – See above.

nft(*w*) *tpw* … – Passive *sḏmw.f.*

wnn mn – An (active) participle + a stative. This is not a prior circumstance but a habitual one, hence the appropriateness of "normally." This is an example in which the habitual or durative meaning of the geminating form *wnn* seems to work, whereas in many other cases, especially in the *sḏm.f,* it seems to me entirely understandable as a manner nominalization and the habitual "imperfective" meaning often seems illusory.

mn.f – Circumstantial *sḏm.f.*

mn.f … *pw* – Nominal *sḏm.f* as "that" clause, "it means that he suffers …"

šwt<*y*>*.f*<*y*> – To be understood as a dual.

stw – This is a stative, as per *Grundriss,* which I am taking as a stative of result.

The use of circumstantial forms is notable and can serve as an instructive example of the use of multiple forms to express circumstantiality and provide the syntax typical of those forms. Circumstantial forms were first explicitly and consistently identified as a real category of Egyptian verb forms by Polotsky in *Egyptian Tenses*.

Medical Commentary

Type of Injury

This is a case of thoracic wall blunt trauma producing chest wall cartilaginous and bone injury, but without symptoms suggesting major cardio-respiratory involvement. Dislocation of the ribs can occur anteriorly, at the costo-chondral junction, or at the costal cartilage with its separation from the sternum,[268] and more infrequently posteriorly, at the costo-vertebral junction. The sternocostal joints articulate with the sternum via their costal cartilages. The first rib attaches to the sternal manubrium. Ribs two to seven attach to the body of the sternum by synovial joints, and, as such, they have a joint capsule. The sternocostal joints from the eighth to tenth ribs are simple gliding synovial articulations without a defined capsule. The costochondral joints are hyaline cartilaginous joints, with the rib's periosteum forming a continuous layer with the perichondrium of the cartilage. The interchondral joints between the sixth and the ninth costal cartilages are classified as plain synovial joints, while the joint between the ninth and tenth cartilages is a fibrous joint (Visual Index II).[269]

Any, or several of these joints, can be dislocated by blunt trauma to the chest. Dislocation that occurs at the sternum can produce separation of one or more of the costal cartilages, including the interchondral cartilage. Dislocations between the rib and its costal cartilage involve tearing of their periosteum and perichondrium, often producing upward rib displacement, overriding the next rib.

The symptoms and signs of sternocostal dislocation are readily detected on physical examination by the local pain and deformity over the side of the sternum. Frequently these dislocations are not evident today on routine chest x-rays. In the early post-injury period ice, compression, and possible manipulation of the dislocated rib can be attempted. The chest is wrapped with an elastic bandage, keeping the patient at rest and administering analgesics. Sternocostal dislocations associated with multiple rib fractures could be part of a "flail chest,"[270] in which the stability and normal respiratory motion of the rib cage is dangerously disrupted.

Today, blunt chest trauma is the consequence of motor vehicle accidents, and contact sports, most frequently in football, hockey, basketball, boxing, and wrestling.

Ancient Medical Methodology and Knowledge

On physical examination, the abnormal appearance of the injured chest wall is clear: "... how you find the ribs of his chest (is): bent / arched forward, their heads being reddened." Chest-wall deformity is evident and the

268. "Joints and Ligaments of the Thorax: Gross Anatomy," Patrick W. Tank, (ed.) Department of Anatomy, University of Arkansas for Medical Sciences. Online: http://anatomy.uams.edu/anatomyhtml/joints_thorax.html.

269. Keith L. Moore and Arthur F. Dalley, *Clinically Oriented Anatomy* (5th ed.; Philadelphia: Lippincot Williams & Wilkins, 2006), 86–90.

270. There is paradoxical chest movement upon inspiration. One panel of the thoracic wall moves independently from the rest, making the patient unable to breathe effectively; see D. B. Hoyt, R. Coimbra, and J. Acosta, "Management of Acute Trauma," in Townsend and Evers, *Sabiston Textbook of Surgery*, 496.

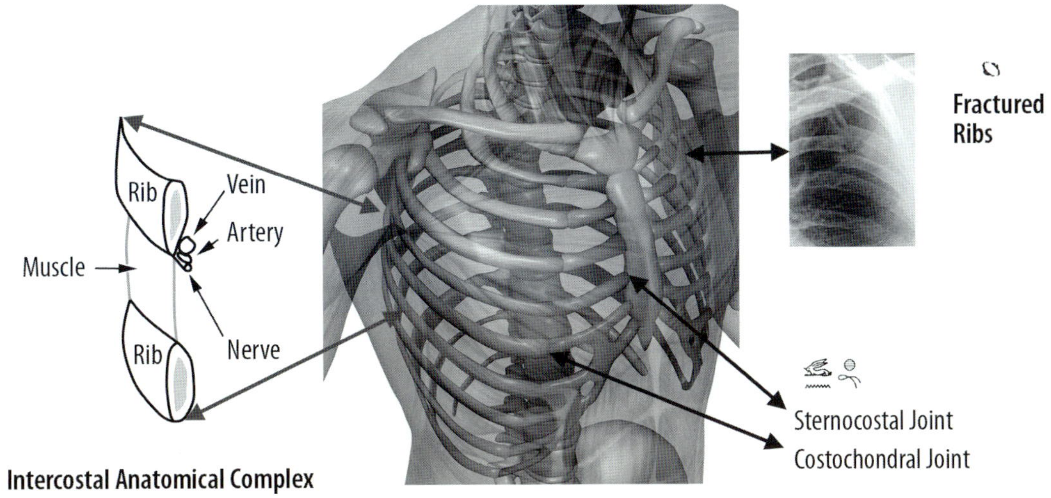

Fig. 39. Chest wall cartilagenous and bone injuries.
Center image courtesy of PHOTO RESEARCHERS, 307 Fifth Ave., New York, NY 10016.

irritated and stretched skin over the protruding rib "heads"[271] is red. The anatomical pathology of the dislocation is accurately described in Explanation A as: "… the heads of the ribs of his chest having been detached, that are normally fixed in his chest."

The patient's primary symptom of pain on the sides of his chest/flanks is explained by the disruption that has occurred at the intercostal anatomical complex: "he suffers from their displacements in his chest, so that they are surging in the flesh of both sides of his chest … it means 'his two flanks'" (fig. 39). The pain is described in Explanation B as "surging," depicting quite accurately its electric shock-like nature. This pain follows the distribution of the intercostal nerves in the chest and abdominal walls injured by the trauma, and made worse by every breath and by any chest motion.[272]

The pivotal part of the treatment for rib dislocations in ancient Egypt was binding of the chest. It is presumed that the initial application of powdered alum to the chest wall would have provided anti-inflammatory relief. Binding the chest with honey followed until the patient healed. The beneficial effects, presumed by the ancient Egyptian physician, of topical applications of honey to unbroken skin are, to us, uncertain.

In ancient Egypt these types of injuries would have been frequent in falls from construction scaffolding, chariots, direct blows in warfare, and altercations.

271. It should be noted that our current terminology apparently reverses the ancient Egyptian's concept of what is commonly called the head of the rib. To us, it is the posterior end of the rib, the portion that attaches to the spine. To the ancient Egyptians, the head of the rib was its front end.

272. The reader is directed to appendix 2 for a compilation of the neurological symptoms and signs in the Edwin Smith Papyrus.

CASE #44:
Open Comminuted Rib Fractures
(Plate XV:6–9)

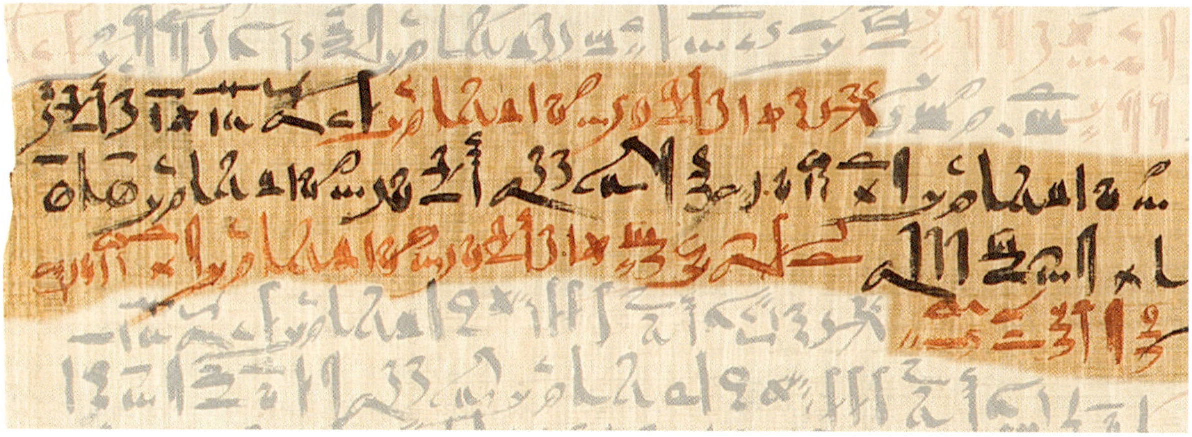

Courtesy New York Academy of Medicine.

6. 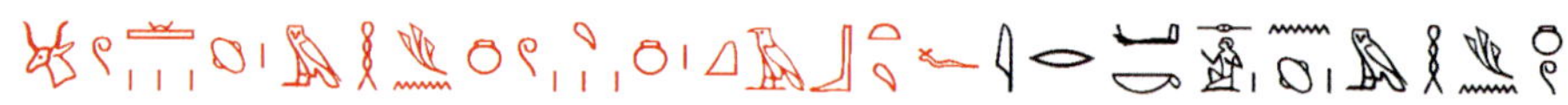

7. 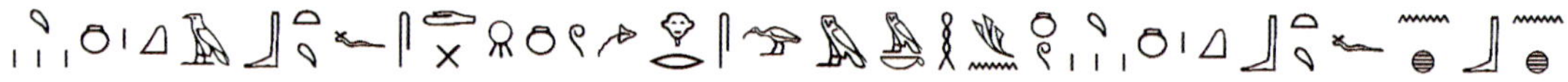

8. 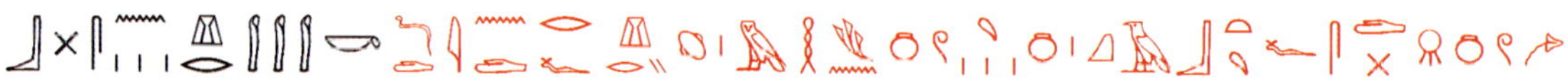

9. 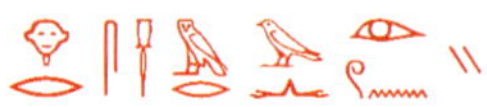

Transliteration

6§ … *šsꜣw ḥsb m ḥnw nw ḳꜣbt.f ir ḫꜣ.k s n ḥsb m ḥnw*

7§ *nw ḳꜣbt.f sḏ wbnw ḥr.s gmm.k ḥnw nw ḳꜣbt.f nẖbẖb.sn*

8§ *ẖr dbꜥw.k ḏd.in.k r.f ẖry ḥsb m ḥnw nw ḳꜣbt.f sḏ wbnw*

9§ *ḥr.s mḥr n irw.ny*

Translation

Title:

Necessary knowledge and skills for a fracture in the ribs of his chest:

Examination:

If you should examine a man for a fracture in the ribs of his chest, a wound having been smashed over it, how you find the rib sections attached to the breastbone of his chest (is): they shifting/crepitating under your fingers.

Diagnosis:

Then you are to say about him: "One having a fracture in the ribs of his chest, a wound having been smashed over it, a medical condition that cannot be handled/dealt with."

Notes

sd(*w*) – Passive *sḏmw.f*, taken as an adverbial/circumstantial form giving an anterior circumstance. It is possible to understand it as an indefinite or unmarked relative following the indefinite antecedent *ḥsb* "a fracture" (see above).

nẖbnẖb[sic]*.sn* – Circumstantial *sḏm.f*. *Grundriss* 7, 1:477 refers us to *nẖbẖb*, which occurs elsewhere in Edwin Smith, though in that entry the authors transliterate the form in this passage as *nẖbnẖb*. See also Faulkner, *CDME*, 138. It is perhaps worth pointing out that the fully reduplicated sesquiliteral type of root "ABCABC" is attested in the Pyramid Texts (Edel, *AG*, sec. 439, 446) as well as later (*Wb*. 2:381).

sd(*w*) – As above.

Medical Commentary

Type of Injury

Case #44 is that of a rib linear fracture (*ḥsb*) which, today, is seen in 10 percent of all traumas, most often produced by blunt chest impact in motor-vehicle accidents. Most of these fractures occur in the chest wall from the fifth to the ninth rib. Often more than one rib is involved (Visual Index II, and fig. 39).

The primary symptom of rib fracture is chest pain, which is aggravated by deep breathing. The process of breathing involves intrathoracic pressure changes created by the diaphragm muscle, which separates the abdominal and chest cavities, and by rib motions resulting from synchronous contractions of the intercostal muscles. The upward and forward movement of the anterior part of the ribs increases the thoracic space. The combined action of all of the respiratory muscles and the ribs generate the necessary intrathoracic pressure gradients needed for inspiration and expiration. In this type of injury, the depth of respiratory excursions is reduced, as is the air volume flowing through the lungs. Upon examination, these patients are in distress due to pain, and shallow breathing contributes to their anxiety.

Upon exploration of the fracture site, there is obvious chest wall deformity and crepitus to the manual exploration of the fractured site. Severe rib fractures can cause a flail chest[273] (defined in Case #43). In that situation, the affected thoracic wall moves independently from the rest of the chest wall, and often in the opposite direction, creating a critical respiratory problem through a lack of oxygen.

273. Hoyt, Coimbra, and Acosta, "Management of Acute Trauma," in Townsend and Evers, *Sabiston Textbook of Surgery*, 496.

The primary treatment objective is pain control, achieved today primarily through medication. While chest binders reduce pain, they are not currently recommended because of frequent respiratory complications[274] seen with their use: reduced ventilation, respiratory decompensation,[275] atelectasis,[276] and pneumonia.

In this case a smash wound has been inflicted over the rib cage fracturing the ribs. We are not quite in agreement with Jungraithmayr and Weder's assessment that in this injury "the dislocation of the rib caused a rupture of the overlying skin creating a wound."[277] The text indicates the presence of a smashing wound over the ribs with their fragments attached to the sternum, shifting under palpating fingers. There is no reference to wound edges, the clearly open chest wall wound in Case #47, or the skin rupture from the inside by a fractured and splintered humerus (Case #37).

Ancient Medical Methodology and Knowledge

In Case #44, the presence of a smash wound (*sd*) over the fractured ribs (*ḥsb*), refers to the contused soft tissues of the chest wall and probably indicates a rib fracture communicating to the outside. Injuries of this sort in ancient Egypt were most likely due to low velocity impact occurring in falls, labor related accidents such as in construction, blows with fists, maces, clubs, kicks, and horse related trauma.

In this case of rib fractures, the Egyptian physician clearly identifies the broken ribs through the primary physical finding of crepitation by palpation of the injured site. Except for describing a smash wound over the fracture site, no other features are given in this case that would suggest a more serious injury.

Our case does not provide a treatment segment or any explanation segment. No chest binding was advocated though it was in the two previous chest wall injuries of lesser severity. Today we would recognize tight binding in cases of rib fractures as being counterproductive, with the possible complications of reduced ventilation, atelectasis (lung lobe collapse) and pneumonia. Their observations perhaps had been the same.

The verdict is "a medical condition that cannot be handled/dealt with." This prognostication appears to address the lack of treatment methods available to the ancient Egyptian physician to create or enhance healing, rather than that the case had lethal consequences. Unquestionably, without infection, as this case appears, many such injuries heal spontaneously.

274. Lennard A. Nadalo and Kory Jones, "Rib Fracture Imaging." Medscape Reference: http://www.emedicine.com/radio/topic609.htm.

275. Hoyt, Coimbra, and Acosta, "Management of Acute Trauma," in Townsend and Evers, *Sabiston Textbook of Surgery*, 496.

276. Collapse of one or more lobes of the lungs.

277. W. Jungraithmayr and W. Weder. "Chest Surgical Disorders in Ancient Egypt: Evidence of Advanced Knowledge," *Annals of Surgery* 255/3 (2012): 607.

CASE #45:
Round "Masses" on the Chest
(Plate XV:9–19)

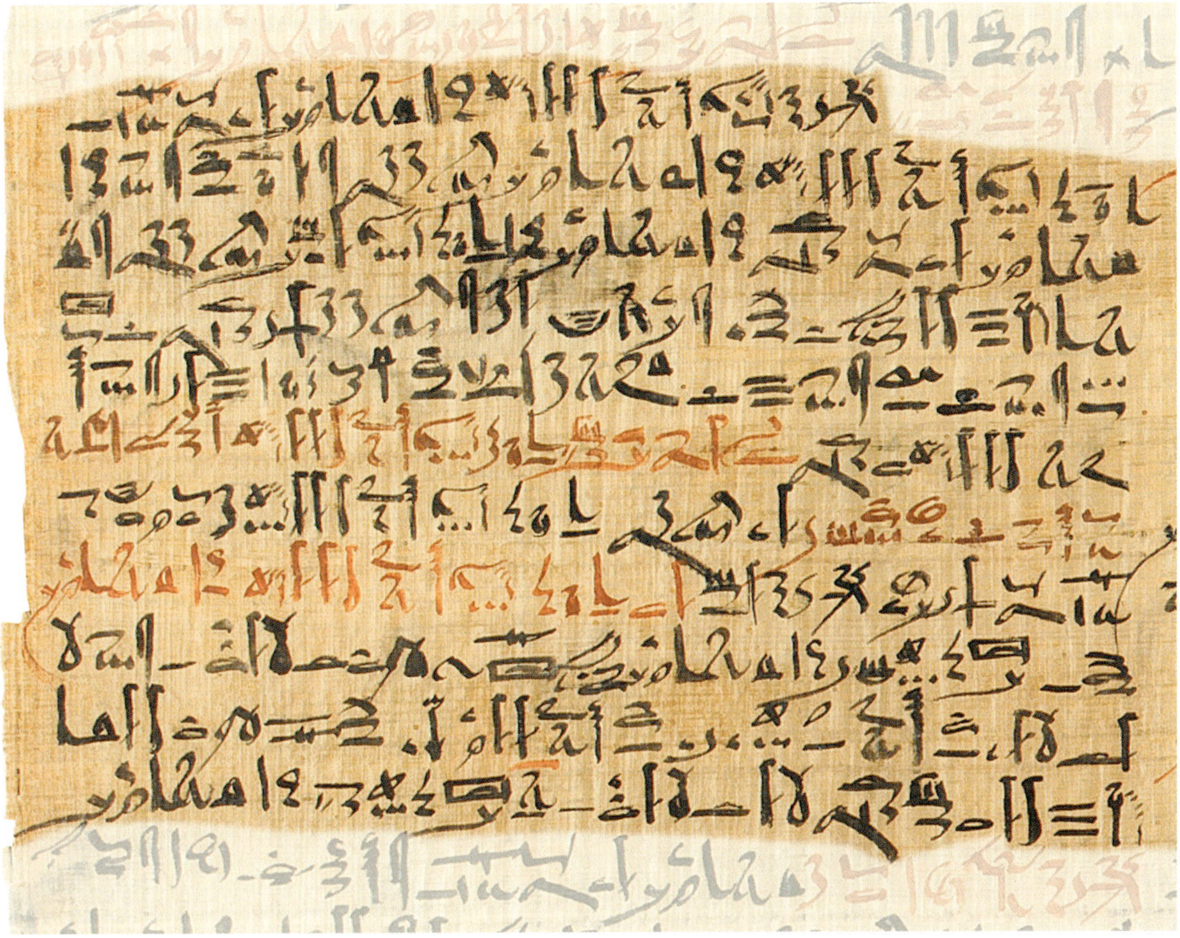

Courtesy New York Academy of Medicine.

9. 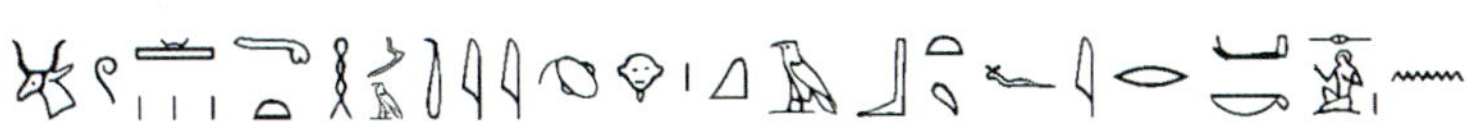

10. 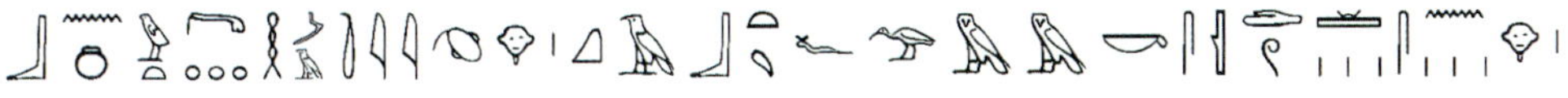

11. 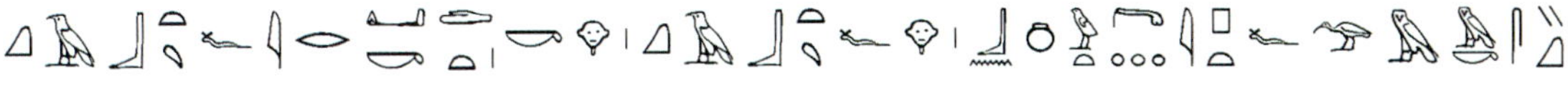

12. 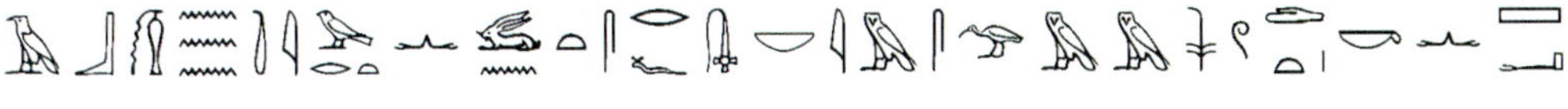

13. 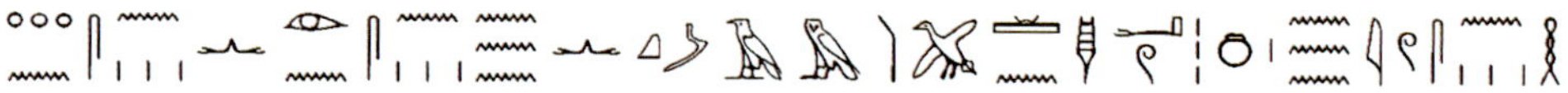

14. 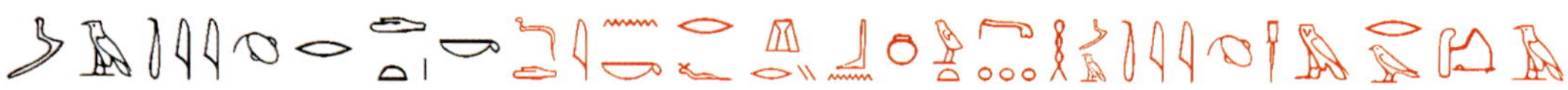

15. 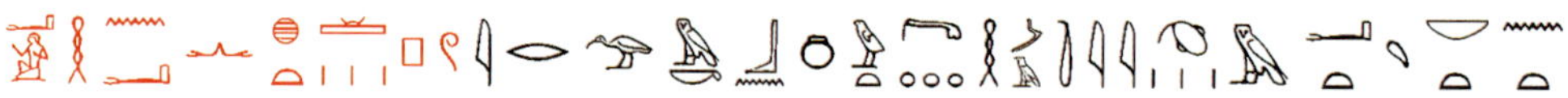

16. 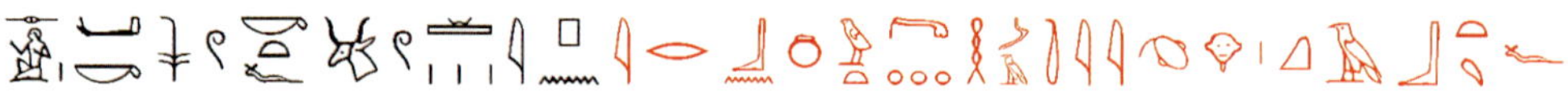

17. 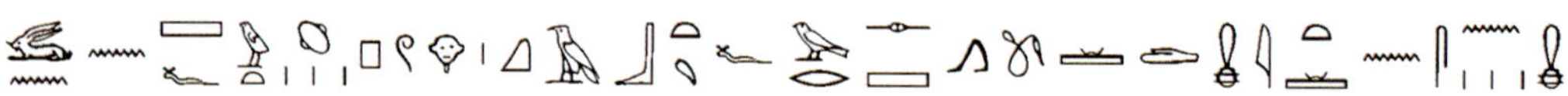

18. 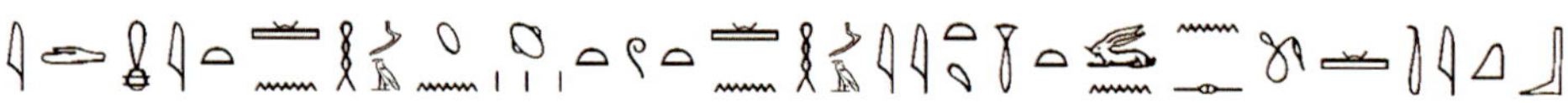

Transliteration

9§ … *šsꜣw bnwt-ḥmꜣ.ty ḥr ḳꜣbt.f ir ḫꜣ.k s n*

10§ *bnwt-ḥmꜣ.ty ḥr ḳꜣbt.f gmm.k skd.n.sn ḥr*

11§ *ḳꜣbt.f ir di.k ḏrt.k ḥr ḳꜣbt.f ḥr bnwt iptf gmm.k sy*

12§ *ḳb.ti wrt n wnt srf nb im.s gmm sw ḏrt.k n šꜥ.*

13§ *n.sn n ir.n.sn mw n ḳmꜣ.n ꜥḥꜥ.w nw mw iw.sn*

14§ *ḥmꜣ.ty r ḏrt.k ḏd.in.k r.f ẖry bnwt-ḥmꜣ.ty mḥr ꜥḥꜣ.i*

15§ *ḥnꜥ n ẖt pw ir gm.k bnwt-ḥmꜣ.ty m ꜥt nbt nt*

16§ *s ḫꜣ.k sw ḫft šsꜣw ipn ir bnwt-ḥmꜣ.ty ḥr ḳꜣbt.f*

17§ *wnn šfwt pw ḥr ḳꜣbt.f wr sš rwḏ dmit n.sn mi*

18§ *dmit ḥmꜣ n wt twt n ḥmꜣyt wꜣḏt wnn.s rwḏ.ti*

19§ *ḳb.ti r-ẖr ḏrt.k mi dmit n nꜣ n šfwt nty ḥr ḳꜣbt.f*

Translation

Title:

Necessary knowledge and skills for spherical masses on his chest:

Examination:

If you should examine a man for spherical masses on his chest,

How you find (is): they having spread on his chest,

and, if you put your hand on his chest, on those masses, (how) you find it (the chest) is very cool, there being no heat at all within it,

and how your hand finds it (is): they not being(?) granular,

neither can they make fluid, nor generate secretions of water,

while they are ball-like to your hand,

Diagnosis:

then you are to say about him: "One who has ball-like masses:

a medical condition I will fight with."

Treatment:

It is nothing/There is no treatment/remedy.

If you find ball-like masses in any bodily part of a man, you should examine him according to these instructions.

Case #45 - Explanation:

As for "ball-like masses on his chest,"

it means, how the swellings on his chest are (is): large, spread out, and hard,

touching them being like touching a ball of bandages, similar to a green fenugreek pea, which is firm and cool under your hand, like

touching these/the swellings that are on his chest.

Notes

gmm.k (first occurrence) – Either an unusual pregnant use of *gmi*, or else an omitted object, *gmm.k* <*sn*> or *gmm.k* <*st*>

sḳd.n.sn – Circumstantial *sḏm.n.f*

n wnt – Existential negation. Hoch notes that existential *nn* can introduce either a main or circumstantial clause and *nn wn* always introduces a main clause (*MEG*, sec. 103); he does not specify whether *n wnt* can be used circumstantially, but Doret (*Narrative Verbal System*, 28 with note 150, also p. 37) describes a somewhat complicated situation. Satzinger considers clauses with *n wnt* subordinate, but Gunn considers them main clauses. Doret states that in Old Egyptian, the circumstantial existential negation is *ny wnt* and gives an example from *Urk.* 1:42. In Middle Egyptian, the explicitly circumstantial negation that corresponds to Old Egyptian *ny* is *n-is*, but on the theory that some examples of Middle Egyptian *n* can be descended from Old Egyptian *ny*, we think that there can be some flexibility in the understanding of *n wnt*, and that this can resolve or reconcile the apparent contradictions between the positions of Satzinger and Gunn. Thus we are taking this clause as a circumstantial. In our extensive study of negative existential constructions, we have not encountered *n-is wnt* as a circumstantial counterpart to *n wnt*.

n šꜥ.n.sn – This form is not listed by Doret (*Narrative Verbal System*, 68, 151) among those that are attested as the adverbial complement or adjunct to a nominal *sḏm.f* or *sḏm.n.f*, but there seems no straightforward alternative in this instance. Hoch accepts a broad ambivalence or bivalence of *n sḏm.n.f*, stating (*MEG*, sec. 108), "As with the other negated clauses, these may be either main or subordinate. When this construction occurs in past time contexts, it is almost always in a circumstantial clause." Despite Hoch's reference to past contexts, which I do not think is very applicable to this passage, I do not think that *n sḏm.n.f* expresses a past tense or anteriority.

ḳmꜣ.n – An elliptical construction for the expected *ḳmꜣ.n.sn*, but one which is paralleled, see Gardiner, *EG*[3], sec. 486.

iw.sn – *iw* + suffix-pronoun is ambivalent, with both independent and circumstantial meaning, as noted earlier.

ir gm.k – This is the true protasis form, not *gmm.k*.

wnn šfwt pw… – Nominal *sḏm.f* of *wnn*, "it means, how the swellings… . are (is)…"

wr, etc. – statives. *rwd* is a possible normal variant and I would hesitate to call it an abbreviated writing.

dmit n.sn … – Nominal (infinitival phrase) + prepositional phrase, not introduced by *iw*; this is a circumstantial, not an independent clause. For *dmi* construed with the preposition *n*, see *Grundriss* 7, 2:979.

wnn.s … – Circumstantial *sḏm.f* of *wnn* as an indefinite or unmarked relative after the indefinite antecedent *ḥmꜣyt wꜣḏt*.

nꜣ n šfwt nty ḥr ḳꜣbt.f – *nty* introduces a marked relative clause modifying the definite antecedent *nꜣ n šfwt*. *nꜣ n* "these" can probably already be understood as the definite article "the" (Gardiner, *EG*[3], sec. 112, "already before Dyn. XVIII").

Though I think that the syntactic patterns can be accommodated in a Standard Theory model, some of the examples in this case can be seen as pushing the limits of Polotsky's syntax more than previous cases, or as entering a gray area.

Medical Commentary

Type of Injury

The chest masses described in Case #45 are:

- Multiple in number
- Widespread in the chest, but can occur elsewhere at any body part
- Their shape is round, ball-like (like a ball of bandages)
- Their consistence is firm, hard
- They are not hot to the touch, or produce heat inside
- They do not make fluid
- They do not produce a secretion
- They are shaped like a fenugreek pea (slightly pear-shaped)

From the physical and behavioral characteristics of these masses, we can eliminate common bacterial abscesses, tubercular, actinomycotic, or fungal abscesses.

Bacterial abscesses are hot. Tuberculous abscesses are usually single, cold, soft, and their size varies from a small olive to a large mass filled with purulent content. The abscess eventually ruptures externally, leaving an open sinus tract.

Cutaneous Actinomycosis, a chronic granulomatous infection caused by *Actinomyces israelli* (a gram-positive microaerophilic bacterium), would be manifested by nodular, erythematous (reddish) swollen lesions that eventually drain into fistulae, yielding "sulfur"-colored granules. We cannot find an acceptable clinical correlation to the negative finding in the examination section of this case: "they not being(?) granular." unless it refers to the lack of presence of "sulfur"-colored granules in an actinomycotic abscess.

Sporotrichosis is a fungal infection caused by *Sporothrix schenckii.* It usually infects the skin but also grows along lymph nodes and vessels. It produces multiple nodular, skin lesions, that as they enlarge would resemble abscesses, and later rupture leaving chronic ulcerations. Nocardiosis[278] is an infection produced by Nocardia asteroides genus, a filamentous gram positive bacteria that can produce systemic infections, with a cutaneous form in 10 percent of such cases. It presents as firm, tender, and warm subcutaneous nodules that later become movable, compressible, and eventually ulcerate.

Less easily mistaken for the masses described in Case #45 are lipomas, parasitic cysts, tuberous sclerosis, and cutaneous tuberculosis, each of which lack several of the qualities attached to these masses.

The characteristics of the multiple masses in Case #45 distinguish them from the above entities, and suggest the likelihood of their being of neoplastic origin. Benign tumors would be more likely than malignant, because there is in our case no evidence of ulcerations or of hemorrhage. Benign multiple neoplasms such as neurofibromas present in von Recklinghausen's disease/Neurofibromatosis 1 (NF1) need to be considered.

Neurofibromas are nerve sheath tumors that can develop in the skin, subcutaneously, anywhere along peripheral nerve fibers. NF1 is a very common autosomal genetic disorder with an incidence of 1:3000–4000 people,[279] affecting all ethnic groups. On genetic basis Nicola K. Ragge[280] proposes that NF-1 is an ancient disease. NF1 originates from a genetic mutation, or translocation from the centromeric region of the long arm of chromosome 17,[281] at band 17q11.2.[282] The NF1 gene mutation rate is very high and has penetrance of 100 percent. Cutaneous and subcutaneous neurofibromas can be from a few to several thousand and generally continue to develop throughout the patient's life. Most neurofibromas are benign, but cause various degrees of damage to the nerves themselves and to adjacent structures. Neurofibromas also occur in the intraspinal and the intracranial space and affect the cardiovascular, gastrointestinal, musculo-skeletal, endocrine, and central nervous systems. Although NF1 is a disorder that may affect any organ in the body, its cutaneous visible features are the most apparent. "Caffe-au-lait spots"[283] are associated with the Neurofibromatosis 1 syndrome and today are part of our diagnostic criteria for NF1. Tumors in Neurofibromatosis 1 are benign neoplasms, with only 5 percent turning malignant.

Although not all skin lesions or symptoms of NF1 systemic involvement are recorded in this case, it remains the strongest diagnostic entity to be considered in Case #45. Neurofibromas are indeed multiple, widespread, can occur at any bodily part, their shape is mostly round or ovoid, they can be firm or hard, they are not hot to the touch, they do not make fluid, or generate secretion.

There is no cure today for NF1, but tumors can be removed if the masses are rapidly growing, become painful, or produce weakness or numbness. Microsurgical procedures are carried out under electrophysiological intraoperative monitoring to assess the nerve status in real time, providing invaluable input to the surgeon as the tumor resection proceeds.

I conclude that Case #45 is most likely Neurofibromatosis NF1.

---

278. "Nocardiosis." Online: http://www.dermaamin.com/site/atlas-of-dermatology/13-n/1010-nocardiosis-.html.

279. A. N. Khan and I. Turnbull, "Neurofibromatosis Type 1 Imaging." Medscape Reference: http://emedicine.medscape.com/article/342500-overview.

280. N. K. Ragge and F. L. Munier, "Ancient Neurofibromatosis," *Nature* 368 (1994): 815. Online: http://ghr.nlm.nih.gov/condition/neurofibromatosis-type-1.

281. "Neurofibromatosis." Online: http://ghr.nlm.nih.gov/condition/neurofibromatosis-type-1.

282. "NF1." Genetics Home Reference. Online: http://ghr.nlm.nih.gov/gene/NF1.

283. Term referring to skin light-brown discoloration, usually present as birthmarks, often seen as part of the Neurofibromatosis F1 syndrome.

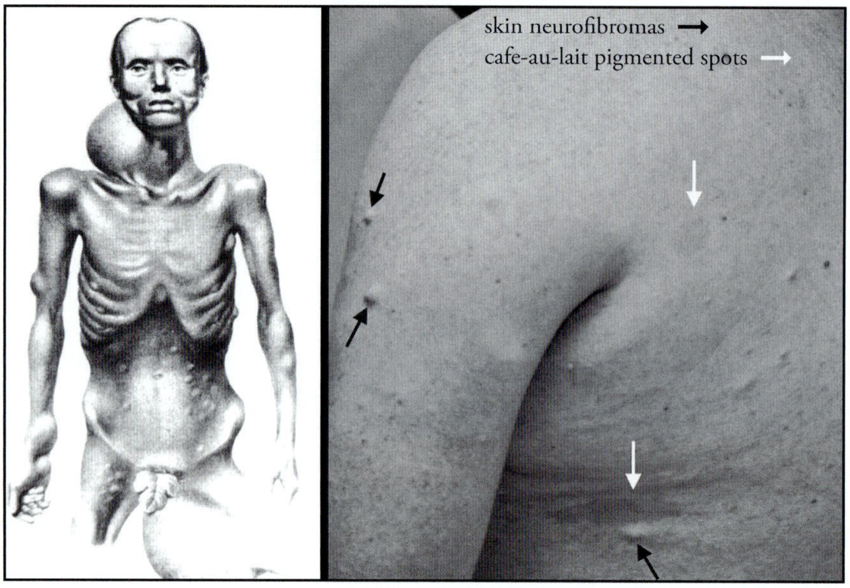

Fig. 40. Left: From Robert William Smith, *A Treatise on the Pathology, Diagnosis and Treatment of Neuroma* (Dublin: Hodges & Smith, 1848), plate 1. Right: Skin neurofibromas and "caffe-au-lait spots" in neurofibromatosis 1.

Ancient Medical Methodology and Knowledge

The ancient Egyptian physicians give precise features of identification of the masses in Case #45 differentiating these from masses associated with infection, such as in Cases #39 and #41. Case #45 relates to multiple tumors. It is of interest that once arrived to the diagnosis, the ancient physician declares his intention to fight with the medical condition, but his treatment segment states: "It is nothing/there is no treatment/remedy." He did not use the verdict "a medical condition that cannot be handled/dealt with." This could be interpreted as his understanding that the condition is best managed by "no treatment."

This puzzling situation in Case #45 is reminiscent of the treatment warning pronounced in Ebers Papyrus #873, a situation that refers to ball-like tumors of the *mtw*, probably neurofibromas,[284] where the treatment states: *imi.k wḏy ꜥ r mitt nw pw iꜣt ꜥt m-ꜥ.f*, "Don't you strike a hand against the like of it, this is the injury of a body part by means of it." Similarly, in Ebers #876, in the surgical treatment consisting of cauterization of varicose or arteriovenous fistulas, a warning is issued to the surgeon in case he encounters lesions resembling those in #873: "Don't you strike a hand against the like of any of these, it means 'head to the ground.'" Injury to the nerves would have resulted in severe pain and further compromise of neurological function, to leave these alone would be most logical. The parallel of this recommendation "not to treat" is also consistent with Case #45 as a case of Neurofibromatosis 1.

Finally, we need to observe that the ancient Egyptian physician recommended: "If you find ball-like masses in any bodily part of a man, you should examine him according to these instructions." This indicates that the physician must examine the patient with consideration of the characteristics described in order to reach a differential diagnosis and to determine if there should be any treatment given for ball-like masses.

284. Gonzalo M. Sanchez and T. Siuda, "Ebers Papyrus Case #873 - A Probable Case of Neurofibromatosis," *The South Dakota Journal of Medicine* 55/12 (2000): 529–35. (A misunderstanding of this article occurred in Paula Veiga, *Oncology and Infectious Diseases in Ancient Egypt: The Ebers Papyrus' Treatise on Tumors 857–877 and the Cases Found in Ancient Egyptian Human Material* [Saarbrücken: Müller, 2009], 37).

CASE #46:
Possible Keratinous/Epidermoid Cyst of the Chest
(Plate XV:20–XVI:16)

Courtesy New York Academy of Medicine.

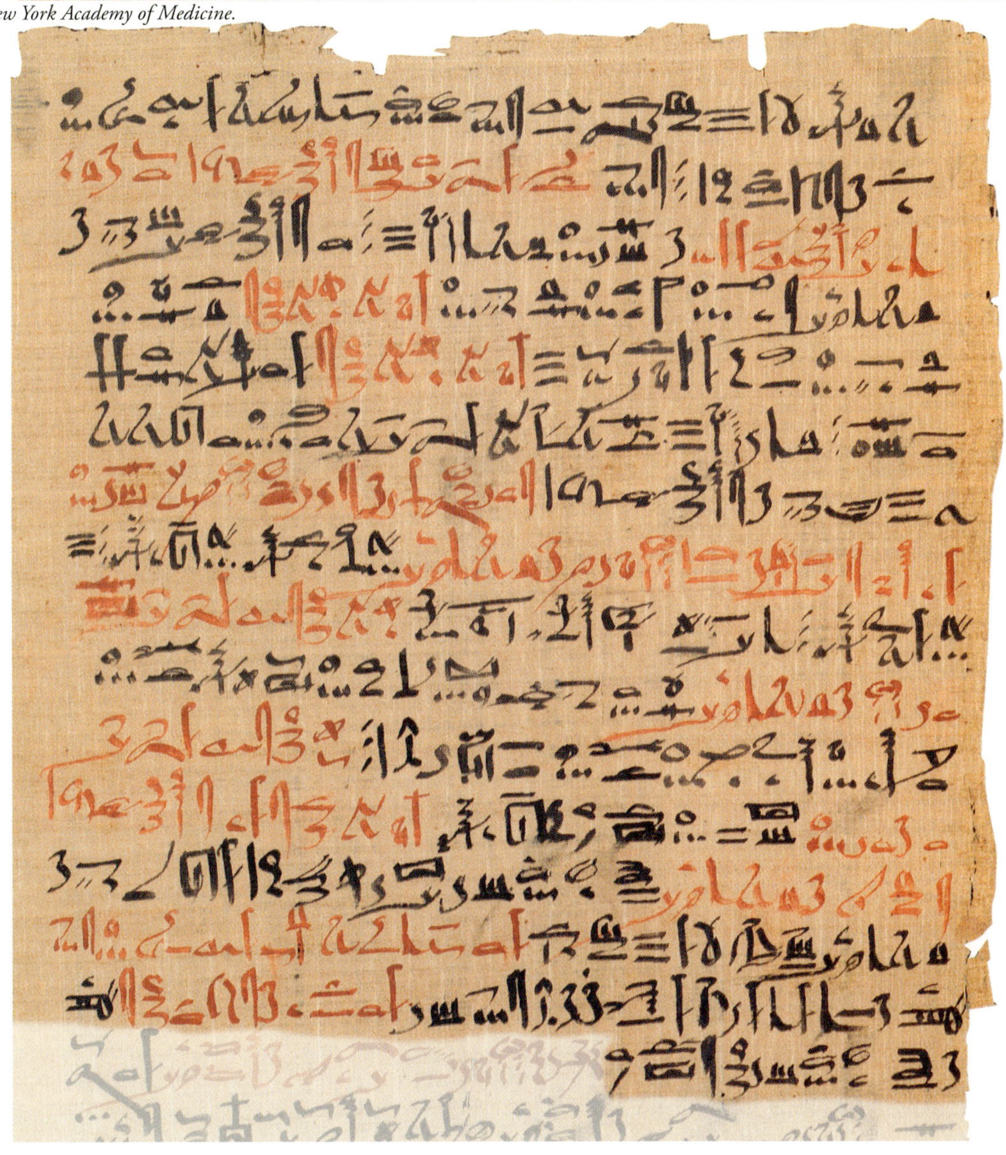

20. 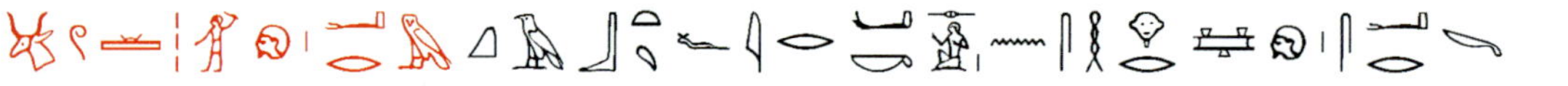

21. 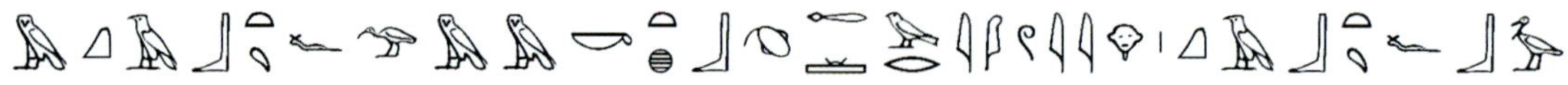

1. 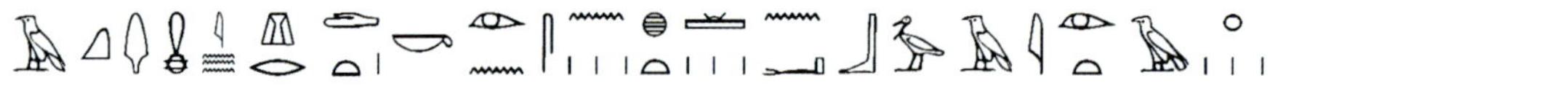

2. 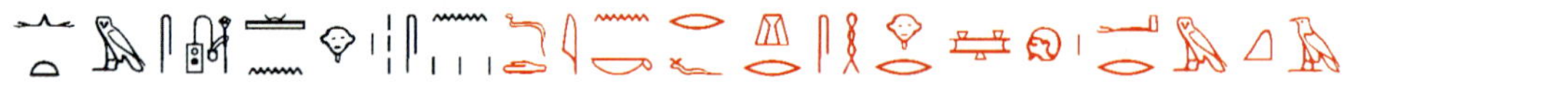

3. 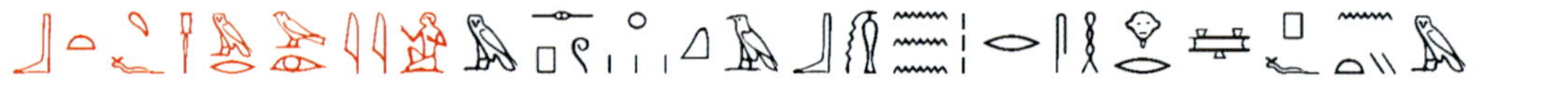

4. 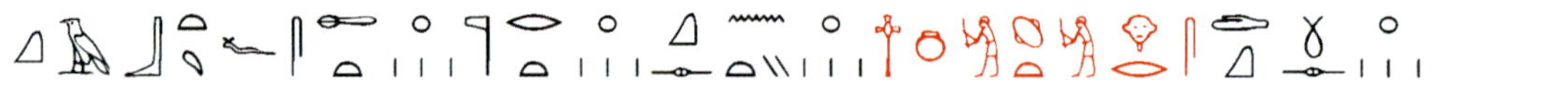

5. 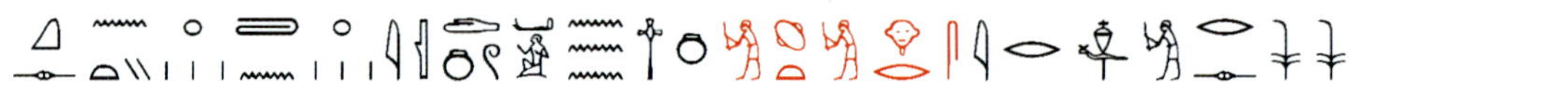

6. 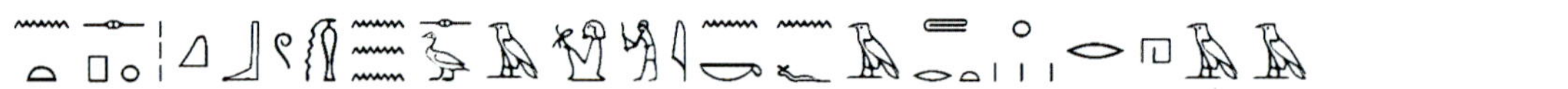

7. 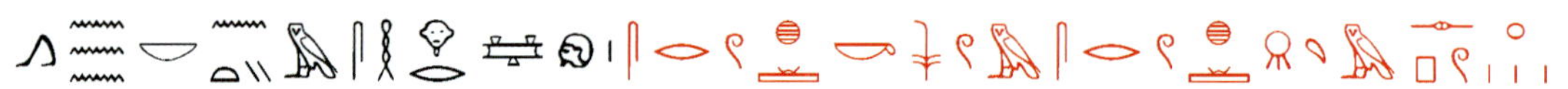

8. 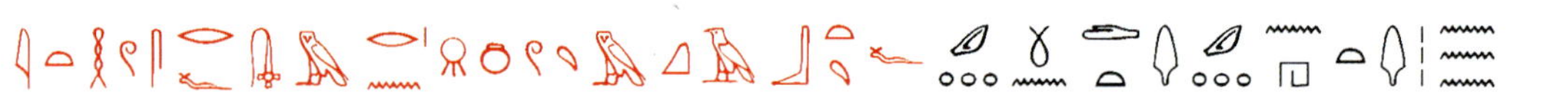

9. 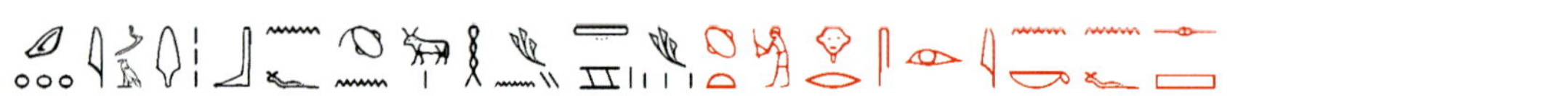

10. 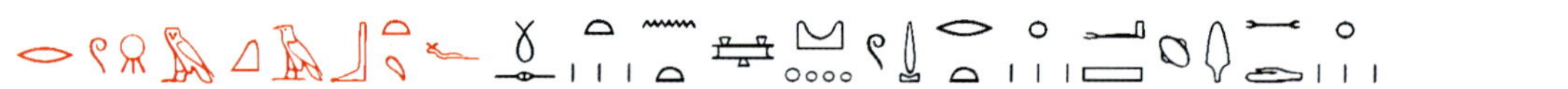

11. 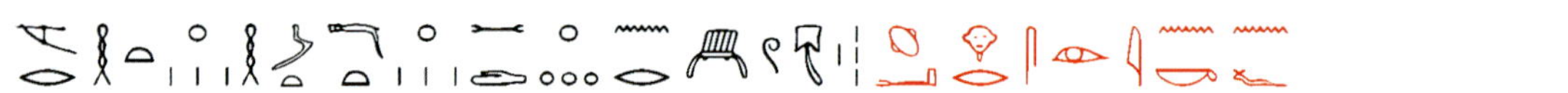

12. 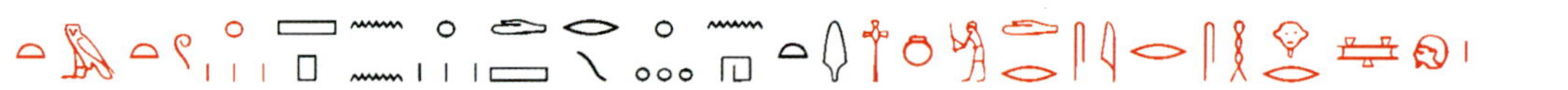

13. 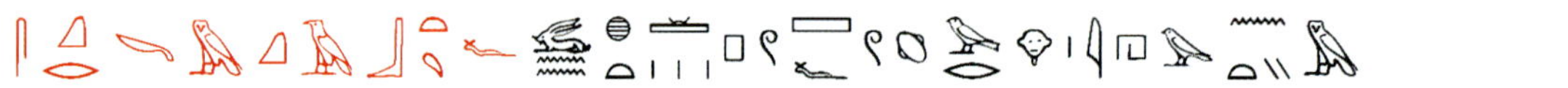

14. 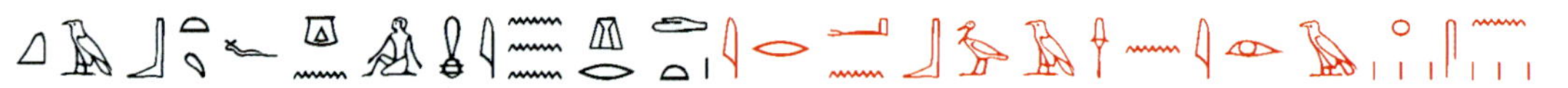

15. 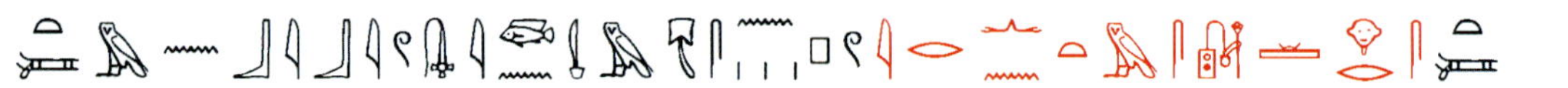

16. 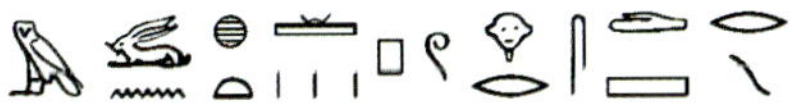

Transliteration

20§ *šsꜣw sḥr tp <s> ꜥr m ḳꜣbt.f ir ḫꜣ.k s n sḥr tp sꜥr*

21§ *m ḳꜣbt.f gmm.k ṯḫb ꜥꜣ wr išwy ḥr ḳꜣbt.f bꜣḳ*

1§ *mi mw ẖr ḏrt.k ir.n.sn ḫt n ꜥbꜣ irtyw*

2§ *n tms ḥrw.sn ḏd.in.k r.f ẖr<y> sḥr tp ꜥr m*

3§ *ḳꜣbt.f mḥr iry.i m spw ḳbw r sḥr pf nty m*

4§ *ḳꜣbt.f sẖt nṯrt ḳsnty nḏ wt ḥr.s dḳ šs*

5§ *ḳsnty dbn iḳdw mw nḏ wt ḥr.s ir ḫsf r.s nn nt*

6§ *spw ḳbw sꜣ.in.k nfꜣ pẖrt r hꜣꜣ*

7§ *mw nb nty m sḥr tp srwḫ.k sw m srwḫ wbnw m spw*

8§ *itḥ srf m rꜣ n wbnw m ḳꜣbt.f ḏrḏw šnḏt ḏrḏw nht mw*

9§ *ḏrḏw imꜣw bnf n iwꜣ ḥni-tꜣ wt ḥr.s ir.in.k n.f sšrw*

10§ *n wbnw m ḳꜣbt.f šst nt wꜣḏw ḏꜣrt ꜥš ꜥḏ*

11§ *mrḥt ḥmꜣt ꜥḏ nrꜣww wt ḥr.s ir.in.k n.f*

12§ *tmtw špnn dšr nht nḏ dr.s ir sḥr tp*

13§ *sḳr m ḳꜣbt.f wnn ḫt pw šfw wr ḥr ih nty m*

14§ *ḳꜣbt.f gn mi mw ẖr drt. ir n ꜥbꜣ n irtyw.sn*

15§ *tm nbibi.w inm.sn pw ir nn tms ḥr.s tm*

16§ *wn ḫt pw ḥr.s dšr*

Translation

Uncomplicated

Title:

Necessary knowledge and skills for a cyst (with) a head, which has arisen in his chest.

Examination:

If you should examine a man for a cyst which is caused to arise/stricken/inflicted(?) in his chest,

how you find the swelling (is): very large, protruding on his chest, being oily like fluid under your hand,

they having made something clammy/shiny(?) of nature/coloring/surface appearance,

and their faces cannot be ruddy,

Diagnosis:

then you are to say about him: “One who has a cyst (with) a head, arisen in his chest.

a medical condition which I will handle/deal with,

Treatment:

with cooling medicines for that cyst that is in his chest.”

sẖt seeds, natron, and *ḳsnty* mineral,

grind. Bandage (along) with it.

Calcite powder, *ḳsnty* mineral, builder’s mortar, and water,

grind. Bandage (along) with it.

Infected

Treatment:

If these cooling medications contend against it (?) (or, If these cooling medications are brought into contact with it?), you should delay (or restrain, or carefully avoid using) those prescriptions, until all the fluid which is in the abscess (with) the head descends,

and you should treat him with the wound treatment with medications for drawing out the heat from the mouth of a wound in his chest:

leaves of acacia, leaves of sycamore, water, leaves of *im3* trees, ox bile, and land rushes.

Bandage (along) with it.

Then you make him a desiccant <for the wound> in his chest:

powder of malachite, carob (seeds), fir (resin), grease, northern natron salt, and fat of ibexes.

Bandage (along) with it.

Then you make for him a powder of poppy, flax seeds, and sycamore.

Grind and apply to it.

Explanation A:

As for a cyst (with) a head stricken/inflicted(?) in his chest, it means: How the thing is (is) greatly swollen over the injury that is in his chest, being “soft,” like fluid under the hand.

Explanation B:

As for “shiny/clammy(?) of their nature/coloring/surface appearance,” it means that their skin is not hot.

Explanation C:

As for “there being no redness on it,” it means the things on it are not reddened.

Notes

sḥr tp – *tp* seems to be an attributive. It is probably most likely a genitival construction, "a mass of a head," but I have wondered very inconclusively whether it should be understood as an appositive, "a mass, (i.e.) a head/ peak."

ḳsnty mineral seems to be absent from Aufrère, *L'univers minéral dans la pensée égyptienne.*

ꜥr in the title can be understood either as an active participle or as a stative.

sꜥr – This can also be understood either as an active participle or a stative. The closest identifiable Egyptian etymology would seem to refer this to *sꜥr* "cause to arise or ascend" (Faulkner, *CDME*, 214). *Grundriss* 7, 2:721 lists the present writing of *sꜥr* with the general/uncertain category meaning "injury" (in brackets highlighting its generality and uncertainty). *Grundriss* notes that in the title only *ꜥr* appears, and that in the explanation, *sḳr* is used to describe or paraphrase *sꜥr. Grundriss* 7, 2:805–6 provides a cross-reference to *sḳr*. I am using an inclusive or compromise translation which is frankly tentative, "caused to arise/stricken/inflicted."

bꜣḳ is clearly a stative and part of the adverbial complement of the manner nominalization *gmm.k*.

ir.n.sn – Circumstantial *sḏm.n.f.*

n ꜥbꜣ or *nꜥbꜣ(?)* – First let us consider readings that would regard *n* and *ꜥbꜣ* as two separate words. *ẖt n ꜥbꜣ* can be taken as an attributive genitive construction. Explanation B is a little more difficult to reconcile with this; we would have to regard the scribe's citation as the attributive/adjectival segment *n ꜥbꜣ* whereas the entire phrase *ẖt n ꜥbꜣ* might be more expected, though this is inconclusive. *Grundriss* takes both of these occurrences as comprising two words, *n ꜥbꜣ* with the negative *n*. Especially in the examination, negative *n ꜥbꜣ irtyw* would have to be an *n sḏm.f* construction, a past negative, which makes less sense here, though in the explanation it would be *n sḏm.n.f*, which would be more understandable. If, on the other hand, *nꜥbꜣ* is taken as one word, as proposed by Breasted, it need not be merely an ad hoc reading or "shot in the dark," but can be explained as a derivation from *ꜥbꜣ* with the *n*-prefix, perhaps with an intensified meaning; for the *n*-prefix, out of an extensive literature an informative citation is Ward, *The Four Egyptian Homographic Roots B-3*, 19–21. My inclinations or suggestions for the meaning of *nꜥbꜣ* as a derivative of *ꜥbꜣ*, though they are tentative and do not involve any proof or rigorous demonstration, are as follows. (1) I think that the meaning "shiny, shininess" goes along with Breasted's "clamminess"—that is, moist with perspiration. (2) I think that this does not contradict the lack of redness (examination) or the lack of heat (explanation). There is an incongruity, also, in the prescription of agents to draw out heat from a wound and application of cooling medicines while the explanation states that heat is absent.

ir ḫsf... – The alternative in parentheses follows *Grundriss* 7, 2:786, in which case the verb form would be a passive *sḏmw.f*, which is also found as a nominal form and can thus follow *ir*. This passage is not entirely clear to me. The demonstrative phrase *nn n{t}* does not mean "those of the," but simply "those."

r hꜣꜣ mw – *r* + nominal *sḏm.f.*

tmtw – following *Grundriss* in understanding powder, not paste.

d + r + s – *d(w) r.s* "Apply to it."

wnn ẖt – Manner nominalization.

tm (both occurrences) – The negation of the manner nominalization (as distinguished from the negation of an adverbial complement or the negation of the nexus between the two; see Gilula, review of *Die negativen Konstruktionen im Alt- und Mittelägyptischen*, 212–13), or otherwise put, the manner nominalization of the negative verb *tm*.

I consider the rendition of this case to be one of the most, if not the most tentative or preliminary that I have undertaken so far. There are passages that are not clear to me even if I think that the words are identified correctly, and which I think will be affected by the medical implications of the translation. I have not gotten to the bottom of the lexicographical identification of a number of the ingredients. This will certainly be a continuing discussion.

Medical Commentary

Type of Injury

Case #46 describes an enlarging lesion in the soft tissues of the chest (Visual Index II) that has neither the characteristics of a tumor, or of a typical bacterial purulent abscess. Dr. Arno Luckhard (Breasted's medical consultant) considered the possibility of abscesses in the so-called cool category (*Edwin Smith*, 407), the *Grundriss* considers this lesion as some sort of a growth, and Dr. W. Benson Harer[285] suggested it to be an enlarged keratinous cyst, also known as epidermal cyst and sebaceous cyst. Based on the characteristics of this lesion, the authors concur with the diagnosis of an inflamed keratinous or epidermal cyst in Case #46. The second section of Case #46 seems to deal with the same entity being infected, we have subtitled it as Case #46b.

The lesion described in Case #46 has the following characteristics:

Physical:

- It has developed on an injury site on the chest: "a cyst (with) a head arisen in his chest"; "over the injury that is in his ... chest"; "As for a cyst (with) a head stricken/inflicted(?) in his chest"
- It is very large and protruding: "the thing is (is) greatly swollen"
- Its consistency is soft, "being oily like fluid under your hand"; "being 'soft' like fluid under the hand"
- "They having made something clammy/shiny(?) of nature/coloring/surface appearance," is further detailed in explanation B: "it means that their skin is not hot." (glowing? sebaceous cyst?; *Grundriss* 7, 1:456)
- "and their faces cannot be ruddy"

Therapeutic: It is first treated with "cooling medicines," and if it does not respond to treatment it needs to be treated as an abscess (Case #46b).

A keratinous or epidermoid cyst is a closed sac located below the surface of the skin that has a lining resembling the uppermost part of a hair follicle. Its appearance is as flesh-colored to yellowish, firm, round nodules of variable size. A central pore (called punctum) may be present, being obvious in the cyst's skin surface. A thick whitish material can sometimes be expressed through the punctum. Although it is difficult to reconcile fully all of the physical characteristics given in the description of the lesion in Case #46 with an epidermoid cyst, it is arguable that the examination statement "they having made something clammy/shiny of nature" refers to the whitish material forming the cyst. Explanation B relates the words "clammy/shiny" to the skin not being hot. Both bacterial abscesses and epidermoid cysts can be filled with whitish-appearing material. A bacterial abscess is filled with pus, and its skin is red and hot. An epidermoid cyst cheesey content material is also white, but its covering skin is not hot, though it can appear shiny as it is being stretched. Moreover, an Epidermoid cyst can become secondarily infected. A keratinous or epidermal cyst may form after skin trauma, particularly after crushing injuries. "A sac of cells is created into which a protein called keratin is secreted."

The word *sḫr* is characterized by *Grundriss* (7, 2:786) as: "The morbid appearance on an injury." On palpation a keratinous cyst is usually soft, nontender, movable, and painless. The cyst being filled with semi-solid, cheese-like material could be compared to the feeling of a rubber or leather bag that has been filled with oil. Upon discharge, this grayish-white material is foul smelling.

Keratinous cysts usually do not interfere with daily activities unless they become large and inflamed, or infected. In that case, the cyst should be surgically excised. If the cyst is inflamed, but small, today, some physi-

285. Personal discussion with Dr. W. Benson Harer during his critical review of this manuscript. 10/16/2008.

cians would first inject it with steroids to reduce the swelling. But, if acute inflammation is present and the cyst is large, it may be initially treated by drainage, then by complete excision.

The entire cyst wall and punctum need to be removed, or the lesion may recur. Although at this stage a keratinous cyst may be infected, this does not have to be so to show acute inflammation if it is large enough and has often being bruised, squeezed, or irritated because of its anatomical location in the body. Once surgical treatment is undertaken, antibiotic coverage is obligatory.

Once the cyst has become acutely inflamed or it is infected, surgical drainage and excision are necessary.

Ancient Medical Methodology and Knowledge

The Egyptian physician gives key clinical features to indicate the nature of this lesion, which we believe are consistent with the diagnosis of a keratinous or epidermal cyst, such as: "they having made something clammy/shiny(?) of nature/coloring/surface appearance." As noted in the previous section, it is uncertain if the ancient Egyptian physician is referring to the stretched skin covering the cyst, or to the cyst's contents. Distended skin over the cyst could be characterized as appearing shiny, although lack of redness "on their faces" indicates there are no signs of acute infection.

The initial treatment is by using cooling medications, which is concordant with the treatment of a large, inflamed cyst, not necessarily hot or clearly infected. The field of ancient pharmacology is now being systematically studied, primarily by the KNH Centre for Biomedical Egyptology, University of Manchester, directed by A.R. David.[286] At this stage, however, the identification of some ingredients is uncertain and assessments of the effectiveness of the remedies listed in this document remain limited and conjectural.

In contrast with Case #41, at the start of this case we do not have clear evidence of infection. The prescription is to use "cooling" medicines over the large mass. Initially the mix consists of natron, as a powerful dehydrating and anti-inflammatory agent, used to reduce swelling, *s̱ḫt* seeds (apparently a type of barley)[287] and *ḳsnty* (analgesic?), which is an unknown mineral. The latter two ingredients are still unknown. Next to be used on the wound is a mix of builder's mortar,[288] calcite powder, water, and *ḳsnty* mineral. This combination has antimicrobial properties with the formation of calcium hydroxide. The mechanism of action is related to the effect of high pH on bacterial cytoplasmic membrane, producing chemical injury to organic components and transport mechanisms. According to Estrela, et al. these effects were similar on aerobic, anaerobic, Gram-positive and Gram-negative bacteria.[289] Calcite powder is also a sclerotic agent that induces a local inflammatory response, leading to a fibrotic process. The above medications are primarily intended to reduce the bulk of the mass/cyst. Potential benefit from the initial treatment of the ancient Egyptian's "cooling medications" is related to the dehydrating and anti-inflammatory topical agents with antiseptic properties within the ingredients. It is easy to defend their use in treatment of an enlarging, painful cyst, whether or not it is hot.

Once it is determined that there is resistance to these medications, with the implication of this mass/cyst being infected (Case #46b) the treatment protocol requires drainage of the mass and pharmacologically changes to one similar to the treatment for an infected chest wound in Case #41.

286. A. R. David, "The Pharmacy in Ancient Egypt Project at the KHN Centre for Biomedical Egyptology," in Cockitt and David, *Pharmacy and Medicine in Ancient Egypt*, 1–5.

287. R. Germer, *Handbuch der altägyptischen Heilpflanzen*, 122.

288. Lucas, *Ancient Egyptian Materials and Industries*, 534, identifies the principal componenets of ancient Egyptian gypsum mortar as gypsum sand (Hydrated calcium sulphate), calcium carbonate, magnesium carbonate, and oxides of aluminum and iron.

289. C. Estrela, J. D. Pecora, M. D. Souza-Neto, C. R. Estrela, L. L. Bammann, "Effect of Vehicle on Antimicrobial Properties of Calcium Hydroxide Pastes," *Brazilian Dental Journal* 10/2 (1999): 63–72. Online: http://www.ncbi.nlm.nih.gov/pubmed/10863391.

The topical prescriptions, with their specific purposes are to be used sequentially. The first purpose is to draw out the heat from the mouth of the wound, then to desiccate it.

For drawing out the heat from the mouth of the wound, the prescription includes a mixture of anesthetic (sycamore leaves[290]), antimicrobial (leaves of *im3* tree[291] and ox bile[292]), an astringent and demulcent (acacia leaves[293]), and mixed with land rushes.

Lastly, astringent medications were applied over the opened and drained cyst to desiccate the wound. This prescription calls for malachite powder (a powerful antimicrobial[294]), northern salt, and carob seeds (strong astringent mix) with grease and fat of ibex. Then poultices with a mix of poppy[295] and sycamore leaves[296] (a powerful local analgesic/anesthetic) are applied and bandaged to the wound in powder form. The poppy seeds also have anti-inflammatory properties.

It is of interest to compare the treatment protocols in Cases #41 (an infected chest wound), and Case #46b, an infected keratinous cyst. Although not identical, the similarities of the substances used for "drawing the heat" in each case are striking.

	"Drawing the heat"	
from the open wound (Case #41)		**from the open cyst (Case #46)**
im3 tree leaves and ox bile	antimicrobials	*im3* tree leaves and ox bile
leaves of willow	analgesic	sycamore leaves
zizyphus leaves	astringent	acacia leaves
zizyphus leaves	demulcent	acacia leaves
ground rushes		land rushes
ḳsnty		water

For Drying/Desiccating the open wound/cyst the substances are practically identical.

290. An anesthetic comparable to Xylocaine; S. G. Zaku, F. A. Abdulrahaman, P. A. Onyeyili, O. C. Aguzue, and S. A. Thomas, "Photochemical Constituents and Effects of Aqueous Root-Bark Extract of *Ficus sycomorus* L. (Moracaea) on Muscular Relaxation, Anaesthetic and Sleeping Time on Laboratory Animals," *African Journal of Biotechnology* 8/21 (2009): 6004–6. Online: http://www.academicjournals.org/AJB/abstracts/abs2009/2Nov/Zaku%20et%20al.htm.

291. Aufrère, "Plants, Gardens and Horticulture"; Abdel-Sattar, et al. "Antimicrobial Activity of Extracts of Some Plants," 00. See also Maerua crassofolia Forssk Prelude Medicinal Plants Database. Online: http://www.africamuseum.be/collections/external/prelude/view_mu?id=225592.

292. Alan F. Hoffman and Lars Eckmann, "How Bile Acids Confer Gut Mucosal Protection against Bacteria," *Proceedings of the National Academy of Sciences of the United States of America* 103/12 (2006): 4333–34. Online: http://www.ncbi.nlm.nih.gov/pmc/articles/PMC1450168/. A. I. Prieto, F. Ramos-Morales, and J. Casadesus, "Bile-Induced DNA Damage in *Salmonella enterica*," *Genetics* 168 (2004): 1787–94. M. Begley, C. G. Gahan, and C. Hill, "The Interaction between Bacteria and Bile," *FEMS Microbiology Reviews* 29/4 (2005): 625–51. Online: http://www.ncbi.nlm.nih.gov/pubmed/16102595. Alan F. Hoffman and Lars Eckmann, "How Bile Acids Confer Gut Mucosal Protection against Bacteria," *Proceedings of the National Academy of Sciences of the United States of America* 103/12 (2006): 4333–34. Online: http://www.ncbi.nlm.nih.gov/pmc/articles/PMC1450168/.

293. An astringent and demulcent (soothing) that, by its viscidity, it covers and sheathes surfaces; "Acacia Nilotica," Botanical.com: http://www.botanical.com/botanical/mgmh/a/acaci006.html#med.

294. In addition to Guido Majno's malachite powder and bacterial growth research, there are numerous citations in the ancient literature on the use of copper compounds to prevent and treat infections. "Medical Uses of Copper in Antiquity" (Copper Development Association, Inc.: http://www.copper.org/publications/newsletters/innovations/2000/06/medicine-chest.html) cites the Greeks sprinkling copper oxide and copper sulfate powder on fresh wounds to prevent infection. And in more recent times, there is reference to the fact that copper workers in Paris were immune to the cholera epidemics of 1832, 1849, and 1852.

295. M. Krajnik, Z. Zylicz, F. Finlay, J. Luckza, A. A. van Sorge, "Potential Use of Topical Opioids in Palliative Care Report of 6 Cases," *Pain* 80 (1999): 121–25.

296. Zaku, et al., "Photochemical Constituents and Effects of Aqueous Root-Bark Extract," 6004–6.

Drying the wound Case #41		**Desiccating the open cyst Case #46**
malachite powder	antibacterial	malachite powder
frit	antibacterial	resin?
carob	astringent	carob
wšbt (alum?)	astringent – antiseptic	
poppy	analgesic	poppy
sycamore	anesthetic	sycamore
carob	demulcent	carob
fat of ibex	vehicle	fat of ibex
natron	osmotic	northern salt
poppy	anti-inflammatory	poppy

CASE #47:
A Slash Wound in the Armpit
(Plate XVI:16–XVII:15)

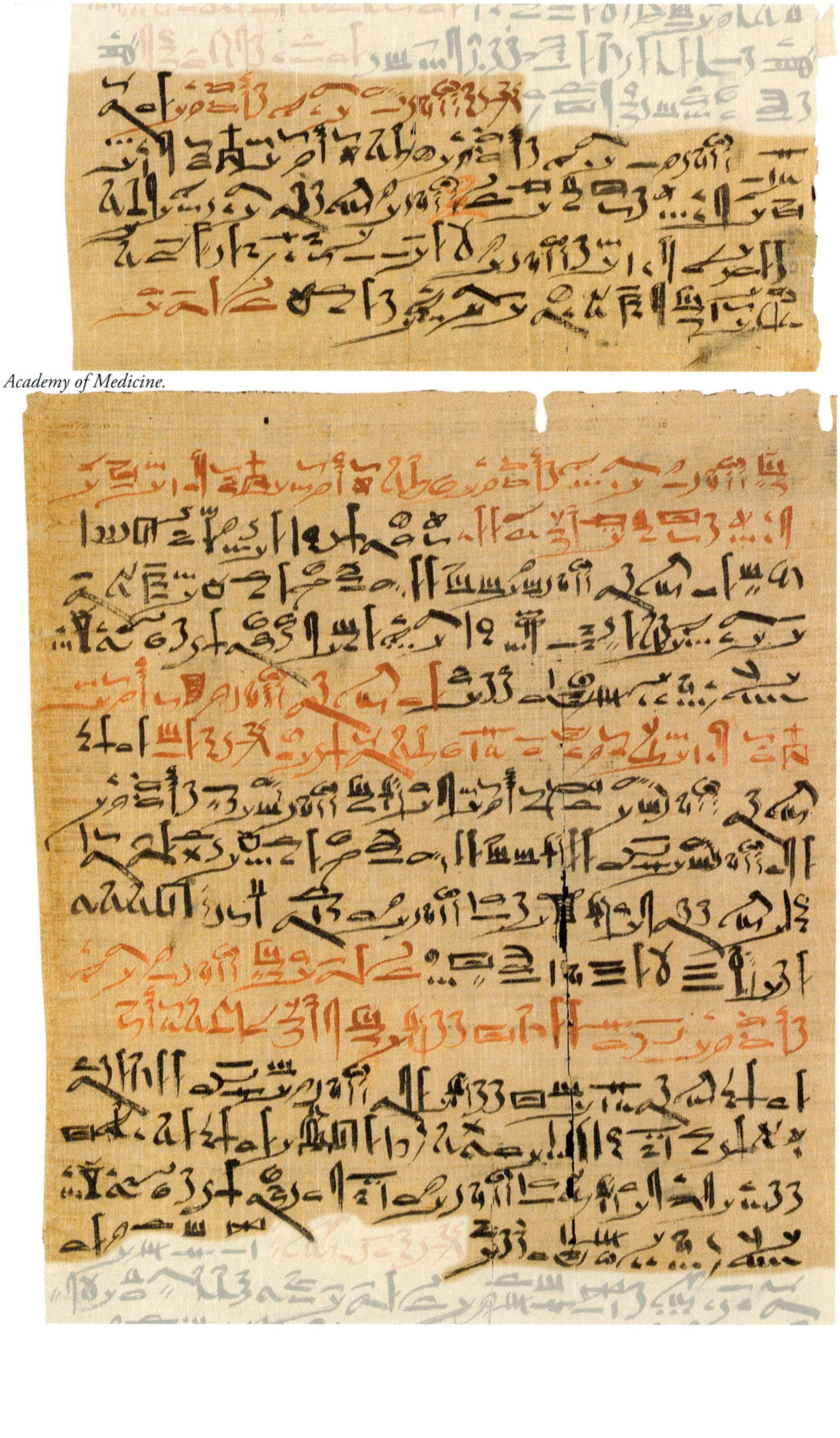

Courtesy New York Academy of Medicine.

16.
17.
18.
19.
20.
1.
2.
3.
4.
5.
6.
7.
8.
9.
10.
11.
12.
13.

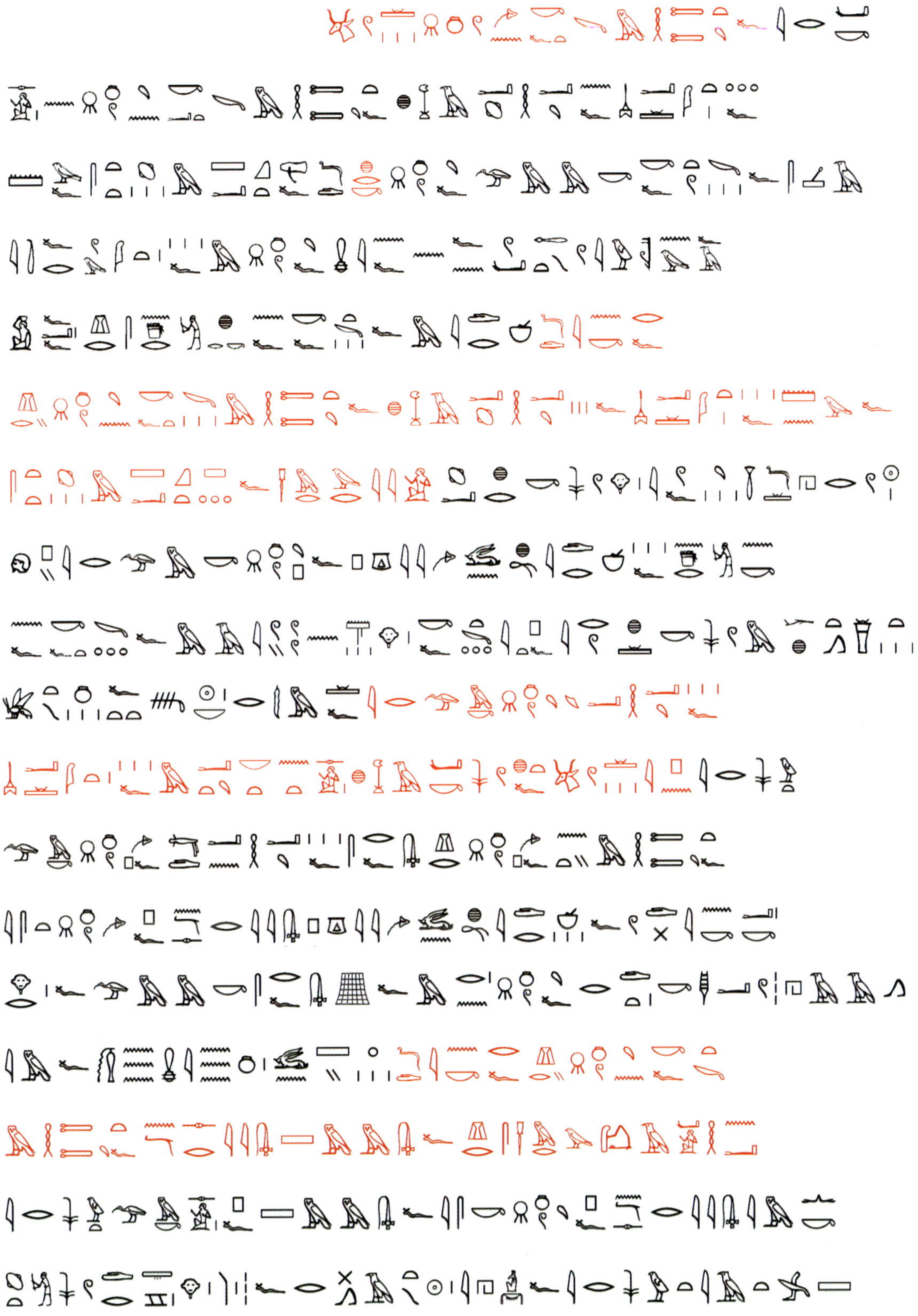

14. 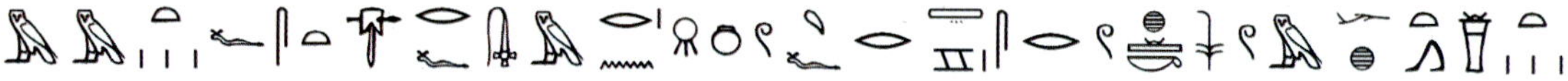

15. 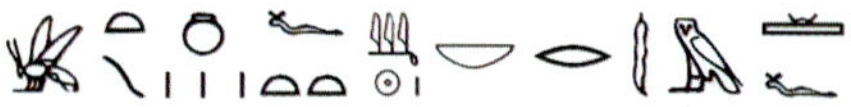

Transliteration

16§ … *šsꜣw wbnw-n-kft m ḥṯṯ.f ir ẖꜣ.k*
17§ *s n wbnw-n-kft m ḥṯṯ.f ḫꜣꜥ ḥꜥw.f wḏꜥ šwt.f*
18§ *mn.f stwt mšꜥḳt.f {ḏd.ḫr.k} <ḏꜥr.ḫr.k> wbnw.f gmm.k kfwt.f sꜣ.ti*
19§ *frw šwt.f m wbnw.f mi nfnfn ꜥꜣt iw ḳsn fꜣ.f*
20§ *ꜥ.f ẖr-s nḏr.ḫr.k n.f kft.f m idr ḏd.in.k r.f*
1§ *ẖry wbnw-n-kft m ḥṯṯ.f ḫꜣꜥ ḥꜥw.f wḏꜥ šwt.f mn.f*
2§ *stt m mšꜥḳt.f mḥr iry.i wt.ḫr.k sw ḥr iwf wꜣḏ hrw*
3§ *tpy ir gm.k wbnw pf pgy wnḫ idrw.f nḏr.<i>n.k*
4§ *n.f kft.f m ꜣiwy n ḥbsw ḥr kftw iptf srwḫ.k sw m-ḫt <m> mrḥt*
5§ *bit ftt rꜥ nb r nḏm.f ir gm.k wbnw-<n>-ḳrḏn ḫꜣꜥ ḥꜥw.f*
6§ *wḏꜥ šwt.f m ꜥt nbt nt s ẖꜣ.k sw ḫft šsꜣw ipn ir swt*
7§ *gm.k wbnw pf šd.n ḥꜥw.f srf ẖr wbnw pf nty m ḥṯṯ.f*
8§ *isṯ wbnw pf nsry pgy wnḫ idrw.f wd.in.k ꜥ.k*
9§ *ḥr.f gmm.k srf nš.f m rꜣ wbnw.f r ḏrt.k ꜥḥꜥ.w hꜣꜣ*
10§ *im.f ḳb mi mw wnšy ḏd.in.k r.f hry wbnw-n-kft*
11§ *m ḥṯṯ.f nsry šmm.f ẖr-s mḥr ꜥḥꜣ.i ḥnꜥ*
12§ *ir swt gm.k s pf šmm.f isk wbnw pf nsry im.k*
13§ *wt sw <w>d <sw> r tꜣ ḥr mniw.f r swꜣ ꜣt ih.f ir swt iꜣṯ*
14§ *šmmt.f st srf m rꜣ n wbnw.f r tꜣ srwḫ.k sw m-ḫt <m> mrḥt*
15§ *bit ftt rꜥ nb r nḏm.f*

Translation

Uncomplicated

Title:

Necessary knowledge and skills for a slash wound in his armpit:

Examination:

If you should examine a man for a slash wound in his armpit:

whose flesh has been laid back/flayed open, the side of whose rib cage has been severed, while he suffers from shooting pains in his shoulder blade,

{you have to say} <You should investigate> his wound.

How you find his slash wound(s?) (are): displaced so that he is weak/faint(?),

its sides (being) in his wound, even as how/the way a linen cloth is unrolled(?),

and it is painful when he raises his arm because of it,

you have to draw tight for him his slash wound(s?) with thread/stitching.

Diagnosis:

Then you are to say about him: One who has a slash wound in his armpit,

whose flesh has been laid back/flayed open, its sides have been severed,

while he suffers shooting pain in his shoulder blade—

a medical condition which I will handle/deal with.

Treatment:

You have to bandage it (along) with fresh meat the first day.

First Alternative Course: Wound Dehiscense

Examination:

If you find that wound opened up, its threads having been loosened,

Treatment:

you should draw together his slash wound(s?) for him with two cloth binding bandages on those slash wounds,

and you need to treat it/him afterward <with> ointment and honey and a dressing every day until he/it is well.

Treatment of similar wounds:

If you find a wound, his flesh having been removed/whose flesh has been removed and its sides have been severed, in any body part of a man, you should examine it/him according to these necessary knowledge and skills.

Second Alternative Course: Infected Wound

Examination:

If, however, you find that wound whose flesh has removed/taken(?) heat/fever under that wound which is in his armpit,

while that wound is inflamed-hot/infected and open,

its stitches/sutures having been loosened,

then you should lay your hand on it.

How you find the heat (is): flowing/issuing from the mouth of his wound into your hand,

the secretions that descend from it pouring out like grape juice,

Diagnosis:

then you are to say about him: "One who has a slash wound in his armpit, which is inflamed-hot/infected, he being febrile as a result of it—

a medical condition I will fight with."

Treatment:

If, however, you find that man being feverish, while that wound is inflamed-hot/infected, you should not bandage him/it.

Lay (him) down on his mooring post/bed until the critical period of his injury passes.

Third Alternative Course: Improving Wound Infection

Examination:

If, however, his fever abates(?), the heat shooting away/dissipating from the mouth of his wound to the ground (i.e., completely gone?),

Treatment:

you should treat it/him afterwards <with> ointment and honey and a dressing every day until it/he is well.

Notes

wbnw n kft – Can be understood as attributive genitive, see earlier notes.

ḫꜣꜥ(w) ḥꜥw.f wḏꜥ(w) šwt.f – I take these as parallel clauses. I identify them as passive *sḏmw.f* forms used as indefinite or unmarked relatives following the indefinite antecedent "a man."

mn.f – Circumstantial *sḏm.f.*

kft or *kfwt*(?) – I am very willing to entertain the possibility of the plural strokes or markers indicating multiple slash wounds, but I do not know whether a consistent understanding is possible, so I am using a question mark in the absence of clear grammatical agreement. Support is found in the form of the plural demonstrative *iptf* after one occurrence, "those slash wounds," where I do not use a question mark.

frw or *r fw*(?) – This is a crux; Breasted, who read *r fw*, remarked that the text is corrupt here. It seems impossible to get a clear meaning from the text as it stands. Neither *frw* nor *fw* is listed in *Grundriss* 7. Very tentatively, I suggest that what we have here is to be read *frw* and that *fr* + "evil bird" determinative is related to, or a variant of, *fn*, "to be weak, faint" (Faulkner, *CDME*, 98). Thus I propose to read this as a stative, which I take as a stative of result, "so that he is weak/faint." For possibly analogous alternation, see *knḥ* "dark," *knḥw* "darkness" (Faulkner, *CDME*, 286), *grḥ* "night" (Faulkner, *CDME*, 290), and *gng* as a variant of *grg* (Faulkner, *CDME*, 290).

šwt.f m wbnw.f – Circumstantial clause, not independent.

mi nfnfn ꜥꜣt – I take as *mi* + passive *sḏmw.f* as a nominal form. I use a question mark because Faulkner does (*CDME*, 131).

iw ḳsn(w) – *iw* + impersonal stative, see above.

f3.f – Circumstantial *sḏm.f.*

pgy wnḫ(w) idrw.f – stative and passive *sḏmw.f.*

ḫ3ᶜ – the blade + ayin, or strong-arm determinative without the stick, are a writing of *ḫ3ᶜ* "remove," as per *Grundriss* 7, 2:647, though in that font the blade sign is a little different. Cf. *Wb.* 3:227. The verb form here is a passive *sḏmw.f.*

šd.n ḥᶜw.f srf – Grammatically, despite the apparent graphic nature of the verb *šdi*, which can mean "cut out, remove etc.," it is extremely difficult and unlikely for the form to mean "whose flesh has been removed," because as a relative form, the sense of the verb would have to be active, not passive (cf. Gardiner, *EG*[3], sec. 388), and "his flesh" would have to be the subject of the *affirmative* sense of the verb, "whose flesh removes(?)," which is in fact how we have taken it. It is possible to rationalize the former sense by taking *šd* as a passive participle and the *n* + *ḥᶜw.f* as a qualifying noun construction (a topic I talk about in "Problems of Adjectival Constructions in Old and Middle Egyptian," sec. IV), but it is convoluted and not the natural way for such a sequence to be parsed; in effect it is a "long shot." Thus we follow *Grundriss* 7, 2:875 in taking *ḥᶜw* as the subject or actor-expression of the relative form. However, it is not at all clear how the verb *šdi* is to be understood here. Does it mean something like "whose flesh has absorbed fever?"

nsry pgy – Statives.

wnḫ(w) idrw.f – Passive *sḏmw.f.*

nš.f – Circumstantial *sḏm.f.*

h33 – Active participle.

ḳb(w) – Stative.

nsry – Stative.

šmm.f – Circumstantial *sḏm.f* (2ae gem. verb).

i3t (*i3ṯ*) – The *Grundriss* listing (7, 2:20) indicates sufficient uncertainty regarding the precise meaning that I think a question mark is called for.

r t3 – Some translators take this in the present context as "entirely" or similar, but I think a question mark is still called for.

Medical Commentary

Type of Injury

Case #47 is an extensive slash wound to the soft tissues of the chest wall inflicted from the side (Visual Index II, and fig. 41), probably with the arm in an elevated position, produced by a sword or axe thrust. The deep gash this patient sustained peeled off muscles from the rib cage and reached the shoulder blade: "whose flesh has been laid back/flayed open, the side of whose rib cage has been severed." The physical appearance of the slashed wound is graphically described: "its sides (being) in his wound, even as how/the way a linen cloth is unrolled(?)."

In this kind of wound, the affected chest wall and axillary muscles are the latissimus dorsi, the teres major, the rhomboid major, and the infraspinatus. Primary symptoms are pain and impairment of shoulder motion, particularly in extension, due to latissimus dorsi muscle injury. The brachial plexus and major axillary vessels could also be involved.

There are today approximately 300,000 cases of open chest wounds in the U.S. per year of which 70 percent penetrate into the cavity, posing a serious threat to life. Penetrating injuries to the chest cavity, which,

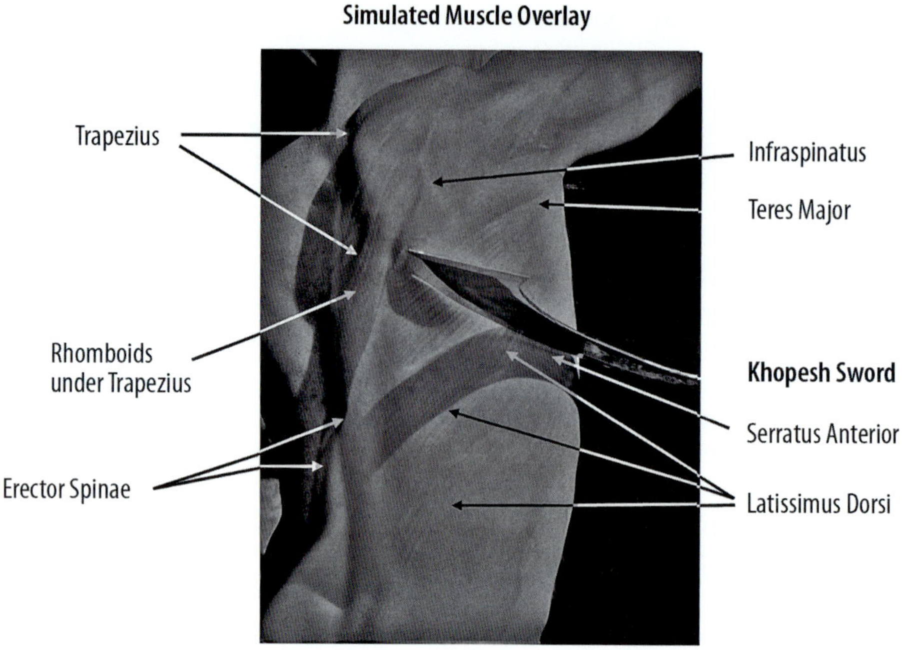

Fig. 41. Posterior lateral torso musculature slash wound.

from ancient times to the beginning of the First World War were almost inevitably fatal,[297] are not presented in the Edwin Smith Papyrus. Our Case #47 was considered by the ancient Egyptian physician to be a treatable injury.

The treatment today for superficial injuries to the chest wall that do not penetrate the chest cavity consists in thorough cleansing and debridement from all foreign matter and nonviable tissue with proper attention to major nerve or vascular structure involvement. The wound would be closed in layers with temporary drains, which are often left in the wound for a few days. If the wounds are grossly infected, or the patient is over twelve hours from his injury, the wound may be left open for five to seven days and closed then, or may be allowed to heal by secondary intention.[298] All of these patients require coverage with broad spectrum antibiotics. Tetanus toxoid is given if it has been over ten years from the last booster tetanus shot.

The alternative courses given in Cases #47b, c, and d, respectively, relate to wound dehiscence, wound infection, and wound inflammation without development of infection. The potential for wound complications are related to tissue trauma, incomplete tissue layer apposition, wound closure technique, and materials used.[299] Wound infection is the most common complication of laceration repair due to accidental introduction of bacteria at the time of trauma and/or the length of time before wound repair. R. F. Eldich, et. al. have established that 100,000 bacteria per gram of tissue (105) constitute an infective inoculation and that wounds over five hours

297. Survival examples of chest-penetrating injuries in antiquity cited by Salazar refer to Alexander the Great's surviving his most serious wound sustained in India, 326 and the story of Gorgias's who was shot in the lung, "still carrying the arrowhead in his chest a year and a half later." In Salazar, *The Treatment of War Wounds in Graeco-Roman Antiquity*," 13–14. Another reference to survivors of penetrating chest injuries is in "Coan Prenotions, Lungs 422," *Hippocrates* (vol. 9; ed. and trans. Paul Potter; LCL 509; Cambridge, MA: Harvard University Press, 2010), 209. It refers to wounded individuals who later developed empyemas.

298. To heal by secondary intention means to allow the wound to heal by granulation tissue from depth to surface.

299. Trott, *Wounds and Lacerations*, 297–33.

old grew >10^6 bacteria per gram of tissue (cited by Trott).[300] Today the treatment of an infected wound involves removal of all the suture material, drainage, wound irrigation, and exploration for foreign materials. The patient would receive appropriate antibiotic therapy and the wound would be cleansed daily and covered with sterile gauze. Afterwards, the wound is allowed to close by secondary intention. Cosmetically important body areas would likely require plastic surgery once the infection is cleared.[301]

Ancient Medical Methodology and Knowledge

This type of injury would have most likely occurred in war. The Edwin Smith Papyrus most surely was used as a text by the military physicians known to be attached to combat units. The type of weapons in ancient Egypt capable of producing an injury as in Case #47 would have primarily included the khopesh sword (fig. 41), and the broad-bladed axe (Visual Index III).

In addition to a detailed description of the wound, the physician singles out the symptom of pain produced by arm motion:[302] "and it is painful when he raises his arm because of it." The extensive soft-tissue chest-wall traumatic separation considered in Case #47a, would have been accompanied by considerable blood loss and pain, easily explaining the patient's faintness from hypovolemic shock. Concern over major blood loss would prompt immediate wound closure following the examination. After the wound was sutured, fresh meat dressings were applied the first day and held in place with bandages. The prognosis: "a medical condition which I will handle/deal with" reflects the ancient physician's confidence in successfully treating an uncomplicated thoracic-wall slash wound.

Case #47 includes three possible clinical courses. Case #47b is wound dehiscence where the stitches have become loose and the slashed area has reopened. The second clinical course, Case #47c, is one in which the wound has developed infection. The third course, Case #47d, is one in which a wound that had some possible signs of infection, has actually improved. The appropriate treatments are prescribed for each of these eventualities.

Simple wound dehiscence in Case #47b could result from tissue swelling, serous or bloody fluid collections. Excessive tissue tension by improper suturing technique produces wound ischemia, increased inflammation, and necrosis. The suture material itself can be a potential contributor to tissue edema. Treatment in this case consisted in the approximation of the dehiscent wound margins by reinforcing these with taping, which, as previously noted in this document (Cases #2, #10, #14, and #27), probably consisted of adhesive taping strips. In addition to producing even tension across the wound, and not contributing to deep infection, taping has proven effective in closing flap lacerations,[303] as is the case here. The same treatment instructions were generalized to the treatment of similar wounds occurring in any other part of the body.

The infection in Case #47c is evidenced by the wound being hot to the examiner's touch and the wound opening up with its stitches being loose. The patient is febrile and secretions are flowing out of the mouth of his wound: "pouring out like grape juice." Although exhibiting clear signs of infection, the wound drainage is at this stage characterized more serous and bloody, than purulent. A large flap of detached soft tissues would easily form a large pocket, in which serous fluid or blood could accumulate. Wound infection developing in Case #47c has changed the verdict to: "a medical condition I will fight with," indicative of uncertainty about the treatment success. The ancient Egyptian physician's recommendation not to bandage an infected wound is consistent with

300. Ibid., 29.
301. Ibid., 272–73.
302. The reader is directed to appendix 2 for a compilation of the neurological symptoms and signs in the Edwin Smith Papyrus.
303. Trott, *Wounds and Lacerations*, 213.

the purpose of avoiding purulent pockets being trapped. The main objective in such a case is to allow the wound to drain free. This type of patient was placed at rest, in a recumbent position, cared for and supported on his bed under observation and support until the critical period of his injury passes. Although not specified in Case #47, the detailed management of wound infections as implemented in Case #41 (an infected wound of the chest) would likely be used here.

After the first day of treatment of the uncomplicated chest wound in Case #47a, and as primary treatment in Case #47d (a wound infection that does not clearly develop, or improves), the wound care protocol of daily applications of honey dressings standardized throughout the Edwin Smith Papyrus was implemented.

CASE #48:
Wrenching/Sprain in the Vertebral Column in the Lower(?) Back/Disc Injury
(Plate XVII:15–19)

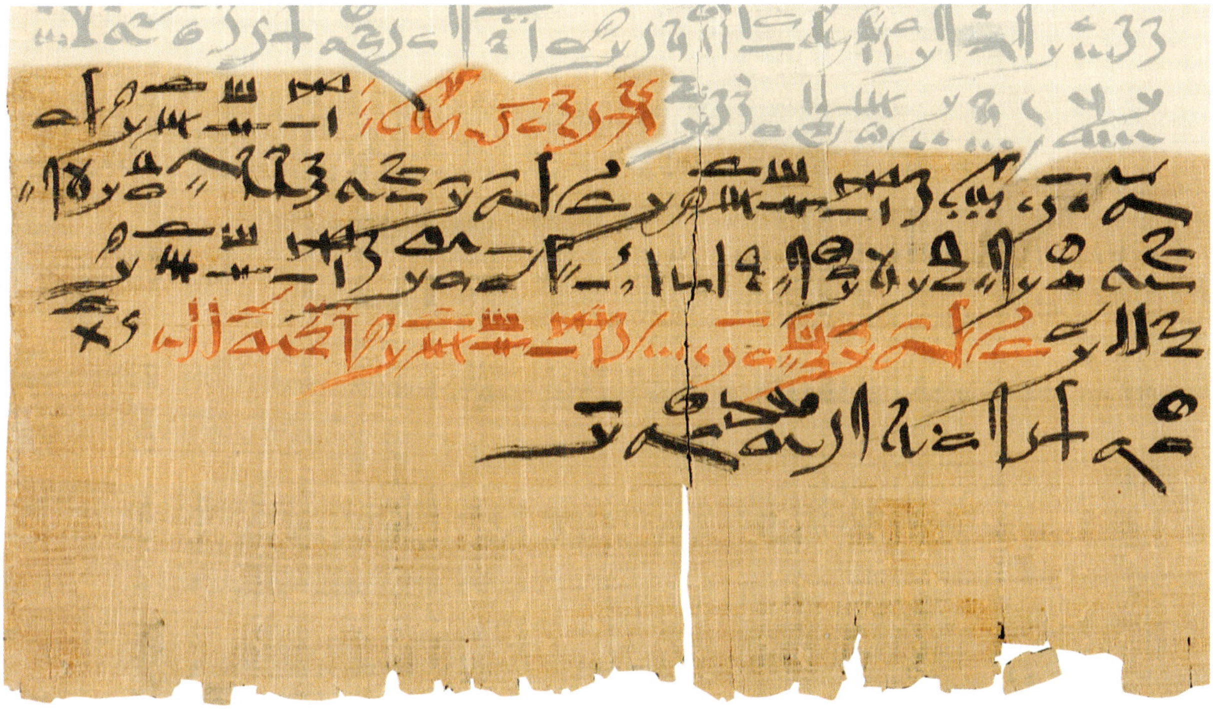

Courtesy New York Academy of Medicine.

15. 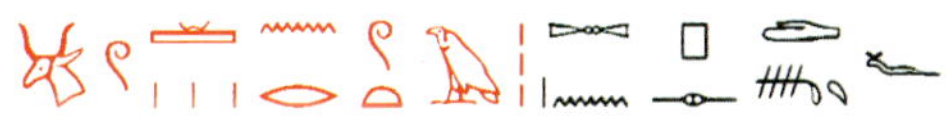

16. 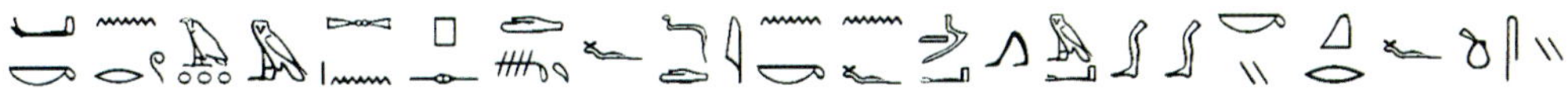

17. 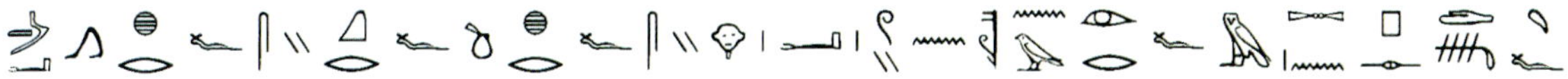

18. 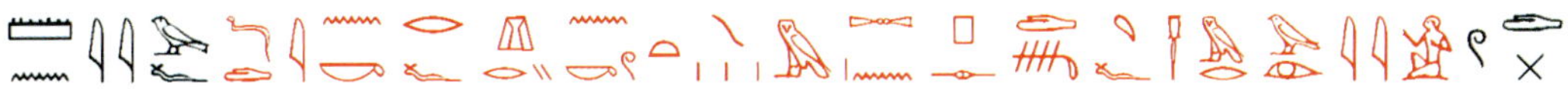

19. 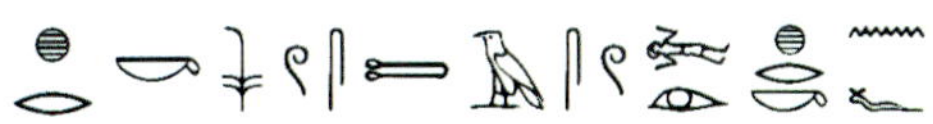

Transliteration

15§ *… šs3w nrwt ṯs n psḏ.f ỉr*

16§ *ḫ3.k nrwt m ṯs n psḏ.f ḏd.ỉ n.k n-f m3ꜥ mꜥ wꜥrty.ky ḳrf sy*

17§ *m3ꜥ.ḫr.f sy ḳrf.ḫr.f sy ḥr-ꜥwy n ḳsn ỉrr.f m ṯs psḏ.f*

18§ *mny.f ḏḏ.ỉn.k r.f ẖry nrwt m ṯs psḏ.f mḥr ỉry.ỉ wd*

19§ *ḫr.k sw sṯ3s.w ỉr.ḫr.k nf …*

Translation

Title:

Necessary knowledge and skills for a wrenching/sprain in the vertebral column in his lower(?) back.

Examination:

If you should examine a wrenching/sprain in the vertebral column of lower(?) back,

then you are to say to him: "Please/now extend your legs."

"Contract it."

Then he must extend it.

He has to contract it immediately because of the pain that it makes/produces in the vertebral column of his lower(?) back from which he suffers.

Diagnosis:

Then you are to say concerning him, "One who has a wrenching/sprain in the vertebral column of his lower(?) back,

a medical condition which I will handle/deal with."

Treatment:

You must lay him so that he is stretched out/prostrate and you must prepare for him …

Notes

psd, psḏ – Walker (*Studies in Ancient Egyptian Anatomical Terminology,* 269) defines this word as "upper back." However, the diagnostic tests seem to apply to the lower back. I am keeping a question mark because I do not think that a comprehensive lexical study has been done that would demonstrate the general meaning "lower back" for this word.

m3ꜥ, ḳrf – Imperatives.

m – I think it preferable to translate with both of Allen's suggested glosses (*ME*, 459), "please, now," so as to avoid conveying the impression that the particle has a special connotation of politeness, which is not really known. I think that all that can be said is that it is a reinforcer of the imperative. As I have suggested in earlier notes, choosing a one-word translation equivalent for a particle is arbitrary and often misleading; Gilula was especially outspoken about this ("Sinuhe B 255," *Journal of Near Eastern Studies* 35 [1976]: 25–28).

irr.f, mny.f – Relative forms. Note that both of these forms have the additional explicit actor-expression which is one of the necessary criteria for identifying a relative form.

sꜣꜣsw – stative. I think it is best taken as a stative of result. If one analyzes examples such as the present passage according to Noam Chomsky's transformational grammar (a type of analysis that has been done by Callender, Junge, and other Egyptologists), it may well be that something approximating to a pseudo-verbal clause or Subject-stative sequence appears in the "deep structure" level of the analysis, but in the surface structure this is not the case, and the pronoun (in this case *sw*) acts more as an antecedent than a subject. In the surface structure I do not think that the pronoun and the stative are clause-mates.

Medical Commentary

Type of Injury

The injury in case #48 (Visual Index II) is a wrenching/sprain in the *psḏ* region of the vertebral column. This *nrwt* injury addressed also in Case #30 as a sprain injury of a cervical intervertebral disc,[304] refers now to the spinal column below the neck, an area that includes the thoracic, the lumbar spine and the lumbo-sacral junction. The reader is directed to Case #30 for further information on this type of case and for Dr. Walker's excellent summary. Because the Edwin Smith Papyrus is generally considered to be a practical didactic document dealing with common injuries, it is overwhelmingly likely that Case #48 is that of a lumbar disc herniation. Statistics show that 90 percent of all herniated discs occur in the lower lumbar spine and only 1 to 2 percent in the thoracic spine.[305]

In contrast to the circumferential support of the thoracic and pelvic spines afforded by the rib cage and the pelvic bones, the lumbar spine is unsupported and particularly vulnerable to injury in the bipedal stance when subjected to overload and torque strains producing repeated injuries to the lumbar intervertebral discs. Heavy work and injuries to the lower back would have been extremely frequent in ancient Egypt. Clinically, a patient with a lumbar disc herniation would have low back and leg pain. Discogenic pain originates from pain generators present in the disc capsule and the corresponding facet joints. Leg pain arises from compression and stretching of the local nerve root(s).

Of utmost importance is that the sole clinical information provided in Case #48 is testing by leg movements for provocation of pain down the leg resulting from neural compression. This is the most sensitive test for a lumbar disk herniation.[306] Case #48 has been singled out in the medical literature as being the first description of the test known as the "Lasègue sign," a clinical procedure that stretches the sciatic nerve. Because of the disc herniation, the mobility of the nerve is already restricted and further stretching of the sciatic nerve roots by this maneuver causes leg pain. The Lasègue's test begins with the patient in a recumbent supine position. Each lower extremity is tested in turn from a starting flexed position of both the hip and the knee. The examiner then proceeds to extend the patient's knee by gradually raising the heel. A positive test is the production, or the increase

304. In Case #30: "about 'wrenching/rending,' as pertains to an intervertebral joint; each (vertebra: *ts*) is (still) in its place." In Case #30 the word *ʿty* is used to designate the joint where injury has occurred. This is a term that applied only to "nonsynovial joints," those joints that have no joint space. In the spine, these joints are the intervertebral discs.

305. John Campbell, "Herniated Discs of the Thoracic Spine: An Unusal Cause of Back Pain," Yahoo Voices: http://www.associatedcontent.com/article/1352269/herniated_discs_of_the_thoracic_spine.html?cat=5.

306. Kamran Sahrakar, and Martin Melicharek, "Lumbar Disc Disease." Medscape Reference: http://emedicine.medscape.com/article/249113-overview.

of leg pain. In the supine position with the legs extended, the lower lumbar spine and the sacrum are in moderate extension. By flexing the lower extremities at the hip and the knees, lumbar extension is reduced and tension on the compromised sciatic is diminished. In agreement with Sahrakar and Melicharek,[307] there are many other testing methods to examine evidence of sciatic nerve root tension, but the basis for all is the straight-leg raising test. This specific test for a lumbar herniated disc is the only one prescribed in Case #48.[308] We agree on clinical grounds with John F. Nunn[309] and other authors[310] that Case #48 is a lumbar disc injury.

We respectfully disagree with the 1988 proposal of Hughes that Case #48 is an incomplete spinal cord lesion implying a thoracic or L-1 level spinal injury.[311] The thoracic spine and the rib cage form a rigid structure to the level of T-7, the last level of individually fused ribs and most thoracic disc herniations occur below that, because more flexion is allowed. The papyrus, however, does not describe for us the typical signs and symptoms of thoracic disc herniation, such as chest wall or abdominal, inguinal, and lumbar pain associated with the distribution of the affected thoracic nerve root. The papyrus has described in prior cases, such as Case #43 and Case #47, shooting pain in the flank with rib dislocations and thoracic wall slashing injuries (Case #47), but nothing of the like is recorded in this case. Due to the fact that the spinal cord ends approximately at L-1 level, and it occupies a much larger proportion of the spinal canal in the thoracic spine, thoracic disc herniations can produce spinal cord injury with weakness of the lower extremities and bladder or bowel control problems in up to 30 percent of the patients.[312] Again, although in Cases #31 and #33 the papyrus documents descriptions of the effects of spinal cord injury, nothing of the like is recorded in Case #48.

Regarding the anatomical implications of the word *psḏ*, we must stress that most Egyptian anatomical terminology was derived from butchery practices and that our concept of dividing the human spine as cervical, thoracic, lumbar, sacral and coccyx does not have to apply to the ancients. There are various ancient Egyptian terms applied to the spine below the neck. The thoracic spine has been specifically named *mkꜣt*. The term *mkꜣt* is somewhat interchangeable with *psḏ*. The word *psḏ* is interpreted as "the back bone," "the spinal column,"[313] and, therefore, probably refers to the entire spine of the trunk. The word *pḥwy* is mostly associated with the pelvic structures and the body's "bottom," probably including the sacrum. The word *sꜣ* appears to be more generic, referring to "posterior" or "inferior" surfaces on any body part.[314] In Walker's opinion, the ancient Egyptians conceptualized the body as separate functional anatomical units working as a corporation.[315] Although the word *ẖt* is the general term for the entire torso, it has been proposed that it most likely refers to the anterior portion of the torso, with *psḏ* and *iꜣt*[316] being more specific anatomical terms for the "back of the torso,"[317] with *psḏ* often found in anatomical apposition to *ẖt*. The thoracic and the lumbar spines both are part of the posterior aspect

307. Ibid.

308. The reader is directed to appendix 2 for a compilation of the neurological symptoms and signs in the Edwin Smith Papyrus.

309. Nunn, *Ancient Egyptian Medicine*, 180.

310. Van Middendorp, Sanchez, and Burridge, "The Edwin Smith Papyrus: A Clinical Reappraisal." By proposing Case #48 of the Edwin Smith Papyrus is a possible description of Lasegue's sign, Buchanan and Kean ("Possible Description of Lasègue's Sign in the Edwin Smith Surgical Papyrus," *Clinical Rheumatology* 2 [1987]: 296) tacitly accept this case is a lumbar disc herniation.

311. J. T. Hughes, "The Edwin Smith Surgical Papyrus: An Analysis of the First Case Reports of Spinal Cord Injuries," *Paraplegia* 26 (1988): 79.

312. R. S. Rohde and J. D. Kang, "Thoracic Disc Herniation Presenting with Chronic Nausea and Abdominal Pain," *The Journal of Bone and Joint Surgery (American)* 86 (2004): 379–81.

313. Rainer Hannig, *Die Sprache der Pharaonen: Großes Handwörterbuch Ägyptisch–Deutsch (2800–950 v. Chr.)* (Mainz: von Zabern, 2006), 295

314. For information on: *sꜣ*, see Cases #1 and #8.

315. Walker, "Egyptian Medicine and the Gods," 83.

316. Note that the term *iꜣt* does not occur in the Edwin Smith Surgical Papyrus but is included in this discussion to provide a fuller explanation of the ancient Egyptian concept of spinal architecture.

317. Walker, *Studies in Ancient Egyptian Anatomical Terminology*, 107.

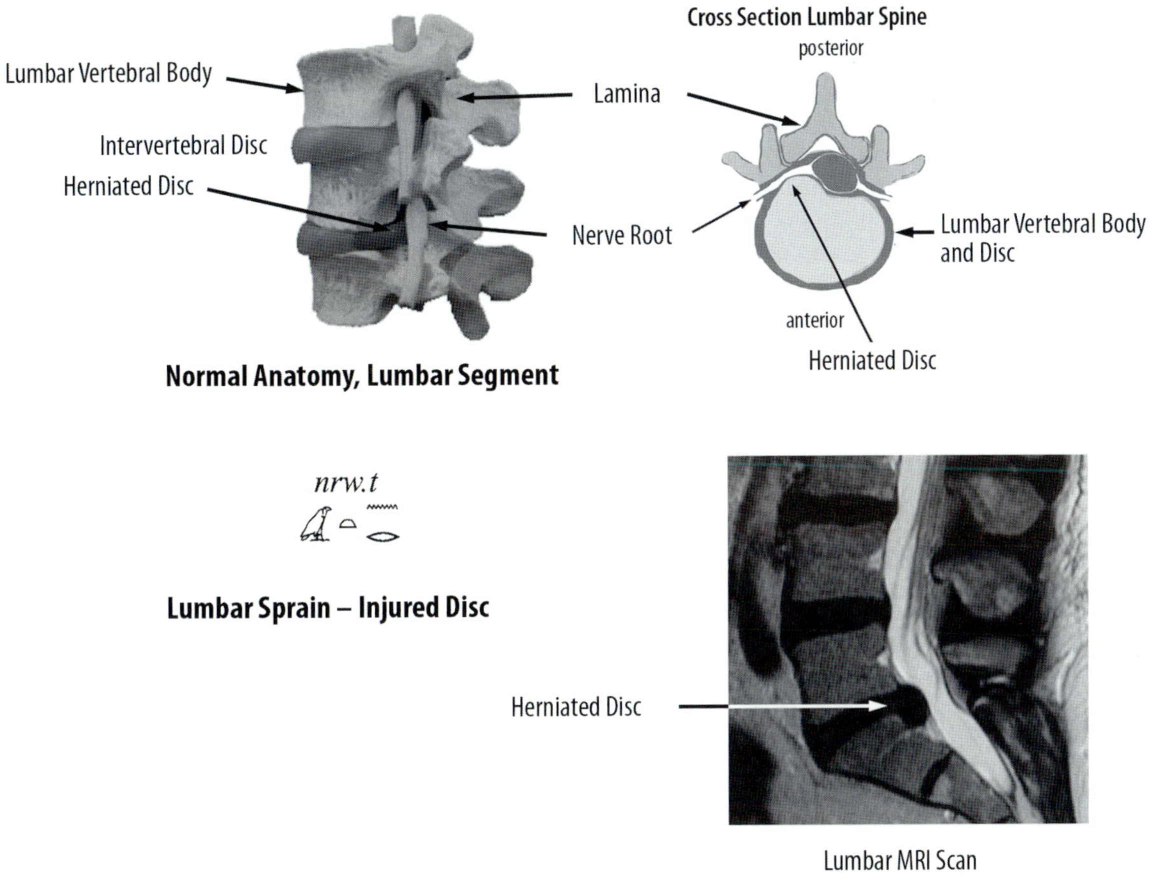

Fig. 42. Lumbar anatomy and herniated disc.

of the trunk. We have no detailed linguistic basis to adjudicate the word *psḏ* to the lower vertebral spine, but clinical information in Case #48 leads us to confidence that it is a lumbar herniated disc.

Today, the clinical diagnosis of a lumbar herniated disc requires appropriate history, positive findings of back pain and sciatic nerve root irritation including positive straight leg raising weakness and numbness, and reflex abnormalities in the corresponding nerve root distribution to the anatomical area compromised by the disc herniation. The investigation would also require radiological assessment of the lumbo-sacral spine and imaging studies, most often by MRI Scan. If conservative treatment fails, the patient may be treated by surgical decompression of the nerve roots with removal of the offending herniated disc fragments (fig. 42).

Ancient Medical Methodology and Knowledge

From the texts of both Case #48 and Case #30, it is obvious that the Egyptian physicians were experienced with problems related to spine pain and disc disease. The clinical information in Case #48 includes description of clinical techniques used to diagnose lower back problems, particularly with the intervertebral discs. There is no indication in the text of Case #48 being a spinal fracture, an infection, or a tumor.

The clinical leg maneuver performed by the ancient Egyptian physicians in Case #48 does not exactly correspond to our classic Lasègue. The testing carried out in Case #48 begins with a recumbent patient who, to begin with, must have had his legs in a flexed position, since the first command given to him is to extend both his legs. The testing proceeds by having the patient contract one of his legs (flex it). Next, he must extend his leg again, but, by doing so "he has to contract it immediately because of the pain that it makes/produces in the vertebral column of his lower(?) back from which he suffers." Although the text clearly states that the pain produced by this testing method is in the spinal column, the fact that the patient's pain caused by extending the leg immediately improved upon flexing it, again, points to sciatic nerve stretch causing this response.

There are few references in remote antiquity that can be considered related to the lower back and associated leg pain. One such source is from the Middle Assyrian and Babylonian period *'āšipu's* (physician's) diagnostic and prognostic handbook, redacted by Esagil-kīn-apli (1068–1047 BC) and translated with commentary by Scurlock and Anderson.[318] This text describes leg pain that could be sciatic in nature (11.60, 11.61) and severe back pain attributed to a slipped disc or sciatica: "It bites with the bite of a wolf; it leaps with the leap of an Elamite dog…"

To the ancient Egyptian physician's credit, we stress that in Case #48 he clearly identified the "wrenching/sprain" lesion to the intervertebral disc and provided the single most sensitive test for diagnosing a lumbar disk herniation. Nonetheless, it is unfortunate that the Edwin Smith Papyrus ends mid-sentence in the treatment segment of this case, leaving us with an unfinished case and many questions.

In Breasted's words: "It appears that the scribe laid down his reed pen midsentence and never completed the document."

318. J. Scurlock and B. R. Anderson, *Diagnoses in Assyrian and Babylonian Medicine: Ancient Sources, Translations, and Modern Medical Analyses* (Urbana: University of Illinois Press, 2005), 257–58.

Appendix 1
Open and Closed Injuries in the Edwin Smith Papyrus

Open injuries:

Lacerations	Case #1	Scalp
	Case #18	Temporal Area
	Case #24	Mandible
	Case #37a	Humeral Fracture
	Case #44	Rib Fractures
Perforating wounds	Case #3	Skull
	Case #15	Maxilla-Zygoma
	Case #19	Temporal Area
	Case #36	Lip
	Case #28	Anterior Neck
	Case #29	Posterior Neck
	Case #40	Chest, Sternum
Cutting wounds with clear margins ("lips")	Case #2	Scalp
	Case #10	Frontal Area
	Case #14	Nose
	Case #23	Ear
	Case #27	Chin
	Case #41	Chest
	Case #47b	Chest Wall
Cutting wounds with "a mouth" (variant of above)	Case #9	Frontal Area
	Case #20	Temporal Area
Extensive open wounds	Case #4	Braincase
	Case #5	Braincase
	Case #6	Braincase
	Case #7	Frontal Bone and Sinus
	Case #37b	Humeral Piercing
Fracture	Case #47	Chest Wall
Secondary opening due to infection	Case #39	Chest Wall
	Case #41	Chest Wall
	Case #46	Chest Wall

Closed injuries:

Braincase without and with bone fragmentation	Cases #8a&b	
Braincase	Case #21	Temporal Area
Braincase	Case #22	Temporal Area
Craniofacial injuries with brain damage	Case #13	Nasal Area
	Case #17	Temporal Area
Maxilla-Zygoma	Case #16	
Nasal injuries	Cases #11, #12	
Mandibular dislocation	Case #25	
Cervical sprain/Disc injury	Case #30	
Cervical dislocation	Case #31	
Cervical compression fracture	Case #32	
Cervical burst fracture	Case #33	
Clavicular dislocation	Case #34	
Clavicular fracture	Case #35	
Humeral fracture	Case #38	
Traumatic Costochondritis	Case #39	
Lumbar sprain/Disc injury	Case #48	

Appendix 2
Neurological Symptoms and Signs in the Edwin Smith Papyrus

Case	Type of Injury	Symptoms and Signs	Comments on Neurologically Related Findings
3	*thm* Open	Meningismus	Neck stiffness from subarachnoid hemorrhage in Explanations B and C. Sign of severe head injury.
4	*pšn* Open fracture Elevated	Meningismus Skull base fracture	Bleeding from the nose and the ears are symptoms of base of skull fractures. Signs of severe head injury.
5	*sd* Open fracture Depressed	Meningismus Skull base fracture	Signs of severe head injury. Description of depressed skull fragments on exam.
6	*sd* Open fracture Depressed, dura laceration	Exposed brain Cerebrospinal fluid leaking	Description of torn meningeal covering (Dura). Description of appearance of the brain surface and its pulsating motion. Description of cerebrospinal fluid leaking
7	*thm* Frontal cutting wound with compound skull fracture penetrating the Frontal air sinus	Depressed level of consciousness Meningismus Skull base fracture	Signs of severe head injury with penetration of the frontal air sinus.
7	*thm* First Alternative Course: Infection–*tiȝ* Tetanus	Facial paralysis and symptoms of tetanus	Same patient has developed full-blown tetanus, and symptoms of cephalic tetanus. Complicating infection is directly attributed to the head wound.
8a	*sd* Closed cranial vault fracture	Oculomotor nerve paralysis Spastic hemiparesis Meningismus Skull base fracture	Probable VI nerve abducens oculomotor nerve paralysis. This case has passed the acute stage, as development of spasticity takes several weeks.
13	*sd* Closed, cranio-facial injury	Torpor	Significant brain contusion accompanies this type of injury.
17	*sḏ* Closed, cranio-facial injury	Torpor	Significant brain contusion accompanies this type of injury.
19	*thm* Open	Orbital injury Meningismus	Penetrating injury has caused orbital damage and meningismus.

Case	Type of Injury	Symptoms and Signs	Comments on Neurologically Related Findings
20	*thm* Open left frontotemporal fracture	Orbital injury Skull base fracture Meningismus Motor Aphasia Stupor	Penetrating injury has caused orbital and nasal roof damage. Aphasia indicates damage to the left cerebral hemisphere.
21	*pšn* Closed temporal fracture	Skull base fracture Hyperacusia	Fracture to the petrous–mastoid areas of the temporal bone has damaged the facial nerve, with signs of stapedius nerve branch paralysis.
22	*sd* Closed temporal fracture	Meningismus Skull base fracture Aphasia Stupor	Penetrating injury has caused orbital and nasal roof damage. Injury to the left temporal area has aphasia.
31	*wnḫ* Closed cervical vertebral dislocation	Quadriplegia, incontinence and ileus from the cervical spinal cord injury	Signs of complete spinal cord injury with detailed explanation of the mechanism of vertebral injury.
33	*sḥm* Closed cervical burst fracture Head injury	Quadriplegia, spinal cord injury Aphasia Stupor	Signs of complete spinal cord injury with detailed explanation of the mechanism of vertebral injury.
43	*wnḫ* Closed rib dislocation	Intercostal nerve pain	Neurogenic pain from dislocated ribs described as shooting pains in his sides.
47	*kft* Open chest wall slashing injury	Pain from latissimus dorsi muscle injury	Pain when raising the arm due to major slash wound to the muscles of the chest wall
48	*nrwt* Closed lumbar sprain	Low back/sciatic pain on Laségue maneuver testing	Classic symptom of sciatic nerve being compressed as the leg is raised in the stretched position.

Appendix 3
Case Type and the Verdict III: "This is a Medical Condition that Cannot be Handled/Dealt With"

Case	Type of Injury	Symptoms /Signs	**Why verdict III? No effective treatment available at that time.**
5	*sd* Open fracture Depressed	Meningismus Skull base fracture	With signs of severe head injury and *depressed skull fragments* into the skull, the Egyptian physicians could not directly treat.
6	*sd* Open fracture Depressed Dura laceration	Exposed brain Cerebrospinal fluid leaking	A severe head injury with *dura laceration, exposing the brain surface and leaking spinal fluid*, was trauma the Egyptian physicians could not directly and effectively treat.
7	*thm* First Alternative Course: Infection, *tiꜣ*	Facial paralysis and Symptoms of Tetanus	This is the same patient with a Frontal Cutting wound with compound skull fracture penetrating the Frontal air sinus, who now has developed Tetanus. This complicating infection is directly attributed to the head wound.
8a	*sd* Closed cranial vault fracture	Oculomotor nerve paralysis Spastic hemiparesis Meningismus Skull base fracture	This is a *closed head injury at the sub-acute state*. The patient has residual oculomotor nerve paralysis and spastic hemiparesis. A neurological state for which the Egyptian physicians could not directly and effectively treat.
8b	*sd* Closed cranial vault fracture		This is a *severe closed head injury with extensive bone comminution*, transmitting pulsations through the skin. A condition for which no direct treatment was possible.
13	*sd* Closed, cranio-facial injury	Torpor	The major *craniofacial disruption* has impacted the brain from below producing alteration of the level of consciousness. The Egyptian physicians could do nothing to treat it directly.
17	*sd* Closed, cranio-facial injury	Torpor	Significant *brain contusion accompanies this type of craniofacial traumatic separation*. The Egyptian physicians could do nothing to directly treat it, but used the sitting position and local wound care.
20	*thm* Open left frontotemporal fracture	Orbital injury Skull base fracture Meningismus Motor Aphasia, Stupor	*Penetrating injury* has caused orbital and nasal roof damage. *Aphasia* indicates damage to the left cerebral hemisphere. The Egyptian physicians could do nothing to treat it directly.

Case	Type of Injury	Symptoms /Signs	Why verdict III? No effective treatment available at that time.
22	*sd* Closed temporal fracture	Meningismus Skull base fracture Aphasia, Stupor	Penetrating injury has caused orbital and nasal roof damage. *Injury to the left temporal area has aphasia.* The Egyptian physicians could do nothing to treat it directly.
24	*ḥsb* Open jaw fracture	Jaw comminuted fracture. The patient has fever from it	The verdict here does not necessarily imply a lethal situation, but rather *complex with bone fragmentation* inside an open wound, now probably infected. The Egyptian physicians could not treat it directly.
31	*wnḫ* Closed cervical vertebral dislocation	Quadriplegia, Incontinence and Ileus from the cervical spinal-cord injury.	Neurological signs of *spinal cord transection.* No effective treatment is available even today.
33	*sḥm* Closed cervical burst fracture Head injury	Quadriplegia, spinalcord injury. Aphasia Stupor	Neurological signs of *spinal cord transection.* No effective treatment is available even today. Aphasia from accompanying severe head injury. No available treatment existed for either injury.
37b	*ḥsb* Humeral fracture	Piercing through from the inside out.	Serious complication with *major tissue laceration,* but not automatically lethal. The verdict expresses the fact that the Egyptian physician could do nothing to cure this injury effectively.
44	*ḥsb* Rib fractures	Multiple ribs fractured with a wound over. The only finding is bone crepitation over the ribs being examined.	Although an open *chest wound would be potentially lethal if it had penetrated the cavity,* no symptoms or signs of respiratory difficulties are given. The verdict III here simply reflects an injury for which no effective treatment existed.

Appendix 4
Medical Considerations regarding Nasal Anatomical Terminology

Three important terms are used in this papyrus to refer to nasal anatomical terminology. Their analysis in the medical context suggests the interpretations assigned to these words by the current authors:

- *fnḏ* = Nose
- *msdty.fy* = [Nostril], nostrils - nasal cavities
- *šrt* = Nasal walls

fnḏ = Nose

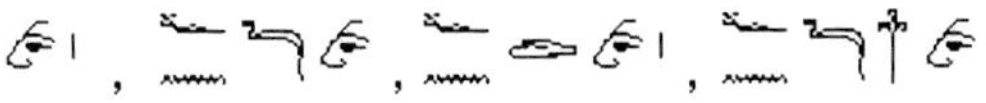

fnḏ is used as the term for nose, referring to its pillar (septum; Cases #11, #26); its chamber (roof of the nose; Case #12); the site of smash in/burst fracture (Case #13); the site of perforation (Case #14); the structure to affix rolled bandages to, from the inside, and from the outside (Cases #11, #12). It appears in:

Case #11, Fracture of the Nasal Septum
Hieratic Plate V
Ln. 10, Necessary knowledge and skills for a fracture in the pillar of his nose...
Ln. 11, If you examine a man for a fracture in the pillar of his nose,...
Ln. 13, "... they having restricted (sic) his nose ..."
Ln. 14, "As for 'the pillar of his nose': it is the upper top of his nose / top of his nose which is above down to its side and on the upper part of his nose within his nose in the midst of his two
Ln. 15, ... nostrils/nasal cavities."
This is the definition of the nasal septum [*iwn n fnd*].
Ln. 15, As for "his two nostrils/nasal cavities," (these are) the two sides of his nose reaching/penetrating to his cheek...

Case #12, Nasal Comminuted Depressed Fracture
Hieratic Plate V
Ln. 16, Necessary knowledge and skills for a fracture in the chamber / vault of his nose:
Ln. 16, If you examine a man for a fracture in the chamber / vault of his nose...
Ln. 21, ...(a fracture) in the chamber / vault of his nose, it is in the middle of his nose...

Case #13, Closed Comminuted Nasal Fracture with Basilar Skull Fracture and Cerebral Contusion
Hieratic Plate VI
Ln. 3, Necessary knowledge and skills for a crushed fracture in his nose:

Ln. 4, If you examine a man for a crushed fracture in his nose, you must place your hand on his nose on …

Case #14, Perforating Wound in[to] the Interior of his Nasal Walls
Hieratic Plate VI
Ln. 14, … (to the inside) of his nose," according …

Case #26, … Upper Lip Full Thickness Slash Wound …
Hieratic Plate IX
Ln. 8, … (as) far as the column of his nose.

msdty.fy = [Nostril], Nostrils - Nasal Cavities (It Is Not *šrty.fy*) (Figs. 10a, 10c, 11, and 12)

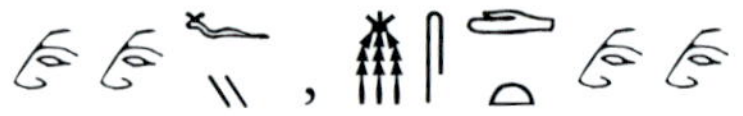

It is the site from which blood comes out through the nostrils from the nasal cavities in severe head injuries to the cranial convexity with secondary, but indirect, fractures of the anterior cranial base (Cases #4, #5, #6, #7, #8, #22). Bleeding through the nostrils - nasal cavities is also described in direct stab penetration of the temporal area that reach the nasal chamber Case #20. In Case #11, the term *msdty.fy* is anatomically defined, serving also as reference for the description of the nasal septum. Furthermore, in Case #11 the term for nostrils is used to indicate a site from which active bleeding is seen and the area from which coagulated blood inside the nose must be extracted. It appears in:

Case #4, Head Injury with Open, Displaced, Elevated Skull Fracture
Hieratic Plate II:2–11
Ln. 4, … while he bleeds from both his nostrils/nasal cavities and his ears…
Ln. 6, Diagnosis: … (while he bleeds from) both his nostrils/nasal cavities and ears…
This case is an anterior skull base fracture with convexity injury and no direct nasal injury, but with bleeding from facial orifices.

Case #5, Head Injury with Open, Comminuted, Depressed Skull Fracture
Hieratic Plate II
Ln. 13, … while he bleeds from both his nostrils/nasal cavities …
This case is an anterior skull base fracture with convexity injury. No direct nasal injury, bleeding from facial orifices.

Case #6, Head Injury with Open Comminuted, Depressed Skull Fracture and Dura Laceration
Hieratic Plate II
Ln. 22, … while he gives blood from both his nostrils/nasal cavities, …
This case is an anterior skull base fracture with convexity injury. No direct nasal injury, bleeding from facial orifices.

Case #7, Frontal Stab Wound with Open Skull Fracture. Penetrating the Frontal Air Sinus
Hieratic Plate III

Ln. 4, … while he bleeds from his nostrils/nasal cavities…

Ln. 6, … while he bleeds from both his nostrils/nasal cavities…

This case is an anterior skull base fracture with convexity injury. No direct nasal injury, bleeding from facial orifices.

Case #8, Closed Head Injury with Comminuted Skull Fractures
Hieratic Plate IV

Ln. 9, … while he bleeds from his nostrils/nasal cavities and from his ears …

This case is an anterior skull base fracture with convexity injury and no direct nasal injury, but with bleeding from facial orifices.

Case #11, Fracture of the Nasal Septum
Hieratic Plate V

Ln. 11, … he has bled from both his nostrils/nasal cavities …

Ln. 12, …Then you must place two swabs of cloth, saturated with oil, within both his nostrils/nasal cavities …

Ln. 14, As for "the pillar of his nose": it is the upper top of his nose / top of his nose which is above down to its side and on the upper part of his nose within his nose in the midst of his two nostrils/nasal cavities …

This is the definition of the nasal septum [*iwn n fnd*].

Ln. 15, As for 'his two nostrils/nasal cavities," (these are) the two sides of his nose reaching/penetrating to his cheek, down to the back of his nose, leaving the upper part of his nose …

This is the definition of nostril - nasal cavities [*msdty.fy*]

This case is a direct nasal injury.

Case #12, Nasal Comminuted Depressed Fracture
Hieratic Plate VI

Ln. 2, As for "every eel of blood which has knotted/coagulated inside both of his nostrils/nasal cavities …

Ln. 3, … it means that the clotted blood inside both of his nostrils/nasal cavities is like the eel that exists in water.

This case is a direct nasal injury.

Case #20, Temporo-Zygomatic Stab Wound with Skull Perforation and Basilar Skull Fracture
Hieratic Plate VII

Ln. 24, … while he bleeds from both of his nostrils/nasal cavities …

Hieratic Plate VIII

Ln. 4, … since he bleeds from both his nostrils/nasal cavities …

This case is an indirect anterior skull base fracture with temporal convexity perforating injury. Direct nasal injury is likely. Bleeding is from facial orifices.

Case #22, Closed Head Injury, Temporo-Zygomatic Area with Comminuted Fracture and Basilar Skull Fractures
Hieratic Plate VIII

Ln. 11 …Then the blood comes down, out of his nostrils/nasal cavities …

Ln. 13 … while he bleeds from both of his nostrils/nasal cavities and both of his ears …

This case is an anterior skull base fracture with closed temporal injury. No direct nasal injury, but bleeding through the facial orifices (nostrils - nasal cavities).

šrt = Nasal Walls 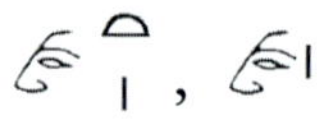

The ancient Egyptian word *šrt* appears in Case #13 for the first time in this papyrus. On the basis of all its applications in the Edwin Smith Papyrus we conclude its meaning is "nasal walls." This interpretation of the word *šrt* is similar, but not identical to Brawanski's "nose wing/nose shell."[1]

The anatomical integrity of the nasal walls can be directly disrupted in major skull fractures in which actual separation of various forms occur at the skull base and the facial bones (Cases #13, #17, #21). The anatomical integrity of the nasal walls can also be disrupted by direct penetration through its anterior cartilaginous and thin bone structure (Case #14). The nasal walls may produce active bleeding (Cases #13, #17, #21) and blood clot formation (Case #14). It appears in:

Case #13, Closed comminuted Nasal Fracture with Basilar Skull Fracture and Cerebral Contusion
Hieratic Plate VI
Ln. 5, … while he is bleeding from his nasal walls and from his ear on his side…
Ln. 6, … One who has a crushed fracture in his cheek, while he bleeds from his nasal walls, from his ear, …
Craniofacial fractures open but away from the nose, with disruption of skull base.

Case #14, Perforating wound in[to] nasal walls
Hieratic Plate VI
Ln. 7, … necessary knowledge and skills for a wound into his nasal walls …
Ln. 9, … One who has a wound in his nasal walls …
Ln. 11, … coagulated inside his nasal walls …
Ln. 13, As for 'a wound in his nasal walls, *pierced* …

Case #17, Cranio-Facial injury with open Maxillo–Zygomatic Fractures and Basilar Skull Fractures Anterior and Middle Fossa
Hieratic Plate VII
Ln. 3, … while he is bleeding from his nasal walls and from his ear …
Ln. 4, … while he bleeds from his nasal walls, from his ear …
Craniofacial fractures disrupt the skull base, forming part of the "walls" of the nose, i.e., the roof of the nasal cavity.

Case #21 - Closed Head Injury with Temporo-Zygomatic Displaced Fracture and Basilar Skull Fractures into the Mastoid Area with Hyperacusis
Hieratic Plate VIII
Ln. 7, … time he bleeds from his nasal walls and from his one ear…
Ln. 8, One who has a split in his temple / zygomatic area while he bleeds from his nasal walls and his ear …

1. Brawanski, "Mittelgesichtsverletzungen im Pap. Smith (Fälle 9–14)," 53.

Source of Confusion with the Nasal Terminology

Breasted's opinion was that the Egyptian scribe committed a number of mistakes in Case #13. In our opinion, there were no scribal errors in this section. Breasted, however, presumed an error in the use of the word *fnḏ* "nose," believing that the scribe meant "nostril." He also proposed the use of the word *šrt* to designate the nostril. Considering that it has been clearly established in Case #11 by Breasted himself that the Egyptian term for 'nostril' is *msd.ty* his proposed textual changes to the original script of Case #13 have created some confusion.

We cannot accept Breasted's (*Edwin Smith*, 252) translation of the title reading: "Instructions concerning a smash in his nostril." This would imply an injury only to the tissue forming the nostril's boundaries, a trivial injury, when clearly it is not.

Case #13 is, in actuality, a severe head injury producing a cranio-facial disruption of enough severity to result in a nasal closed comminuted fracture, a base of skull fracture, or a cerebral contusion.

Breasted's substitution of = nose for nostril appears in the first line of Case #13 under the Examination (*Edwin Smith*, 254). This is followed by a description of severe local tissue damage, and hemorrhage "while he discharges blood from his nostril." Breasted elected to use the Egyptian word *šrt* meaning "nostril" for . While nosebleeds are reported in simpler injuries than in Case #13, the use of *šrt* here and in subsequent appearances in the Edwin Smith Papyrus, only occurs in severe trauma cases in which there has been violation of the structural integrity of the nasal walls.

The authors believe that the word *šrt* , also written , refers to the structures forming the nasal walls, of which the external soft tissues of the nose are part (in this we agree with Breasted). Disruption of the nasal wall anatomy would be seen in major skull fractures in which actual separation occurred between the skull base and the facial bones. Examples of such injuries are found in Cases #13, #17 and #21. Direct disruption of the structural integrity of the nasal wall would also occur with direct penetration, as shown in the stab wound of Case #14.

Active bleeding and intra-cavitary clot formation are present in Cases #13, #14, #17, and #21.

There are several examples of the word *šrt* outside this papyrus, cited by Breasted, in which the translation "nasal walls" makes more sense than "nostril," that is, "Give me that sweet breath that is in thy two nostrils" would be better translated as "Give me that sweet breath that is inside the nose" (*Edwin Smith*, 253). The amount of air in the nostril per se would be insignificant!

We also disagree with Breasted's translation wherein he perceived another scribal error (*Edwin Smith*, 254–55) in line 5, plate VI. We translate the original text in Case #13 as follows: "and while assuredly, he bleeds from his nasal walls , from his ear and from his mouth because of that crushed fracture."

Here, Breasted changed the original word *rꜣ* = "mouth," for *gs* = "side," it seems, in order to conform the text to his presumption that bleeding just from one ear had to be paired with bleeding from only one side of the nose. Breasted's textual changes resulted in the following translation with which we must disagree: "while at the same time he discharges blood from his nostril (and) from his ear, on the side of him having that smash."

On clinical grounds this above change to the original scribal text of Case #13 is unwarranted and not supported by medical understanding. The original text in Case #13 as written is medically sound. The cranio-facial skull base disruption occurring in this case would produce bleeding from the mouth and the nose; whether from one nostril, or both, is irrelevant. The source of hemorrhaging is from the roof of the mouth and the nose, and the disrupted nasal structures. Bleeding from the ear is indicative of fracture of the petrous portion of the temporal bone which forms part of the skull base and houses all the ear structures. The temporal bone communicates to the outside through the external auditory canal (fig. 4). Bleeding from only one ear in Case #13 would merely indicate a unilateral petrous bone fracture resulting from an asymmetric disruption of the skull base.

Appendix 5
Edwin Smith's Handwritten Manuscript

With nothing but Breasted's brief remarks to guide us, we knew that Edwin Smith's attempted translation of the papyrus that bears his name was a considerable achievement, but we were not prepared for the tour-de-force of Smith's remarkable breadth of vocabulary, grasp of syntax, and overall systematic approach. In this appendix we present, along with this brief introduction, a transcription of the handwritten document (strictly speaking, of a digitized positive version of the photostat of the handwritten document), and the facsimile plates of the text from which we worked. Our reading is frankly preliminary and provisional at a number of points, as Mr. Smith's handwriting is not always easy to read and some words continue to defy decipherment at least on our part. The reader is urged to compare the plates with our transcription and perhaps propose corrections to the present transcription. Meanwhile, this is the best we have to offer.

It is with some diffidence that we make available a document that has not only never been published but, as best as we can determine, has seldom even been seen. It seems to have been regarded as a lost obscure curiosity or quaint set of marginalia not quite belonging to the main thrust of investigation of the papyrus by well-known scholars such as Breasted, Allen, the authors of the *Grundriss* and others cited in these pages. We have come away from our encounter with this manuscript with a very different impression. Our observations in this work will be brief and we will mainly give Smith the opportunity to speak for himself; we hope to expand on this in future publications.

One of the first things that struck us as we read Smith's translation was how many passages are startlingly accurate or at least contain what might be called flashes of accuracy. Thus we had a sensation of déjà vu reading about the foot sinking into the field, "there is a softening (crushing) of what is under," and also inter alia "If there be opposition to such cooling tinctures." Speaking of skull fragments he translates "and its thrust discharges within his head," a noteworthy approximation of modern translations including ours. These examples could be multiplied many times.

The degree of accuracy with what is not at all a general or banal vocabulary but is highly specific and detailed cannot fail to impress the reader. This is the case with terminology regarding bandages and other equipment, some at least of the anatomical terminology and likewise of the remedies prescribed, and various verbs denoting what has happened to the patient and what the physician must do. He understands the key word *mtw* as referring to veins, ducts, muscles, and members. He has to be credited with formidable powers of intuition and inference.

Not only in the case of lexicon but also with respect to verb forms Smith is often commendably on target, as with his frequent translation of the *sḏm.ḫr.f* as "thou must" and his translation of the negative of ability, for example, "He cannot open his mouth." While he plainly does not command the full syntactic arsenal of present-day grammarians, he is adept at framing a coherent and flowing discourse with subordinate clauses. One of the most striking discoveries that we have made in reading Smith's document is that his rendition of the *gmm.k* clauses is closer to our identification as manner nominalizations (which of course had not yet been proposed and would not be for many decades), in that he quite consistently takes them as statements, not as continuations of a conditional protasis: "If thou take, ... thou findest"! The collocation *ir swt gm.k* is aptly rendered "Now if thou find." Of course, as has already been noted, the nature of the papyrus as a hieratic text makes Smith's accomplishment all the more impressive; he seems to have been at home in the cursive script and to have scarcely dropped a stitch in his understanding of its signs and ligatures.

One significant feature of Smith's translations is that even his errors often proceed from the correct recognition of an Egyptian word. Frequently he translates the Master Physician reminding his apprentice to "place earth on its fingers"—his understanding of *d(w)* (etc.) *r tꜣ ḥr mniw.f*, "place him on the ground on his bed under observation and support." Note the writing of *mniw* and its similarity to "fingers." One case in which he seems to have been led astray by rudimentary notions of Egyptian grammar and also by then-popular Euroamerican medical practices is his understanding of bleeding from the nose and ears as a medical treatment not a sign of the injury. He seems to take the *.f* in *di.f* as an object rather than a subject, "cause him." He misses the precise sense of the references to the soft crown of an infant's skull though he is definitely playing in the right ballpark and one wants to cheer him on. Another observation is that he accords far more prominence to pathogens and parasites than does any modern reading of the papyrus, thus making more ambiguous the nature of the trauma treatise as overwhelmingly a manual of trauma as such.[1] In these, as in some other respects, he did go astray and his understanding of the papyrus was incomplete, but how could it have been otherwise? Sometimes despite a flawed translation, he drew the correct inference, as in his clear understanding that the third verdict, which he translated "the ailing will not recur," was an unfavorable one; cf. his comment at XXXI 9.12 below.

In summation, we do not think we are exaggerating when we say that it was after all fitting for Edwin Smith to be the first Egyptologist to translate the papyrus that bears his name. Thus two Masters encountered each other, a master physician and a master scholar, though the fruits of that encounter have waited a long time to see the light of day.[2]

Transcription[3]

Transcribed by Edmund S. Meltzer

Note The constant terms used in this pap(yrus) have a variety of meanings acc to context:

Sore, includes boils wounds lesions red or with pus.
wound, i.e. of a cutting instrument are incision, something to spread, cover & to
parasite, also has sense of to beat, bruise
Abrasion, deter'ant [determinative?] of a thorn or pointed instrument prick, thrust pierce itching
rupture, also way to branch out spread
lesion is also a disease caused by foreign [*illegible word*] may even be parasites
invade the word interchanges with rupture and invasion in different authors and same text

0.18 Concerning a sore ~~that breaks out~~ on his head, near the bone, infected the brain, ... on exploring his sore,

1. For the use of words such as "germs" and "virus," which today have specific bacteriological and microbiological meanings, in the time of Edwin Smith and even much earlier, see Lois N. Magner, *A History of Medicine* (New York: Marcel Dekker, 1992).

2. Some of these comments are included in "Edwin Smith Speaks, and His Papyrus Lives," presented by the authors at the annual meeting of ARCE in Providence, RI, April 2012.

3. The transcription given here is complete, including the Verso, which we are not translating in this edition. Notes and question marks in brackets [ ] are those of the authors.

III . . . . his shoulder he fails in the supporting of his neck, say to him . . . . his skull, & who fails to hold up his neck, the ailing is human in raw (meat) the first day to his sore, do not cicatrize it, put earth . . . . . afterwards cerate, honey & soap every day till he recovers. . . . . The abrasion diminishing in its extent is, the ~~rupture~~ abrasion is like the contents [*illegible word*] of the gourd (drinking vessel probably the colocynth?) . . . . . his not being strong in his arms and his shoulder. . . . . he may recover his strength in his shoulder, his failing in the supports of his neck is that the sustaining (muscle) during it(?) his attack seems to retire from his neck and his neck must fail on account of it. The placing earth on his fingers is the giving it in the routine of his prescriptions instead of making for it(?) (regular) prescriptions. (or testifies no prescription is made for it.)

1.2 IV Concerning sore that is ~~gathering~~/[*illegible word*] on his head, near the bone, and rupture of his cranium if thou take one with a boil gathering on his head, near the bone and rupture of his cranium, thou must explore his boil, thou findest the things of a secretion, under the fingers, which will move (or gripe) considerably, it is the secretion of the virus that is in it, cause him to bleed from his nostrils and his ears, till he is failing in thc supports of his neck, and does not find his strength in his arms and his shoulder. Say to him having sore of ~~gathering~~/[*illegible word*] on his head near the bone, and [*illegible word*]/rupture of his cranium, bleeding him from his nostrils and his ears, till he can not sustain his neck, it is an ailing I am contending with (I or perhaps one, is contagious) Now if thou find one whose cranium is ruptured/affected, do not cover it, place earth on its fingers to assuage the violence of his attack, it is a sedative application, it was prepared in the brick yard, when thou knowest he is coming to things, thou must place cerate (or ointments) on him, to mollify his neck and his forearms. do so to every one thou findest whose cranium is ruptured/affected (x or he ought to sit, make for him two guards of clay till thou know how he comes on)

The rupture of his cranium, between the membrane and the membrane of his cranium, are scraps fixed to the parts of his head not falling to the earth. (rupture or bruise)

The secretion of virus that is on him, is the abundance of ichor that is in the affection is bearing upwards.

Thy knowing he is coming to things, is to say thou knowest his death is imminent whatever is done (but) the ailing I contend against . .

1.11 V Concerning sore gathering, on his neck, ~~a gash~~/an abbrasion [(*illegible word*)] on his cranium, on taking one so affected, this must explore his his (sic) sore, thou findest this ~~gash~~/[*illegible word*] on his cranium a pit of moisture with thy fingers, gathering the virus in it, bleed him to syncope, and say to him affected (as described) on his failing the supports of his neck & shoulder the ailing does not recur

Smith ms. p. 2

do not cicatrice it, put earth on its fingers to pass the season of his attack.

The abrasion on his cranium; the cranium is pierced in the bone, showing in this thrust the softness within his cranium, the removal of the contents of the sore will declare the thrust within; his cranium contains a considerable mass of softness within his cranium.

VI.1.18 Concerning sore of wound on his head near the bone, abrasion in his cranium & emitting a corrupt matter on his cranium: on taking one (so affected) thou must explore his sore, thou findest in the abrasion that is on his cranium, mites such as appear in (old or) rotting vessels, things to be scrutinised individually under thy fingers, as when arranging the brow of an infant for its bandages, it will manifest on the scrutiny of this and that under thy fingers all the corrupt matter on his cranium; bleed him from his nostrils till the supports of his neck fail, the ailing does not recur thou must dress this sore with cerate, do not cicatrise it, do not put linen on it until thou knwest how he comes on.

The abrasion on his cranium with corrupt matter on his cranium, a great thrust penetrating his cranium, his scalp is a mass of its corruption and its thrust discharges within his head,

The mites manifest in rotting vessels, the vessels such as the boatman drags he does not abandon it till the greater part of it is a mass like maggots so to say they are like the mites in pimples (or nits of rit) insert [or insect??] rit seems to be any parasite

VII.2.2 Concerning sore of a wound on his head, near the bone, infesting with germs(??) his cranium (the meaning is clear, Pau never nits, maggots as according to the origin) thou must explore his sore, which will move considerably, cause him to lift up his face, he can scarcely open his mouth tho his heart yearns to speak, if thou give him a potion, his lips will fall, the dirt will not fall, bleed him from his nostrils & ears to syncope. Say to him having (as first described) the muscles of whose limbs are bound, on bleeding him to syncope, the ailing I contend with. Now if thou find one the muscles of whose lifting & upper jaws are bound, cause to be made for him hot things to cure him, its (or his) mouth must open, and thou must cover it with cerate honey & soap till thou knowest how he comes on.

And if thou find one whose limbs are affected and feverish because of this sore, which has ~~Pau~~/germs on his cranium, suppose it be one whose tooth is affected because of this sore, place thy hand on him thou findest his nose a stream of mucus, the members of his neck turgid, his face discolored and his teeth & spine, this odor of the crown of his head is like the castings of wild goats, his mouth is bound, his eye brows reach up and his face is like the things of the weeper: say to him having sore of a wound on his head, near the bone, whose cranium is infected with ~~Pau~~/germs, whose tooth is affected, whose mouth is bound and who fails, the supports of his neck & shoulder, the ailing will not recur.

And if thou find one who has cleansed himself of his ~~Pau~~/germs, there is ground for hoping cause to be made for him a stick of wood freed from the covering (bark) to be placed on his mouth, cause to be made for him a draught of hyoscianus, his treatment is to be seated between shields of brick till thou knowest how he comes on.

(See no. IV. Shield of brick may mean, hospital or brick yard as in IV either or neither translation may be right!)

The troop of nasty things on, between the membrane and the membrane of his cranium are the germs of insects.

The being bound in the cord of his jaws, is an indication, the posterior veins (muscles) of his hook (apophysy) fixed in the posterior motors of his jaws (temporalis), not obtaining a bearing, has not force to open his mouth during the attack. The muscle (cord) of his

Smith ms. p. 3

lifting jaw is the members attached to the back part of his jaws as mentioned, the cord is a sort of band (Note, the whole of this papyrus shows that the egyptians [sic] had no dictionary and no fixed meaning to the words and, being excessively figurative, the author has to explain the words used, and the explanation is often as difficult to understand as the text from not knowing what attribute of the root employed is present to his imagination, the roots of Egyptian words were always nouns. Many of which are lost.)

His nose flowing with mucus, is that the interior of his head is purging and diminishing like a brook of things. (The brooks filled from the river lessen as they proceed by absorption)

The members of his neck turgid is, the members (veins) of his neck are lifted up and hard because of this attack.

His face discolored is a redness of the matter on it like the sanies of the seeds of the cactus.

The odor of the crown of his head like the casting of wild goats is the odor within his horns is like that of the voidings of the wild goats.

The crown of his head over & between his horns (temples) abounding with his putrescence is a collection on his crown.

His mouth bound, his eye brows ambitious and his face like the things of the weeper is that he cannot open his mouth, his speech is halting and his eyebrows now a statil[?] upwards now a cowering downwards as when one who cannot is about to weep who has cleansed the germs putting[??] hope is his brightness (sc. cleanliness enlightenment) has a power to destroy the enemy by means of confidence.

VIII.3.5. Concerning pricking on his cranium on the skin of the head; if thou take one with pricking on his cranium on the skin of his head not having any thing upon it thou must explore his sore, thou findest virus gathering about the pricking that is on his cranium and his eye inflamed on account of it; when his lower part partakes of the irritation on his cranium, he walks lightly in his slipper, when his lower part partakes of this irritation on his cranium, thou determinest then that the irritation is entering from above by the not sheathing of the head of the process of his forearm and what turns his thumb within his hand, bleed him from his nostrils and ears to syncope the ailing will not recur. [Approximately one line crossed out.] Prescribe his resting from his charge till thou knowest how he comes on, and if thou find this pricking on his cranium like those mites appearing in rotten vessels; things that, on an investigation of this and that under thy fingers, like as when arranging the crown of an infant for his bandages, manifest in him on investigating this and that by thy fingers, all the putrid things in his cranium, bleed him to syncope the ailing does not recur.

The pricking on his cranium, on the skin of his head, not having any sore (lesion) on it, is the pricking of germs on his cranium, the adjacent parts of his head are sound.

His walking delicately in his slipper tells that his walking in his slipper is weakening, there is no pleasure in it for him, to walk is tiresome and stumbling, the heads of his toes are compressed by the belly of his slipper passing over them and crowding the parts which tells him to be careful of it.

The irritation entering from above to his lower part in this attack is, the juice enters from above to his lower part in this disease. (juice or torture, figure from the wine press, the grapes being in a sort of long bag, which was twisted to express the juice).

The entering from above is the breath of the god of the arch or death and the entrance is to acquire his limbs.

The unsheathing of the head of the process of his fore arm and not turning his thumb within his hand, tell that he is unable to place this head of the process of his fore arm so that he cannot turn his thumb within his hand.

Smith ms. p. 4

IX.3.19 Concerning sore on the front of his face pricking the integument of his cranium if thou take one with sore on the front of his face pricking the integument of his head, thou must prepare for him the egg of the ostrich, kneaded with serate to place on the mouth of his sore, and afterwards thou must prepare for him the egg of the ostrich kneaded and made as a styptic; there is a blister, thou must make for him a covering for it of the skin of the physician [! – ESM], thou must dress it <u>three days</u> (or on the 3d day) thou findest the fascise of the integument milky like the egg of the ostrich.

A.4.1 Words of magic on this prescription. Off, critic whose food is sore infesting the paths that contain the blood dedicated to Horus, there is no place for the mouth of the Djin, nor for the waster of this (my) cheek, now the defiler of the member, I am the Genius, the Son of Osiris is saved.

.3 Afterwards thou must ferment for him the juice of milfoil, cerate & honey heated and fermented to be applied to him.

The covering of the skin of the physician is a bandage, the body servant must be ready to apply it with the prescription for sore on the front of his face.

X.4.5 Concerning sore on his eyebrow, if thou take one with sore on his eyebrow near the bone, thou must explore his sore which is making its coverings like an ear (husk scab) Say to him the lesion on his eyebrow the ailing is human.

Then husking it with raw meat the first day if thou find this sore dislocating its husks, thou must make for it pads apply them with cerate and honey every day till he recovers.

The pads of cloth are a double bandage of cloth ~~applied~~ given on the lips of the sore to compress and cause the union one to one (one to the other)

XI 4.10 Concerning lesion in the apex of his nose, if thou take one with lesion in the apex of his nose, his nose is invading the area [written over "face"] of his face, secreting the virus that is in it, bleed him from his nostrils, say to him having lesion in the apex of his nose the ailing is human, thou must pull for him fragments of cloth and put the fragments of cloth smeared with cerate, within his nostrils and put on its fingers to draw out its virus, though must put on it guards of cloth heading (plugging?) with them his nose and apply to it afterwards cerate, honey and soap several days till he recovers.

The apex of his nose is the head, the upper part of his ~~nasal cavity~~ nose, will in its place, in the upper part of his nose and within his nose, in the interior of the shell of his nostrils

The shell of his nostrils is the heels of his nose, the road to his breast, well in the back part of his nose and sheathing the upper part of his nose.

XII 4.16 Concerning lesion in the septum of his nose. If thou take one with lesion in the septum of his nose thou findest his nose expressing and invading his face and secreting the virus that is in it. Say to having &c the ailing is human, cause it to turn its socket drawing out what is in his nostrils with rolls of cloth, that every impurity of the blood bound up within his nose may go out, but afterwards thou must put fragments of cloth smeared with cerate, placed in his nostrils, thou must put on it guards of cloth covered [sic] it and apply to it afterwards cerate, honey and soap every day till he recovers.

The lesion in the septum of his nose is within his nose well in the back part of the road between his eyebrows. [half a line crossed out.]

His nose expressing and invading his face is, that his nose is catarrhous and will altogether corrode his breasts in the same manner as his face is invaded by it, unless he contrives that the members (ducts) of every integument be freed from the ichor by which his face is seen to be invaded.

Smith ms. p. 5

Every impurity of the blood that is bound in his nostrils is the fermenting of the blood that is within his nostrils, the type of the impurity being watery.

XIII 5.3 Concerning abrasion in his nose, if thou take one with abrasion in his nose, put thy hand on his nose where this abrasion is which throbs under thy fingers; let him render blood from his nose, his ear and his mouth on account of this abrasion, he can scarcely open his mouth on account of this abrasion, he can scarcely open his mouth on account of it; he is dumb. Say to him having the abrasion in his nose the ailing will not recur, (lit "the ailing does not make two")

XIV 5.7 Concerning sore on his nose, if thou take one with sore on his nose discharged/ing and find lips on this sore that will impede (the flow) thou must make for him this sore a sort of husk (i.e. cicatrize it). Say to him having the sore on his nose, discharged, the ailing is human. Thou must make for it rolls of cloth and draw out every impurity of the blood bound up in his nose, cover it with raw meat the first day and when its husks are dislocated, take away the raw meat from it, & cover it with cerate honey and soap every day till he recovers.

The sore on his nose discharged is, the weakening of the lips of his sore and working into his nose, so to say paying for the strings that are weak.

XV 5.14 Concerning parasites on his breast, If thou take one with parasites on his heart and find a virus secreting dark and feverish in his breast. Say to him (&c.) the ailing is human, thou must cover it with a plaster, apply to it afterwards cerate honey and soap every day till he recovers.

XVI 5.18 Concerning rupture (or bruise) on his breast, If (&c) thou find virus and a discolored secretion about this rupture, say to him having (&c.), the ailing is human, thou must cover it with raw meat the first day, cause him rest to draw out its virus, apply to it afterwards cerate, honey and soap every day till he recovers.

XVII 6.1 Concerning abrasion on his heart, If (&c) thou place thy hand on his breast where this abrasion is ~~which~~ it throbs under thy fingers, let him be bled from his nose, ear and the part having that irritation, let him yield blood from his mouth, he can scarcely open his mouth on account of it, say to him (&c) & who is dumb the ailing will not recur. Cover it with raw meat the first day, he ought to sit to draw out its virus, apply to it afterwards cerate (of, &c.) goose and soap every day till he recovers. (abrasion here seems not forcible enough, thrust or tear of a pointed instrument is the root, I fail to seize an english (sic) word comprehensive enough for this and about a dozen other affections.)

XVIII 6.7 Concerning sore on his temporalis, If thou take one with sore on his temporalis that is not a wound, let it be a boil near the bone, on exploring his sore thou findest his temporalis sound not having rupture, parasites or abrasion on it: say to him having sore on his temporalis, the ailing is human, cover it with raw meat the first day and apply afterwards cerate, honey & soap every day till he recovers.

The sore that has no wound tho it is near the bone, is a sore of an inferior kind near the bone, the non appearance of wound on it tells that it will decline there being no lips to his sore.

His temporalis is in two parts and is thrown down from his eye to the bosom of his ear, to the back part of upper jaw.

XIX 6.14 Concerning parasites on his temporalis, if thou take one with parasite on his temporalis, a sore on it, when thou seest his sore say to him, Strength is (not) in thy forearm, *he can scarcely make a little circuit with it around his neck, his eye is cloudy in the part under the irritation (construction forced, may be read "The strength of thy arm fails, little can he arrange his neck) Say to him having parasite on his tempralis and fails to support his neck the ailing is human, put something on its fingers during the attack, & apply cerate honey & soap every day till he recovers.

Smith ms. p. 6

His eyes cloudy is a purulent redness of his eyes like the matter of the safflower, and [*illegible word*] the the taking away the contents by the body servant from him having the wretched bloodshot eyes like an eye that is behind its hope.

XX 6.22 Concerning sore on his temporalis, near the bone & parasites on his temporalis If thou take (such an one) his eyes being cloudy, bleed him from his nostrils less than falling, if thou put thy fingers on the mouth of this sore it will move (gripe) considerably, if thou introduce his failing to him, he will not speak to thee, a great tear falls from his eyes, he will snatch his hand to his face often, he rubs his eyes with his hand like a child not knowing what he does; Say to him having (&c) bleeding him from his nostrils till he fails in the supports of his neck and who is dumb the ailing will not recur. Now when thou findest such an one who is dumb (from the disease) he ought to sit bending down his head with cerate & the fruit of the colocynth on his ears.

XXI 7.6 Concerning a bruise on his temporalis , if thou take such an one & find virus secreting about that bruise, bleed him from his nose and his ear, the one near that bruise he can scarcely hear a word on account of it, say to him (&c) bleeding him from his nose and the ear under this irritation the ailing I contend against, put something (?hemlock) on its fingers, till thou knowest how he comes on.

XXII 7.9 Concerning abrasion (laceration) of his temporalis, ... put thy finger on his condyle and thy finger behind his hinge joint, blood must fall from his nostrils and from within his ears on account of this abrasion, it must be drawn out with fragments of cloth that thou may see its foramina within his ears, if thou speak to him he is mute, he can not speak, say to him . . . . who is mute and faint away the ailing will not recur.

Behind his hinge is the back part of his lower jaw, the hinge is behind it and his temporalis, like as the thumb makes a hinge, there is no difference in the circumstances. (the spaces & dots . . . . indicate repitions as in the previous [*illegible word*])

The seeing the foramina within his ears, there are little things in the foramina that will be espied held on the fragments of cloth on causing it is fall to draw out what is in the passage of the ear.

His being dumb is that the tongue is weak and speechless, as if on the point of going up (an euphemism for dying). [faint or washed out but legible:] I know the feeling of going up(!)

XXIII 7.18 Concerning sore on his ear, If thou take one with sore in his ear, destroying to the mouth its limbs, let the things belonging to his ear be taken as the limbs, thou must make for it a husk, behind the passage of his ear, say . . . . the ailing is human, when thou findest the sore dislocating its husks, that are on the lips of his sore, make for it pads of cloth to be rendered behind his ear, smear it afterwards with cerate, honey and soap, every day till he recovers.

XXIV 7.22 Concerning lesion on his lower jaw. . . . put thy hand on it and find this lesion throbbing under thy fingers, say to him . . . . the sore abrasion is on him a poison is operating in him and impurity consuming him on account of it, the ailing will not recur.

XXV 8.2 Concerning dislocation of his jaw, If thou take one whose jaw is dislocated, thou findest his mouth open, he can not close his mouth, place thy finger on back of the apophysis of his lower jaw and within his mouth, thy thumb under his condyle cause them to fall to their sockets, Say to him having dislocation of the jaw, the ailing is human, and cover it with a plaster & honey every day till he recovers.

XXVI 8.6 Concerning sore on his lip, If thou take one with sore on his lip discharging within his mouth, cover his sore quite to the apex of his nose and make that sore to husk, (cicatrize)

Smith ms. p. 7

Say to him . . . . the ailing is human, after husking it cover it with raw meat the first day, apply to it afterwards cerate & honey every day till he recovers.

The sore on his lip discharging within his mouth; the lips of his sore are sluggish, the working into his mouth is called the discharge (lit. payment) for sluggishness

XXVII 8.13 Concerning sore of a wound on his condyle, ... near the bone, thou must explore his sore, if thou find his bone sound having no rupture nor parasite on it, say to him . . . . . the ailing is human, put on it a napkin (or holders) on that wound and cover it with raw meat the first day, apply afterwards ointment of goose grease & soap every day till he recovers

XXVIII 8.18 Concerning sore on his sternum, . . . discharging on his larynx, if he drinks water its taste must go out by the mouth of his sore and is very acrid, he is feverish on account of it; thou must make the sore to husk, Say to him . . . . the ailing ~~is human~~ I contend against; cover it with raw meat the first day and apply to it afterwards cerate honey and soap every day till he recovers. and if thou find him feverish on account of this sore, add to it dry soap on the mouth of his sore, placing earth on its fingers till he recovers.

XXIX 9.3 Concerning sore of wound (cut) on the band of his neck, ... near the bone with parasite on the band of his neck, if thou examine this sore, it will move (gripe?) considerably and there is not found feeling in him in his forearms nor his shoulder, Say to him the sore on his neck near the bone with parasite on the band of his neck, & [~~illegible letter~~] failing in the supports of his neck, the ailing I contend against. Thou must cover it with raw meat the first day and afterwards put earth on its fingers to pass the period of his attack. (There seems an omission of the bleeding formula.)

XXX 9.8 Concerning moving (gripe) in the band of his neck. . . . say to him feel with thy forearm and thy shoulder, he can scarcely make seen the appearance of it, say to him having moving in the band of his neck, the ailing is human. Thou must cover it with raw meat the first day and afterwards apply afterwards [sic – ESM] a plaster of goose (or fly) every day till he recovers (strain or rheumatism?) [Strain seems to be written over Sprain – ESM]

The moving, is said of the binding of the condyles, they are in their sockets. (the figure is [*illegible word*] act of the vulture, perhaps griping)

XXXI 9.12 Concerning dislocation of the band of his neck, ... thou findest it attenuating him in his arms and his legs on account of it and his member is stiff on account if it, urine falls from his member without his knowing it, his flesh will receive the aura and his eyes are cloudy.

The dislocation of the band of his neck is near his atlas (pivot) causing the attenuation of his arms and legs and if the interior band of his neck be dislocated, there is no retention manifest in his bladder, Say to him having dislocation of the band of his neck, attenuating his legs and arms, and weakness of his urine the ailing will not recur. (It was hardly necessary to say this when the neck was so dislocated!)

The dislocation of the band of his neck is said of what is between the band of his neck and its second the limbs upon it are sound, but as we say things will be dislocated from what keeps, when one is separated from its second.

The non retention manifest in his urinary passage, is that his member hardened because of the spleen that is in the back part of his member so to say it cannot (or has no) guard nor bolt on the apparatus, the lower part will not sustain nor the upper

The weakening of his urine is a falling of urine for his member has no defense to hold what is in it (defense, crocodile, sleeping, a thrust at the watchmen who generally sleep at their post)

Smith ms. p. 8

XXXII 10.1 Concerning paralysis of the band of his neck . . . . . . his face is fixed and he cannot turn his neck, Say to him, feeling in thy joints and thy forearms can not be found, it chases from him his feeling in his joints and his forearms. Say to him having paralysis of the band of his neck the ailing is human. Cover it with raw meat the first day. Then thou must take (off) its coverings and place ointments on it to stimulate his neck, cover it with poultices and apply afterwards goose (or fly) every day and he ought to rest till he recovers

The paralysis in the band of his neck is said of a softening of the band of his neck within his neck, as when a foot wanders in the field there is a softening (crushing) of what is under.

XXXIII 10.9 Concerning twisting of the band of his neck . . . . thou findest him turning one band upon its second let him be drunk (blind or paralyzed) he [written over and] can not speak. its turning is as if upset, causing the band to be twisted on its second: thou findest it attenuating his arms and his legs on account of it. Say to him heavily[?] . . . . the ailing will not recur.

The twisting of the band of his neck, is said of the turning of the band of his neck on its second, one enters upon one (i.e. the other) without obtaining a bearing (literally not taking account)

Its turning on it upside down causing the band to be turned on its second is that it turns and falls on its head, locking the band of his neck on its second.

XXXIV 10.17 Concerning dislocation of his shoulder-head, if thou take one dislocating his shoulder head & find his forearms pendant, the head of his shoulder head opposing its face, say to him . . . . the ailing is human. Thou wilt turn their sockets, and cover them with pads of cloth and apply to them afterwards cerate & honey several days till he recovers, and if thou find his shoulder head abraded on account of it and discharging within the ailing is human.

The dislocation of his shoulder head is the retraction of the heads of the ligaments fixing their heads in the upper bone of his shoulder near his throat, having the limbs of his shoulder head on it, they are the limbs on his scapula, there are two members (veins or muscles) under it one on the left and one the right of his throat where his scapula takes them from his body.

XXXV 11.3 Concerning lesion on his shoulder head, if thou take one with lesion on his shoulder head, or find his shoulder head attacking and restraining its fellow say to him . . . . the ailing is human put him on his back placing the things of the shoulder in its harness/adjustments, thou must pass from his forearms to lift his shoulder head that this lesion may turn in its home: make for him a pair of pillows of cloth and put one of them inside his arm and the other under his arm, cover it with poultices and offer to it afterwards honey every day till he recovers. (probably a sprain

XXXVI 11.8 Concerning lesion on his arm . . . . finding his arm attacking and restraining its fellow say to him . . . the ailing is human, put him on his back, placing the things of his shoulders in (or between) its adjustments, thou must pass from his arms to lift his arm, to turn the lesion in (or from) its home: make for him a pair of rolls of cloth and place for him one of them inside his arm and the other of them under his arm: & cover it with poultices, apply afterwards honey every day till he recovers.

XXXVII 11.14 Concerning lesion on his arm and a sore on it . . . . abraded, thou findest this lesion throbbing under thy fingers. Say to him . . . . . the ailing I contend against. Make for him a pair of rolls of cloth, cover it with poultices and apply after ointments & goose & soap every day till thou knowest how he comes on. And if thou find the sore that is on the lesion yielding blood from it and a discharge within his sore, say to him having (as described) the ailing will not recur.

XXXIX 11.21 Concerning rupture on his arm . . . . . virus secreting/gathering about this rupture on his arm say to him . . . . the ailing is human. Cover it with poultices and apply to it after honey every day, till he recovers.

Smith ms. p. 9

XXXIX 12.3 Concerning cyst & irritation on his shoulder . . . . and <u>spots</u> forming in them with pimples on his shoulders which will cause discoloration. Let there be a burning of as many as thy hand shall find. Say to him having cysts and irritation in his shoulders who has made guests of pimples and the lesion, the ailing is human. With a needle, thou must cauterize for him on his shoulder on those his cysts being on his shoulder, and apply to it some of the applications for sore; do not wait for it to penetrate itself, nor for their forming the things of his sore, the hole of every sore appearing on his shoulder is the making a penetration of itself.

The cysts and irritation on his shoulder are things that are ichorish passing on his shoulder on account of his attack, they will make pimples and red things on his shoulder so to say they are like the things of point (architectural) that indicate pimples.

(The point in egyptian archit: resembles the louse and the word translated pimples is in many places if not all a parasite including fleas(?) but as yet I prefer my reading).

xl 12.12 Concerning sore on his shoulder, ... washing to the bone with parasite & scale on his shoulder, hold the scale on his shoulder with thy fingers, it will move (gripe) greatly Say to him . . . . the ailing is human; thou must cover it with raw meat the first day and apply to it afterwards cerate goose and soap every day till he recovers

The scale on his shoulder is on the upper part of his shoulder and is like what is manifest on the lizard.

xli 12.18 Concerning fever from sore on his shoulder . . . . suppose this sore inflamed; heat will purge [x in margin] its spleen from the mouth of this sore to thy hand: discolored are two lips of this sore, if the person be feverish on account of it, its flesh must not be taken away, cover, without taking (it) away, this sore, the skin of which will slough, the matter that is in the mouth of this sore is a caustic fluid, their sanies[?] raises piramids [sic], to drop (fall) after the manner of the gum (or pine) trees. Say to him having fever from sore on his shoulder, who is hot & feverish on account of it the ailing is human: Thou must prepare for him cooling tinctures to draw the inflammation from the mouth of the sore,

Ears of olives, dates & figs apply it

Ears of amomeron, rennet, Sodom apple, & figs, apply it

And thou must prepare tinctures for the vesication of the sore; Alabaster of the gryst, alum, <u>mites of cheese</u>? mix & cover with it

Salt of the north, fat of the ibex, knead and cover with it; make for him styptics, <u>nettles</u>? <u>rubrum</u>? gall, onion and ears of the sycamore, cover with it

If the same things appear on any of the processes, treat them according to these prescriptions.

The fever from sore on his shoulder & inflammation is that the sore on his shoulder is working upwards from the bed, and the heat is tall that goes out from it its lips are red, its mouth is open, and bespeaks the taking away the contents of his sore, it is ichorish in the highest degree, and this heat is said to be tall. (or as we say it's a high fever)

The purging by heat of his sore is that the heat purges (cleansed what is going around within his sore, completely

The discoloration of its lips is that the lips are red like the matter of the cactus

The not taking away its flesh, and covering, is not taking away the surrounding flesh on account of the fever that is on, that is on its flesh (sic)

And the causing to be burned its spleen on the mouth of his sore by thy hand, is the going out of fire (or [x in margin] heat) from the mouth of his sore <u>to</u> thy hand, as to say, the spleen is the thing that goes out on the ground.

xlii 13.17 Concerning motions (or griping, in the members of his shoulder, if thou take one who fails in the members of his shoulder, without dislocation or lesion of it; there may be one failing in these things, oh how it moves (gripes) say to him . . . the ailing is human, cover it with poultices, and apply afterwards honey & soap every day till he recovers

Smith ms. p. 10

The members of his shoulder are the bones of his shoulder, having a glans like what is manifest in the prepuce of the glans (not intelligible unless referring to the process of condyle of his shoulder)

xliii 13.22 Concerning dislocation of the members of his shoulder, . . . thou findest the members of his shoulder nosing (prominent) and discoloring their heads, suppose he be one who fails in the odor of his glands; <u>Say to him</u> . . . . <u>the ailing is human</u>. Thou must cover it with poultices and apply after honey every day till he recovers.

[Marginal notation: Red] <u>The discoloration of the members of his shoulder is</u> the retraction of the heads of the members of his shoulder that are fixed on his shoulder

His failing, in the odor of his glands is the failing in the puttings (reservoirs) in his shoulder (and axilla) that discharge by means of its glands.

Its glands (feathers) are its kidneys (or tonsils)

xliv 14.6 Concerning lesion on the members of his shoulder . . . . . with an abrasion sore on it, thou findest the members of his shoulder throbbing under thy fingers, say to him . . . . the ailing will not recur.

xlv 14.9 Concerning saline cysts upon his shoulder . . . . . thou findest them working on his shoulder, if thou place thy hand on his shoulder, on these his cysts, thou findest them very cold, there is no warmth in them, and thy hand finds there is no nourishment in them, they do not make water, nor will stations for water be discovered and they are saline to thy hand. Say to him having the saline cysts, the ailing I contend against, they are nothing. If thou find saline systs on any member of one, thou treatest him according to this prescription.

The saline cysts on his shoulder are ichors on his shoulder in excess, pussing beyond the growth of the receptacles for them, or when keeping salt in pouches which are of fresh bladder, it increases and is cold to thy hand, so does the receptacle of the ichor which is on his shoulder.

xlvi 14.20 Concerning clearing the way upwards (i.e. rising) and irritation on his shoulder if thou take one (as described . . .) thou findest a great quantity of virus secreting in his shoulder and yielding (Freeing it) like water under thy hand, they will make heaps of sanies, (but) their faces are not discolored, Say to him . . . . the ailing is human. ~~Some tinctures (remedies)~~

Some cooling tinctures for this rise that is on his shoulder

Poppy, the ash, and figs; knead and cover with it

Paste of alabaster? figs, lime of the builder and water, knead and cover with it

If there be opposition to such cooling tinctures, thou servest him certain prescriptions, to discharge all the water that is in the rising.

Thou appliest to it according to the applications for sores, and tinctures to draw the heat from the mouth of a sore on his shoulder.

Ears of acacia, ears of sycomore [sic], water, ears of amoraum[?], rennet of the cow and Sodom apple, cover with it and make for him a blister on his shoulder

Alabaster of the quarry, onions, fir, fat, cerate, sea salt, and fat of the ibex.

Cover with it, and make for him styptics.

Gourd rubrum & sycomore [sic] knead and apply it

The rising and irritation on his shoulder are things very ichorish on account of the attack that is in his shoulder, yielding like water under thy hand

The heaping of their sanies is that their skins do not perspire

And the non discoloration of their faces is, that they have nothing of redness

Smith ms. p. 11

xlvii 15.16 Concerning sore, a wound on his throat . . . . . . covering its limbs and visiting its glands, so that he fails in the odor of his adjustments, his sore tells thee, and thou findest its wounds restraining and fouling his glands by his sore, it will be like a great nose, he can scarcely lift his [sic] on account of it, thou must form for him on his wounds a husk, and say to him, . . . the ailing is human. Cover it with raw meat the first day and when thou findest this sore softening declining and dislocating its husks, thou must form for it and its' [sic] wounds pads of cloth for those its wounds and apply to it afterwards cerate, honey and soap every day till he recovers.

If thou find this sore covering its limbs and visiting its glands on any member of one thou treatest it according to this prescription.

But if thou find it a sore affecting its limbs with burning on account of this sore that is on his throat, suppose this sore burning, declining and dislocating its husks, put thy hand on it thou findest heat is imparted from the mouth of his sore to thy hand, the heaps (drops) falling from it cold like the water of hops. Say to him having sore of warmth on his throat with feverish heat on account of it, the ailing I contend against. And if thou find one who is feverish, let this sore burn, do not cover it, put earth on its fingers to pass the period of his attack; and if his fever be heavy, draw out the heat from the mouth of his sore with earth and apply to it afterwards cerate, honey and soap every day till he recovers.

xlviii 16.15 Concerning motions (gripings) the band of his back (spine) if thou take one vulturing on the band of his spine, say to him straighten thy legs, and retract them, he must straighten them and retract them with his hands, he can scarcely do it with the band of his back, he fails. Say to him . . . . the ailing is human; thou must put him on his back and make for him —— [sic]

Here ends abruptly the face of the papyrus, on the back are found five more pages, the work of two different hands and the first part mere magical bosh [sic!] with four [? – looks like "five" with "four" written over it] receipts of not much value [sic!] – In all this translation I have endeavored in all critical words to give the same signification throughout.

[Smith's translation of the verso follows; cf. Allen, *AM*, 106–16; Breasted, *Edwin Smith*, 467–507.]

B 17.1 Prayer to avert the breath of the dews, the evil season, Oh Glowing face, within the orbit, so thou art called from within Sais, flourishing as Asra[4] in the land.

[Following paragraph has a marginal bracket and marginal note reading "parenthetical the Hyades also Divisions"]

Elethya, partaking of earth and heaven, (thy) Father not pioneering [sic], if thou attach noxious secretions on me, attach them, I live I am sound in as much as I am the law which is first, the Elder Horus of those in Heliopolis The second is Isis the third is Nebthis. I have the staff which is grasped by Horus the son of Hecate [Sekhmet – ESM]; the Support of supports, son of the Hyades; Competitor son of Hathor the Mistress of creation brooding upon the waters. — (Hyades or Pleiades confounded by some there were 7 of these)

Thou art the pilot of Firmament, thou art transported in the cutter, thou wilt save me from every noxious insect operating in the body, in the season when the breath of every wind is pestiferous. Horus the second, the scion of Hecate attacks my flesh, life is not.

[Marginal note: "red," with double vertical line in margin indicating the following passage:] Written on the feathers of the vulture (or ostrich?) to give strength to one, let it be placed in his amulets, wherever he may be going, let them (the words) be amulets for the year to put away pests in the season of noxious dews.

(Asra sometimes Osiris* is the maker of home & Humanity; Horus = Existence; Isis = Nature; Nebtis = Womanhood; Hathor = Home; Hecate seems [*two illegible words*] poison vendor [*several illegible words*] witch wizzard [sic]; Hows that a quack;

Smith ms. p. 12

C Another to avert the breath of noxious insects of the Hyades, Demi gods and Messengers of Hekate; Avaunt ye Hyades, let not your breath reach me on passing over the passages of the inundation against me, I am Horus passing from the bowels of Hecate (or red Hag), Horus the 2d scion of Hag, I am Unity in Duality, I die not at all.

Said by one on the basil (or tree) when it goes out on high, it surrounds his house (he or) it will not die from the dews of the noxious seasons. (or noxious annual dews)

4. What Smith transcribes "Asra" and correctly identifies as Osiris is the writing of the name "Osiris" with the solar disk instead of the eye; see T. DuQuesne, "Osiris with the Solar Disk," *Discussions in Egyptology* 60 (2004) 21–25.

D Another, charms against the noxious annual seasons. I despise what goes out from Thapis the nursery god going out in Heliopolis, the people and the gods, the Genii and the Necromancers, there are two paths (open) to me, I despise them

E Another, I am sound in the path, the transgressor strikes me, let him; I am safe, I have seen the great Inundation and Heat which are as it were put against me, I go out from the Inundation, I will escape.

F Likewise another It is strictly commanded, thou shalt not pluck out this my heart nor this my pancardium (the whole system of veins &c). No, Hag thou canst not pluck out my Kidneys(?) nor can Osiris, by any means, be deprived of things sacred by those in Pi (Buto?); the earth is clean. The Eye of Horus does not take account in Pi of any Genius male or female nor any dead male or female (dead probably an [illegible word] necromancer) manifested in the form of various beasts, but taken by the crocodile, stung by the snake they waste away:

Annihilation does not steal into his reception room: The Hyads are those who follow the seasons (or time servers) and those holding to trifles, Horus the 2d scion of Hag causes their flesh not to live. (The Hyads therefore are blasting winds & silly prophets)

Said concerning Hag the sister of Osiris and Draco, written with written with dragons blood on the band of the burnoose and placed on one on his throat, to avoid giving entrance to the asses of the Beneficent, I exult over the scion of falsehood, the amulets of life are Wisdom upon me and within, I escape dispersion.

Note, the Sister in the house of one informing one that the season is unlucy [sic] (or very evil). (there seems an error here of f for t)

G ~~Prayer for the purification of the fly. Prayer for a certain one under my finger. Prayer for~~ Prayer for purification, cause him to say a prayer for this person, my fingers are held on the mouth. (??)

G Prayer for the little calf coming out of the belly of his mother. This son enters this belly of his, and having entered will go out alive, guard him to the earth, on the earth his seed will not fail his belly, let there go out his seed reconed [sic] not Darkness (a clumsy expression for innumberable?)

H Prayer for the purification of every thing from the noxious dews, and lessen the heat of the messengers of Hecate. And avert the Hyads (blasts) of Duality. Let not the Fate of the Inundations pass before me nor behind me his breath. I am Horus in the bowels of Hecate, I am Horus of Hecate. I am Unity of the Fair one. I shall not die at all, I am Law, I am daughter the son of Duality; when they fall upon me who are among the Cajolers, when they fall upon me, or come near me, I am Satan [sic! – this seems to be Smith's rendering of the word *nsw* or *nswt* meaning "King," which early Egyptologists read "suten" or "seten."] in his fascination.

One says this prayer on a wreath bound with the things of basil, woven in the border of the cloak, making them abound with things (here probably fingers) to disperse the noxious dews and avert the passing by the Hyads (blasts) on any thing edible likewise in the reception halls. (or store rooms for clothing)

Smith ms. p. 13

I Another; Wheat for me, it is an abomination for my Servants to rule me, or for the bowels to rule me and absorb my attention; I look out for my fowls: for Horus the second scion of Hecate to be on my flesh is the destruction of life

One says of this prayer, he will take wheat shocks in his hand

xlix.19.13 If thou take one who fails in her private month, that does not come with the nitrous passages, and find things in the upper part of her cyst, thou must say, there is a clot of blood in her womb, thou must make for her, aloes 1/5 cerate ⅛ sweet beer ½ heated (boiled) to drink four days. and make for her that she may discharge the blood, pitch, bile, cohol and sweet dragons blood, made as one thing, paint her pudendum with it abundantly: thou must make horse-ear (or horse chestnut) as an ointment, it is to stop her secretion; thou must cover her and paint her posteriors with it abundantly thou must prepare the dragons blood with kuphi (an incense) to hold between her legs Cause it to enter hot to hold to her flesh.

l 20.3 Prescriptions to cause to turn the complexion (or hair) Honey 1, red nitre 1, basalt 1, knead on one thing and paint with.

li.20.6 Another to beautify the face, paste of alabaster 1, paste of nitre 1, sea salt 1, honey 1, grind as one thing and paint with (for paste take flour)

lii.20.9 Chapter from a book of secrets, to cause the old man to appear as a youth, Fetch a quantity of Melilot very much also two Cads (the Cad is 18 galls) Separate the portion and place to dry, when they are thoroughly dry, the portion is pounded as corn is pounded, and the protion is well sifted (winnowed the practice is & was to throw into the air the wind carrying off the light parts the heavy falling). That the seeds contained in it remain, every form of the portion is treated (thrown) so as to cause the flour (or dust light things) to ~~fall~~ be caught in a hold (store house), the flour is one cad, treat in like manner all that appears as seeds, make two heaps, one of the seeds another of the catching making them equal. Reserve a portion and make one portion with water making an extract with the water and place the portion in a new Sebec (an earthen cooking pot) on a fire that burns steadily, thou knowest how it is cooking partly by the evaporation of the contained water, is dryness, partly by becoming like the dry catching, keeping in water cause the portion to become an extract, then let it cool, placing the portion in a trough, washing it at the fountain, washing the portion thoroughly, thou knowest the washing partly by its taste, tasting the water that is in the trough there is no contamination in it

Make the portion that is dry pass through the cloth of the adorners it must be kept dry, knead the portion in a mortar, Attend to the reserved portion in water made like a delicate extract place the portion in a sebec on the fire that burns steadily the cooking is known by the going out of the froth of cerate, let some one pour in the cerate that goes out let the froth be taken away and placed in a gourd when it thickens (or scales) and the charge is covered, penetrate its scale and pour the aforesaid cerate placed on the veil (in lace) in the upper part of that gourd afterwards place the portion in a jar of big stone.

Horus, grant the person to put away mucus from the head, and if there be defect in the limbs may there go out a beautifying of the complexion, putting away the germs of every deficiency, every abrasion and every fever appearing on the limbs. it is a true phylactery often times.

liii 21.11 If thou see one failing in his behind, he stands and sits with difficulty, the joints of his legs being very large: thou must prepare for him a prescription, cerate osysites (or cheese) and the ear of acacia knead the portion and heat as one thing, annoint [sic] the lap of the burnoose with it, and place it on the behind that he may convalesce speedily –

Note The Constant terms used in this pap have a variety of meanings acc to context.
Sore, includes boils wounds lesions ... as with us.
wound, i.e. of a cutting instrument an incision, sometimes to spread, cover, & to compress.
parasite, also has sense of to beat bruise
abrasion, also act of a thorn or pointed instrument prick, thrust pierce itching.
rupture also means to branch out spread.
lesion is also a disease caused by foreign substances may even be parasites,
invade the word interchanges with rupture. and abrasion in different authors & same text

0.18 Concerning a sore on his head, near the bone, infested the
III brain, ... on exploring his sore ..... his shoulder, he fails in the supports of his neck,
Say to him ..... his skull, to who fails to hold up his neck, the ailing is human.
in raw (meat) the first day to his sore, do not cicatrize (?) it. put earth .... afterwards
cerate, honey & soap every day till he recovers. .... the abrasion diminishing in its extent
is, the abrasion is like the contents of the gourd, (drinking wine probably the colocynth ?) .....
his not being strong in his arms and his shoulder ..... he may recover his strength in his
1.1 shoulder, his failing in the supports of his neck is that the sustaining (muscle) during this
his attack seems to retire from his neck and his neck must fail on account of it.
The earth on his fingers is the giving it in the routine of his prescriptions, instead
of making for him (regular) prescriptions. (or "testifies no prescription is made for it")

1.2 IV Concerning sore that is around on his head, near the bone, and rupture of his cranium, if thou
take one with a boil gathering on his head, near the bone and rupture of his cranium, thou
must explore his boil, thou findest the things of a secretion, under thy fingers, which will
move (or gripe) considerably, it is the secretion of the virus that is in it, cause him to
bleed from his nostrils and his ears till he is failing in the supports of his neck
and does not find his strength in his arms and his shoulder. Say to him having
sore of wound on his head near the bone, and rupture of his cranium, bleeding him
from his nostrils and his ears, till he can not sustain his neck, it is an ailing I
am contending with (I or perhaps one, i.e. contagious) Now if thou find one whose
cranium is ruptured, do not cover it, place earth on its fingers to assuage the violence
of his attack,[x] it is a sedative application it was prepared in the brick yard. when
thou knowest he is coming to things, thou must place cerate (or ointments) on him
to mollify his neck and his forearms, do so to every one thou findest whose cranium
is ruptured (x or he ought to sit; make for him two guards of clay till thou knowest how he comes on)
The rupture of his cranium, between the membrane & the membrane of the cranium
are scraps fixed to the parts of his head not falling to the earth. (rupture or bruise)
The secretion of virus that is on him, is the abundance of ichor that is in the affection
is bearing upwards.
Thy knowing he is coming to things, is to say thou knowest his death is imminent
whatever is done (but) the ailing I contend against.

1.11 V. Concerning sore gathering on his head, an abrasion (or thrust) on his cranium, on taking one so
affected, thou must explore his his sore thou findest this [illegible] on his cranium a pit
of moisture under thy fingers, gathering the virus in it, bleed him to syncope, and say
to him affected (as described) on his failing the supports of his neck & shoulder the ailing does not
recur

do not cicatrise it, put earth on its fingers to pass the season of his attack. thrust
The abrasion on his cranium; the cranium is pierced in the bone, showing in this gash
the softness within his cranium, the removal of the contents of the sore will declare
the thrust within; his cranium contains a considerable mass of softness within his
cranium.

VI. 1.18 Concerning sore of wound on his head near the bone, abrasion in his cranium & emitting
a corrupt matter on his cranium; on taking one (so affected) thou must explore his
sore, thou findest by the abrasion that is on his cranium, mites such as appear in (old
or) rotting vessels, things to be scrutinised individually under thy fingers, as when
arranging the brow of an infant for its bandages. It will manifest the scrutinizing
of this and that under the fingers all the corrupt matter on his cranium; bleed
him from his nostrils till the supports of his neck fail, the ailing does not recur
thou must dress this sore with cerate, do not cicatrise it, do not put linen on it
till thou knowest how he comes on.
The abrasion on his cranium with corrupt matter on his cranium, a great thrust pen-
etrating his cranium, his scalp is a sack of its corruption and its thrust discharges
within his head,
The mites manifest in rotting vessels, the vessels such as the boatman drags
he does not abandon it till the greater part of it is a mass like maggots,
so to say they are like the mites in pimples (a nits of rit) [illegible]
rit seems to any [illegible]
VII 2.2 Concerning sore of a wound on his head, near the bone, infesting with
germs his cranium (the meaning is clear, Pau means nits, maggots or decaying [illegible]
thou must explore his sore which will move considerably, cause him to lift up his
face, he can scarcely open his mouth tho his heart yearns to speak, if thou give
him a potion, his lips will fall, the dirt will not fall. bleed him from his
nostrils & ears to syncope. Say to him having (as first described) the muscles of whose
limbs are bound, on bleeding him to syncope, the ailing I contend with: Now
if thou find one the muscles of whose lifting & upper jaws are bound, cause to be made
for him hot things to cure him, its (or his) mouth must open, and thou must
cover it with cerate honey & soap till thou knowest how he comes on.
And if thou find one whose limbs are affected and feverish because of this sore
which has germs on his cranium, suppose it be one whose tooth is affected because
of this sore, place thy hand on him thou findest his nose a stream of mucus,
the members of his neck turgid, his face discolored and his teeth & spine, the
odor of the crown of his head is like the castings of wild goats, his mouth is
bound, his eye brows reach up and his face is like the things of the weeper:
Say to him having sore of a wound on his head, near the bone, whose cranium is
infested with germs, whose tooth is affected, whose mouth is bound and who fails,
the supports of his neck & shoulder, the ailing will not recur.
And if thou find one who has cleansed himself of his germs, there is ground for hope,
cause to be made for him a stick of wood freed from the covering (bark) to be placed
on his mouth, cause to be made for him a draught of hyoscyamus, his treatment
is to be seated between shields of brick till thou knowest how he comes on.
[see no IV. shields of brick may mean, hospital or brick yard as in IV either or neither
translation may be right.]
The troop of nasty things on, between the membrane and the membrane of his cranium
are the germs of insects.
The being bound in the cord of his jaws, is an induration of the posterior veins (muscles)
of his hook (apophysis) fixed in the posterior sutures of his jaws (temporalis), not obtaining
a bearing, has not force to open his mouth during his attack. The muscle (cord) of his

lifting jaw is the members attached to the back part of his jaws as mentioned, the cord
is a sort of band
(Note, the whole of this papyrus shews that the egyptians had no dictionary and no fixed
meaning to the words used, being excessively figurative, the author has to explain the
words used, and the explanation is often as difficult to understand as the text from
not knowing what attribute of the root employed is present to his imagination, the
roots of Egyptian words were always nouns. many of which are lost.)
His nose flowing with mucus, is that the interior of his head is purging & diminishing
like a brook of things. (the brooks filled from the river lessen as they proceed by absorption)
The members of his neck turgid is, the members (veins) of his neck are lifted up and hard
because of this attack
His face discolored is a redness of the matter on it like the sanies of
the seeds of the cactus.
The odor of the crown of his head like the casting of wild goats is the odor within his horns
is like that of the voidings of the wild goats.
The crown of his head over & between his horns (temples) abounding with his putres-
cence is a collection on his crown.
His mouth bound, his eyebrows ambitious and his face like the things of the weeper is
that he cannot open his mouth, his speach is halting and his eyebrows now a snatch
upwards now a cowering downwards as when one who cannot is about to weep
Who has cleansed the germs putting hope is his brightness (i.e. cleanliness enlightenment)
has a power to destroy the enemy by means of confidence.

VIII 3.5 Concerning pricking on his cranium on the skin of head; if thou take one
with pricking on his cranium on the skin of his head not having any thing upon
it thou must explore his sore, thou findest virus gathering about the pricking
that is on his cranium and his eye enflamed on account of it; when his lower
part partakes of the irritation on his cranium, he walks lightly in his slipper,
when his lower part partakes of this irritation on his cranium thou determinest
then that the irritation is entering from above by the not sheathing of the
head of the process of his forearm and what turns his thumb within his hand, bleed
him from his nostrils and ears to syncope the ailing will not recur. Prescribe his resting
from his charge till thou knowest how he comes on, and if thou find this
pricking on his cranium like those mites, appear in rotten vessels; things, that, on an
investigation of this and that under thy fingers, like as when arranging the crown
of an infant for his bandages, manifest in him on investigating this and that by
thy fingers, all the putrid things on his cranium, bleed him to syncope the ailing
does not recur.
The pricking on his cranium on the skin of his head not having any sore (lesion)
on it, is the pricking of germs on his cranium, the adjacent parts of his head are sound
His walking delicately in his slipper tells that his walking in his slipper is weak-
ening there is no pleasure in it for him, to walk is tiresome and stumbling, the
heads of his toes are compressed by the belly of his slipper passing over them
and crowding the parts which tells him to be careful of it.
The irritation entering from above to his lower part in this attack is, the juice
enters from above to his lower part in this disease. (juice or torture, figure from the wine
press, the grapes being in a sort of long bag which was twisted to express the juice).
The entering from above is the breath of the god of the arch or death and the
entrance is to acquire his limbs.
The unsheathing of the head of the process of his fore arm and not turning his thumb
within his hand, tell that he is unable to place this head of the process of his fore
arm so that he cannot turn his thumb within his hand.

IX 3.19 Concerning sore on the front of his face pricking the integument of his cranium
if thou take one with sore on the front of his face pricking the integument of his
head, thou must prepare for him the egg of the ostrich, kneaded with cerate
to place on the mouth of his sore, and afterwards thou must prepare for him
the egg of the ostrich kneaded and made as a styptic; there is a blister, thou
must make for him a covering for it of the skin of the physician, thou
must dress it three days (or on the 3d day) thou findest the fasciae of the
integument milky like the egg of the ostrich.
A 4.1 Words of magic on this prescription. Off, critic whose food is sore infesting
the paths that contain the blood dedicated to Horus, there is no place for the
mouth of the Djin, nor for the waster of this (my) cheek, nor the defiler of the
member, I am the Genius, the Son of Osiris is saved.
3 Afterwards thou must ferment for him the juice of milfoil, cerate & honey
heated and fermented to be applied to him
The covering of the skin of the physician is a bandage, the body servant must
be ready to apply it with the prescriptions for sore on the front of his face.
X 4.5 Concerning sore on his eyebrow, if thou take one with sore on his eyebrow near
the bone, thou must explore which is making its coverings like an ear
(husk scab); say to him the lesion on his eyebrow the ailing is human,
Then husking it with raw meat the first day if thou find this sore dislocating
its husks, thou must make for it pads apply them with cerate and honey
every day till he recovers.
The pads of cloth are a double bandage of cloth given on the lips
of the sore to compress and cause the union one to one (one to the other)
XI 4.10 Concerning lesion in the apex of his nose, if thou take one with lesion in
the apex of his nose, his nose is invading of his face, [illegible]
the virus that is in it, bleed him from his nostrils, say to him having lesion
in the apex of his nose the ailing is human, thou must pull for him frag-
ments of cloth and put the fragments of cloth smeared with cerate, within his
nostrils and put on its fingers to draw out the virus, thou must put on it
guards of cloth heading (plugging?) with them his nose and apply to it afterwards
cerate, honey and soaps several days till he recovers.
The apex of his nose is the head, the upper part of his nose, well in its
place, in the upper part of his nose and within his nose, in the interior of the shell
of his nostrils
The shell of his nostrils is the heels of his nose, the road to his breast, well in
the back part of his nose and sheathing the upper part of his nose.
XII 4.16 Concerning lesion in the septum of his nose. If thou take one with lesion in the septum of
his nose thou findest his nose expressing and invading his face and secreting the virus
that is in it. say to him having &c the ailing is human, cause it to burn its socket
drawing out what is in his nostrils with rolls of cloth, that every impurity of the blood
bound up within his nose may go out, but afterwards thou must put fragments of cloth
smeared with cerate, placed in his nostrils, thou must put on it guards of cloth covered
it and apply to it afterwards cerate, honey and soaps every day till he recovers.
The lesion in the septum of his nose is within his nose well in the back part [illegible]
the road between his eyebrows.
His nose expressing and invading his face is, that his nose is catarrhous and will alto-
gether corrode his breasts in the same manner as his face is invaded by it, unless he contrive
that the members (ducts) of every integument be freed from the ichor by which his face is
seen to be invaded.

Every impurity of the blood that is bound in his nostrils is the fermenting of the blood
that is within his nostrils, the type of the impurity being watery.

XIII 5.3 Concerning abrasion in his nose, if thou take one with abrasion in his nose, put thy
hand on his nose where this abrasion is which throbs under thy fingers; let him ren-
der blood from his nose, his ear and his mouth on account of this abrasion, he can
scarcely open his mouth on account of it; he is dumb. Say to him having the
abrasion in his nose the ailing will not recur. (lit "the ailing does make two")

XIV 5.7 Concerning sore in his nose, If thou take one with sore on his nose discharged and find
lips on this sore that will impede (the flow) thou must make for him this sore a sort of
husk (i.e. cicatrize it). Say to him having the sore on his nose, discharged, the ailing
is human. thou must make for it rolls of cloth and draw out every impurity of
the blood bound up in his nose, cover it with raw meat the first day and when
its husks are dislocated, take away the raw meat from it, & cover it with cerate
honey and soap every day till he recovers.

The sore on his nose discharged is, the weakening of the lips of his sore and working into
his nose, so to say paying for the things that are weak.

XV 5.14 Concerning parasites on his breast, If thou take one with parasites on his breast and find a
virus secreting dark & feverish on his breast. Say to him (&c) the ailing is human, thou
must cover it with a plaster, apply to it afterwards cerate honey and soap every day
till he recovers.

XVI 5.18 Concerning rupture (or bruise) on his breast, If (&c) thou find virus and a discolored se-
cretion about this rupture, Say to him having (&c), the ailing is human, thou must
cover it with raw meat the first day, cause him rest to draw out its virus, apply
to it afterwards cerate, honey and soap every day till he recovers.

XVII 6.1 Concerning abrasion on his breast, If (&c) thou place thy hand on his breast where this
abrasion is it throbs under thy fingers, let him be bled from his nose, ear and
the part having that irritation, let him yield blood from his mouth, he can
scarcely open his mouth on account of it, Say to him (&c) & who is dumb the ailing
will not recur. Cover it with raw meat the first day, he ought to sit to draw
out its virus, apply to it afterwards cerate (of the) goose and soap every day till
he recovers. (abrasion here seems not forcible enough, thrust or tear of a pointed
instrument is the root, I fail to sieze an english word comprehensive enough for this
and about a dozen other affections.)

XVIII 6.7 Concerning sore on his temporalis, If thou take one with sore on his temporalis that is
not a wound, let it be a sore near the bone, on exploring his sore thou findest
his temporalis sound not having rupture, parasites or abrasion on it; say to him
having sore on his temporalis, the ailing is human. cover it with raw meat
the first day and apply afterwards cerate honey & soap every day till he recovers

The sore that has no wound tho it be near the bone is a sore of an inferior kind
near the bone, the non appearance of wound on it tells that it will decline
there being no lips to his sore.

His temporalis is in two parts and is thrown down from his eye to the bosom
of ear, to the back parts of upper jaw

XIX 6.14 Concerning parasites on his temporales, If thou take one with parasite on his tempo-
ralis, a sore on it, when thou seest his sore say to him, strength is (not) in thy fore
arm, he can scarcely make a little circuit with it around his neck, his eye is
cloudy in the part under this irritation (construction forced, may be read "the strength
of thy arm fails, little can he arrange his neck") Say to him having parasite on
his temporalis and fails to support his neck, the ailing is human, put something on
its fingers during his attack, & apply cerate honey & soap every day till he recovers

His eyes cloudy is a purulent redness of his eyes like the matter of the safflower, and bespeaks
the taking away the contents by the body servant from him having the wretched bloodshot
eyes like an eye that is behind its hope.

XX 6.22 Concerning sore on his temporalis, near the bone & parasites on his temporalis If thou
take (such an one) his eyes being cloudy, bleed him from his nostrils less than falling,
if thou put thy fingers on the mouth of this sore it will move (gripe) considerably,
if thou introduce his failing to him, he will not speak to thee, a great tear
falls from his eyes, he will snatch his hand to his face often, he rubs his eyes
with his hand like a child not knowing what he does; Say to him having (&c)
bleeding him from his nostrils till he fails in the supports of his neck and who is dumb
the ailing will not recur. now when thou findest such an one who is dumb (from the
disease) he ought to sit bending down his head with cerate & the fruit of the colo-
cynth on his ears.

XXI 7.6 Concerning a bruise on his temporalis, if thou take (such an one) & find virus secreting
about that bruise, bleed him from his nose and his ear, the one near that bruise
he can scarcely hear a word on account of it, say to him (3) bleeding him from his nose
and the ear under this irritation the ailing I contend against; put something
(? hemlock) on its fingers, till thou knowest how he comes on.

XXII 7.9 concerning abrasion (laceration) of his temporalis, ... put thy finger on his
condyle and thy finger behind his hinge joint, blood must fall from his nostrils
and from within his ears on account of this abrasion, it must be drawn
out with fragments of cloth, that thou may see its foramina within
his ears, if thou speak to him he is mute, he can not speak, say to
him .... who is mute and faint away the ailing will not recur
Behind his hinge is the back part of his lower jaw, the hinge is behind it and
his temporalis, like as the thumb makes a hinge, there is no difference in the
circumstances. (the spaces & dots .... indicate repetitions as in the previous parts)
The seeing the foramina within his ears, there are little things in the foramina
that will be espied held on the fragments of cloth on causing it to fall to draw
out what is in the passage of the ear
His being dumb is that the tongue is weak and speechless, as if on the point
of going up. (an euphemism for dying).

XXIII 7.18 Concerning sore on his ear, If thou take one with sore in his ear, destroying to
the mouth its limits, let the things belonging to his ear be taken as the limits, thou
must make for it a husk, behind the passage of his ear, say .... the ailing
is human, when thou findest the sore dislocating its husks that are on the
lips of his sore, make for it pads of cloth to be rendered behind his ear, smear
it afterwards with cerate, honey and soap, every day till he recovers.

XXIV 7.22 Concerning lesion on his lower jaw .... put thy hand on it and find this sore abrasion is on him
lesion throbbing under thy fingers, say to him .... impurity consuming him on account of it, the
a poison is operating in him and
ailing will not recur.

XXV 8.2 Concerning dislocation of his jaw, If thou take one whose jaw is dislocated, thou findest
his mouth open, he can not close his mouth, place thy fingers on back of the
apophysis of his lower jaw and within his mouth, thy thumb under his condyle
cause them to fall to their sockets, Say to him having dislocation of the jaw, the ailing
is human, and cover it with a plaster of honey every day till he recovers.

XXVI 8.6 Concerning sore on his lips, If thou take one with sore on his lips, discharging within his mouth
cover his sore quite to the apex of his nose, and make that sore to husk, (cicatrize)

Say to him .... the ailing is human, after husking it, cover it with raw meat the
first day, apply to it afterwards cerate & honey every day till he recovers.
The sore on his lip discharging within his mouth; the lips of his sore are sluggish
the working into his mouth is called the discharge (lit payment) for sluggishness

XXVII 8.13 Concerning sore of a wound on his condyle, ... near the bone, thou must explore his
sore, if thou find his bone sound having no rupture nor parasite on it, say to him
.... the ailing is human, put on it a napkin (or holders) on that wound and cover it
with raw meat the first day, apply afterwards ointment of goose grease & soap every
day till he recovers

XXVIII 8.18 Concerning sore on his sternum, ... discharging on his larynx, if he drink water
its taste must go out by the mouth of his sore and is very acrid, he is feverish
on account of it; thou must make the sore to husk, Say to him .... the ailing
~~is human~~ I contend against; cover it with raw meat the first day and apply to
it afterwards cerate honey and soap every day till he recovers. And if thou
find him feverish on account of this sore, add to it dry soap on the mouth
of his sore, placing earth on its fingers till he recovers.

XXIX 9.3 Concerning sore of wound (cut) ~~on~~ the band of his neck, ... near the bone with parasite
on the band of his neck, if thou examine this sore, it will move (gripe?) considerably
and there is not found feeling in him in his forearms nor his shoulder, say to him
the sore on his neck near the bone with parasite on the band of his neck, ~~&~~ ~~a~~ failing
in the supports of his neck, the ailing I contend against. Thou must cover it with
raw meat the first day and afterwards put earth on its fingers to pass the period
(There seems an omission of the bleeding formula)
of his attack.

XXX 9.8 Concerning movings (gripe) in the band of his neck .... Say to him feel with thy forearm
and thy shoulder, he can scarcely make seen the appearance of it, Say to him
having moving in the band of his neck, the ailing is human. Thou must cover
it with raw meat the first day and afterwards apply afterwards (sic) a plaster
(Strain or rheumatism?)
of goose (or fly) every day till he recovers
The movings is said of the binding of the condyles, they are in their
(The figure is drawn act of the vulture perhaps griping)
sockets.

XXXI 9.12 Concerning ^dislocation^ of the band of his neck, ... thou findest it attenuating him in his arms
and his legs on account of it and his member is stiff on account of it, urine falls
from his member without his knowing it, his flesh will receive the air,
and his eyes are cloudy. ~~.....~~
The dislocation of the band of his neck is near his atlas (pivot) causing the atten-
uation of his arms and legs and if the interior band of his neck be dislocated, there
is no retention manifest in his bladder, Say to him having dislocation of the band
of his neck, attenuating his legs & arms, and weakness of his urine the ailing will not
recur (It was hardly necessary to say this when the neck was so dislocated!)
~~The~~ dislocation of the band of his neck is said of what is between the band of his
neck and its second, the limbs upon it are sound, but ~~as~~ we say things will be
dislocated from what keeps, when one is separated from its second.
The non retention manifest in his urinary passage ~~is~~ that his member hardened
because of the spleen that is in the back part of his member, so to say it cannot
(he has no) guard nor bolt on the apparatus, the lower part will not sustain nor the
upper
The weakness of his urine is a falling of urine for his member has no defense to hold
what is in it
(defense, crocodile, sleeping, a thrust at the watchmen
who generally sleep at their posts)

8

XXXII 10.1 Concerning paralysis of the band of his neck .... his face is fixed and he cannot
turn his neck, say to him, feeling in thy joints and thy forearms can not be found, it
chases from him his feeling in his joints and his forearms. Say to him having paralysis
of the band of his neck the ailing is human. Cover it with raw meat the first day.
then thou must take (off) its coverings and place ointments on it to stimulate his neck,
Cover it with poultices and apply afterwards goose (or fly) every day, he ought to rest
till he recovers

The paralysis in the band of his neck is said of a softening of the band of his neck
within his neck, as when a foot wanders in the field there is a softening (crushing)
of what is under.

XXXIII 10.9 Concerning twisting of the band of his neck .... thou findest him turning one band
upon its second let him be dumb (blind or paralyzed) can not speak. its turning is
as if upset, causing the band to be twisted on its second; thou findest it attenuating
his arms and his legs on account of it. Say to him having .... the ailing will not ...
The twisting of the band of his neck, is said of the turning of the band of his neck
on its second, one enters upon one (ie the other) without obtaining a bearing (literally
not taking account)

Its turning on it upside down causing the band to be turned on its second is
that it turns and falls on its head, locking the band of his neck on its second.

XXXIV 10.17 Concerning dislocation of his shoulder-head, if thou take one dislocating his shoulder head
& find his forearms pendent, the head of his shoulder head opposing its face, say to him
.... the ailing is human. Thou wilt turn their sockets, and cover them with
pads of cloth and apply to them afterwards cerate & honey several days till he
recovers, And if thou find his shoulder head abraded on account of it and dischar-
ging within the ailing is human.

The dislocation of his shoulder head is the retraction of the heads of the ligaments
fixing their heads in the upper bone of his shoulder near his throat, having
the limbs of his shoulder head on it, they are the limbs on his scapula, there
are two members (veins or muscles) under it one on the left and on the right of his
throat where his scapula takes them from his body.

XXXV. 11.3 Concerning lesion on his shoulder head, if thou take one with lesion on his shoulder head, &
find shoulder head attacking and restraining its fellow say to him .... the ailing is human
put him on his back placing the things of the shoulder in its adjustments (harness), thou
must pass from his forearms to lift his shoulder head that this lesion may
turn in its home; make for him a pair of pillows of cloth and put one of them
inside his arm and the other under his arm, cover it with poultices and
apply to it afterwards honey every day till he recovers. (probably a sprain

XXXVI 11.8 Concerning lesion on his arm ... finding his arm attacking and restraining its fellow
say to him .... the ailing is human, put him on his back, placing the things of his
shoulder in (or between) its adjustments, thou must pass from his arms to lift
his arm, to turn the lesion in (or from) its home: make for him a pair of rolls
of cloth and place for him one of them inside his arm and the other of them under
his arm; & cover it with poultices, apply afterwards honey every day till he recovers.

XXXVII 11.14 Concerning lesion on his arm and a sore on it .... abraded, thou findest this
lesion throbbing under thy fingers. Say to him .... the ailing I contend against
make for him a pair of rolls of cloth, cover it with poultices and apply after
ointment & goose & soap every day till thou knowest how he comes on. and if
thou find the sore that is on the lesion yielding blood from it and a discharge
within his sore, say to him having (as described) the ailing will not recur.

XXXVIII 11.21 Concerning rupture on his arm .... viscus gathering (separating) about this rupture on his
arm say to him .... the ailing is human. Cover it with poultices and apply to it
after honey, every day, till he recovers.

XXXIX 12.3 Concerning cyst & irritation on his shoulder .... and spots forming in them with
pimples on his shoulder which will cause discoloration. Let there be a burning of
as many as thy hand shall find. Say to him having cysts and irritation in his shoulder
who has made guests of pimples and the lesion, the ailing is human. With a needle,
thou must cauterise for him on his shoulder on those his cysts being on his
shoulder and apply to it some of the applications for sore; do not wait for
it to penetrate itself, nor for their forming the things of his sore, the hole
of every sore appearing on his shoulder is the making a penetration of itself
The cysts and irritation on his shoulder are things that are ichorish passing on his shoulder
on account of his attack, they will make pimples and red things on his shoulder
so to say they are like the things of point (architectural) that indicate pimples.
(the point in egyptian archit. resembles the louse, and the word translated pimples is
in many places ?, not all a parasite including fleas?) but as yet I prefer my reading).
XL 12.12 Concerning sore on his shoulder, ... washing to the bone with parasite scale on his shoulder;
hold the scale on his shoulder with thy fingers, it will move (gripe) greatly. Say to him ...
the ailing is human; thou must cover it with raw meat the first day and apply to
it afterwards cerate goose and soap every day till he recovers
The scale on his shoulder is on the upper part of his shoulder and is like what is
manifest on the lizard.
XLI 12.18 Concerning fever from sore on his shoulder ...... suppose this sore inflamed; heat
× will purge its spleen from the mouth of this sore to thy hand: discolored are the
lips of this sore, if the person be feverish on account of it, its flesh must not
be taken away, cover, without taking (it) away, this sore, the skin of which will slough,
the matter that is in the mouth of this sore is a caustic fluid, their sanies
raises piramids, ~~falling~~ to drops (fall) after the manner of the gum (or juice) trees.
Say to him having fever from sore on his shoulder who is hot & feverish on account
of it the ailing is human: thou must prepare for him cooling tinctures to draw
the inflamation from the mouth of the sore,
Ears of olives, dates & figs apply it
Ears of amomum, rennet, sodom apple, & figs, apply it
and thou must prepare tinctures for the vesication of the sore;
Alabaster of the gorge? alum, mites of cheese? mix & cover with it
Salt of the north, fat of the ibex, knead and cover with it; make for him
styptics, nettles? rubrum? gall, onion and ears of the sycomore, cover with it
If the same things appear on any of the processes, treat them according to these pre-
scriptions.
The fever from sore on his shoulder & inflammation is that the sore on his shoulder
is working upwards from the bed, and the heat is tall that goes out from it
its lips are red, its mouth is open, and bespeaks the taking away the contents of his
sore, it is ichorish in the highest degree, and the heat is said to be tall. (or as we
say 'tis a high fever)
The purging by heat of his sore is that the heat purges (cleanses) what is going around
within his sore, completely
The discoloration of its lips is that the lips are red like the matter of the cactus
The not taking away its flesh. and covering is not taking away the surrounding
flesh on account of the fever that is on, that is on its flesh (sic)
And the causing to be burned its spleen from the mouth of his sore by thy
× hand is the going out of fire (or heat) from the mouth of his sore to thy hand,
so to say, the spleen is the thing that goes out on the ground.
XLII 13.17 Concerning motions (or griping; ~~of the members~~ of his shoulder, if thou take one
who fails in the members of his shoulder, without dislocation or lesion of it; there
may be one failing in these things, oh how it moves (gripes) Say to him ... the ailing is
human, cover it with poultices, and apply afterwards honey & soap every day till he recovers

· The members of his shoulder are the bones of his shoulder, having a glans.
· like what is manifest in the prepuce of the glans. process or condyle of the shoulder (not intelligible unless referring to the
XIII 13.22 Concerning dislocation of the members of his shoulder, ... thou findest the members of his
shoulder rising (prominent) and discoloring their heads, suppose he be one who fails
in the odor of his glands; say to him ... the ailing is human: thou must cover
it with poultices and apply after honey every day till he recovers
The dislocation of the members of his shoulder is the retraction of the heads of the
red members of its shoulder that are fixed on his shoulder
His failing in the odor of his glands is his failing in the puttings (reservoirs) in his
shoulder (axilla) that discharge by means of its glands.
Its glands (feathers) are its kidneys (or tonsils)
XIV 14.6 Concerning lesion on the members of his shoulder .... with an abrasion sore on
it, thou findest the members of his shoulder throbbing under thy fingers, say to him
.... the ailing will not recur.
XV 14.9 Concerning saline cysts on his shoulder .... thou findest them working on his
shoulder, if thou place thy hand on his shoulder, on these his cysts, if thou findest
them very cold, there is no warmth in them, and thy hand finds there is
no nourishment in them, they do not make water, nor will elations for
water be discovered and they are saline to thy hand. Say to him having
the saline cysts, the ailing I contend against; they are nothing. If thou find
saline cysts on any member of one, thou treatest him according to this prescrip-
tion.
The saline cysts on his shoulder are ichorous on his shoulder in excess, passing
beyond the growth of the receptacles for them, as when keeping salt in
pouches which are of fresh bladder, it increases and is cold to thy hand, so
does the receptacle of the ichor which is on his shoulder.
XVI 14.20 Concerning clearing the way upwards (i.e. rising) and irritation on his shoulder
if thou take one (as described ...), thou findest a great quantity of virus secreting
in his shoulder and yielding (freezing it) like water under thy hand, they
will make heaps of sanies, their faces are not discolored, say to him
... the ailing is human. Some tinctures (cosmetics)
Some cooling tinctures for this rise that is on his shoulder
Poppy, the ash, and figs; knead and cover with it
Paste of alabaster: figs, lime of the builder and water, knead & cover with it
If there be opposition to such cooling tinctures, thou servest him certain prescrip-
tions, to discharge all the water that is in the rising.
thou appliest to it according to the applications for sores, and tinctures to
draw the heat from the mouth of a sore on his shoulder.
Ears of acacia, ears of sycomore, water, ears of amomum; rennet of the cow
and Sodom apple, cover with it and make for him a blister on his shoulder
Alabaster of the ..., onions, fir, fat, cerate, sea salt, and fat of the ibex.
cover with it, and make for him styptics
gourd, redbrum & sycomore knead and apply it
The rising and irritation on his shoulder are things very ichorish on
account of the attack that is in his shoulder, yielding like water under thy
hand
The heaping of their sanies is that their skins do not perspire
and the non discoloration of their faces is, that they have nothing of redness

XLVII 15.16. Concerning sore, a wound on his throat ..... covering its limbs and visiting
its glands, so that he fails in the odor of his adjustments if his sore tells thee and
thou findest its wounds restraining and fouling his glands by his sore
it will be like a gnat nose, he can scarcly lift his on account of it, thou
must form for him on his wounds a husk, and say to him, in the
ailing is human. Cover it with raw meat the first day and when thou find-
est this sore declining and dislocating its husks, thou must form
for it and its wounds pads of cloth for those its wounds and apply to it
afterwards cerate, honey and soap every day till he recovers.
If thou find this sore covering its limbs and visiting its glands on any member
of one thou treatest it according to this prescription.
But if thou find it a sore affecting its limbs with burning on account of this
sore that is on his throat, suppose this sore burning, declining and dislocating
its husks, put thy hand on it thou findest heat is imparted from the mouth
of his sore to thy hand, the heaps (drops) falling feverish cold like the water
of hops. Say to him having sore of wound on his throat with feverish heat
on account of it, the ailing I contend against. And if thou find one who is
feverish, let this sore burn, do not cover it, put earth on its fingers to pass
the period of his attack; and if his fever be heavy, draw out the heat from
the mouth of his sore with earth and apply to it afterwards cerate, honey and
soap every day till he recovers.

XLVIII. 16.15. Concerning motions (gripings) the band of his back (spine) if thou take one
vulturing on the band of his spine, say to him straighten thy legs, and
retract them, he must straighten them and retract them with his hands
he can scarcly do it with the band of his back, he fails. Say to him
... the ailing is human; thou must put him on his back and
make for him —

Here ends abruptly the face of the papyrus, on the back we find
five more pages, the work of two different hands and the first part
mere magical bosh — with some receipts of not much value —
In all the translation I have endeavored in all critical words to give the same
signification throughout.

B 17.1 Prayer to avert the breath of the dews of the evil season. Oh Glowing face, within
the orbit, so thou art called from within Sais flourishing as Asra in the land.
Elethya, partaking of earth and heaven, (thy) father not pioneering, if thou
attach noxious secretions on me, attach them, I live I am sound
in as much as I am the law which is first, the Elder of those in Heliopolis
The second is Isis the third is Nebthis. I have the staff which is grasped by Horus
the son of Hecate; the Support of supports, son of the Hyades; Competitor son
of Hathor the Mistress of creation brooding upon the waters. — (Hyads or Pleiads confounded by some those win of stars)
Thou art the pilot of Firmament, thou art transported in the cutter, thou wilt save
me from every noxious insect operating in the body, in the season when the breath
of every wind is pestiferous. Horus the second, the scion of Hecate attacks my flesh,
life is not.
Written on the feathers of the vulture (or Ostrich?) to give strength to one. let it
be placed in his amulets, wherever he may be going, let them (the words) be amulets for
the year to put away pests in the season of noxious dews.
(Asra sometimes Osiris is the maker of home = Humanity; Horus = Existence; Isis = Nature; Nebthis
= Womanhood; Hathor = Home; Hecate ... poison venom ... Horus the 2 a quack;

parenthetical — the Hyads also Diviners

red

C Another, to avert the breath of noxious insects of the Hyades, Demi gods and Messengers of Hecate; Avaunt ye Hyads, let not your breath reach me on passing over the passages of the inundation against me, I am Horus passing from the bowels of Hecate (or ~~red~~ Hag); Horus the 2d scion of Hag, I am Unity in Duality, I die not at all.

Said by one on the ~~[illegible]~~ basil (a tree) when it goes out on high, it surrounds his house (he or) it will not die from the dews of the noxious seasons. (or noxious annual dews)

D Another, charms against the noxious annual seasons. I despise what goes out from ~~[illegible]~~ Thapis of the nursery god going out in Heliopolis, the people and the gods, the Genii and the necromancers, there are two paths (open) to me, I despise them

Another, I am sound in the path, the transgressor strikes me, let him; I

E am safe, I have seen the great Inundation and Heat which are as it were put against me, I go out from the Inundation, I will escape.

Likewise another It is strictly commanded, thou shalt not pluck out this my

F heart nor this my pancardium (the whole system of veins &c). No, Hag thou canst not pluck out my kidneys (?) nor can Osiris, by any means be deprived of things sacred by those in Pi (Buto?); the earth is clean. The Eye of Horus does not take account in Pi of any Genius male or female nor any dead male or female (dead probably as also necromancer) manifested in the form of various beasts, but taken by the crocodile, stung by the snake they waste away: Annihilation does not steal into his reception room: the Hyads are those who follow the seasons (or time servers) and those holding to trifles, Horus the 2d scion of Hag causes their flesh not to live. (the Hyads therefore are blasting winds & silly prophets)

Said concerning Hag the sister of Osiris, and Draco, written with dragons blood on the band of the ~~cottar~~ burnose? and placed on one on his throat, to avoid giving entrance to the asses of the Beneficent, I exult over the scion of falsehood, the amulets of life are Wisdom upon me and within. I escape dispersion. Note, the Sister in the house of one inform one that the season is unlucky (or very evil). (there seems an error here of any sort?) ~~Prayer for a certain one~~ [illegible]

~~Prayer for the purification of the fly.~~

~~Prayer for~~ Prayer for purification, cause him to say a prayer for this person, my fingers are held on the mouth. (?)

Prayer for the little calf coming out of the belly of ~~his~~ mother. This son

G entering this belly of his, and having entered will go out alive, guard him to the earth, on the earth his seed will not fail his belly, let there go out his seed recorded not Darkness (a clumsy expression for innumerable?)

H Prayer for the purification of every thing from the noxious dews, and lessen the heat of the messengers of Hecate. ~~And~~ Avert the Hyads (blasts) of Duality. Let not the Fate of the Inundations pass before me nor behind me his breath. I am Horus in the bowels of Hecate, I am Horus of Hecate, I am Unity of the Fair one. I shall not die at all, I am Law, I am daughter the son of Duality; when they fall upon me who are among the Cajolers, when they fall upon me, or come near me I am Satan in his fascination.

One says this prayer on a wreath bound with the things of basil, woven in the border of the cloak, making them around with things (here probably fringes) to disperse the noxious dews, and avert ~~the passing~~ by the Hyads (blasts) on any thing edible likewise in the reception halls. (or store rooms for clothing)

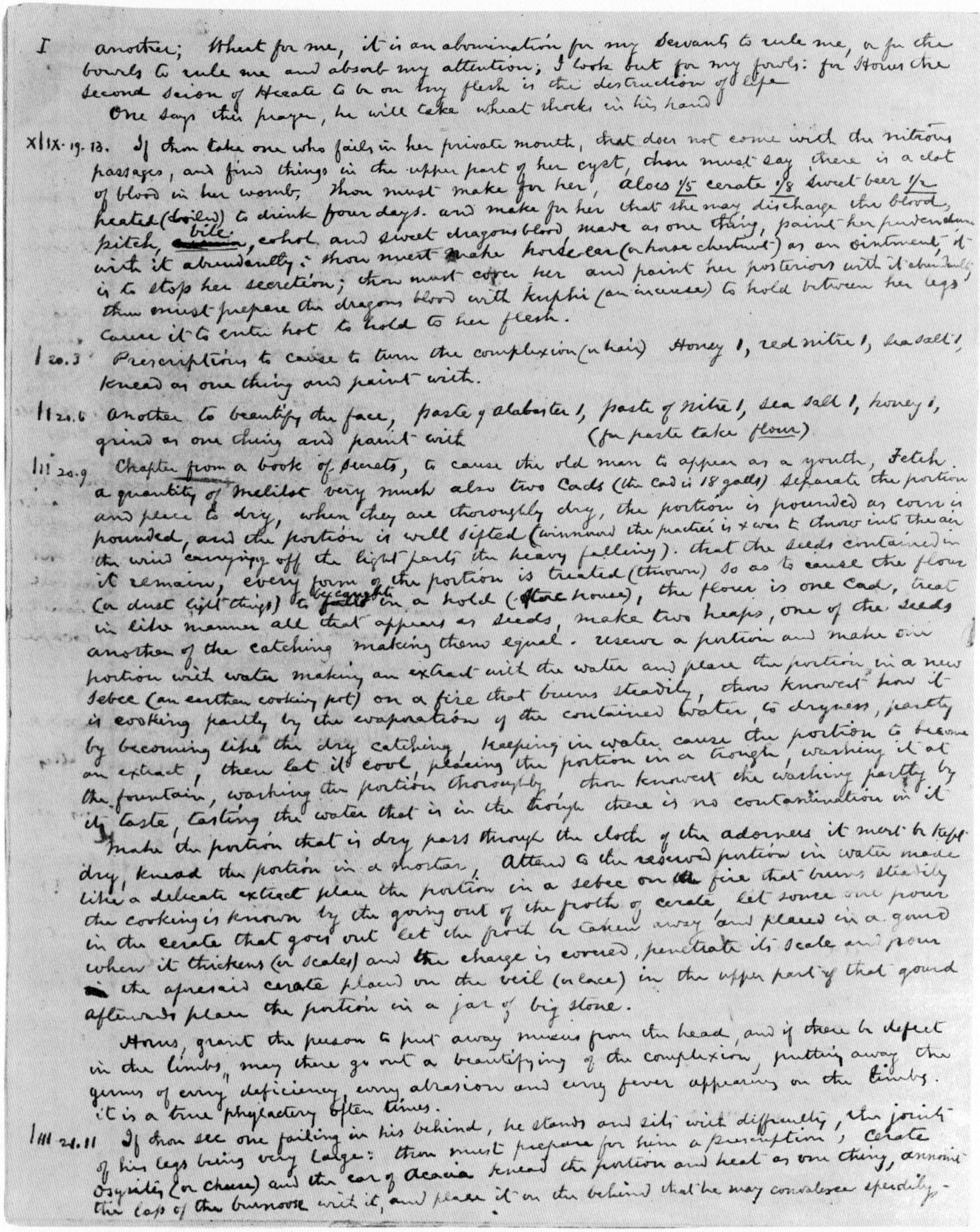

I another; Wheat for me, it is an abomination for my servants to rule me, or for the bowels to rule me and absorb my attention; I look but for my fowls: for Horus the second scion of Hecate to be on my flesh is the destruction of life

One says this prayer, he will take wheat shocks in his hand

X|IX. 19. 13. If thou take one who fails in her private mouth, that does not come with the nitrous passages, and find things in the upper part of her cyst, thou must say there is a clot of blood in her womb, thou must make for her, aloes 1/5 cerate 1/8 sweet beer 1/2 heated (boiled) to drink four days. and make for her that she may discharge the blood, pitch, bile, cohol and sweet dragons blood made as one thing, paint her pudendum with it abundantly: thou must make horse ear (or horse chestnut) as an ointment, it is to stop her secretion; thou must cover her and paint her posteriors with it abundantly; thou must prepare the dragons blood with kuphi (an incense) to hold between her legs cause it to enter hot to hold to her flesh.

| 20.3 Prescriptions to cause to turn the complexion (or hair) Honey 1, red nitre 1, sea salt 1, knead as one thing and paint with.

|| 20.6 another to beautify the face, paste of alabaster 1, paste of nitre 1, sea salt 1, honey 1, grind as one thing and paint with (for paste take flour)

||| 20.9 Chapter from a book of secrets, to cause the old man to appear as a youth, Fetch a quantity of melilot very much also two cads (the cad is 18 galls) separate the portion and place to dry, when they are thoroughly dry, the portion is pounded as corn is pounded, and the portion is well sifted (winnowed the practice is x was to throw into the air the wind carrying off the light parts the heavy falling). that the seeds contained in it remain, every form of the portion is treated (thrown) so as to cause the flour (or dust light things) to be caught in a hold (store house), the flour is one cad, treat in like manner all that appears as seeds, make two heaps, one of the seeds another of the catching making them equal. reserve a portion and make one portion with water making an extract with the water and place the portion in a new sebec (an earthen cooking pot) on a fire that burns steadily, thou knowest how it is cooking partly by the evaporation of the contained water, to dryness, partly by becoming like the dry catching, keeping in water cause the portion to become an extract, then let it cool, placing the portion in a trough, washing it at the fountain, washing the portion thoroughly thou knowest the washing partly by its taste, tasting the water that is in the trough there is no contamination in it

Make the portion that is dry pass through the cloth of the adorners it must be kept dry, knead the portion in a mortar, attend to the reserved portion in water made like a delicate extract place the portion in a sebec on the fire that burns steadily the cooking is known by the going out of the froth of cerate, let some one pour in the cerate that goes out let the froth be taken away and placed in a gourd when it thickens (or scales) and the charge is covered, penetrate its scale and pour the aforesaid cerate placed on the veil (or lace) in the upper part of that gourd afterwards place the portion in a jar of big stone.

Horus, grant the person to put away mucus from the head, and if there be defect in the limbs, may there go out a beautifying of the complexion, putting away the germs of every deficiency, every abrasion and every fever appearing on the limbs. it is a true phylactery often times.

|||| 21.11 If thou see one failing in his behind, he stands and sits with difficulty, the joints of his legs being very large: thou must prepare for him a prescription, cerate annointing (or cheese) and the ear of acacia knead the portion and heat as one thing, annoint the cap of the burnoose with it, and place it on the behind that he may convalesce speedily.

Works Cited

Abbaspour-Fard, M. H., B. Emadi, and M. H. Aghkhani, "Fertility Recognition of Ostrich Egg Using Physical Properties," *Journal of Applied Sciences* 10 (2010): 1405–12. Online: http://scialert.net/fulltext/?doi=jas.2010.1405.1412&org=11.

Abdel-Sattar, Essam, Fathalla M. Harraz, and Sabah H. El-Gayed. "Antimicrobial Activity of Extracts of Some Plants Collected from the Kingdom of Saudi Arabia," *Journal King Abdulaziz University: Med. Sci.* 15/1 (2008): 25–33. Online: http://malsuraihi.kau.edu.sa/Files/320/Researches/52140_22272.pdf.

Allen B. L., R. L. Ferguson, T. R. Leheman, and R. P. O'Brien, "A Mechanistic Classification of Closed Indirect Fractures and Dislocations of the Lower Cervical Spine," *Spine* 7 (1982): 1–27.

Allen, James P. *The Art of Medicine in Ancient Egypt*. New York: The Metropolitan Museum of Art. New Haven: Yale University Press, 2005.

———. *Middle Egyptian: An Introduction to the Language and Culture of Hieroglyphs*. 2nd rev. edition. Cambridge: Cambridge University Press, 2010.

Allman, Fred L., "Fractures and Ligamentous Injuries of the Clavicle and Its Articulation," *Journal of Bone and Joint Surgery, American Volume* 49/4 (1967): 774–84.

Anaya, D. A., and E. P. Dellinger, "Necrotizing Soft-Tissue Infections: Diagnosis and Management," *Clinical Infectious Diseases* 44/5 (2007): 705–10.

Anderson, D. G., and A. R. Vaccaro, "Classification of Lower Cervical Spine Injuries." Pages 651–59 in *The Cervical Spine*. Edited by Charles R. Clark. 4th Edition. Philadelphia: Lippincott Williams & Wilkins, 2005.

Anonymous, "Case of a Bite of a Rattlesnake," *The North American Medical and Surgical Journal* 11 (1831): 227–28.

Argenson, C., F. de Pereti, A. Ghabris, P. Eude, J. Lovet, and I. Hovorka, "Classification des Lesions Traumatiques du Rachis Cervical Inferieur," *Maîtrise Orthopédique* 61 (1997): http://www.maitrise-orthop.com/viewPage.do?id=86.

Asencio, J. A., S. Chahwan, W. Forno, "Penetrating Esophageal Injuries: Multicenter Study of the American Association for the Surgery of Trauma," *Journal of Trauma* 50/2 (2001): 289–96.

Aufrère, Sydney H., "Plants, Gardens and Horticulture in Their Relationship to Egyptian Culture and Cosmology." Online: http://www.clusiusstichting.nl/aufrere.html.

———, *L'univers minéral dans la pensée égyptienne*. 2 vols. Cairo: IFAO, 1991.

Badawy, A., "The Ideology of the Mastaba Tomb in Egypt," *Journal of Near Eastern Studies* 15 (1956): 180–83.

Bardinet, Thierry, *Les papyrus médicaux de l'Égypte pharaonique*. Lyon: Fayard, 1995.

———, *Dents et mâchoires dans les représentations religieuses en la pratique médicale en Égypte ancienne*. Studia Pohl, Series Maior 15. Rome: Pontifico Istituto Biblico, 1990.

Barrera, Jose E., and Stephen G. Batuello, "Mandibular Body Fractures." Medscape Reference: http://emedicine.medscape.com/article/869123-overview.

Barrett, George, Catherine Williams, and David Thomas, "Delayed Presentation of a Penetrating Neck Injury: Diagnostic and Management Difficulties with Retained Organic Material," *Journal of the Royal Society of Medicine Short Reports* 1/2 (2010): 19. Online: http://www.ncbi.nlm.nih.gov/pmc/articles/PMC2984346/.

Begley, M., C. G. Gahan, and C. Hill, "The Interaction between Bacteria and Bile," *FEMS Microbiology Reviews* 29/4 (2005): 625–51. Online: http://www.ncbi.nlm.nih.gov/pubmed/16102595.

Bellakhdar, J., "Médecine traditionelle et toxicology ouest-serharienne, contribution à l'ètude de la pharmacopèe marocaine." Prelude Medicinal Plants Database: http://www.metafro.be/prelude/view_mu?id=225592.

Bergman, A., J. Yanai, J. Weiss, D. Bell, and M. P. David, "Acceleration of Wound Healing by Topical Application of Honey," *The American Journal of Surgery* 145 (1983): 374–76.

Bietak, M., and E. Strouhal, "Die Todesumstände des Pharaos Seqenenre (17. Dynastie)," *Annals des Naturhistorischen Museums in Wien* 78 (1974): 45–50.

Bleck, T. P., "Clostridium Tetani (Tetanus)." Pages 2537–43 in *Principles and Practice of Infectious Diseases*. 5th edition. Edited by Gerald L. Mandell, John E. Bennett, and Raphael Dolin. 2 vols. Philadelphia: Churchill Livingstone, 2000.

Budras, Klaus-Dieter, and Robert E. Habel, *Bovine Anatomy: An Illustrated Text*. Hannover: Schlütersche Verlagsgesellschaft, 2003.

Borghouts, J. F., "The Evil Eye of Apopis," *Journal of Egyptian Archaeology* 59 (1973): 114–50.

———, *Egyptian: An Introduction to the Writing and Language of the Middle Kingdom*. 2 vols. Leuven: Peeters, 2010.

Brawanski, A., "Die Fälle 1–8 des Papyrus Edwin Smith," *Studien zur altägyptischen Kultur* 29 (2001): 7–39.

———, "Mittelgesichtsverletzungen im Pap. Smith (Fälle 9–14)," *Studien zur altägyptischen Kultur* 35 (2006): 43–60.

———, "Die Wirbelsäulenverletzungen des Papyrus Edwin Smith (Fälle 29–33)," *Studien zur altägyptischen Kultur* 32 (2004): 59–80.

Breasted, James Henry, *The Dawn of Conscience*. New York: Scribner, 1933.

———, *The Development of Religion and Thought in Ancient Egypt*. New York: Scribner, 1912. Repr. New York: Harper & Row, 1959.

———, "The Edwin Smith Papyrus: Some Preliminary Observations." Pages 385–429 in *Recueil d'études égyptologiques dédiées à la mémoire de Jean-François Champollion*. Paris: Champion, 1922.

———, *The Edwin Smith Surgical Papyrus*. 2 vols. Chicago: University of Chicago Press, 1930.

Buchanan W. W., and W. F. Kean, "Possible Description of Lasègue's Sign in the Edwin Smith Surgical Papyrus," *Clinical Rheumatology* 6/2 (1987): 296.

Budge, E. A. Wallis, *Osiris: The Egyptian Religion of Resurrection*. 2 vols. New Hyde Park, NY: University Books, 1961.

Burns, J. L., and S. J. Blackwell, "Plastic Surgery." Pages 2141–43 in *Sabiston Textbook of Surgery*. 18th edition. Edited by Beauchamp Townsend and Mattox Evers. Philadelphia: Elsevier, 2008.

Buttaravoli, Philip M., and Thomas O. Stair, *Common Simple Emergencies*. Bowie, MD: Brady Communication Co., 1985. Online: http://www.ncemi.org/cse/cse0402.htm.

Bytchenko, B., "Microbiology of Tetanus." Pages 28–29 in *Tetanus: Important New Concepts*. Edited by R. Veronesi. Amsterdam: Excerpta medica, 1981.

Callender, J. B., *Studies in the Nominal Sentence in Egyptian and Coptic*. Near Eastern Studies 24. Berkeley and Los Angeles: University of California Press, 1984.

Campbell, J. M., and A. R. David. "The Application of Archaeobotany, Phytogeography and Pharmacognosy to Confirm the Pharmacopoeia of Ancient Egypt 1850–1200 BC." Pages 20–29 in *Pharmacy and Medicine in Ancient Egypt*. Edited by Jenefer Cockitt and Rosalie David. BAR International Series 2141. Oxford: Archaeopress, 2010.

Černý, J. "Language and Writing." Pages 196–219 in *The Legacy of Egypt*. Edited by J. R. Harris. 2nd ed. Oxford: Oxford University Press, 1971.

Chapman, P. H., "Case Seven of the Smith Surgical Papyrus: The Meaning of *tp3w*," *Journal of the American Research Center in Egypt* 29 (1992): 35–42.

Chapman, P. H. and R. Gupta, "Reinvestigation of a Middle Kingdom Head Provides New Insights Concerning Mummification and Its Relationship to Contemporary Anatomic Knowledge and Funerary Ritual," *Journal of the American Research Center in Egypt* 43 (2007): 113–27.

Chaudhry, M., and A. J. Rosh, "Dislocation, Mandible: Treatment & Medication." Medscape Reference: http://emedicine.medscape.com/article/823775-treatment.

Chesnut, R. M., and L. F. Marshall, "Management of Head Injury: Treatment of Abnormal Intracranial Pressure," *Neurosurgery Clinics of North America* 2/2 (1991): 267–84.

Conti, Giovanni, *Studi sul bilitterismo in semitico e in egiziano*. Quaderni de semitistica 9. Florence: Istituto di linguistica e di lingue orientali, Università di Firenze, 1980.

Cooper R. A., E. Halas, and P. C. Molan, "The Efficacy of Honey in Inhibiting Strains of Pseudomonas Aureginosa from Infected Burns," *Journal of Burn Care & Rehabilitation* 23/6 (2002): 366–70.

Courville, C. B., "Injuries to the Skull and Brain in Ancient Egypt," *Bulletin of the Los Angeles Neurological Society* 14/2 (1949): 53–82.

Crumplin, M. K. H., and P. Starling, *A Surgical Artist at War: The Paintings and Sketches of Sir Charles Bell 1809–1815*. Edinburgh: The Royal College of Surgeons of Edinburgh, 2005.

Dagi, T. F., "The Management of Head Trauma." Pages 289–313 in *A History of Neurosurgery*. Edited by Samuel H Greenblatt. Park Ridge, IL: American Association of Neurological Surgeons, 1997.

Dammak, I., F. B. Ben Adballah, S. Boudaya, L. Keskes, S. Besbes, A. El Gaied, H. Attia, H. Turki, and B. Hentati, "Effects of Date Seed Oil on Normal Human Skin in vitro," *European Journal of Dermatology* 17/6 (2007): 516–29.

David, A. R., "The Pharmacy in Ancient Egypt Project at the KHN Centre for Biomedical Egyptology." Pages 1–5 in *Pharmacy and Medicine in Ancient Egypt: Proceedings of the Conferences Held in Cairo (2007) and Manchester (2008)*. Edited by Jenefer Cockitt and Rosalie David. BAR International Series 2141. Oxford: Archaeopress, 2010.

Davies, Nina M., "Birds and Bats at Beni Hasan," *Journal of Egyptian Archaeology* 35 (1949): 13–20.

Davison, Steven P., Brooke N. Bosley, and Henry D. Sandel, "Ear Reconstruction and Salvage Procedures." Medscape Reference: http://emedicine.medscape.com/article/1288828-overview.

Dawson, W. R., *Charles Wycliffe Goodwin, 1817–1878: A Pioneer in Egyptology*. Oxford: Oxford University Press, 1934.

de Buck, Adriaan, *Egyptian Readingbook: Exercises and Middle Egyptian Texts*. 3rd ed. Leiden: Nederlands Instituut voor het Nabije Oosten, 1970.

von Deines, Hildegard, Hermann Grapow, and Wolfhart Westendorf, *Übersetzung der medizinischen Texte*. Vol. 4/1 of *Grundriss der Medizin der alten Ägypter*. Berlin: Akademie, 1958.

von Deines, Hildegard, and Wolfhart Westendorf, *Wörterbuch der Medizinischen Texte*. Vol. 7 of *Grundriss der Medizin der alten Ägypter*. 2 vols. Berlin: Akademie, 1961–62.

Depuydt, Leo, *Conjunction, Contiguity, Contingency*. Oxford: Oxford University Press, 1993.

———, *Fundamentals of Egyptian Grammar*. Norton, MA: Frog, 1999.

———, "The Standard Theory of the 'Emphatic' Forms in Classical (Middle) Egyptian: A Historical Survey," *Orientalia Lovaniensia Periodica* 14 (1983): 13–54.

Dev, V. R. , et al. "Nasal Fracture Surgery Treatment & Management." Medscape Reference: http://emedicine.medscape.com/article/1283709-treatment.

Doret, E. "La forme *sḏm.n.f* Narrative," *Bulletin de la Société d'Egyptologie de Genève* 2 (1979): 13–22.

———, *The Narrative Verbal System of Old and Middle Egyptian*. Cahiers d'Orientalisme 12. Geneva: Patrick Cramer, 1986.

Dupoirieux, L. "Ostrich Eggshell as a Bone Substitute: A Preliminary Report of Its Biological Behaviour in Animals – A Possibility in Facial Reconstructive Surgery," *British Journal of Oral and Maxillofacial Surgery* 37/6 (1999): 467–71.

DuQuesne, T. "Osiris with the Solar Disk," *Discussions in Egyptology* 60 (2004): 21–25.

Ebeid, Nabil I., *Egyptian Medicine in the Days of the Pharaohs*. Cairo: General Egyptian Book Organization, 1999.

Edel, E., *Altägyptische Grammatik*. 2 vols. Analecta Orientalia 34/39. Rome: Pontifico Istituto Biblico, 1955/1964.

———, "Die Herkunft des neuägyptisch-koptischen Personalsuffixes der 3. Person Plural *-w*," *Zeitschrift für ägyptische Sprache und Altertumskunde* 84 (1959): 17–38.

Efem, S. E. E. "Clinical Observations on the Wound Healing Properties of Honey," *British Journal of Surgery* 75 (1988): 679–81.

Ekpa, O. D., and R. U. B. Ebana, "Comparative Studies of Mmanyanga, Palm and Coconut Oils: Anti-Microbial Effects of the Oils and Their Metallic Soaps on Some Bacteria and Fungi," *Global Journal of Pure and Applied Sciences* 1/2 (1996): 155–63.

Ekwenye, U. N., and C. A. Ijeomah, "Antimicrobial Effects of Palm Kernel Oil and Palm Oil," *King Monkut s Institute Technology Laudkrabang Science* 5 (2005): 502–5.

Elsberg, C. A., "The Anatomy and Surgery of the Edwin Smith Surgical Papyrus," *Journal of Mount Sinai Hospital* 12 (1945): 141–51.

Erman Adolf, and Grapow, Hermann, *Wörterbuch der ägyptischen Sprache*. 5 vols. Leipzig: Hinrichs, 1926–1931.

Estes, J. W., *The Medical Skills of Ancient Egypt*. Canton, MA: Science History Publications, 1993.

Estrela, C., J. D. Pecora, M. D. Souza-Neto, C. R. Estrela, L. L. Bammann, "Effect of Vehicle on Antimicrobial Properties of Calcium Hydroxide Pastes," *Brazilian Dental Journal* 10/2 (1999): 63–72. Online: http://www.ncbi.nlm.nih.gov/pubmed/10863391.

Faulkner R. O., *A Concise Dictionary of Middle Egyptian*. Oxford: Griffith Institute Asmolean Museum, 1962. Repr. Frome and London: Butler & Tanner, 1996.

———, "*dw, wdi, rdi*," *Journal of Egyptian Archaeology* 45 (1959): 102.

Filer, J. M., "Head Injuries in Egypt and Nubia: A Comparison of Skulls from Giza and Kerma," *Journal of Egyptian Archaeology* 78 (1992): 281–85.

———, "Ancient Egypt and Nubia as a Source of Information for Cranial Injuries." Pages 48–73 in *Material Harm: Archaeological Studies of War and Violence*. Edited by John Carman. Glasgow: Cruithne 1997.

Foster, J. L. *Thought Couplets in* The Tale of Sinuhe. Münchener Ägyptologische Beiträge 3. Frankfurt: Lang, 1993.

Friedman, F. D., "The Root Meaning of Ax: Effectiveness or Luminosity," *Serapis* 8 (1985): 39–46.

Frölich, Franz Hermann, *Die Militärmedicin Homers*. Stuttgart: Enke, 1879.

Gabay, Jeffrey, Gadi Borkow, Joseph Mishal, Eli Magen, Richard Zatcoff, and Yonat Shemer-Avni, "Copper Oxide Impregnated Textiles with Potent Biocidal Activities," *Journal of Industrial Textiles* 35/4 (2006): 323–35. Online: http://jit.sagepub.com/content/35/4/323.short.

Gabriel R. A., "War in the Ancient Word 2500 B.C.E.–1453 C.E." Page 24 in *The Great Armies of Antiquity*. Wesport, CT: Praeger, 2002.

Gardiner, Alan H. *Egyptian Grammar*. 3rd edition. Oxford: Oxford University Press/Griffith Institute, 1957.

Gee, J., "Fronted Adverbials," *Bulletin of the Egyptological Seminar* 18 (2008): 83–90.

Germer, R. *Handbuch der altägyptischen Heilpflanzen*. Phillipika: Marburger Altertumskundliche Abhandlungen 21. Wiesbaden: Harrassowitz, 2008.

Ghalioungui, Paul, *Magic and Medical Science in Ancient Egypt.* Amsterdam: Israël, 1963.

Gilula M., review of H. Satzinger, *Die negativen Konstruktionen im Alt- und Mittelägyptischen. Journal of Egyptian Archaeology* 56 (1970): 205–14.

———, "Sinuhe B 255," *Journal of Near Eastern Studies* 35 [1976]: 25–28.

———, "The Stative Form of the Verb *sḏm* 'to hear'," *Journal of the American Research Center in Egypt* 14 (1977): 37–40.

Goedicke, H., "The Scribal Palette of Athu (Berlin Inv. Nr. 7798)," *Chronique d'Égypte* 63 (1988): 42–56.

Goldwasser, O., "On Dynamic Canonicity in Late-Egyptian: The Literary Letter and the Personal Prayer," *Lingua Aegyptia* 1 (*Proceedings of the Second International Conference on Egyptian Grammar (Crossroads II) Los Angeles, October 17–20, 1990* (1991): 129–41.

Goodrich, J. T., "Cervical Spine Surgery in the Ancient and Medieval Worlds," *Neurosurgical Focus* 23/1 (2007): 2–4.

———, "History in Spine Surgery in the Ancient and Medieval Worlds," *Neurosurgical Focus* 16/1 (2004): 2.

Gordon, B. L., *Medicine through Antiquity.* Philadelphia: Davis, 1949.

Grapow, Hermann, *Die Medizinischen Texte in hieroglyphischer Umschreibung Autographiert.* Vol. 5 of *Grundriss der Medizin der Alten Ägypter.* Berlin: Akademie, 1958.

Griffiths, J. Gwyn, "The Relative *Nty* with Generic Reference," *Journal of Egyptian Archaeology* 54 (1968): 60–66.

Grmek, Mirko D., *Diseases in the Ancient Greek World.* Baltimore: Johns Hopkins University Press, 1989.

Grmek, Mirko D., ed., *Western Medical Thought from Antiquity to the Middle Ages.* Trans. Antony Shugaar. Cambridge, MA: Harvard University Press, 1998.

Gurdjian, Elisha S. *Head Injury from Antiquity to the Present with Special Reference to Penetrating Head Wounds.* Springfield, IL: Thomas, 1973.

———, *Impact Head Injury.* Springfield, IL: Thomas, 1975.

van Gurp, G., T. J. Hutchison, and W. A. Alto, "Arrow Wound Management in Papua New Guinea," *Journal of Trauma* 30/2 (1990): 183–88.

Halioua, Bruno, *La médecine au temps des pharaons.* Paris: Liana Levi, 2002.

Hannig, Rainer, *Grosses Handwörterbuch Deutsch–Ägyptisch.* Mainz: von Zabern 2000.

———, *Die Sprache der Pharaonen: Großes Handwörterbuch Ägyptisch–Deutsch (2800–950 v. Chr.).* Mainz: von Zabern, 2006.

Helgason, C. M., "Commentaries on the Significance for Modern Neurology of the 17th Century B.C. Surgical Papyrus," *Canadian Journal of Neurological Sciences* 14 (1987): 560–63.

Hoch, J. E., *Middle Egyptian Grammar.* SSEA Publications 15. Mississauga, Ontario: Benben, 1996.

Hodge, C. T., "Afroasiatic S-Causative," *Language Sciences* 15 (1971): 41–43.

Hoffman, Alan F., and Lars Eckmann, "How Bile Acids Confer Gut Mucosal Protection against Bacteria," *Proceedings of the National Academy of Sciences of the United States of America* 103/12 (2006): 4333–34. Online: http://www.ncbi.nlm.nih.gov/pmc/articles/PMC1450168/.

Horrax, G. *Neurosurgery: An Historical Sketch.* Springfield, IL: Thomas, 1952.

Houlihan, Patrick F., *The Birds of Ancient Egypt.* Warminster: Aris & Phillips, 1986.

Hoyt, D. B., R. Coimbra, and J. Acosta, "Management of Acute Trauma." Pages 477–97 in *Sabiston Textbook of Surgery.* 18th edition. Edited by Beauchamp Townsend and Mattox Evers. Philadelphia: Elsevier, 2008.

Hughes, J. T., "The Edwin Smith Surgical Papyrus: An Analysis of the First Case Reports of Spinal Cord Injuries," *Paraplegia* 26 (1988): 71–82.

Hussain, Hidayat, et al., "Chemical Constituents and Antimicrobial Activity of *Salix subserrata,*" *Records of Natural Products* 5/2 (2011): 133–37. Online: http://www.acgpubs.org/RNP/2011/Volume%205/Issue%201/18_RNP-1007-266.pdf.

Jones, F. W., "Some Lessons From Ancient Fractures," *British Medical Journal* (1908): 455–58.

Joy, R. J. T., "Tetanus." Pages 1043–46 in *The Cambridge World History of Human Disease.* Edited by Kenneth F. Kiple. Cambridge: Cambridge University Press, 1993.

Junge, Friedrich, "A Study on Sentential Meaning and the Notion of 'Emphasis' in Middle Egyptian." Pages 189–254 in *Crossroad: Chaos or the Beginning of a New Paradigm.* Edited by G. Englund and P. J. Frandsen. CNI Publications 1. Copenhagen: Carsten Niebuhr Institute, 1986.

———, *Emphasis and Sentential Meaning in Middle Egyptian.* Göttinger Orientforschungen 20. Wiesbaden: Harrassowitz, 1989.

———, "How to Study Egyptian Grammar and to What Purpose. A Summary of Sorts," *Lingua Aegyptia* 1 (*Proceedings of the Second International Conference on Egyptian Grammar (Crossroads II) Los Angeles, October 17–20, 1990* (1991): 389–426.

Jungraithmayr, W., and W. Weder, W. "Chest Surgical Disorders in Ancient Egypt," *Annals of Surgery,* 255/3 (2012): 607.

Kammerzell, Frank, "Augment, Stamm und Endung. Zur morphologischen Entwicklung der Stativkonjugation," *Lingua Aegyptia* 1 (*Proceedings of the Second International Conference on Egyptian Grammar (Crossroads II) Los Angeles, October 17–20, 1990* (1991): 389–426.

———, "Norm, Relikt oder Fiktion? Zweifel an der Existenz einer morphologisch-syntaktischen Kategorie 'indikativ-perfektisches *sḏm=f*' im M[ittel]äg[yptischen]," *Göttinger Miszellen* 102 (1988) 41–57.

Jungraithmayr, W., and W. Weder, "Chest Surgical Disorders in Ancient Egypt." *Annals of Surgery*, 255/3 (2012): 165–99.

Kaye, A. S., "The Nature of the Root in Semitic and Egyptian." Pages 93–111 in *Festschrift in Honor of the Twenty-Fifth Anniversary of California State University, Fullerton*. Edited by J. Kalir. Fullerton, CA: California State University, 1984.

Keith, L. Moore, and Arthur F. Dalley. *Clinically Oriented Anatomy*. 5th Edition. Philadelphia: Lippincot Williams & Wilkins, 2006.

Khalil, N., M. N. Elwany, and J. D. Miller, et al. "Transcranial Stab Wounds: Morbidity and Medicolegal Awareness," *Surgical Neurology* 35 (1988): 294–99.

Khan, A. N., and I. Turnbull, "Neurofibromatosis Type 1 Imaging." Medscape Reference: http://emedicine.medscape.com/article/342500-overview.

Kilgour, F. G., "Locating Information in an Egyptian Text of the 17th Century B.C.," *Journal of the American Society for Information Sciences* 44/5 (1993): 292–97.

Krajnik, M., Z. Zylicz, F. Finlay, J. Luckza, A. A. van Sorge, "Potential Use of Topical Opioids in Palliative Care Report of 6 Cases," *Pain* 80 (1999): 121–25.

Kroeber, B., "Die Neuägyptizismen vor der Amarnazeit." PhD dissertation, Tübingen, 1970.

Lakshminarayanan, R., R. Manjunatha Kini, and S. Valiyaveettil. "Investigation of the Role of Ansocalcin in the Biomemineralization in Goose Eggshell Matrix," *Proceedings of the National Academy of Sciences* 99/8 (2002): 5155–59. Online: http://www.pnas.org/content/99/8/5155.full.

Lawless, M. W., "Midshaft Humerus Fractures." Medscape Reference: http://emedicine.medscape.com/article/1239985-treatment.

Laub, D. R., "Facial Trauma, Mandibular Fractures." Medscape Reference: http://emedicine.medscape.com/article/1283150-treatment.

Leca, A. P., "Maladies Infectieuses, épidémies," *La Médicine Ėgyptienne au Temps des Pharaons*. Paris: R. Dacosta, 1971.

Le Fort, René, "Étude expérimental sur les fractures de la machoire supérieure," *Revue de Chirurgie* 23 (1901): 208–27.

Le Reux, Gordon, "Surgery in Ancient Egypt: A Fresh Dissection of the Edwin Smith Surgical Papyrus." Poster presentation, The Third British Egyptology Congress, 11–12 September 2010. London: The British Museum.

Leestma, J. E., et al. "Impact Injuries to the Brain and Head," *Forensic Neuropathology* (1988): 190–95.

Lefèbvre, Gustave, *Grammaire de l'egyptien classique*. 2nd edition. Cairo: IFAO, 1955.

———, *Essai sur la médecine égyptienne de l'époque pharaonique*. Paris: Presses universitaires de France, 1956.

Leick, G., *The Babylonians: An Introduction*. New York: Routledge, 2003.

Lloyd, A. B., "Once More Hammamat Inscription 191," *Journal of Egyptian Archaeology* 61 (1975): 54–66.

Levy, David B., and Brian S. Gruber, "Neck Trauma." Medscape Reference: http://emedicine.medscape.com/article/827223-overview.

Lucas, A., *Ancient Egyptian Materials and Industries*. 3rd edition. London: Arnold, 1948.

Lucas, A., *Ancient Egyptian Materials and Industries*. 4th edition, rev. and enl. London: Arnold, 1962.

Lukosiunas, A., G. Sabalys, and R. Kubilus, "Prediction of Mandible Traumatic Osteomyelitis," *Stomatoloija, Baltic Dental and Maxillofacial Journal* 5 (2003): 65–69.

Majno, Guido, *The Healing Hand: Man and Wound in the Ancient World*. Cambridge, MA: Harvard University Press, 1975.

Majorga, Oliver, and Natalie P. Higgins, "Nasal Fracture Reduction: Treatment & Medication." Medscape Reference: http://emedicine.medscape.com/article/82831-treatment.

Manassa, Colleen, *The Great Karnak Inscription of Merneptah: Grand Strategy in the 13th Century BC*. Yale Egyptological Studies 5. New Haven: Yale Egyptological Seminar, 2003.

Masdeu, J. C., "Aphasia," *Archives of Neurology* 57 (2000): 892–95.

McDonald, A. "A Metaphor for Troubled Times: The Evolution of the Seth Deity Determinative in the First Intermediate Period," *Zeitschrift für ägyptische Sprache und Altertumskunde* 134 (2007): 26–39.

———, "The Curiosity of the Cat in Hieroglyphs." Pages 361–79 in *Sitting beside Lepsius: Studies in Honour of Jaromir Malek at the Griffith Institute*. Edited by Diana Magee, Janine Bourriau, and Stephen Quirke. Leuven; Walpole, MA: Uitgeverij Peeters en Departement Oosterse Studies, 2009.

———, "Writing as a Weapon in Letters to the Dead." Paper presented at the British Egyptological Conference at the British Museum, 2010.

"Medical Uses of Copper in Antiquity." Copper Development Association, Inc.: http://www.copper.org/publications/newsletters/innovations/2000/06/medicine-chest.html.

Meeks, Dimitri, *Année Lexicographique* 1 (1977), Paris: Impr. de la Margeride, 1980.

Mekhail, A. O., P. M. Steinmetz, and E. C. Benzel, "Subaxial Cervical Spine Burst Fractures." Pages 683–95 in *The Cervical Spine*. Edited by Charles R. Clark. 4th Edition. Philadelphia: Lippincott Williams & Wilkins, 2005.

Meltzer, Edmund S. "Earthquakes in Ancient Egypt with Emphasis on Upper Egypt." Pages 251–73 in *Earthquake Activity and Dam Stability Evaluations for the Aswan High Dam, Egypt* (USAID Project). Walnut Creek: Woodward-Clyde Consultants, 1985.

———, "Hieratic Is Beautiful: Ancient Egyptian Calligraphy Revisited." Pages 293–301 in *Writing Systems and Cognition*. Edited by W. C. Watt. Dordrecht: Kluwer, 1994.

———, "Introduction to Old Coptic Texts of Ritual Power." Pages 13–20 in *Ancient Christian Magic: Coptic Texts of Ritual Power*. Edited by M. W. Meyer and R. Smith. San Francisco: HarperSanFrancisco, 1994.

———, "*Ỉw wn/nn wn* + Indefinite Noun in Old and Middle Egyptian," *Journal of Ancient Civilizations* 5 (1990): 135–50.

———, "The 'Misplaced Letter to the Dead,' and a Stela, Found Again." Paper presented at the annual meeting of the American Research Center in Egypt. Seattle, 2008.

———, "*Nḥ3 n(y) inr* (Wady Hammamat #191): An Earth Tremor?" Paper presented at the annual meeting of the American Research Center in Egypt. New York, 1985.

———, "An Observation on the Hieroglyph " *Journal of Egyptian Archaeology* 56 (1970): 193–94.

———, "Once Again Initial Adverbials and the Standard Theory." Paper presented at the annual meeting of the American Research Center in Egypt. Chicago, 2011.

———, "Participles, Relative Forms and Gemination in Middle Egyptian: A Working Paper," *Lingua Aegyptia* 1 (*Proceedings of the Second International Conference on Egyptian Grammar (Crossroads II) Los Angeles, October 17–20, 1990* (1991): 227–40.

———, "Problems of Adjectival Constructions in Old and Middle Egyptian." PhD dissertation, University of Toronto, 1980.

———, "A Rare Use of *ḏs* + Suffix Pronoun in Middle Egyptian," *Journal of the American Research Center in Egypt* 12 (1975): 33–35.

———, "Wenamun 2, 46," *Journal of the Society for the Study of Egyptian Antiquities* 17 (1987): 86–88.

———, review of Éric Doret, *The Narrative Verbal System of Old and Middle Egyptian. Journal of the American Research Center in Egypt* 27 (1990): 223–24.

———, review of Jürgen Osing, *Die Nominalbildung des Ägyptischen*, *Journal of the American Research Center in Egypt* 15 (1978): 142–45.

Mehta, Samit S., "Biochemical Serum Markers in Head Injury: An Emphaisis on Clinical Utility," *Clinical Neurosurgery* 57 (2010): 134–40.

Mertz, Barbara, *Red Land, Black Land: Daily Life in Ancient Egypt*. 2nd ed. New York: Morrow, 2008.

Miller, R. L., "Tetanus after Cranial Trauma in Ancient Egypt," *Journal of Neurology, Neurosurgery and Psychiatry* 63/6 (1997): 758.

Minagar, A. J. Ragheb, and R. E. Kelly, "The Edwin Smith Surgical Papyrus: Description and Analysis of the Earliest Case of Aphasia," *Journal of Medical Biology* 11 (2003): 114–17.

Moe, Kris S., Patrick Byrne, David W. Kim, and Adele R. Tawfilis. "Maxillary and Le Fort Fractures." Medscape Reference: http://emedicine.medscape.com/article/1283568-overview.

Möller, Georg, *Hieratische Paläographie: Die ägyptische Buchschrift in ihrer Entwicklung von der 5. Dynastie bis zur römischen Kaiserzeit*. Leipzig: Hinrichs, 1927. Repr., Osnabrück: Zeller, 1965.

Moscati, Sabatino, et al. *An Introduction to the Comparative Grammar of the Semitic Languages: Phonology and Morphology*. Wiesbaden: Harrassowitz, 1969.

Moss, C. W., et al. "Gas Chromatography of Bacterial Fatty Acids with a Fused Silica Capillary Column," *Journal of Clinical Microbiology* 28 (1974): 80–85.

Muller, K., "Samuel Birch, the Discreet Pioneer Egyptologist," *The Egyptological Seminar News* 3/1 (Fall 1997/Winter 1998) 1, 3–4.

Nadalo, Lennard A., and Kory Jones, "Rib Fracture Imaging." Medscape Reference: http://www.emedicine.com/radio/topic609.htm.

Namias, N., "Honey in the Management of Infections," *Surgical Infections* 4/2 (2003): 219–26.

"NF1." Genetics Home Reference: http://ghr.nlm.nih.gov/gene/NF1.

"Neurofibromatosis." Genetics Home Reference: http://ghr.nlm.nih.gov/condition/neurofibromatosis-type-1.

"Nocardiosis." DermaAmin. Atlas of Dermatology: http://www.dermaamin.com/site/atlas-of-dermatology/13-n/1010-nocardiosis-.html.

Noffze, M. J., and R. S. Tubbs, "René Le Fort 1869–1951" *Clinical Anatomy* 24 (2011): 278–81.

Nunn, John F. *Ancient Egyptian Medicine*. Norman: University of Oklahoma Press, 2002.

Obaseiki-Elbor, E. E., T. C. Afonya, and A. O. Onyekweli, "Preliminary Report on the Antimicrobial Activity of Honey Distillate," *Journal of Pharmacy and Pharmacology* 35 (1983): 748–49.

Obaseiki-Elbor, E. E., and T. C. Afonya, "In-Vitro Evaluation of the Anticandidiasis Activity of Honey Distillate (HY-1) Compared with That of Some Antimycotic Agents," *Journal of Pharmacy and Pharmacology* 36 (1984): 283–84.

Ogdon, Jorge R., *Sharing New Ideas on the Phenomenon of Possession in Ancient Egypt*. Estudios del C.E.A.E. 1/A. Buenos Aires: Centro de Estudios del Antiguo Egipto, 1997.

Oehmichen, Manfred, R. N. Auer, and H. G. König, *Forensic Neuropathology and Associated Neurology*. Berlin: Springer, 2006.

Olivicra, A. L., J. F. Mano, and R. L. Reis, "Nature-Inspired Calcium Phosphate Coatings: Present Status and Novel Advances in the Science of Mimicry," *Science Direct. Current Opinion in Solid State & Materials Science* 7 (2003): 309–18.

O'Neill, O. R., G. Gilliland, J. B. Delashaw, and T. J. Purtzer, "Transorbital Penetrating Head Injury with a Hunting Arrow," *Surgical Neurology* 42/6 1994): 494–97.

Pahor, A. L., "Ear Nose and Throat in Ancient Egypt." *The Journal of Otolaryngology and Otology* 106 (1992): 863–73.

Parker, Richard A., *A Saite Oracle Papyrus from Thebes*. Brown Egyptological Studies 4. Providence: Brown University Press, 1962.

Parry, A. D., P. R. Chadwick, D. Simon, B. Oppenheim, and C. N. McCollum, "Leg Ulcer Odour Detection Identifies Beta-Haemolytic Strepto-coccal Infection," *Journal of Wound Care* 4/9 (1995): 404–6.

Partridge Robert B., "Weapons and Military Equipment." Pages 21–73 *Fighting Pharaohs: Weapons and Warfare in Ancient Egypt.* Manchester, U.K.: Peartree Publishing, 2002.

Peacock, Z. S., P. H. Chapman, R. Gupta, and L. B. Kaban, "Replication of Ancient Egyptian Osteotomies of the Facial Skeleton: Insights into the Mummification Process," *International Journal of Oral Maxillofacial Surgery* 40/11 (2011): 1301–6.

Polotsky, Hans Jacob, "Ägyptische Verbalformen und ihre Vokalisation," *Orientalia* 33 (1964): 267–85.

———, *Egyptian Tenses.* Israel Academy of Sciences and Humanities Proceedings 2/5. Jerusalem: Central Press, 1965.

———, "Les transpositions du verbe en égyptien classique," *Israel Oriental Studies* 6 (1976): 1–50.

Potter, Paul, *Hippocrates*, vol. 9. Edited and Translated by Paul Potter. LCL 509. Cambridge, MA: Harvard University Press, 2010.

Prieto, A. I., F. Ramos-Morales, and J. Casadesus, "Bile-Induced DNA Damage in Salmonella enterica," *Genetics* 168 (2004): 1787–94.

Quack, J. F., "Zum Lautwert von Gardiner Sign-List U 23," *Lingua Aegyptia* 11 (2003): 113–16.

Ragge, N. K., and F. L. Munier, "Ancient Neurofibromatosis," *Nature* 368 (1994): 815. Online: http://ghr.nlm.nih.gov/condition/neurofibromatosis-type-1.

Ralston, B. L., "Compound Elevated Fractures of the Skull," *Journal of Neurosurgery* 44 (1976): 77–79.

———, "Medical Reinterpretation of Case Four of the Edwin Smith Surgical Papyrus," *Journal of Egyptian Archaeology* 63 (1977): 116–21.

Rangel-Castilla, Leonardo, and Jaime Gasco, "Closed Head Trauma." Medscape Reference: http://emedicine.medscape.com/article/251834-overview.

Redford, Donald B., *Pharaonic King-Lists, Annals, and Day-Books*. Mississauga: Benben, 1986.

———, *Egypt, Canaan, and Israel in Ancient Times*. Princeton: Princeton University Press, 1992.

Revis, D. R., Jr., "Clostridial Gas Gangrene." Medscape Reference: http://emedicine.medscape.com/article/214992-overview.

Ritner, Robert K., "The Cardiovascular System in Ancient Egyptian Thought," *Journal of Near Eastern Studies* 65/2 (2006): 99–102.

———, *The Mechanics of Ancient Egyptian Magical Practice*. Studies in Ancient Oriental Civilization 54. Chicago: The Oriental Institute of the University of Chicago, 1993.

Rohde, R. S., and J. D. Kang, "Thoracic Disc Herniation Presenting with Chronic Nausea and Abdominal Pain." *The Journal of Bone and Joint Surgery (American)* 86 (2004): 379–81.

Ropper, A. H., D. O'Rourke, and S. K. Kennedy, "Head Position, Intracranial Pressure and Compliance." *Neurology* 23 (1982): 1288–91.

Rosner, M. J. et al., "Cerebral Perfusion Pressure, and Head Elevation," *Journal of Neurosurgery* 60 (1986): 636.

Ross, A. T., and D. J. Becker, "Nasal and Septal Fractures." Medscape Reference: http://emedicine.medscape.com/article/878595-overview.

Rubino, L. J., M. W. Lawless, and B. P. Kleinhenz, "Clavicle Fractures." Medscape Reference: http://emedicine.medscape.com/article/1260953-overview.

Rudzinski, John P., "Sternoclavicular Joint Injury." Medscape Reference: http://www.emedicine.com/emerg/topic783.htm.

Sahrakar, Kamran, and Martin Melicharek, "Lumbar Disc Disease." Medscape Reference: http://emedicine.medscape.com/article/249113-overview.

Salazar, Christine F., *The Treatment of War Wounds in Graeco-Roman Antiquity*. Studies in Ancient Medicine 21. Leiden: Brill, 2000.

Sanchez, Gonzalo M., "A Neurosurgeon's View of the Battle Reliefs of King Sety I: Aspects of Neurological Importance," *Journal of the American Research Center in Egypt* 27 (2000): 143–65.

———, "Injuries in the Battle of Kadesh," *KMT* 14/1 (2003): 58–65.

Sanchez, Gonzalo M., and T. Siuda, "Ebers Papyrus Case #873 - A Probable Case of Neurofibromatosis," *The South Dakota Journal of Medicine* 55/12 (2000): 529–35.

Sandison, A. T., "Evidence of Infective Disease," *Journal of Human Evolution* 1/2 (1972): 213–24.

Sanford, J., "Tetanus - Forgotten But Not Gone," *New England Journal of Medicine* 332 (1995): 812–13.

Satzinger, H., "Die Protasis *ir sḏm.f* im älteren Ägyptisch," *Lingua Aegyptia* 3 (1993): 121–35.

Schenkel, W., "Die Farben in ägyptischer Kunst und Sprache," *Zeitschrift für ägyptische Sprache und Altertumskunde* 88 (1963): 131–47.

———, "Das Ende des narrativen *sdm.t=f*," *Göttinger Miszellen* 4 (1973): 23–28.

Scurlock, J., and B. R. Anderson, *Diagnoses in Assyrian and Babylonian Medicine: Ancient Sources, Translations, and Modern Medical Analyses*. Urbana: University of Illinois Press, 2005.

Shashlaie, K., D. J. Chang, J. T. Anderson, "Nonmissile Penetrating Spinal Injury," *Journal of Neurosurgery: Spine* 4 (2006): 400–409. Online: http://thejns.org/doi/pdf/10.3171/spi.2006.4.5.400.

Smith, H. S., P. Johnson, and J. Barr, review of H. J. Polotsky, *Collected Papers*, *Journal of Semitic Studies* 18 (1973): 129–44.

Smith, Jesse E., and Carlos L. Perez, "Nasal Fracture Imaging." Medscape Reference: http://www.emedicine.com/radio/topic468.htm#section~introduction#section~introduction.

Smith, Robert W., *A Treatise on the Pathology, Diagnosis and Treatment of Neuroma*. Dublin: Hodges and Smith, 1849.

Smythe, W. R., S. I. Reznik, J. B. Putnam, Jr., "Lung (Including Pulmonary Embolism and Thoracic Outlet Syndrome)." Page 1729 in *Sabiston Textbook of Surgery*. 18th Edition. Edited by Beauchamp Townsend and Mattox Evers. Philadephia: Elsevier. Philadelphia, 2008.

Solbrig, M. V., "Tetanus," *Neurology in Clinical Practice* 2 (2000): 1340–42.

Stiefel, M., A. Shaner, and S. D. Schaefer, "The Edwin Smith Papyrus: The Birth of Analytical Thinking in Medicine and Otolaryngology," *The Laryngoscope* 116 (2006): 182–88.

Stiver, S. I., and G. T. Manley, "Prehospital Management of Traumatic Brain Injury," *Neurosurgical Focus* 25/4 (2008): 1–11.

Takács, Gábor, *Etymological Dictionary of Egyptian*. Vol. 3: *m-*. Leiden: Brill, 2008.

Talairach, J., and P. Tournoux. *Co-Planar Stereotaxic Atlas of the Human Brain*. Stuttgart: Thieme, 1988.

Thomas, S. A., "Photochemical Constituents and Effects of Aqueous Root-Bark Extract of *Ficus sycomorus* L. (Moracaea) on Muscular Relaxation, Anaesthetic and Sleeping Time on Laboratory Animals," *African Journal of Biotechnology* 8/21 (2009): 6004–6.

Todar, K., "The Genus Clostridium," Todar's Online Textbook of Bacteriology, University of Wisconsin Department of Bacteriology. Online: http://www.textbookofbacteriology.net/Bacillus.html.

Tollefson, T. T., and E. B. Strong, "Zygomaticomaxillary Complex Fractures." Medscape Reference: http://emedicine.medscape.com/article/867687-overview.

Trask, T. W., and R. K. Narayan, "Civilian Penetrating Head Injury," *Neurotrauma* (1996): 868–89.

du Trevon, M. D., and J. R. van Dellen, "Penetrating Stab Wounds to the Brain: The Timing of Angiography in Patients Presenting with the Weapon Already Removed," *Neurosurgery* 13/5 (1992): 905–12.

Trott, Alexander T., *Wounds and Lacerations: Emergency Care and Closure*. 3rd edition. Philadelphia: Mosby, 2005.

Uljas, S., *The Modal System of Earlier Egyptian Complement Clauses*. Probleme der Ägyptologie 26. Leiden: Brill, 2007.

Vallet-Regi, M., and F. Balas,"Silica Materials for Medical Applications," *The Open Biomedical Engineering Journal* 2 (2008): 1–9.

Van Dellen, J. R., and R. Lipschitz, "Stab Wounds of thc Skull," *Surgical Neurology* 10 (1978): 110–12.

Van Middendorp, Joost J., Gonzalo M. Sanchez, and Alwin L. Burridge, "The Edwin Smith Papyrus: A Clinical Reappraisal of the Oldest Known Document on Spinal Injuries," *European Spine Journal* 19/11 (2010): 1815–1823. Online: http://www.springerlink.com/content/vk460l07q7028186/fulltext.pdf.

Veiga, Paula, *Oncology and Infectious Diseases in Ancient Egypt: The Ebers Papyrus' Treatise on Tumors 857–877 and the Cases Found in Ancient Egyptian Human Material*. Saarbrücken: Müller, 2009.

Vender, John R., Jason Miller, Andy Rekito, and Dennis E. McDonnell, "Effect of Hemostasis and Electrosurgery on the Development and Evolution of Brain Turmor Surgery in the Late 19th and Early 20th Centuries." *Neurosurgical Focus* 18/4 (2005): 7. Online: http://thejns.org/doi/pdfplus/10.3171/foc.(2005).18.4.4.

Veronesi, R., and R. Focaccia, "The Clinical Picture." Pages 190–95 in *Tetanus: Important New Concepts*. Edited by R. Veronesi. Amsterdam: Excerpta Medica; 1981.

Vinas, F. C., J. Pilitsis, M. G. Nosko, F. Talavera, R. M. Pluta, P. Zamboni, and R. A. Wyler, "Penetrating Head Trauma." Medscape Reference: http://emedicine.medscape.com/article/247664-overview.

Vycichl, W., "Coptic Dialect Geography Based on Inscriptions," *Enchoria* 8 (1978): 63*/109–65*/111.

Walker, James H., "Egyptian Medicine and the Gods," *The Bulletin of the Australian Centre for Egyptology* 4 (1993): 83–101.

———, *Studies in Ancient Egyptian Anatomical Terminology*, The Australian Centre for Egyptology Studies 4; Warminster: Aris & Phillips, 1996.

Walker, A. Earl, *The Genesis of Neuroscience*. New York: Thieme/AANS, 1998.

Ward, William A., *The Four Egyptian Homographic Roots B-3: Etymological and Egypto-Semitic Studies*. Studia Pohl, Series Maior 6. Rome: Pontifico Istituto Biblico, 1978.

Weber, J., and A. Czarnetzki, "Brief Communication: Neurotraumatological Aspects of Head Injuries Resulting from Sharp and Blunt Force in the Early Medieval Period of Southwestern Germany," *American Journal of Physical Anthropology* 14 (2001): 353–56.

Wente, E. F., "The Syntax of Verbs of Motion in Egyptian." PhD dissertation, University of Chicago, 1959.

Westendorf, Wolfhart, *Papyrus Edwin Smith: Ein medizinisches Lehrbuch aus dem alten Ägypten: Wund- und Unfallchirurgie, Zaubersprüche gegen Seuchen, verschiedene Rezepte*. Bern: Huber, 1966.

———, *Grammatik der medizinischen Texte*. Vol. 8 of *Grundriss der Medizin der alten Ägypter*. Berlin: Akademie, 1962.

———, *Handbuch der altägyptischen Medizin*. 2 vols. HdO 1.36. Leiden: Brill, 1999.

Wilkins, Robert H., *Neurosurgical Classics*. New York: The Harvey Cushing Society, 1965.

Williams, R. J., review of J. B. Callender, *Middle Egyptian*, *Journal of Biblical Literature* 98 (1979) 103–4.

Wilson, John A., *Signs and Wonders upon Pharaoh: A History of American Egyptology*. Chicago: University of Chicago Press, 1964.

Winlock, Herbert E. *The Slain Soldiers of Neb-hep-et-Re Mentu-hotpe*. New York: Metropolitan Museum of Art, 1945.

Wreszinski, Walter, *Atlas zur altaegyptischen Kulturgeschichte*. Leipzig: Hinrichs, 1923.

Zaku, S. G., F. A. Abdulrahaman, P. A. Onyeyili, O. C. Aguzue, and S. A. Thomas, "Photochemical Constituents and Effects of Aqueous Root-Bark Extract of *Ficus sycomorus* L. (Moracaea) on Muscular Relaxation, Anaesthetic and Sleeping Time on Laboratory Animals," *African Journal of Biotechnology* 8/21 (2009): 6004–6. Online: http://www.academicjournals.org/AJB/abstracts/abs2009/2Nov/Zaku%20et%20al.htm.

Zubillaga, Rodríguez I., G. Sánchez Aniceto, J. J. Montalvo Moreno, "Anterior Subcranial Approach: Discussion and Historical Review of the Surgical Technique," *Revista Española de Cirugía Oral y Maxilofacial* 31/1 (2009). Online: http://scielo.isciii.es/scielo.php?pid=S1130-05582009000100001&script=sci_arttext&tlng=en.

General and Medical Index

Page numbers followed by f indicate figures; t indicates tables.

Philological Index

Grammatical Terms and Forms, Palaeography, and Orthography, etc.

These follow English/Roman alphabetization even when Egyptian words are involved.

Egyptian Words

These follow Egyptian alphabetization, such as for instance Faulkner's dictionary. Glosses are only used for disambiguation.

PLATES

I

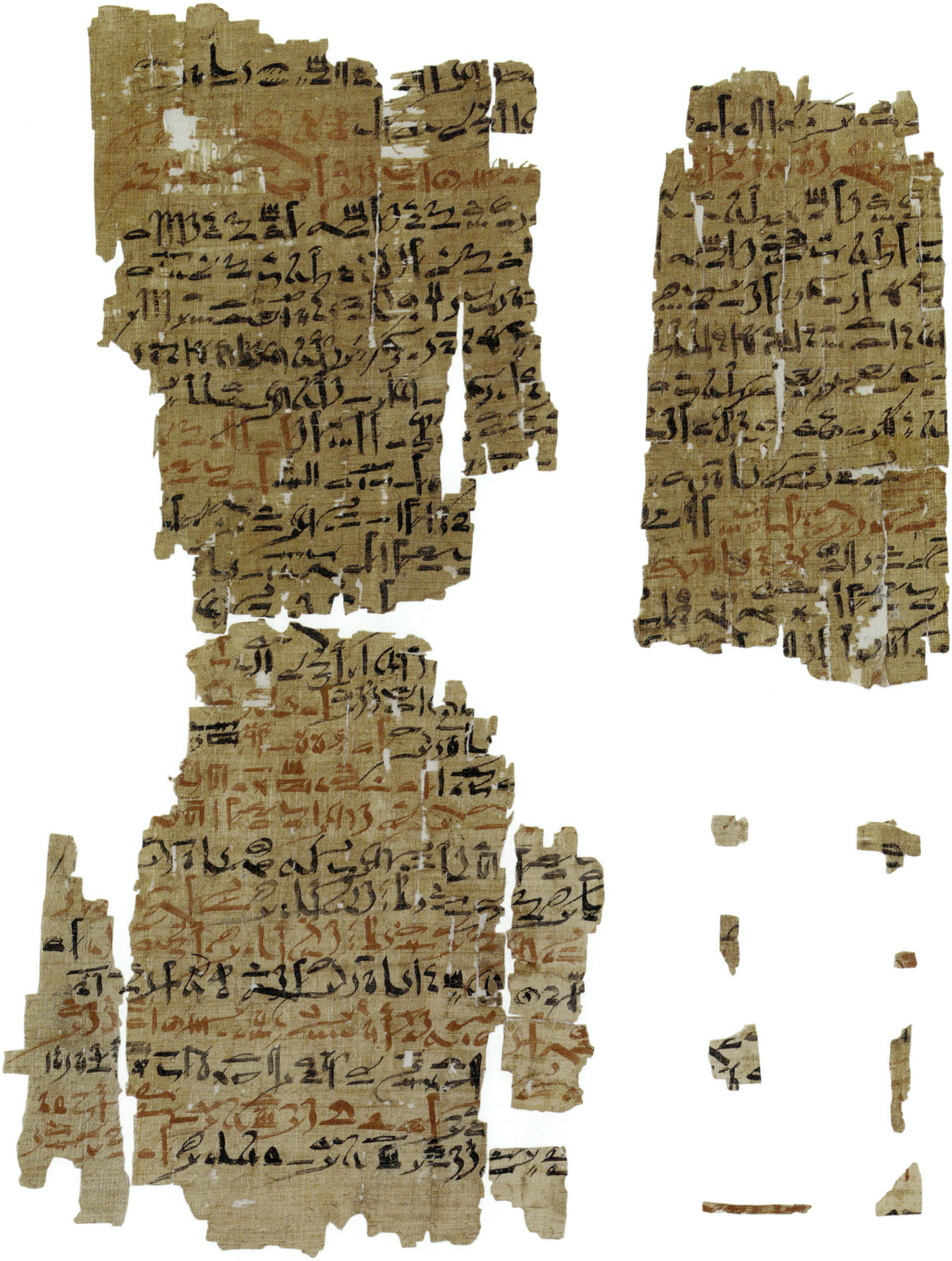

II

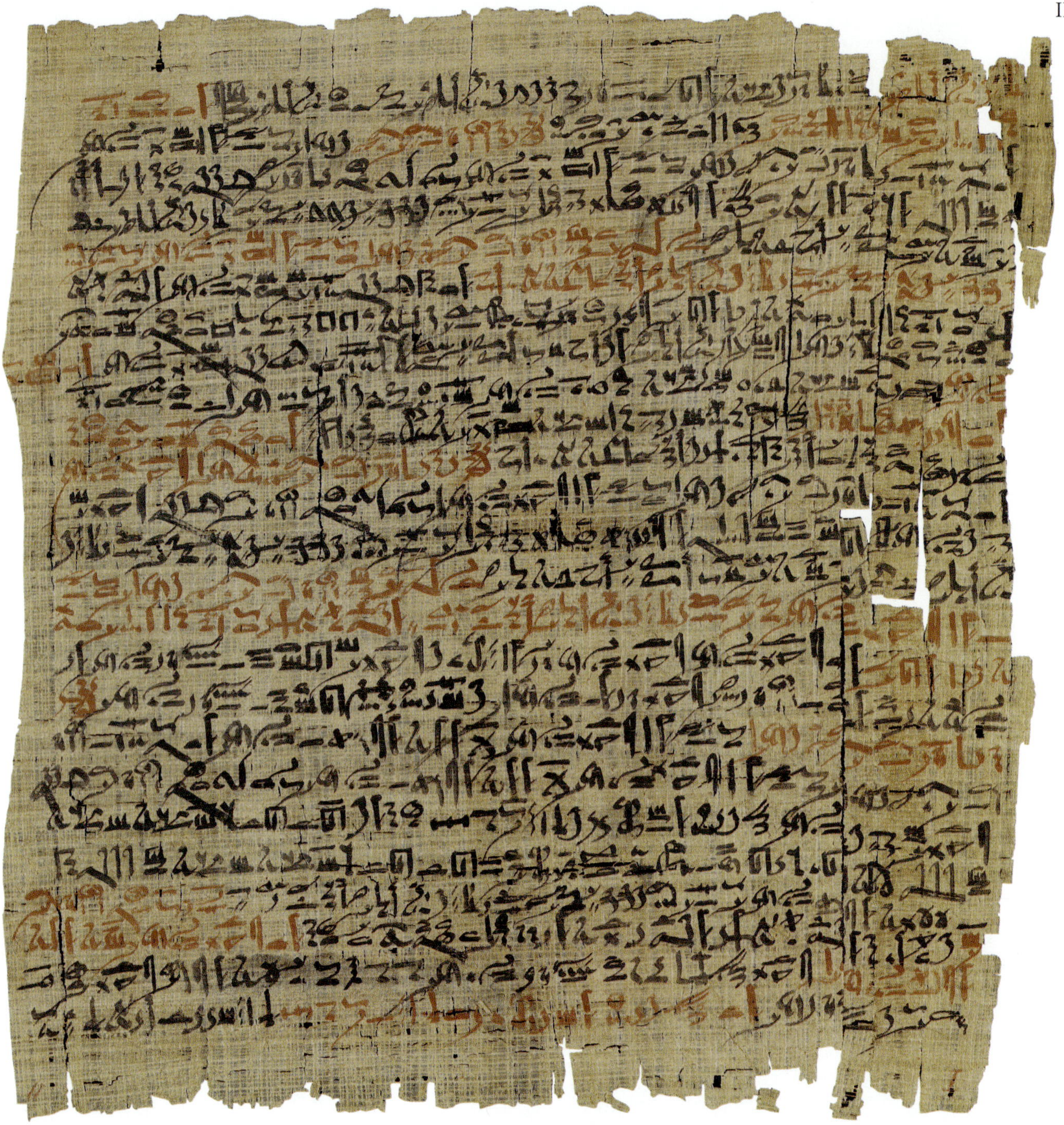

III

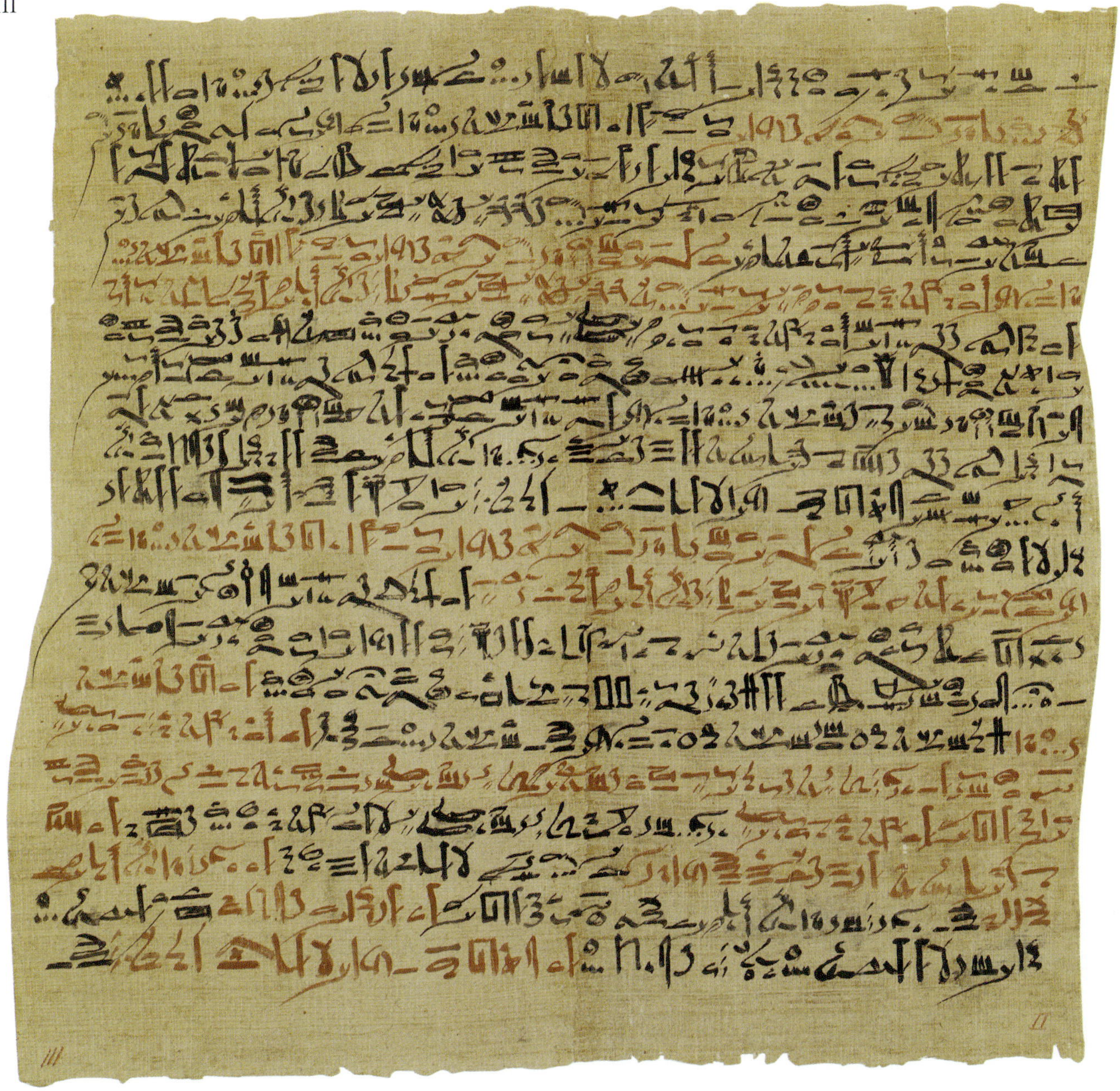

IV

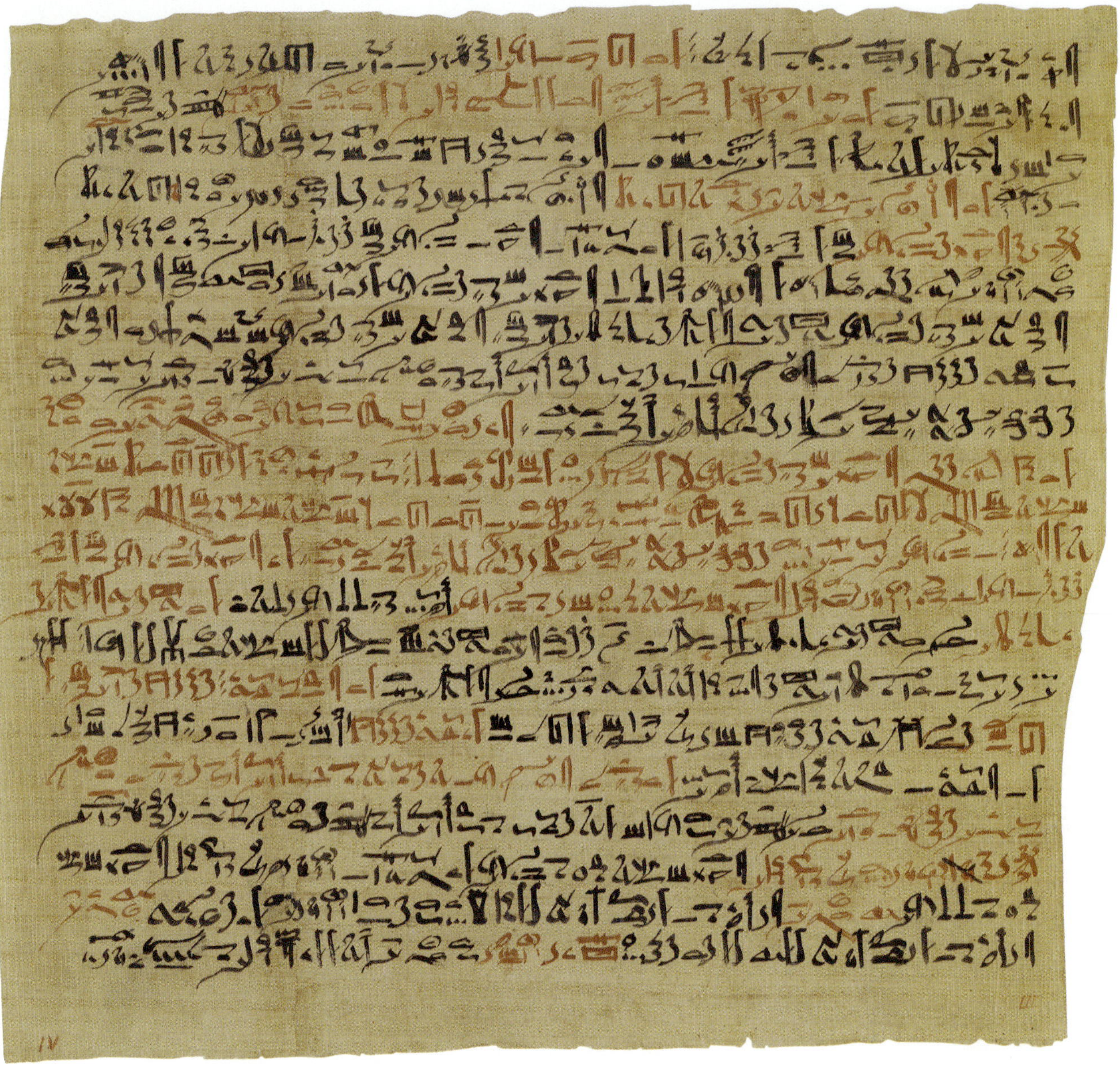

V

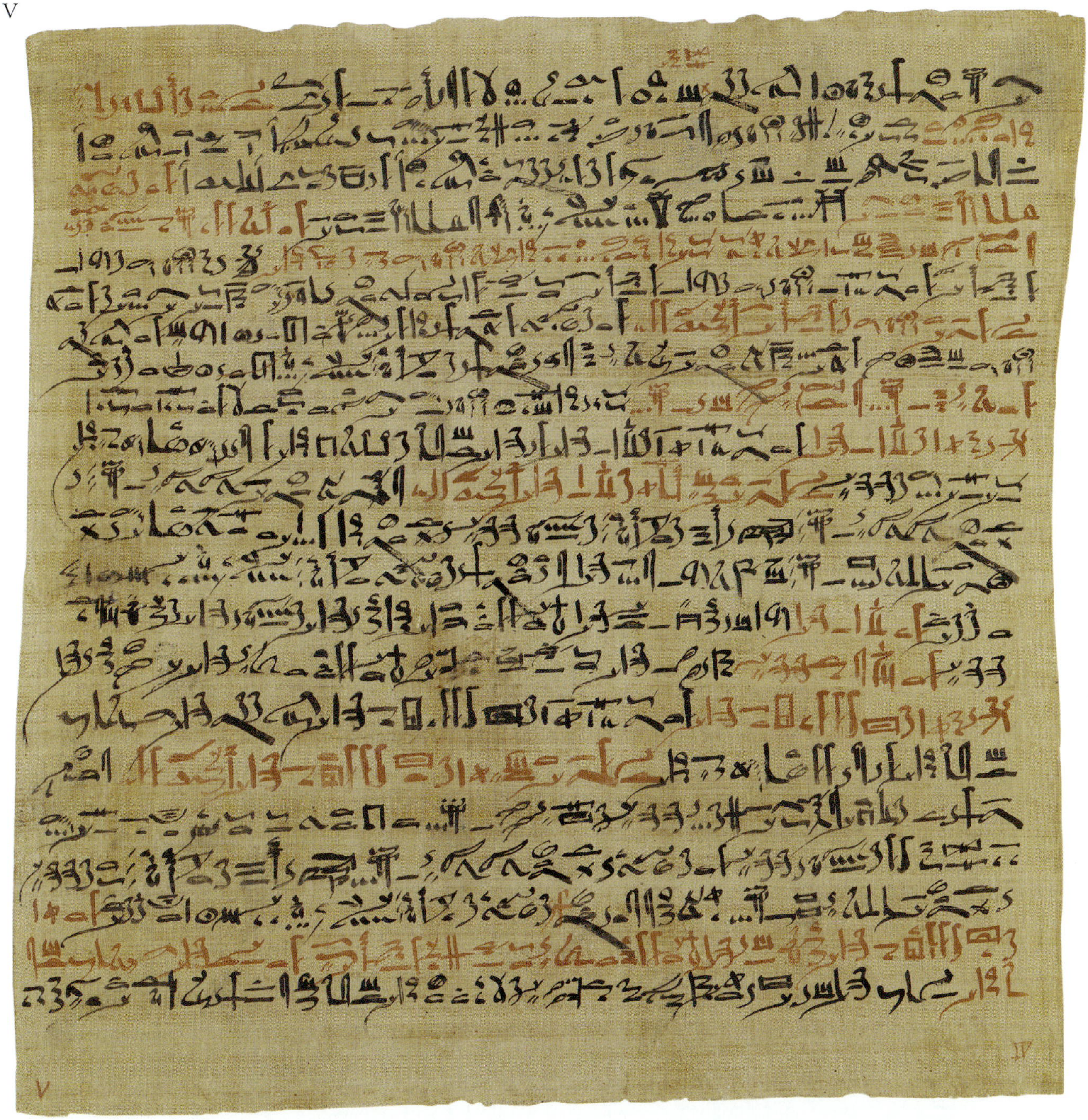

VI–VII

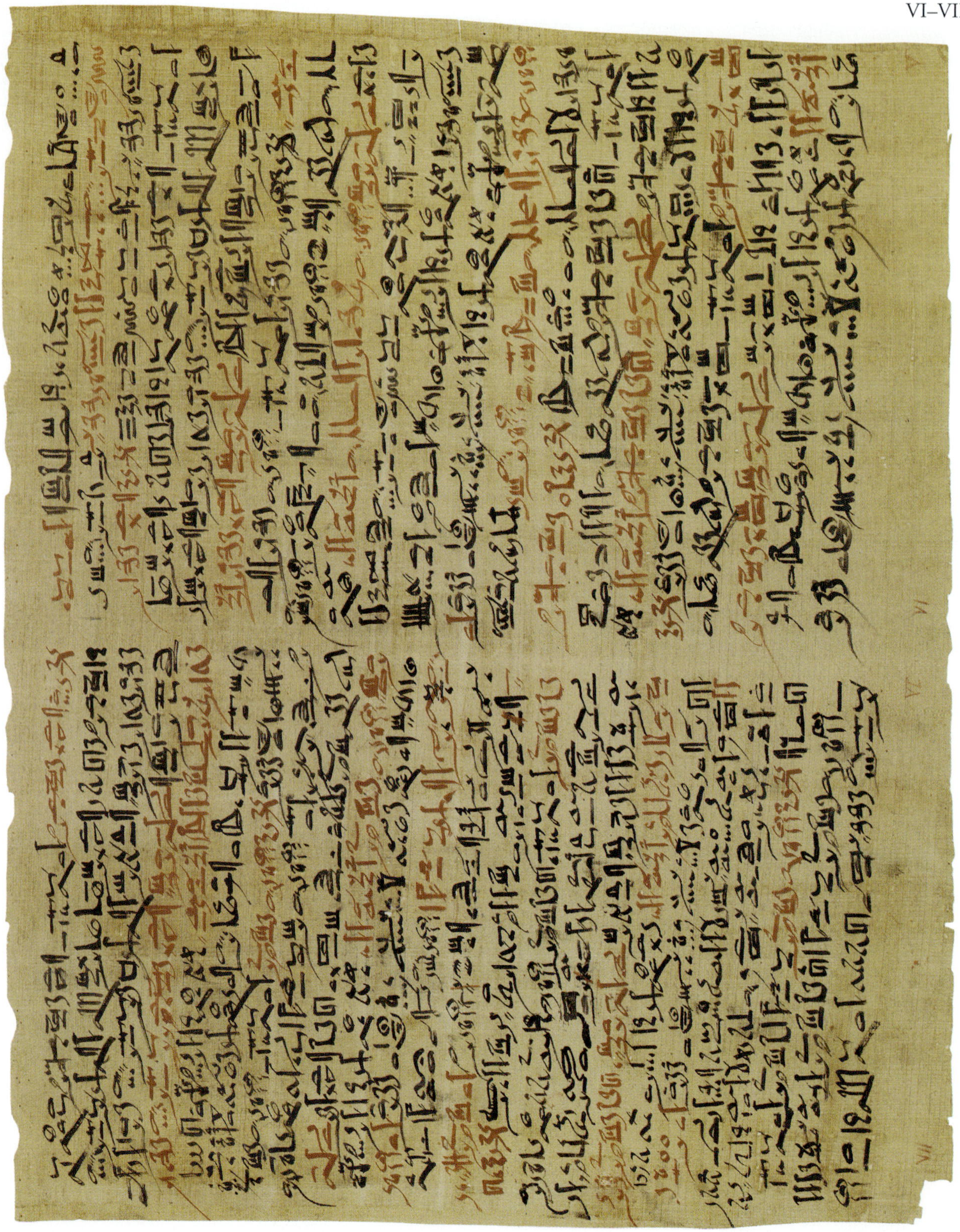

VIII–IX

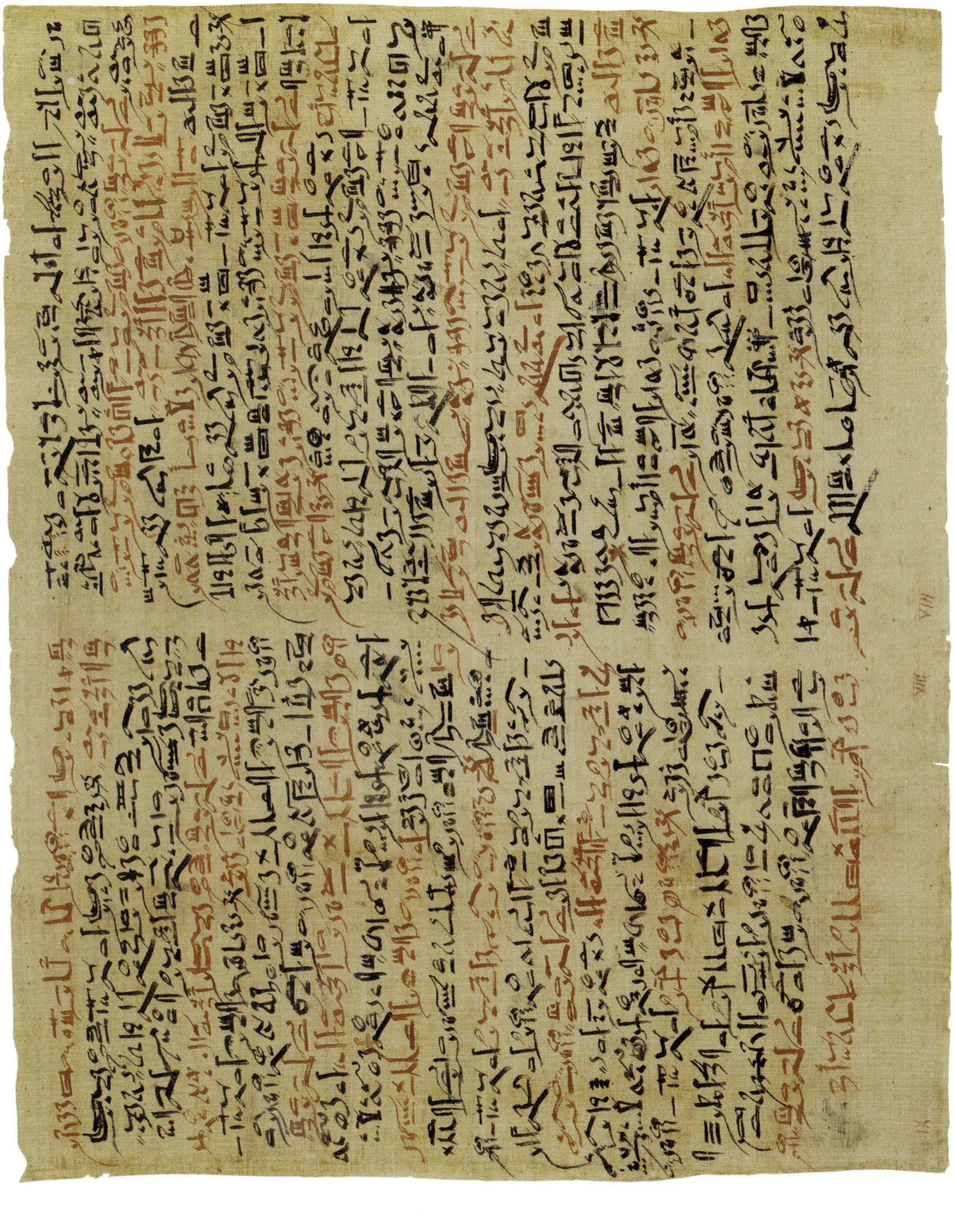

X–XI

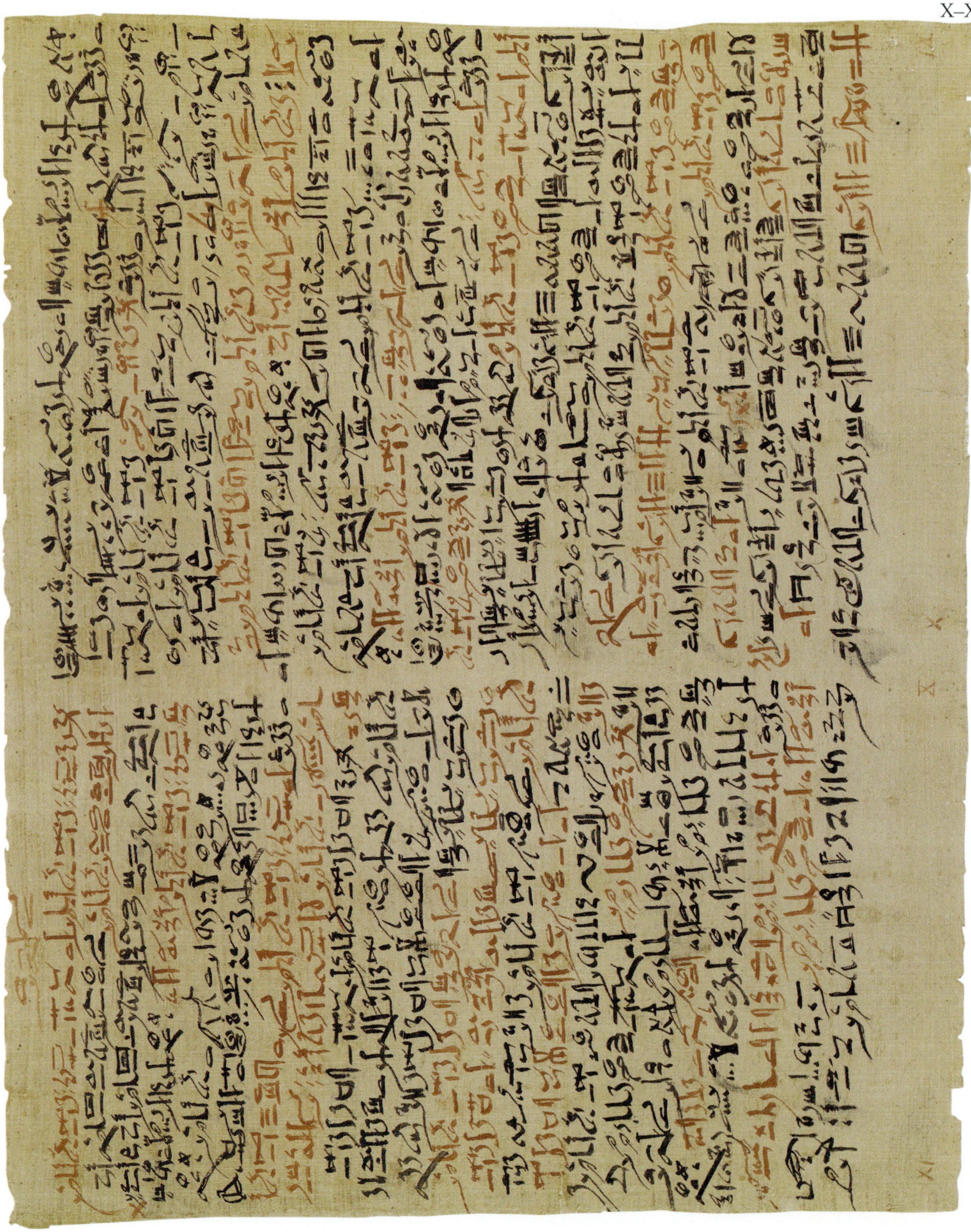

XII–XIII

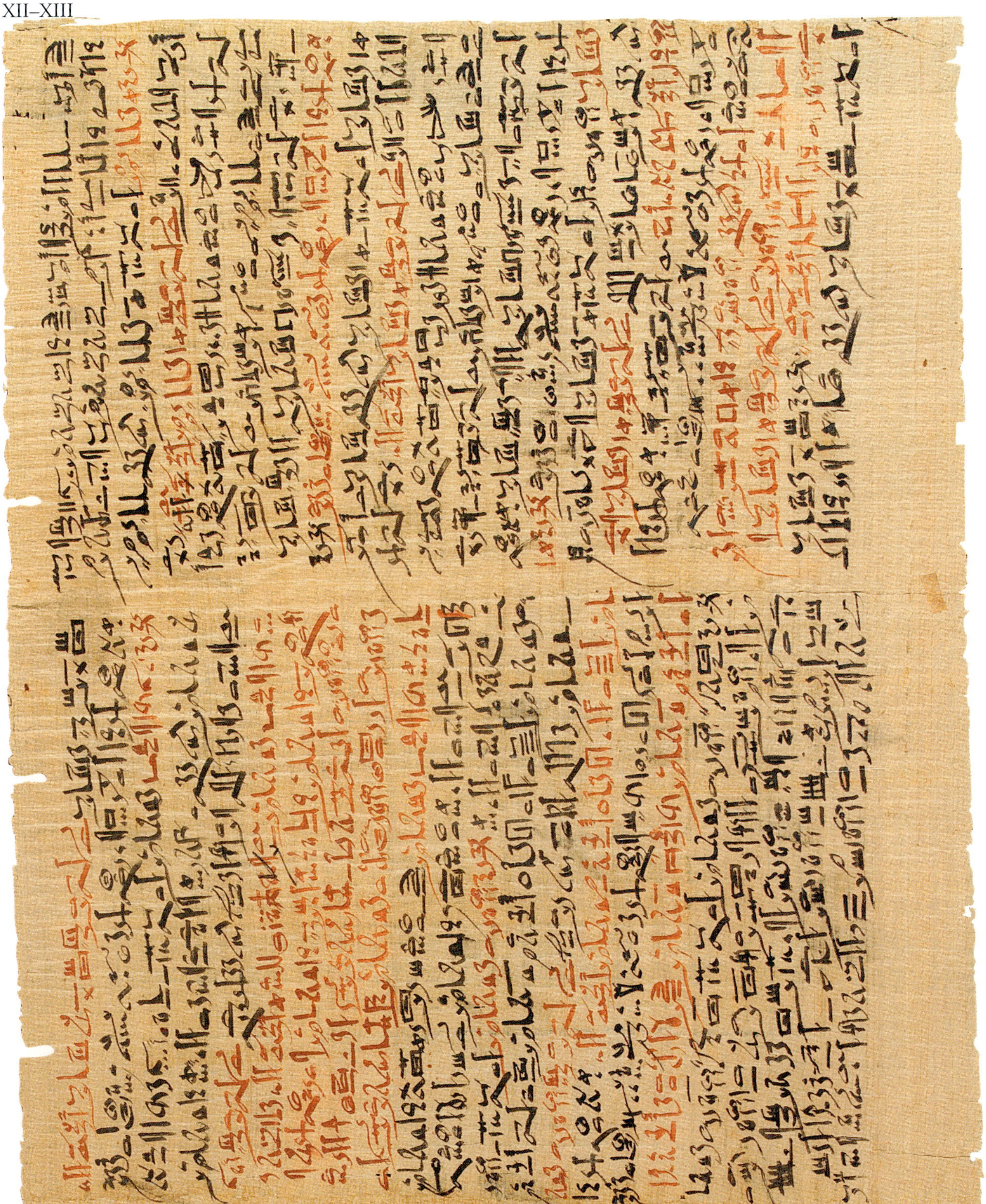

XIV–XV

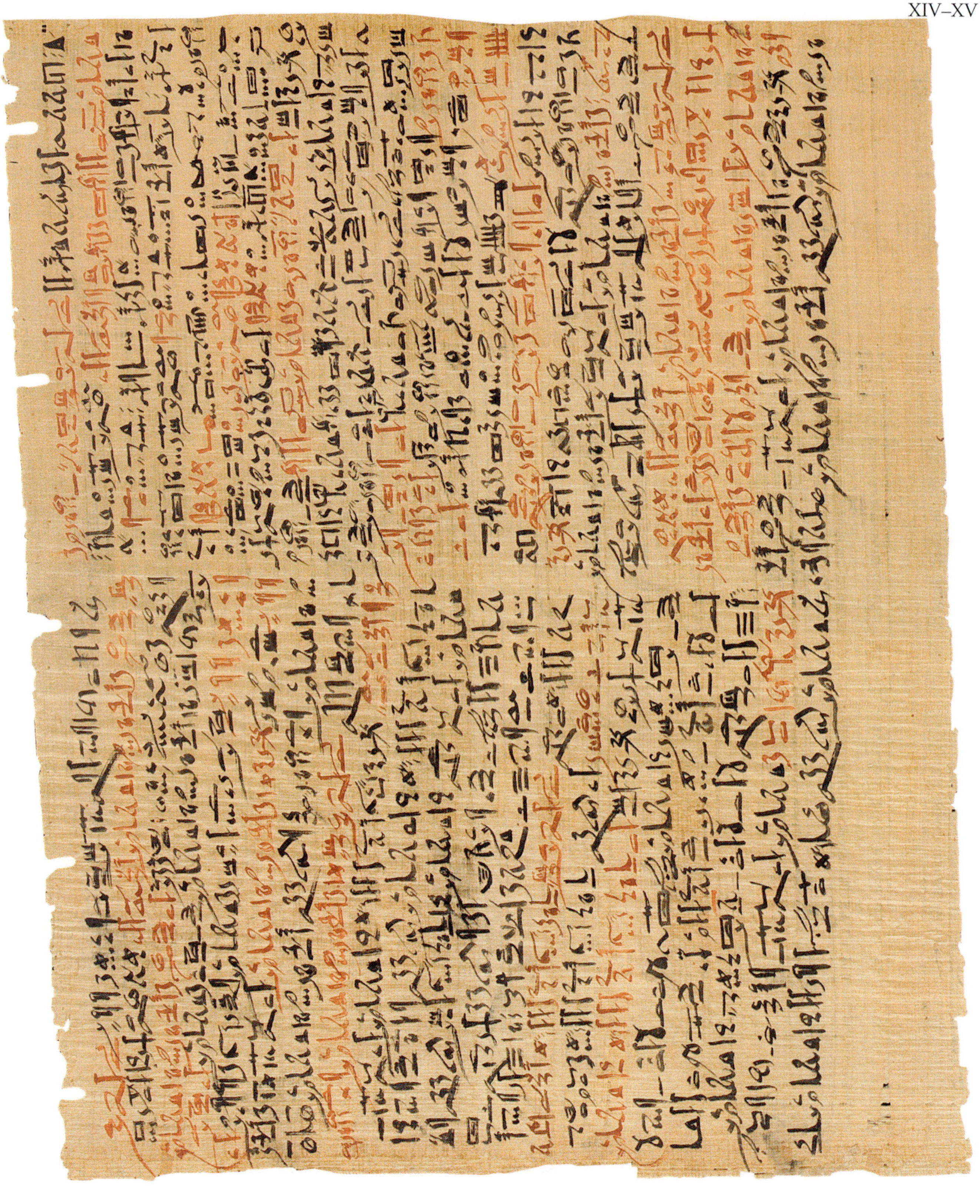

XVI–XVII

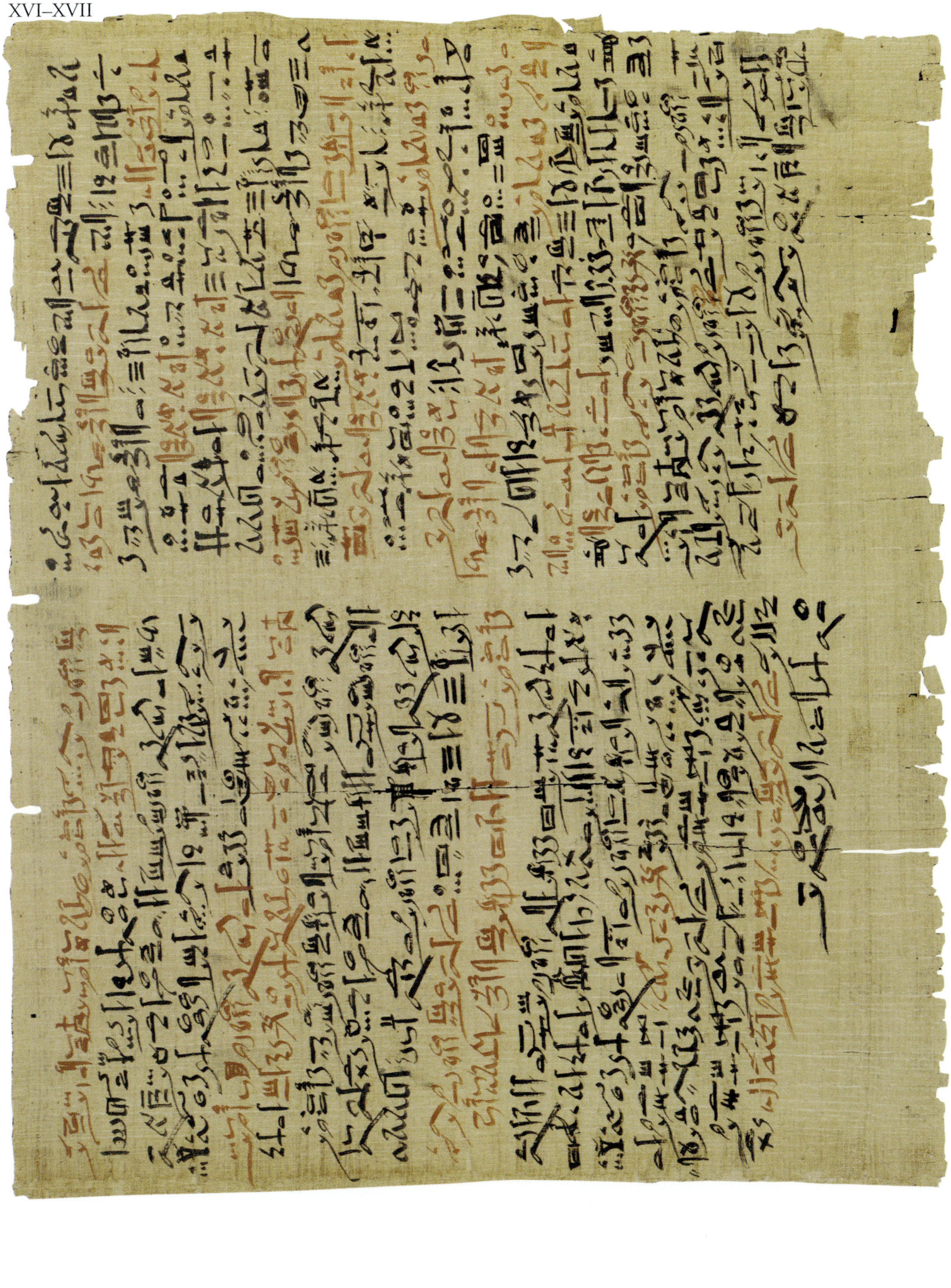